Adrenocortical Carcinoma

Gary D. Hammer · Tobias Else
Editors

Adrenocortical Carcinoma

Basic Science and Clinical Concepts

Springer

Editors
Gary D. Hammer, MD, Ph.D.
Mille Schembechler Professor of Adrenal Cancer
Director – Endocrine Oncology Program
Director – Center for Organogenesis
University of Michigan Health System
University of Michigan

Tobias Else, MD
Department of Internal Medicine
Division of Metabolism, Endocrinology & Diabetes
University of Michigan Health System
University of Michigan

ISBN 978-0-387-77235-6 e-ISBN 978-0-387-77236-3
DOI 10.1007/978-0-387-77236-3
Springer New York Dordrecht Heidelberg London

Library of Congress Control Number: 2010934103

Printed on acid-free paper

Springer is part of Springer Science+Business Media (www.springer.com)

Preface

Adrenocortical carcinoma (ACC) is a disease that most physicians, including many endocrinologists, will rarely, if ever, diagnose or let alone treat during the course of their medical practice. Medical textbooks of endocrinology and oncology rarely dedicate an entire chapter to this disease entity. The pursuit of research and clinical excellence in uncommon diseases is extremely challenging because of a lack of research prioritization, nonexistent treatment guidelines and overall paucity of coordination between researchers and physicians. ACC is one such disease where no infrastructure for a unified research agenda and no consensus treatment guidelines had been developed.

While a number of international meetings over the past two decades have indeed focused on adrenal tumors in the context of hormone excess (Cushing's syndrome, hyperaldosteronism, and pheochromocytoma), few have exclusively catered to the science and clinical care of ACC and those afflicted with the disease. With only a single FDA-approved drug for ACC (mitotane – a derivative of the pesticide DDT), institutional experiences varied widely until recently when historic biases have slowly yielded to data-driven treatment strategies. A large part of the impetus for this push has come from Europe, where the availability of country-wide integrated networks for treatment has allowed a small number of centers in Italy, France, and Germany (among others) to develop specific expertise and specific treatment protocols for this rare disease.

In an attempt to facilitate coordination of global efforts, a consensus conference was organized and held at the University of Michigan in September 2003. At that meeting, an international group of physicians and scientists with research interest and clinical expertise in ACC set up initial guidelines for the diagnosis and treatment of ACC. Three principles emerged. Successful treatment of ACC demands coordinated care in the context of a multidisciplinary team dedicated to the disease. Future therapies for ACC need to be predicated on hypothesis-driven research based on a thorough analysis of tumor biology. Lastly, major advancement in the field demands national and international collaborative networks to facilitate analysis of large datasets and coordinate future clinical trials. The FIRM-ACT (First International Randomized Trial in locally advanced and Metastatic Adrenocortical Cancer Treatment) that coordinated over 35 ACC centers in a single multinational trial set precedence for the actualization of these principles. The Second

International Adrenal Cancer Symposium: Clinical and Basic Science held at the University of Michigan in March 2008 built upon the momentum of the 2003 consensus meeting and the successful development of a large international ACC network through the FIRM-ACT trial.

Over the past decade, the ACC research community has grown to a critical mass with new data emerging in the laboratory and clinic. In times of electronic publications we routinely rely on journal articles and expert reviews on both clinical and research topics. While such publications are informative, when approached by Springer about the possibility of editing such a textbook, we became convinced that the time had come to compile the accumulated clinical and basic science knowledge of 50 years of active research on this rare cancer into a concise medical textbook. The overall goal of this book is therefore to provide definitive reference material for scientists and clinicians, to introduce trainees to concepts of ACC management, and to stimulate further research, future collaborations, and networking.

As opposed to a solitary review article, a textbook with multiple chapters dedicated to discrete topics in the field provides contributors the opportunity to objectively review historic data and detail the current state of clinical care and research accomplishments. While this is a major advantage of a textbook, it is also a major challenge for a book that focuses solely on a rare cancer where data are scant. In editing this book, we tried to ensure that each individual chapter covers well-established knowledge in the area, but also allows room for expert opinion. Lastly, because ACC has been linked to several genetic disorders that usually escape discussion in a focused review of adrenal tumors, the various syndromes will be discussed in their entirety in separate chapters. The 32 Chapters of the 9 Sections are authored by the scientific and clinical leaders in the field.

With publication of this first edition, the editors want to extend special thanks to our colleagues within the ACC community, the contributors, Rachel, Todd and Lesley of the editorial staff at Springer Publishing House, and Lisa K. Byrd of the University of Michigan.

We are hopeful that this first edition of the textbook provides an intellectual platform for the continued coalescence and dissemination of knowledge on ACC in future editions. Both the authors and editors welcome comments and recommendations for improvement in writing or via electronic mail. The editors' and authors' institutional and e-mail addresses are given in the contributor's section.

Ann Arbor, Michigan — Gary Hammer
November 2010 — Tobias Else

Contents

Contributors

Bruno Allolio Department of Internal Medicine I, Endocrine and Diabetes Unit, University of Würzburg, Josef-Schneider-Str. 2, 97080 Würzburg, Germany, allolio_b@medizin.uni-wuerzburg.de

Arianna Ardito Department of Clinical and Biological Sciences, Medicina Interna 1, AOU San Luigi Gonzaga, University of Turin, Regione Gonzole, 10, 10043 Orbassano, Italy, arianna.ardito@gmail.com

Richard J. Auchus Division of Endocrinology and Metabolism, Department of Internal Medicine, UT Southwestern Medical Center Dallas, 5323 Harry Hines Boulevard, Dallas, TX 75390, USA, richard.auchus@utsouthwestern.edu

Anca M. Avram Division of Nuclear Medicine/Radiology, University of Michigan Health System, University of Michigan, 1500 East Medical Center Drive, Ann Arbor, MI 48105, USA, ancaa@umich.edu

Edgar Ben-Josef Department of Radiation Oncology, University of Michigan Health System, University of Michigan, 1500 East Medical Center Drive, Room UHB2C490, Ann Arbor, MI 48109-0010, USA, edgarb@med.umich.edu

Alfredo Berruti Oncologia Medica, Azienda Ospedaliero Universitaria San Luigi, Regione Gonzole, 10, 10043 Orbassano, Italy, alfredo.berruti@gmail.com

Jérôme Bertherat Endocrinology, Metabolism and Cancer Department, Institut Cochin, Descartes University, INSERM U567, CNRS UMR8104, Paris France; Reference center for rare adrenal disorders, Assistance Publique Hôpitaux de Paris, Hôpital Cochin, Paris Descartes University, 27 Rue du Faubourg Saint-Jacques, 75014 Paris, France, jerome.bertherat@cch.aphp.fr

Xavier Bertagna Endocrinology Department, Cochin Hospital, Paris, France; National Network COMETE, INCa, Paris, France; European Network for the Study of @drenal Tumors (ENS@T), 27 Rue du Faubourg Saint-Jacques, 75014 Paris, France, xavier.bertagna@cch.aphp.fr

Felix Beuschlein Department of Medicine, Endocrine Research, University Hospital Innenstadt, Ziemssenstr. 1, 80336 Munich, Germany, felix.beuschlein@med.uni-muenchen.de

Stefan R. Bornstein Department of Medicine, Carl Gustav Carus Medical School, University of Dresden, Fetscherstraße 74, 01307 Dresden, Germany, stefan.bornstein@uniklinikum-dresden.de

James T. Broome Vanderbilt Endocrine Surgery Center, Vanderbilt University, 597 Preston Research Building, 2220 Pierce Ave, Nashville, TN, USA, james.broome@vanderbilt.edu

Maria V. Cicala Division of Endocrinology, Department of Medical and Surgical Sciences, University of Padua, Via Ospedale 105, 35128 Padova, Italy, mariaverena.cicala@unipd.it

Fulvia Daffara Department of Clinical and Biological Sciences, Medicina Interna 1, AOU San Luigi Gonzaga, University of Turin, Regione Gonzole, 10, 10043 Orbassano, Italy, fulviaclaudia@libero.it

Silvia De Francia Department of Clinical and Biological Sciences, Farmacologia, AOU San Luigi Gonzaga, University of Turin, Regione Gonzole, 10, 10043 Orbassano, Italy, silvia.defrancia@unito.it

Michael DeBaun Division of Pediatric Hematology-Oncology, Department of Pediatrics, Washington University School of Medicine, 660 South Euclid Avenue, Box 8067, St. Louis, MO 63110-1093, USA, debaun_m@kids.wustl.edu

Luigi Dogliotti Oncologia Medica, Azienda Ospedaliero Universitaria San Luigi, Regione Gonzole 10, 10043 Orbassano, Italy, luigi.dogliotti@unito.it

Gerard M. Doherty Department of Surgery, University of Michigan Health System, The University of Michigan, 2920 Taubman Center, 1500 East Medical Center Drive, Ann Arbor, MI 48109, USA, gerardd@umich.edu

Tobias Else Department of Internal Medicine – Division of Metabolism, Endocrinology & Diabetes, University of Michigan Health System, University of Michigan, Domino's Farms, Lobby C, Suite 1300, 24 Frank Lloyd Wright Drive, PO Box 451, Ann Arbor, MI 48106, USA, telse@med.umich.edu

Martin Fassnacht Department of Internal Medicine I, Endocrine and Diabetes Unit, University Hospital of Würzburg, Josef-Schneider-Str. 2, 97080 Würzburg, Germany, fassnacht_m@medizin.uni-wuerzburg.de

Anna Ferrero Oncologia Medica, Azienda Ospedaliero Universitaria San Luigi, Regione Gonzole 10, 10043 Orbassano, Italy, anna.ferrero80@gmail.com

Christian Fottner Schwerpunkt Endokrinologie und Stoffwechselerkrankungen, I. Medizinische Klinik und Poliklinik, Universitätsmedizin, Johannes Gutenberg Universität Mainz, Langenbeckstrasse 1, 55131 Mainz, Germany, fottner@endokrinologie.klinik.uni-mainz.de

Paul G. Gauger Department of Surgery, University of Michigan Health System, University of Michigan, 1500 East Medical Center Drive, Ann Arbor, MI 48109, USA, pgauger@umich.edu

Sébastien Gaujoux Endocrinology, Metabolism and Cancer Department, Institut Cochin, INSERM U567, CNRS UMR8104, Paris, France; Department of Digestive and Endocrine Surgery, Assistance Publique Hôpitaux de Paris, Hôpital Cochin, Paris Descartes University, 27 Rue du Faubourg Saint-Jacques, 75014 Paris, France, sebastien.gaujoux@gmail.com

Thomas J. Giordano Departments of Pathology and Internal Medicine, University of Michigan Health System, University of Michigan, 1500 East Medical Center Drive, Ann Arbor, MI 48109, USA, giordano@med.umich.edu

Yvonne E. Groenen Department of Internal Medicine, Máxima Medical Centre, Ds. Th. Fliednerstraat 1, PO Box 90052, 5600 PD Eindhoven, Leiden University Medical Centre, Leiden, The Netherlands, y.groenen@mmc.nl

Stephanie Hahner Department of Internal Medicine I, Endocrine and Diabetes Unit, University Hospital of Würzburg, Josef-Schneider-Str. 2, 97080 Würzburg, Germany, hahner_s@medizin.uni-wuerzburg.de

Gary D. Hammer Endocrine Oncology Program – Comprehensive Cancer Center, Department of Internal Medicine – Division of Metabolism, Endocrinology & Diabetes, Department of Molecular & Integrative Physiology, Department of Cell & Developmental Biology, University of Michigan, 1528 BSRB, 109 Zina Pitcher Pl., Ann Arbor, MI 48109-2200, USA, ghammer@med.umich.edu

Harm R. Haak Department of Internal Medicine, Máxima Medical Centre, Ds. Th. Fliednerstraat 1, PO Box 90052, 5600 PD Eindhoven, Leiden University Medical Centre, Leiden, The Netherlands, h.haak@mmc.nl

Joanne H. Heaton Department of Internal Medicine, Division of Metabolism, Endocrinology & Diabetes, University of Michigan Medical School, 109 Zina Pitcher Place, 1680 BSRB, Ann Arbor, MI 48109, USA, heatonj@med.umich.edu

Ilse G.C. Hermsen Department of Internal Medicine, Máxima Medical Centre, Ds. Th. Fliednerstraat 1, PO Box 90052, 5600 PD Eindhoven, Leiden University Medical Centre, Leiden, The Netherlands, i.hermsen@mmc.nl

Peter J. Hornsby Department of Physiology and Barshop Institute for Longevity and Aging Studies, University of Texas Health Science Center, 15355 Lambda Drive, San Antonio, TX 78245, USA, hornsby@uthscsa.edu

Jennifer Horst Department of Pediatrics, Washington University School of Medicine, Washington University, One Brookings Drive, St. Louis, MO 63130, USA, horst_j@kids.wustl.edu

Hero K. Hussain Department of Radiology, University of Michigan Health System, University of Michigan, 1500 East Medical Center Drive, Ann Arbor, MI 48105, USA, hhussain@med.umich.edu

Lawrence S. Kirschner Division of Endocrinology, Diabetes and Metabolism, Department of Internal Medicine and Department of Molecular Virology,

Immunology and Medical Genetics, The Ohio State University, Columbus Enarson Hall 154 W. 12th Avenue, Columbus, OH 43210, USA, lawrence.kirschner@osumc.edu

Melvyn Korobkin Department of Radiology, University of Michigan Health System, University of Michigan, 1500 East Medical Center Drive, Ann Arbor, MI 48105, USA, korobkin@umich.edu

Anita Kulharya Department of Pediatrics, Pathology and Cytogenetics, Medical College of Georgia, 1120 15th Street, BG-1071, Augusta, GA 30912, USA, akulhary@mail.mcg.edu

David Malkin Division of Hematology/Oncology, Department of Pediatrics, The Hospital for Sick Children, University of Toronto, 555 University Avenue, Toronto, ON M5G 1X8, Canada, david.malkin@sickkids.ca

Franco Mantero Division of Endocrinology, Department of Medical and Surgical Sciences, University of Padua, Via Ospedale 105, 35128 Padova, Italy, franco.mantero@unipd.it

Barbra S. Miller Department of Surgery, University of Michigan Health System, University of Michigan, 1500 East Medical Center Drive, Ann Arbor, MI 48109, USA, barbram@umich.edu

Ina M. Niederle Schwerpunkt Endokrinologie und Stoffwechselerkrankungen, I. Medizinische Klinik und Poliklinik, Universitätsmedizin, Johannes Gutenberg Universität Mainz, Langenbeckstrasse 1, 55131 Mainz, Germany, niederle@1-med.klinik.uni-mainz.de

Jeniel Parmar Department of Physiology, Medical College of Georgia, 1120 15th Street Room CA3091, Augusta, GA 30912, USA, jparmar@students.mcg.edu

Anna Patalano Division of Endocrinology, Department of Medical and Surgical Sciences, University of Padua, Via Ospedale 105, 35128 Padova, Italy, anna.patalano@libero.it

Paola Perotti Oncologia Medica, Azienda Ospedaliero Universitaria San Luigi, Regione Gonzole, 10, 10043, Orbassano, Italy, oncotrial.sanluigi@gmail.com

William Rainey Department of Physiology, Medical College of Georgia, 1120 15th Street Room CA3094, Augusta, GA 30912, USA, wrainey@mail.mcg.edu

Raul C. Ribeiro Department of Oncology, St. Jude Children's Research Hospital, 262 Danny Thomas Place, Memphis, TN 38105, USA, raul.ribeiro@stjude.org

Carlos Rodriguez-Galindo Department of Pediatric Oncology, Dana-Farber Cancer Institute and Children's Hospital, 44 Binney Street, Boston, MA 02115, USA, carlos_rodriguez-galindo@dfci.harvard.edu

Aaron Sabolch Radiation Oncology, University of Michigan Medical School, 1500 East Medical Center Drive, Ann Arbor, MI 48109, USA, sabolch@umich.edu

Wolfgang Saeger Institute of Pathology of the Marienkrankenhaus, Alfredstraße 9, 22087 Hamburg, Germany, saeger.patho@marienkrankenhaus.org

David E. Schteingart Endocrine Oncology Program, Comprehensive Cancer Center, University of Michigan, 1500 East Medical Center Drive, Ann Arbor, MI 48109, USA, dschtein@umich.edu

Britt Skogseid Department of Endocrine Oncology, Uppsala University Hospital, University of Uppsala, Akademiska sjukhuset/Uppsala, SE-751 85, Uppsala, Sweden, britt.skogseid@medsci.uu.se

Paola Sperone Oncologia Medica, Azienda Ospedaliero Universitaria San Luigi, Regione Gonzole 10, 10043 Orbassano, Italy, paola.sperone@email.it

Massimo Terzolo Department of Clinical and Biological Sciences, Medicina Interna 1, AOU San Luigi Gonzaga, University of Turin, Regione Gonzole, 10, 10043 Orbassano, Italy, terzolo@usa.net

Norman W. Thompson Surgery Emeritus Faculty, University of Michigan, Rm 2124C Taubman Health Care Center, 1500 East Medical Center Drive, Ann Arbor, MI 48105, USA, normant@umich.edu

Frédérique Tissier Endocrinology, Metabolism and Cancer Department, Institut Cochin, INSERM U567, CNRS UMR8104, Paris, France; Department of Pathology, Assistance Publique Hôpitaux de Paris, Hôpital Cochin, Paris Descartes University, Rue du Faubourg Saint-Jacques, 75014 Paris, France, frederique.tissier@cch-ap-hop-paris.fr

Matthias M. Weber Schwerpunkt Endokrinologie und Stoffwechselerkrankungen, I. Medizinische Klinik und Poliklinik, Universitätsmedizin, Johannes Gutenberg Universität Mainz, Langenbeckstrasse 1, 55131 Mainz, Germany, mmweber@uni-mainz.de

Holger S. Willenberg Department of Endocrinology, Diabetes and Rheumatology, University Hospital Duesseldorf, Moorenstr. 5, D–40225 Duesseldorf, Germany, holger.willenberg@uni-duesseldorf.de

Barbara Zaggia Department of Clinical and Biological Sciences, Medicina Interna1, AOU San Luigi Gonzaga, University of Turin Regione Gonzole, 10, 10043 Orbassano, Italy, barbara.zaggia@libero.it

Gerard P. Zambetti Department of Biochemistry, St. Jude Children's Research Hospital, 262 Danny Thomas Place, Memphis, TN 38105, USA, gerard.zambetti@stjude.org

Part I
History of Adrenocortical Carcinoma Research and Clinical Care

Chapter 1
The History of Adrenocortical Carcinoma Treatment – A Medical Perspective

David E. Schteingart

Knowledge of the genetic and molecular alterations in adrenocortical carcinoma (ACC) has advanced in the past two decades, as a result of newer laboratory methodology to study mechanisms of oncogenesis and tumor pathophysiology. In contrast, limited progress has been made in our ability to treat and prolong survival in patients with advanced disease. Over the past five decades, a number of reports have summarized the experience of individual medical institutions with ACC; and collectively, based on several thousand cases, there is relative consensus on the epidemiology of ACC, its clinical presentation, criteria for pathological diagnosis, and tumor response to standard cytotoxic chemotherapy. Unfortunately, survival of patients with advanced disease remains poor (Fig. 1.1), and targeted therapies based on new knowledge of the biology of these tumors are only in clinical trial phase. This introduction will attempt to highlight the early experience with mitotane that forms the basis of our current approach to the management of patients with ACC.

Initial publications recognized that ACCs are rare, highly malignant tumors with poor prognosis. It was appreciated that the tumoral production of excessive steroid hormones and coincident metabolic syndromes allow for a more timely diagnosis. In 1961, Soffer et al. [2] detailed several cases of feminizing syndrome associated with large malignant tumors. These patients developed metastases and their life expectancy was just a few months. While aldosterone-producing ACCs were noted to be rare, Cushing's syndrome was the most common clinical presentation in adult patients. Biochemical investigation revealed elevated 17-ketosteroids, but no distinguishing pattern between adrenocortical carcinoma and benign congenital adrenal hyperplasia. At that time, diagnostic tests for adrenal tumors associated with Cushing's syndrome relied on the lack of response to stimulation with ACTH or metyrapone. Assessment of the risk of malignancy was based on the finding

D.E. Schteingart (✉)
Endocrine Oncology Program, Comprehensive Cancer Center, University of Michigan, 1500 East Medical Center Drive, Ann Arbor, MI 48109, USA
e-mail: dschtein@umich.edu

G.D. Hammer, T. Else (eds.), *Adrenocortical Carcinoma*,
DOI 10.1007/978-0-387-77236-3_1,

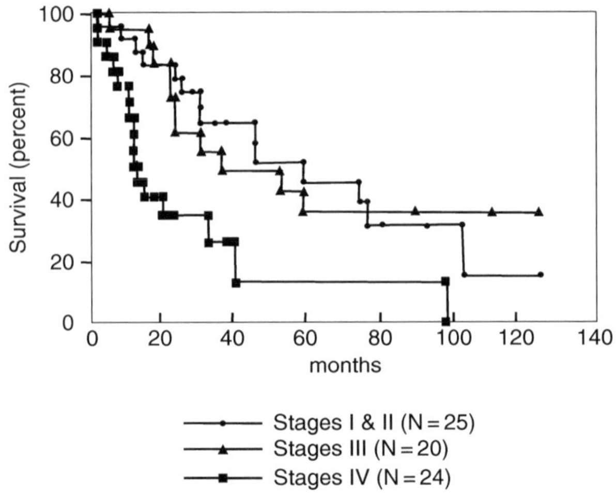

Fig. 1.1 Survival of patients with adrenocortical carcinoma according to stage [1]

of large tumors on a variety of imaging platforms including simple abdominal x-rays, intravenous pyelograms, or procedures with perirenal/retrorectal gas insufflation.

It was accepted over 60 years ago that surgery was the most effective treatment for ACC. As detailed in the accompanying historical section by Thompson, while a variety of surgical approaches were developed and improved upon over the past few decades, the importance of complete resection cannot be overstated. Nonetheless, the ability to safely remove these tumors, especially those associated with Cushing's syndrome, improved only with the availability of glucocorticoids that could be administered easily in stress doses during and following surgery. Cecil in 1932 [3], as quoted by Soffer, reported that 39% of surgical patients died in adrenal insufficiency shock within hours post-operation. The availability of hydrocortisone made surgical resection of adrenal tumors safe. However, as many ACC patients presented with metastatic disease or distant recurrences, additional systemic therapies were necessary. Of the various cytotoxic drugs used, mitotane has been the oldest, with selective activity against ACC. However, acceptance of its use as a pharmacologic agent has been controversial since its initial use. Several chemical compounds derived from DDT were initially tested as adrenalytic agents. These included amphenone, perthane, methylenedianiline, and DDD. Amphenone B (1,2-bis-(*p*-aminophenyl)-2-methyl propane-1) synthesized in 1950 was found to block 11, 17, and 21-hydroxylation of corticosteroids in ACC and cause a decrease in steroid excretion. However, it was associated with severe toxicity. Nelson and Woodward first reported that commercial DDD [2,2-bis(parachlorophenyl)-1,1-dichloroethane] and its ethyl derivative, perthane, can produce adrenocortical atrophy in the dog. Subsequently, mitotane, the o,p′-isomer in the mixture, was found to be active as an adrenolytic agent and useful in the treatment of patients with ACC.

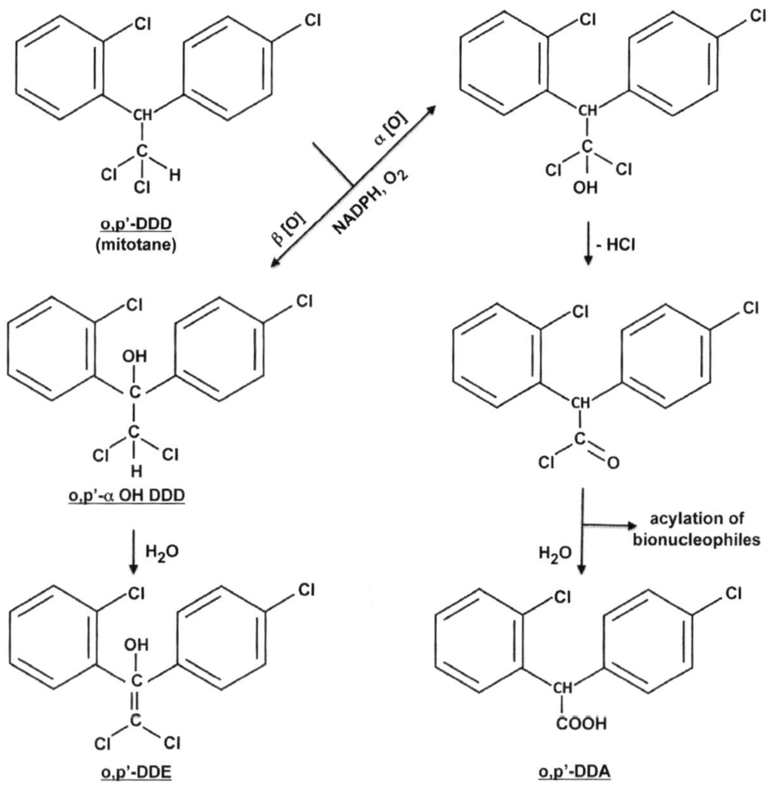

Fig. 1.2 Transformation of mitotane via P450 hydroxylation, dehydrochlorination, and formation of an acyl chloride, a highly reactive species that covalently binds to bionucleophiles within the adrenal cell or converts to the acetic acid derivative, o,p′-DDA or o,p′-DDE

The specificity of mitotane for the adrenal cortex and ACC suggested a requirement for biotransformation of the drug for activity within the adrenal cortex in ways that differ from that which takes place in other extra-adrenal sites. The mechanism of the adrenolytic effects of mitotane involves transformation to an acyl chloride via P450-mediated hydroxylation and covalent binding to specific bionucleophiles (Fig. 1.2). The ability of mitotane to be metabolically transformed and covalently bound determines its pharmacological activity. As a result of the transformation to bioactive mitotane, oxidative damage followed by the formation of free radicals such as superoxide induces lipid peroxidation and, ultimately, cellular death (Fig. 1.3). The metabolic activity of mitotane varies among species, the drug being most effective in dogs and modestly effective in humans. Normal adrenal cortices and adrenal glands of patients with ACTH-dependent adrenocortical hyperplasia are also susceptible to the toxic effects of mitotane (Fig. 1.4), but only 33% of patients with ACC respond. It is likely that different tumors vary in their ability to induce metabolic transformation or initiate free radical production, and as a consequence may express variable sensitivity to mitotane. Substituting the hydrogen on

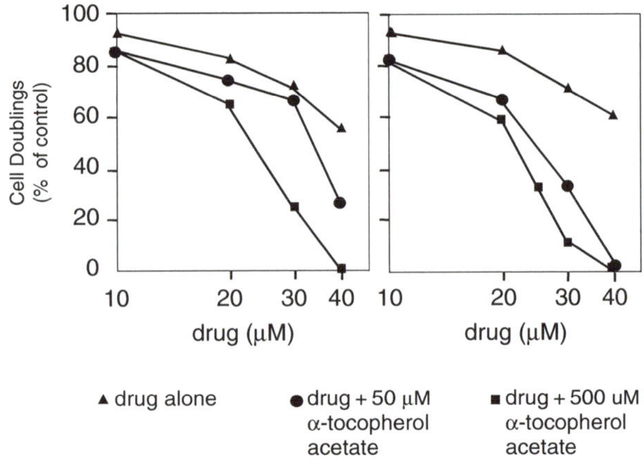

Fig. 1.3 Inhibition by α-tocopherol, an antioxidant of the antiproliferative activity of mitotane

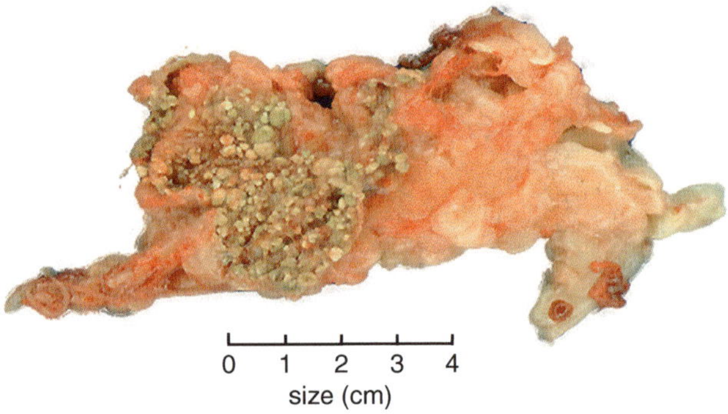

Fig. 1.4 Appearance of the adrenal gland in a patient with ACTH-dependent Cushing's disease, treated with low doses of mitotane for 1 year

the beta carbon by a methyl group blocks the metabolic transformation (Fig. 1.5). Methylated mitotane does not have adrenolytic activity.

Hertz et al. in the mid-1950s, treated 16 patients with Cushing's syndrome due to metastatic ACC with o,p′-DDD, 10 g daily for 2–4 months. Seven patients had radiological evidence of tumor regression and 13 patients had marked decrease in urinary 17-hydroxycorticoids. Clinical remission of Cushing's syndrome was noted in six patients, lasting 4 months to 2 years. Unfortunately, patients experienced severe toxicity [2]. Measurable disease response, overall clinical improvement, and decreases in urinary steroid levels have since been described. The mean survival is short (8.4 months) when the drug is used after the appearance of metastatic disease. Isolated case reports describe impressive remissions and even cures of ACC with mitotane therapy alone. In general, survival appears to depend on the size of the primary lesion and the degree of local and distant extension of the neoplasm at the time of initial surgery.

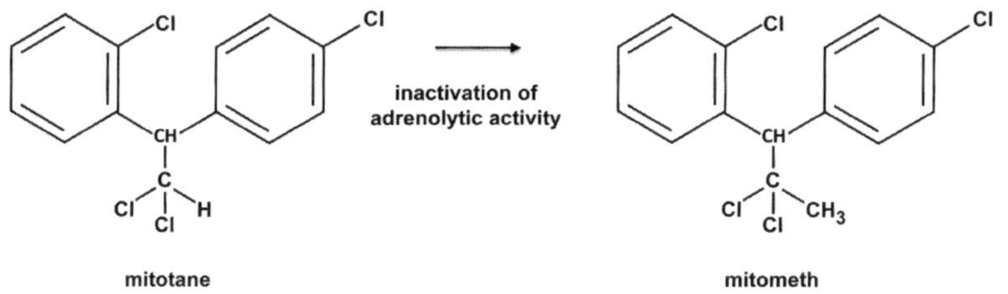

Fig. 1.5 Inactivation of the adrenolytic activity of mitotane by substituting the hydrogen at the β-carbon by a methyl group (mitometh)

In 1967, Eisenstein [4] recommended that patients in whom ACC cannot be completely removed should be treated with o,p′-DDD. Fifteen years later, the concept of post-surgical mitotane therapy was extended to patients following a complete resection but with a high risk of recurrence. In 1982, Schteingart et al. first predicted that the post-surgical use of mitotane would be most effective when instituted early as adjuvant therapy following resection of the primary tumor and before local extension or distant metastases occur [5].

While it was well accepted then that surgery was the most effective treatment for ACC, in 1983, Thompson [6] emphasized the possibility of better treatment outcome with earlier diagnosis and combination of aggressive surgical treatment (including repeated debulking of recurrent disease) and adjuvant treatment with mitotane. In a review of 23 patients treated between 1953 and 1981, six patients had resection of the primary tumor and local radiation therapy without mitotane; mean survival for this group was 10.3 months. In contrast, 17 patients treated with surgery and mitotane therapy had a mean survival of 46.6 months. Longest survival was in the group that received adjuvant treatment before and after surgery for local recurrent tumor, with a mean survival of 74 months.

While mitotane remains the only drug to be selective for treating patients with metastatic ACC, not all agree that its limited efficacy justifies the associated side-effects [7, 8]. Regardless, until new targeted therapies emerge as more effective and selective candidates for ACC, mitotane will remain as an important part of most ACC treatment regimens, with proven results both in the adjuvant setting and in the treatment of advanced disease, by itself or in combination with other cytotoxic drugs (Chapter 22).

The natural history of ACC has not changed dramatically over the past 40 years [9]. In spite of the multiple treatment approaches suggested, life expectancy for patients with ACC has remained constant. However, our experience in the past five decades has taught us that the clinical evolution of these patients varies and some patients can survive for several years with surgical and medical treatment. Therefore, the main tasks for the future are to define those clinical characteristics that are associated with a better prognosis and response to current treatment regimens and to find new therapeutic modalities that may lead to a cure of the majority of ACC patients, whose tumors are unresectable and/or do not respond to available chemotherapies.

Lessons from these early cases include (1) detection and treatment in Stages I and II can be associated with good prognosis; (2) aggressive surgical resection is associated with better outcome; (3) mitotane therapy may be beneficial in extending survival either as adjuvant therapy or given for advanced disease.

References

1. Brennan MF (1987) Adrenocortical carcinoma. CA Cancer J Clin 37:348–365
2. Soffer LJ et al (1961) The human adrenal gland. Lea & Febiger, Philadelphia, PA
3. Cecil HF (1933) Hypertension, obesity, virilism and pseudohermaphroditism as caused by suprarenal tumors. J.A.M.A 100:463
4. Eisenstein AB (1967) The adrenal cortex. Little, Brown and Company, Boston, MA
5. Schteingart DE et al (1982) The treatment of adrenal carcinoma. Arch Surg 117:1142–1146
6. Thompson NW (1983) Adrenocortical carcinoma. In: Thompson NW, Vinik AI (eds) Endocrine surgery update. Grune and Stratton, New York, pp 119–128
7. Luton JP et al (1990) Clinical features of adrenocortical carcinoma, prognostic factors, and the effect of mitotane therapy. N Engl J Med 322:1195–1201
8. Hogan TF et al (1978) *o,p′*-DDD (mitotane) therapy of adrenal cortical carcinoma: observations on drug dosage, toxicity and steroid replacement. Cancer 42:2177–2181
9. Bilimoria KY et al (2008) Adrenocortical carcinoma in the United States. Treatment utilization and prognostic factors. Cancer 113(11):3130–3136

Chapter 2
The History of Adrenocortical Carcinoma Treatment – A Surgical Perspective

Norman W. Thompson

The early history of adrenocortical carcinoma (ACC) is obscure because of the rarity of the disease, confusing nomenclature, inability to diagnose before death, ignorance of its hormonal manifestations, and a vague appreciation of its clinical course. Most reported cases in the 19th century were based on autopsy findings, and the tumors were classified by a variety of terms including hypernephroma, sarcoma, fibromyxosarcoma, and carcinoma. The commonly used term, hypernephroma, was first proposed by Grawitz et al. in 1893 and falsely assumed that tumors arose in rests of adrenocortical tissue within the kidney [1]. This concept was reinforced by Felix Birch-Hirchfield who used it to define benign and malignant tumors of both adrenals and kidneys, some with apparent hormonal disturbances [2]. The designation of hypernephroma for some adrenal tumors persisted in the literature until the 1940s; later it became restricted to what is now referred to as renal cell cancer [3–8].

In 1905, it was stated that no adrenal tumor had been diagnosed before operation or autopsy [9]. None had been suspected on the basis of a hormonal syndrome although an association of virilization and an adrenal tumor found at autopsy was first observed in 1811 [10]. It was not until 1890 that a decrease in virilization was first documented following resection of an adrenal tumor. Cushing's syndrome was not recognized until 1910 but was not associated with an adrenal malignancy until Walters et al. in 1934 described the same syndrome in patients with adrenal tumors and emphasized that the characteristic findings were not exclusively related to pituitary disease [11].

The first tumor operations on the adrenal glands were done to remove "large abdominal swellings" [10]. Knowsly Thornton of London is credited with the first known successful operation to remove an adrenal cancer in 1899 [12]. His patient was a 36-year-old, very hirsute female who was found at operation to have a 20-pound left adrenal tumor. It required a left nephrectomy as well to remove this

N.W. Thompson (✉)
Surgery Emeritus Faculty, University of Michigan, Rm 2124C Taubman Health Care Center, 1500 East Medical Center Drive, Ann Arbor, MI 48105, USA
e-mail: normant@umich.edu

G.D. Hammer, T. Else (eds.), *Adrenocortical Carcinoma*,
DOI 10.1007/978-0-387-77236-3_2, © Springer Science+Business Media, LLC 2011

large tumor. She slowly recovered after developing a subphrenic abscess that spontaneously drained into a bronchus. After dramatic improvement, her hirsutism remised until a recurrence 2 years later caused her death [13]. Thornton, interestingly, was well prepared for this operation, having previously served as Joseph Lister's house surgeon (antiseptic technique) and Spencer Wells' assistant. The latter was a pioneer in the development of hemostats and hemostatic techniques. The first small series was presented by Otto Ramsay later in 1899 who reported three patients operated for large palpable malignant adrenal tumors [14]. In addition, he reviewed a total of 64 other published reports of patients with either carcinomas [15] or sarcomas [13] of the adrenals. The diagnosis was difficult in all and impossible in many. The tumors were found to spread rapidly and the prognosis was considered dismal. Surgery was considered the only hope of temporary relief, but only five patients had been operated and only two with success, Thornton's and another by Howard Kelly in Baltimore with a good result 1 year after excision of a large "fibromyxosarcoma."

From 1905 to 1929, a number of patients were described with what was termed the adrenogenital syndrome and others with adrenal tumors with virilism [5, 16]. Bulloch, in 1905, reported ten girls and two boys who all died within 2 years from malignant adrenal tumors, most with metastases. Most were considered hypernephromas associated with sexual abnormalities, usually in children [10]. In 1921, Collett from Oslo described a 2-year-old with progressive virilization over 18 months who had a palpable tumor of the left adrenal [10]. This was excised after which the hirsutism regressed for 2 years. This was probably the first successful adrenal operation in a child. Other similar cases soon followed and surgical excision seemed to confirm that these tumors caused virilism, perhaps by producing an internal secretion. Although patients with pure adrenal virilism had had tumors successfully removed, several with Cushing's or closely related syndromes had died in "shock" several hours after straightforward operations. At autopsy, their remaining adrenals were found to be atrophic. After 1932, many patients with Cushing's disease (pituitary) were reported. Cushing's syndrome and adrenal virilism were not always clearly distinguished, and the term "suprarenal cortical syndrome" was sometimes used to describe both. Kepler at the Mayo Clinic stressed the frequency of the intermediate forms, especially with ACCs [17]. By 1933 there was clear evidence that the pituitary secreted an adrenocortical factor which was later recognized as ACTH. Whatever the underlying cause, the development of Cushing's syndrome required the presence of the adrenal cortex. Those surgeons including Waltman, Waters, and James Priestly at the Mayo Clinic recognized three main problems: (1) to determine the nature of the adrenal lesion; (2) to relieve the syndrome in patients without adrenal tumors; (3) to prevent operative deaths from adrenal insufficiency. Since 1927, they had been developing an adrenocortical extract and using it perioperatively with some success. In 1934, they reported ten female patients with Cushing's syndrome who had been operated upon, with five having adrenal tumors, four of which were carcinomas. One tumor was palpable, one was seen on x-ray, and three found at operation. Three developed acute adrenocortical failure, and one of them who was treated in 1923 before cortical extract was available died. The other two received cortical extracts and recovered. Three of the five with tumors underwent remission [11]. By 1938, the Mayo group had removed tumors successfully from 16 consecutive patients, most of whom had Cushing's syndrome. Elsewhere, adrenal crises were all too frequent after surgical excision of tumors, and by 1943 more than 80% of such patients were reported to have died [10, 17–20]. The potent preparation of "cortin" at the Mayo Clinic, apparently, was the most important factor allowing their success. The intensive search for the active cortical substance(s) was ongoing from 1927 until its eventual discovery and preparation in 1949.

It was imperative for the management of Cushing's syndrome to have such a preparation whether treatment be pituitary or adrenal surgery. The dismal prognosis for patients with Cushing's syndrome was emphasized by Charles Plotz's paper on the natural history of the disease in 222 patients in 1952 showing a high incidence of cardiovascular disease, psychosis, and osteoporosis. Therapy had been effective in only 5 of their own 33 patients (pituitary irradiation in three and excision of adrenal adenomas in two). The overall mortality was 50% after 5 years from onset. Infections and cardiovascular disease were the most common causes of death. Another 20% died from surgical operations [10].

Between 1930 and the discovery of cortisone in 1949, details of nearly 300 patients with ACC were published [15, 17, 19–22]. Metastases were still often seen initially or soon after operation. The clinical features were in order of frequency, virilism, Cushing's syndrome, and combined Cushing's and virilism. These accounted for 75% and only 25% were apparently without a syndrome. Rarely, feminization was reported. This was first described in 1915, but only 30 additional cases were seen in the next 30 years and all were associated with an adrenal malignancy producing estrogens in excess. In 1930, Anderson described an ACC with fatal hypoglycemia but no other metabolic disturbance [23]. Ten similar cases of Anderson's syndrome were reported in the next 30 years, a few of whom went into remission after tumor removal. Three quarters of the 300 patients reported underwent operation and one-third died postoperatively. The mortality was greatest in those with Cushing's and least in those with nonsecreting tumors. In the surviving group, some had good long-term results, but only when the tumor had been completely excised.

A milestone in the treatment of ACC was the general availability of cortisone after 1950. By 1948, only a few grams were available at the Mayo Clinic. The first patient with Cushing's disease in whom this was used perioperatively was on December 3, 1949. Within a year, 18 patients underwent successful subtotal adrenalectomies there using cortisol pre- and postoperatively [10,15]. Kendall, Hench, and Reichstein received the Nobel Prize in 1950 for the development of cortisone and its use in adrenal surgery as well as in rheumatology. Soon, synthetic analogues of cortisone including prednisone, prednisolone, and dexamethasone became widely available. By 1957, an intravenous preparation of cortisol, hydrocortisone, was used intraoperatively and in urgent situations of adrenal insufficiency. By 1955, Tait and Simpson in London and Reichstein in Basel had isolated and prepared electrocortin, later renamed aldosterone for clinical use as fludrocortisone in 1956 [24]. Thus, surgeons in the 1950s for the first time could operate on patients with ACC and Cushing's syndrome without the danger of acute adrenal insufficiency causing an immediate crisis or early postoperative death. Remission of symptoms and findings followed rapidly in patients with ACCs where excisions were possible. They were usually complete within 1 year. Parallel developments occurred with the introduction of drugs which inhibited adrenocortical tumors from secreting steroids. These included amphenone, metyrapone, and aminoglutethimide in the mid-1960s. These were of some benefit in alleviating symptomatic persistence or recurrences after operations [25].

Many more cases of ACC were reported after 1950. The principal endocrine features in nearly 90% of patients were Cushing's, virilization, a combination of both, feminization and rarely aldosteronism (first case in 1955) [10, 19, 21, 22, 24, 26–31]. Although more women were diagnosed in life, the overall incidence in males was higher. Despite improved diagnostic tests such as urinary steroids, dexamethone suppression test (1960s), and an RIA for ACTH in the mid-1960s, the lag period between the onset of symptoms and the diagnosis was about 8 months. Local invasion and distant metastases at the time of exploration were still frequent. Although there were no good statistics on survival in the 1950s, the general consensus was that most patients died from the disease unless fortunate enough to have been operated before either local invasion was extensive or metastatic disease had occurred. One of the reasons for lack of good data was the rarity of the disease as emphasized by Steiner's 1954 report from the Los Angeles County Hospital [21]. In his study of all autopsies there from 1918 to 1947, only 15 cases of ACC were found, accounting for only 0.2% of all tumors. In 1952, Rappaport in a collective review found a total of 238 hormonal and 34 nonhormonal cases of ACC during the 20-year period from 1930 to 1949 [19]. Wood, in 1957, could find only 27 cases of nonhormonal ACC in the European and American literature from 1923 to 1956 [10]. MacFarlane in 1958 reviewed 55 patients from London teaching hospitals which included 35 with hormonal and 25 with nonhormonal findings [21]. Their average age was 32 years and ranged from infants to 68 years. For those with hormonal symptoms, 80% were less than 40 years of age and 65% with nonhormonal findings were greater than 50 years. The average duration of symptoms before treatment was 13.2 months, 17 months for those with hormonal symptoms but only 10.8 months for those without hormonal symptoms. One-third of all patients had local invasion and all but two of these patients had distant metastases. Overall, 34 of the 55 patients (61.8%) had metastatic disease at diagnosis. The liver was involved in 67%, the lungs in 47%, and local nodes in 44%. For those who were untreated, survival was only 2.9 months for those with nonhormonal findings and 3.8 months for those with hormonal symptoms. MacFarlane was the first to propose an operative staging system based on tumor size, local invasion, nodal and distant metastases. Stage I tumors were 5 cm or smaller without local invasion or metastases, a rare finding as the average tumor size was 12 cm. An operation was performed in 42 of the 55 patients and considered radical and potentially curative in 20 (36.4%). A palliative excision was performed in 12 (22%) patients. The operative mortality was still high at 26% overall but fell from 35% before 1952 to 16.7% after 1952. This was attributed primarily to the availability of cortisone. The 2-year survival was 24% and occurred only in those undergoing radical extirpation and adequate hormone replacement therapy. MacFarlane considered dissection of lymph nodes of limited value and nephrectomy unnecessary unless the kidney was directly involved. London surgeons favored a thoracoabdominal extrapleural approach, resecting the 11th rib to allow maximum exposure.

The next major event in the management of ACC was the introduction of o,p′-DDD (mitotane), an analogue of the insecticide DDT which had previously been found in animal studies to cause adrenocortical atrophy. It was first used clinically in 1960 to treat inoperable or recurrent ACCs. In 1960, Bergenstad reported o,p′-DDD sufficiently effective that the National Cancer Institute sponsored its production and distribution for clinical investigation [3]. Previously, the NCI had reported 38 patients with ACC treated there [30]. In only 18 was it possible to attempt a curative operation, whereas in the others, either a palliative procedure or biopsy was done. They noted a 50% mortality 2 years after first symptoms, and only seven were alive more than 5 years after the onset of symptoms, with only two disease-free. In those in whom a curative operation could not be attempted, the mortality was 70% after 2 years. The causes of death included large pulmonary and abdominal masses causing pneumonia, caval thrombosis, sepsis, and pulmonary embolus. The first major report of the NCI evaluation of o,p′-DDD was by Hutter et al. in 1966 [33, 34]. By then, they had collected 138 previously unpublished cases in which o,p′-DDD was used and compared those with the 48 previously treated and reported cases elsewhere. The average age of their patients was 37.6 years and 92 were female and 43 were males. Cushing's syndrome was found in 59% and virilization in 19%. Local spread was found in 65%, whereas 53% developed pulmonary and 44% liver metastases. Survival was better in females with 52 versus 38 alive 4 years after diagnosis. The median survival after diagnosis for all females was 56 months and only 19 months for males. Mitotane was considered effective in some cases but was of limited value in prolonging survival. The next major report on the use of mitotane in inoperable ACC cases was by Lubitz et al. in 1973 [35]. They reported on 115 patients with inoperable ACC seen between 1965 and 1969. A disease response was seen in 61% of patients treated, lasting an average of 10.3 months. Although 84% had an adverse response to the drug involving the gastrointestinal, central nervous, and dermatological systems, these were all reversible with discontinuance or decrease in drug dosage. They found that 45% showed a favorable clinical response and that elevated steroid levels fell in 85%. Even though there were no cures, the mean duration of life for the entire group was only 8.4 months with treatment. Van Slooten, in 1983, was one of the first to observe that serum level monitoring of mitotane was important [36]. He found that if the serum level was maintained at 14 μg/ml or higher, the survival time at 26.5 months was 50% compared to only 14.5 months if the level was less than 14 μg/ml. Their recommendation was that all patients receiving mitotane should have serum level monitoring and the drug dose adjusted accordingly.

Since then, several large series of ACC patients have been reported and although there had been hope that with the widespread use of a variety of imaging techniques the diagnosis of ACC would be made at an earlier stage, that has not occurred

[26–28, 37, 38]. Luton et al. in reporting 105 patients from France, again found more females than males in a clinical series (75/30) with a mean age of 46 years [38]. Their duration of symptoms was 8.7 months at diagnosis and nearly 70% had endocrine symptoms. When steroid studies were done, 79% were functional. At the time of diagnosis, 30% had distant metastases. Operations were performed in 80% and 59% received mitotane. The median disease-free interval after operation was 12.1 months during which tumor dissemination occurred in 82%. The median survival time was 14.5 months and the 5-year survival was only 22%. They, like others, concluded that mitotane should be used as it did lower hormone levels and was transiently beneficial, particularly when endocrine symptoms were present. Again, survival benefits were not proven.

Since the first patients with ACC were recognized and treated, a radical surgical extirpation remains the only real chance for cure in those patients who do not already have hematogenous spread. In such cases, a number of important surgical principles must be considered in order to increase the possibility of a successful outcome (Table 2.1). Earlier diagnosis, allowing for that option, has not been seen in any large series. Operative mortality has improved because of the recognition and treatment of adrenal insufficiency in those patients with Cushing's syndrome and contralateral adrenal atrophy. Steroid replacement with hydrocortisone and fludrocortisone in patients treated with mitotane has also decreased morbidity. The overall operative mortality has dropped from the pre-1950s level of 30–40% to less than 5% in most reports. Chemotherapy and radiotherapy are traditionally of a very limited value in terms of a curative approach. Mitotane is the only adjunctive therapy currently available, although generally considered to be of only transient benefit. It should be noted, however, that several dozen long-term remissions in patients with distant metastases have been reported [2, 27, 39]. Obviously, the continued failure to detect ACC at an early stage remains a major deterrent to successful therapy. The hope for the future is that new drugs specifically targeted to individual tumors, based on gene profiling, can be developed. Until that day, ACC will remain a most challenging disease for physicians and surgeons to manage.

Table 2.1 Basic principles learned in surgical management of ACC (Figs. 2.1–2.3 are case sketches provided courtesy of the author N. W. Thompson)

1. Adequate steroid preparation and maintenance in patients with Cushing's syndrome or while on long-term mitotane therapy.
2. In case of a high suspicion of an ACC, needle biopsy is contraindicated pre-operatively; spillage of tumor cells will prevent cure (Fig. 2.1a, b).
3. Incisions allowing wide local exposure of the tumor and intra-abdominal metastases, making every effort to avoid rupturing the tumor capsule when it is localized and potentially curable.
4. Avoidance of laparoscopic techniques.
5. Preparation for possible aortopulmonary bypass in cases where tumor extends into the vena cava. This assumes appropriate pre-operative imaging in all patients (Fig. 2.2a, b).
6. Nephrectomy is not beneficial unless kidney or renal vein is invaded (Fig. 2.3).
7. A reoperative procedure is indicated where local recurrence can be excised without excessive risks (see Fig. 2.1).
8. Use of mitotane postoperatively in all patients without anaplastic histopathology providing serum monitoring can maintain serum levels above 14 μg/ml and below 20 μg/ml.

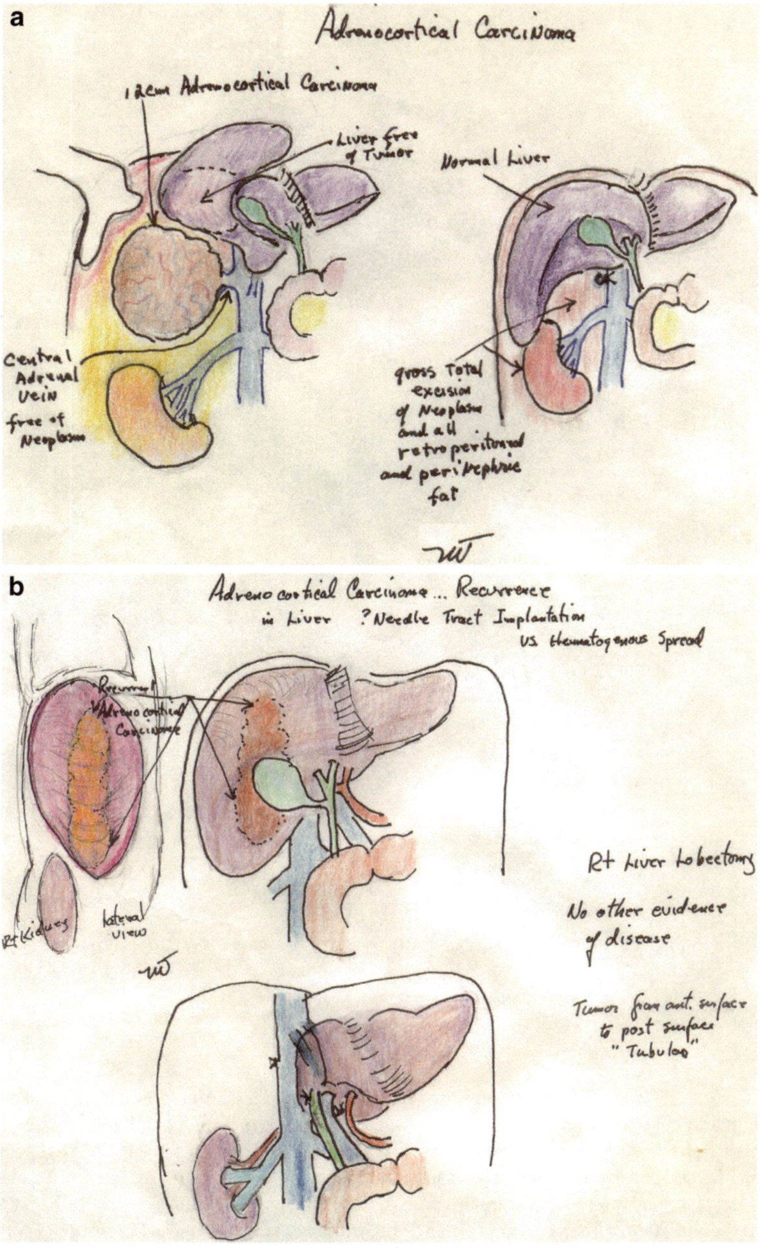

Fig. 2.1 (**a**) A 32-year-old female with large right adrenal ACC mistakenly diagnosed as a hepatic cell adenoma with hemorrhage because of 14-year history of birth control pills, 5-day history of severe right upper quadrant pain, and a percutaneous, transhepatic FNA diagnosis. She was referred for a right hepatic lobectomy. (**b**) Same patient 2 years later with recurrent ACC limited to right lobe of liver along the FNA tract. Following right lobectomy, there was no evidence of recurrence 2 years later

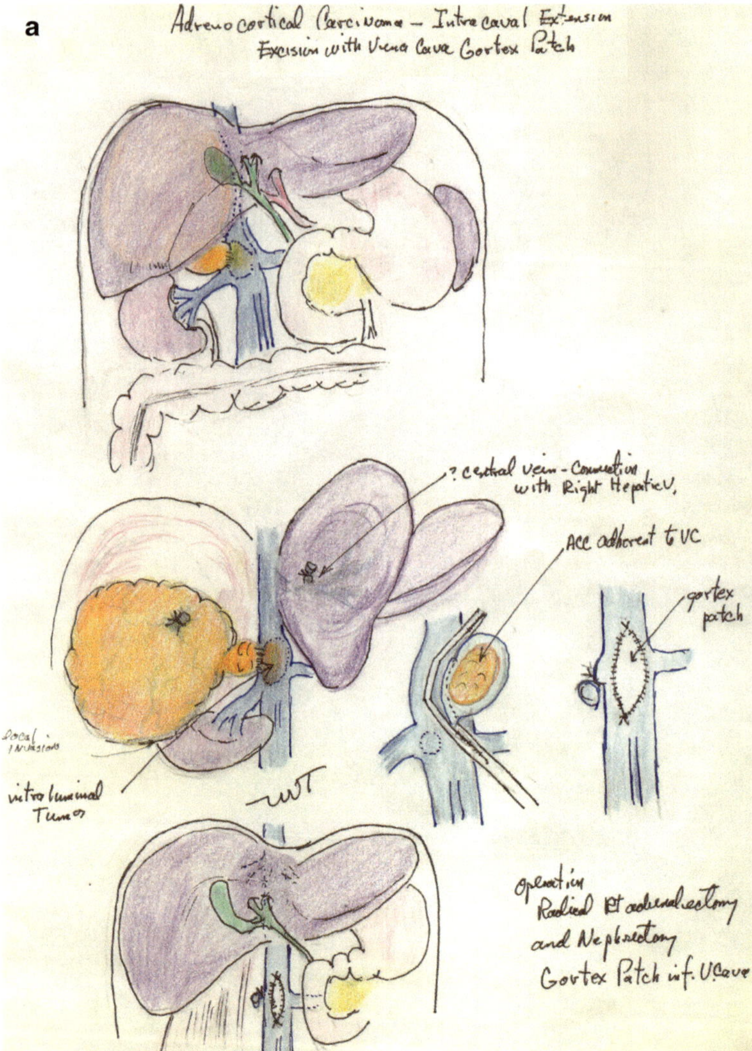

Fig. 2.2 (**a**) A 35-year-old female with nonfunctional ACC and limited extension into the vena cava. Right adrenalectomy and nephrectomy (tumor adherence to kidney) and gortex patch of caval excision site. (**b**) A 40-year-old male 1 year post right adrenalectomy for 11 cm ACC with caval extension. Developed Budd Chiari syndrome and treated with cisplatinum and VP-16. Referred 2 years later for possible operative treatment. No other metastatic disease. With cardiopulmonary bypass and cold arrest, tumor thrombus into right atrium excised and endovenectomy of all tumors in vena cava and both left and middle hepatic veins excised. A pericardial patch was used for the vena cava and distal hepatic veins. The patient had an uneventful course with complete relief of the Budd Chiari syndrome

b

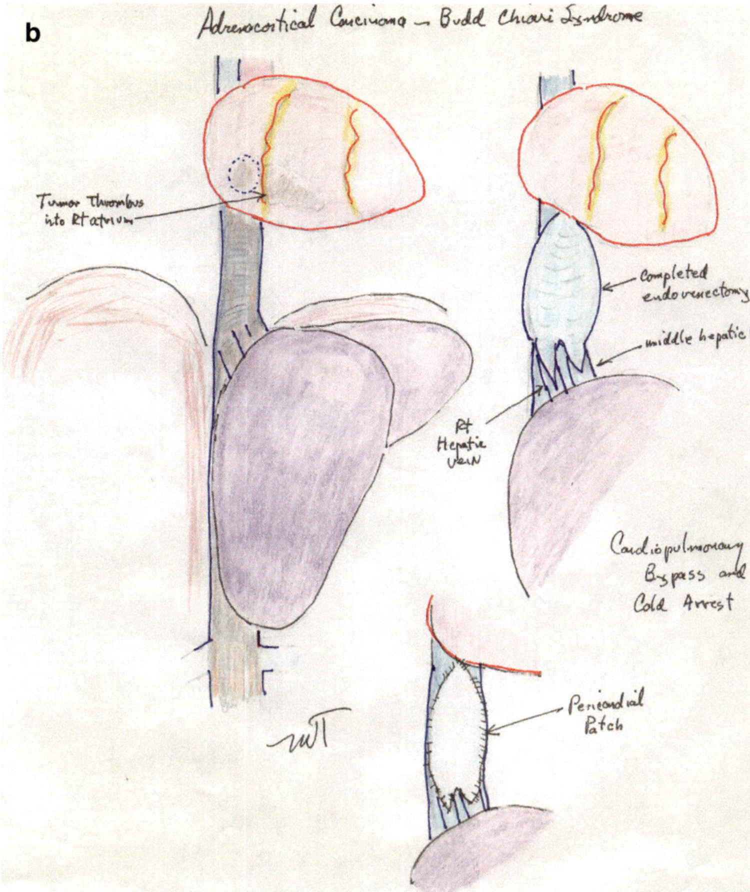

Fig. 2.2 (continued)

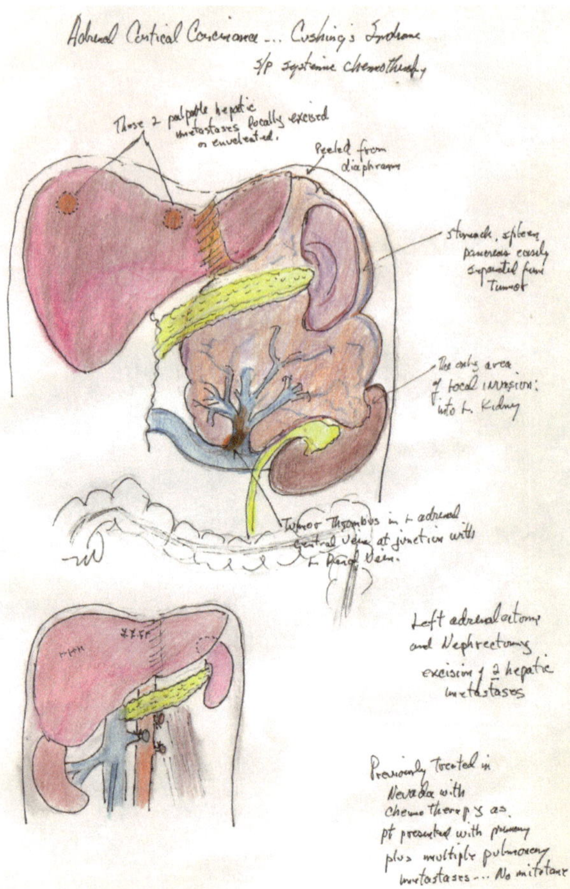

Fig. 2.3 A 47-year-old female with large left adrenal ACC with tumor thrombus into left renal vein. Adrenalectomy, nephrectomy, and excision of two liver metastases resulted in palliation of Cushing's syndrome for 16 months

References

1. Grawitz P (1883) Die sogenannten lipome der niere. Virchow's Archiv Pathol Anal and Klin Med xciii:121–124
2. Rolleston HD (1936) The endocrine organs in health and disease. Oxford University Press, London, pp 301–384
3. Curtis BF (1900) Nephrectomy for suprarenal tumor. Ann Surg 31:759–760
4. Fey B (1926) L'abord du rein par voie thoraco-abdominal. Arch Urol Clin Necker 5:168–178
5. Holmes G (1925) Virilism associated with a suprarenal tumor. Q J Med 18:143–152
6. Kennedy CM, Lister WA (1927) Suprarenal hypernephroma. Lancet 2:739–751
7. Keyser LD, Walters W (1924) Carcinoma of the suprarenal. JAMA 82:87–88
8. Lisser H (1933) Successful removal of adrenal cortical tumor. Trans Associa Am Physicians 48:224–235
9. Richards O (1905) Growths of the kidneys and adrenals. Guy's Hosp Rep 59:217–332

10. Welbourn RB (1990) The history of endocrine surgery. Praeger, New York
11. Walters W et al (1934) The suprarenal cortical syndrome. Ann Surg 100:670–688
12. Thornton JK (1890) Abdominal nephrectomy for large sarcoma of the left suprarenal capsule: recovery. Trans Clin Soc London 23:150–153
13. Robson AWM (1899) Removal of the suprarenal capsule. Br Med J 2:1100–1101
14. Ramsay O (1899) Malignant tumors of the suprarenal gland. Johns Hopkins Hosp Bull nos 94–96:20–29
15. Walters W, Sprague RG (1949) Hyperfunctioning tumors of the adrenal cortex. Ann Surg 129:677–701
16. Broster LB et al (1932) Adreno-genital syndrome: unilateral adrenalectomy. Brit J Surg 19:557–570
17. Kepler EJ, Keating FR (1941) Diseases of the adrenal glands. Arch Int Med 68:1010–1036
18. Murray GG, Simpson G (1929) Virilism due to an adrenal hypernephroma. Lancet 2:734–749
19. Rapaport E et al (1952) Mortality in surgically treated adrenocortical tumors. Postgrad Med 11:325–329
20. Thompson KW, Eisenharatt L (1943) Further consideration of the Cushing's syndrome. J Clin Endocrinol Metab 3:445–452
21. MacFarlane DA (1958) Cancer of the adrenal cortex. Ann R Coll Surg Engl 23:155–162
22. Priestly JT (1952) Lesions of the adrenal glands. Surg Clin N Am 32:1053–1064
23. Anderson HB (1933) Successful removal of adrenal cortical tumor. Trans Associa Am Physicians 48:224–235
24. Thompson NW (1983) Adrenocortical carcinoma.In: Thompson NW, Vinik AI (eds) Endocrine surgery update. Grune and Straton, New York
25. Sahteingart DE et al (1982) Treatment of adrenal carcinomas. Arch Surg 117:1142–1147
26. Cohn K et al (1986) Adrenocortical carcinoma. Surgery 100:1170–1177
27. Icard P et al (1992) Adrenocortical carcinoma in surgically treated patients: a retrospective study on 156 cases by the French Association of Endocrine Surgery. Surgery 112:972–980
28. Kelly WF et al (1979) Cushing's syndrome due to adrenocortical carcinoma. Acta Endocrinologica 91:303–318
29. Lewinsky BS et al (1974) The clinical and pathologic features of "non-hormonal" adrenocortical tumors. Cancer 33:778–790
30. Lipsett MB et al (1963) Clinical and pathophysiologic aspects of adrenocortical carcinoma. Am J Med 35:374–383
31. Richie JP, Gittes RE (1980) Carcinoma of the adrenal cortex. Cancer 45:1957–1964
32. Bergenstall DM et al (1960) Chemotherapy of ACC with *o,p′*-DDD. Ann Int Med 53:672–680
33. Hutter AM, Kayhoe DE (1966) Adrenal cortical carcinoma: clinical features of 138 patients. Am J Med 41:572–580
34. Hutter MM, Jr, Kayhoe DE (1966) Adrenal cortical carcinoma. Results of treatment with *o,p′*-DDD in 138 patients. Am J Med 41:581–589
35. Lubitz JA et al (1973) Mitotane use in inoperable adrenal cortical carcinoma. JAMA 223:1109–1112
36. VanSlooten H et al (1984) The treatment of adrenocortical carcinoma with *o,p′*-DDD: prognostic simplification of serum level monitoring. Eur J Cancer Oncol 20:47–53
37. Hogan TF et al (1978) *o,p′*-DDD (mitotane) therapy of adrenal cortical carcinoma. Cancer 42:2177–2188
38. Lutton JP et al (1990) Clinical features of adrenocortical carcinoma, prognostic factors, and the effect of mitotane therapy. N Engl J Med 322:1195–1201
39. Boven E et al (1984) Complete response of metastasized adrenal cortical carcinoma with o, p′-DDD. Cancer 53:26–29

Part II
Epidemiology, Presentation and Diagnosis

Chapter 3
Epidemiology of Adrenocortical Carcinoma

Martin Fassnacht and Bruno Allolio

3.1 Incidence of Adrenocortical Carcinoma

It is generally accepted that adrenocortical carcinoma (ACC) is a rare disease. However, valid data on the exact incidence and prevalence of ACC are lacking. Adrenal masses are among the most frequent tumors in humans. The vast majority of these tumors are nowadays found incidentally, and the prevalence of these adrenal incidentalomas is estimated as at least 3% in a population over the age of 50 years and increases to as much as 10% in the elderly [1–5]. However, it is well established that about 80% of these incidentally detected adrenal masses represent hormonally inactive adrenal adenomas and only a small minority are ACCs [2, 4, 6]. Data obtained from the National Cancer Institute Survey from the early 1970s estimated an incidence of 1–2 per million population per year, leading to 0.2% of cancer deaths in the United States [7]. A more recent analysis of the SEER database, including data from 12 US states, indicated an annual age-adjusted incidence of 0.72 per million [8, 9]. However, data from the German ACC Registry suggest that the incidence is >1 per million (Fassnacht & Allolio, unpublished data) and may be even higher.

An exceptionally high annual incidence of ACC has been reported for children in southern Brazil, with 3.4–4.2 affected patients per 1 million children vs. an estimated worldwide incidence of 0.3 per 1 million children younger than 15 years [10–12] (see also Chapter 28). Some reports indicate a bimodal age distribution with a first peak in childhood and a second higher peak in the fourth and fifth decade [13]. However, in the German ACC Registry, we do not see an absolute peak in childhood (Fig. 3.1) and the median age is 46 years (range 0.3–86 years). However, based on the low incidence of malignancies in children, in general the incidence of ACC in the German ACC Registry in children below the age of ten may be considered a relative peak (Fig. 3.1).

M. Fassnacht (✉)
Department of Internal Medicine I, Endocrine and Diabetes Unit, University Hospital of Würzburg, Josef-Schneider-Str. 2, 97080, Würzburg, Germany
e-mail: fassnacht_m@medizin.uni-wuerzburg.de

G.D. Hammer, T. Else (eds.), *Adrenocortical Carcinoma*,
DOI 10.1007/978-0-387-77236-3_3, © Springer Science+Business Media, LLC 2011

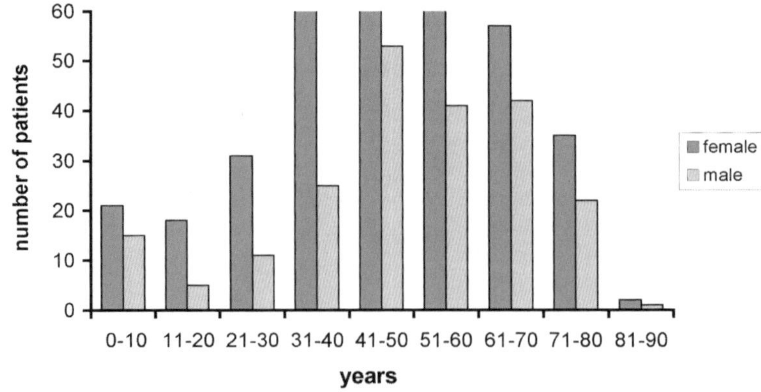

Fig. 3.1 Age and sex distribution at primary diagnosis of ACC in 579 patients. Data from the German ACC Registry (October 2009)

3.2 Risk Factors for Adrenocortical Carcinoma

In most series, women are more often affected than men (ratio 1.5:1; Fig. 3.1) [14–20], leading to the hypothesis that sex hormones may have an influence on ACC tumorigenesis. Interestingly, this female predominance seems to be true only for functional tumors [20, 21]. However, data on the association of risk factors and the development of ACC are rather scarce. The best (although still very limited) data were derived from a case–control study based on the National Mortality Followback Survey, which included a questionnaire sent to the next of kin of almost 20,000 deceased adults in the United States. In this study, 176 patients who died of adrenal cancer (the majority of them suffered most likely from ACC) were compared with 352 controls. Among women, an increased risk for developing ACC was found for ever users of oral contraceptives (hazard ratio = 1.8, 95% confidence interval (CI) 1.0–3.2), especially for those who used them before the age 25 (hazard ratio = 2.5, 95% CI 1.2–5.5). In this context, it is remarkable that in two independent French series a high percentage (9.3 and 5.1%) of female patients with ACC were diagnosed during pregnancy [17, 19]. Furthermore, there is some in vitro evidence that estrogens harbor a proliferative potential for ACC cells [22, 23].

In addition, the above mentioned survey suggested an increased risk for developing ACC in male heavy smokers (hazard ratio 2.0, 95% CI 1.0–4.4), but not in female smokers [24]. The increased risk for male smokers was also seen in another series in 250,000 US veterans [25]. Furthermore, a small study in rats described three ACCs in 80 rats that were exposed to chronic tobacco inhalation in comparison to none in 93 controls [26]. Nevertheless, these epidemiological studies have to be assessed with caution, because in none of the cases ACC was confirmed by histological reports and in some patients adrenal metastases of lung cancer may have been misdiagnosed as ACC. Accordingly, a recent review on tobacco use and cancer causation judged the available evidence for an association of smoking and ACC as too weak to draw firm conclusions [27].

No clear association was found for alcohol use, height and weight, or food consumption patterns in either sex [24]. In addition, there is no evidence that race has an impact on the incidence of ACC [28], although most of the available data stem from series that predominately included Caucasians. There are some case reports that patients with poorly controlled congenital adrenal hyperplasia have a higher incidence of adrenal tumors including ACC [29, 30]. Again, no firm conclusions can be drawn from these observations.

3.3 Stage at Presentation

In early series, the majority of patients were diagnosed with advanced disease. In a meta-analysis by Wooten and King, including more than 600 patients, published between 1952 and 1992, less than one third of the patients had localized disease (stage I or II) and 49% of patients were described as stage IV. In contrast, in more recent studies the percentage of patients in stage I or II is much higher, reflecting earlier diagnosis due to widely available advanced imaging technology [14, 17, 31, 32]. Patients with stage I that were virtually nonexistent in older studies, now account for more than 5% of patients in ACC cohorts, most often presenting with an incidentaloma [16]. Nevertheless, median tumor size is still >11 cm (range 3–40 cm; Fig. 3.2) [15]. Although one would expect an equal distribution between right and left adrenal, some series including the German ACC Registry report a slightly higher frequency of left-sided tumors (ratio 1:1.18–1.25) [14, 20, 33] (Fassnacht & Allolio unpublished results). Bilateral tumors are extremely rare, and it is often not clear whether theses tumors are independent of each other or if one represents a metastasis to the contralateral ACC.

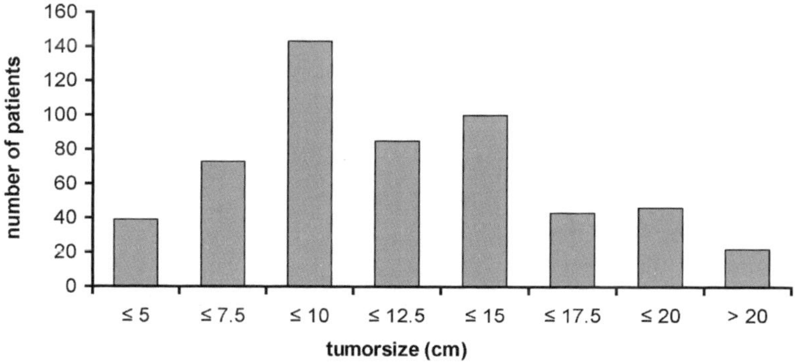

Fig. 3.2 Tumor size at primary diagnosis of ACC in 551 patients. Data from the German ACC Registry (October 2009)

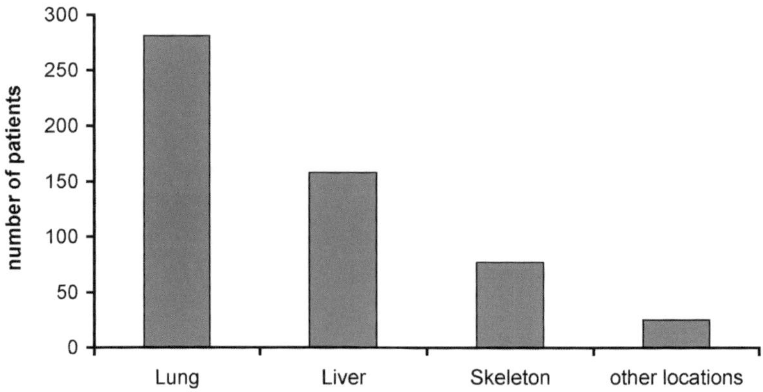

Fig. 3.3 Localization of distant metastases in 376 patients with advanced ACC (at the time of primary diagnosis or during follow-up). Data from the German ACC Registry (October 2009)

Several series have confirmed that liver and lung are the two most frequent sites for metastases [13, 15, 20, 31] (see also Fig. 3.3). In the German ACC Registry, >95% of 376 patients with metastatic disease (at initial diagnosis or during follow-up) had hepatic and/or pulmonary lesions. In only 20 patients (5.3%) metastases were diagnosed in other locations (mainly bone), without concomitant metastatic disease affecting liver or lung. However, bone metastases leading to fractures and pain have been reported as presenting clinical feature in some patients with advanced ACC [34, 35].

3.4 Prognosis of Adrenocortical Carcinoma

As outlined above, ACC-related deaths are rare when calculated on a population basis. However, in affected patients mortality from ACC is substantial. In different series, 5-year overall survival ranged between 16 and 44% [17, 19, 31, 33, 36–40]. However, based on experience with the German ACC Registry, this wide range in 5-year survival and the poor prognosis in some series may be related to a referral bias, as patients cured by surgery may be underrepresented in these series. In our series including 538 patients with follow-up data, the survival rate was 46% (95% CI 41–51%) after 5 years and 38% (32–44%) after 10 years. Prognosis is still mainly depending on tumor stage, and 5-year survival rates were 79% for stage I, 62% for stage II, 50% for stage III, and 17% for stage IV when applying the new ENSAT staging system (Fig. 3.4). Of note, when only patients with stage II who were referred to the German registry within 3 months of primary diagnosis were analyzed, their survival rate after 5 years is >80% (Johanssen, Fassnacht, Allolio unpublished results), again pointing to a relevant referral bias in some series.

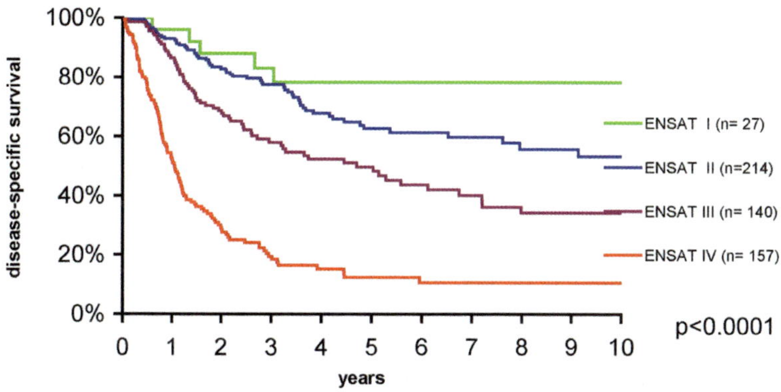

Fig. 3.4 Stage-dependent survival in 538 patients with ACC. Data from the German ACC Registry (October 2009). Of note, in three of six patients in stage I, who died of ACC, violation of the capsule occurred during surgery

3.5 Associated Malignancies

In 1983, Nader et al. reported that 7 out of 74 patients (9.5%) had second primary cancers that were histologically different from ACC. Data from the German ACC Registry confirm this observation: 44 of 423 evaluated patients (10.4%) suffered from a second primary malignancy, including four patients with two different primary tumors. However, no specific pattern of associated tumors could be detected, and up to now no specific germline mutations have been identified in these patients.

References

1. Bovio S et al (2006) Prevalence of adrenal incidentaloma in a contemporary computerized tomography series. J Endocrinol Invest 29(4):298–302
2. Grumbach MM et al (2003) Management of the clinically inapparent adrenal mass (incidentaloma). Ann Intern Med 138(5):424–429
3. Kloos RT et al (1995) Incidentally discovered adrenal masses. Endocr Rev 16(4): 460–484
4. Mansmann G et al (2004) The clinically inapparent adrenal mass: update in diagnosis and management. Endocr Rev 25(2):309–340
5. Song JH et al (2008) The incidental adrenal mass on CT: prevalence of adrenal disease in 1,049 consecutive adrenal masses in patients with no known malignancy. AJR Am J Roentgenol 190(5):1163–1168
6. Terzolo M et al (1997) Prevalence of adrenal carcinoma among incidentally discovered adrenal masses. A retrospective study from 1989 to 1994. Gruppo Piemontese Incidentalomi Surrenalici. Arch Surg 132(8):914–919
7. National-Cancer-Institute (1975) Third national cancer survey: incidence data. DHEW Publ. No. (NIH) 75-787. NCI monograph: 41

8. Golden SH et al (2009) Clinical review: prevalence and incidence of endocrine and metabolic disorders in the United States: a comprehensive review. J Clin Endocrinol Metab 94(6): 1853–1878
9. Kebebew E et al (2006) Extent of disease at presentation and outcome for adrenocortical carcinoma: have we made progress? World J Surg 30(5):872–878
10. Michalkiewicz E et al (2004) Clinical and outcome characteristics of children with adrenocortical tumors: a report from the International Pediatric Adrenocortical Tumor Registry. J Clin Oncol 22(5):838–845
11. Pianovski MA et al (2006) Mortality rate of adrenocortical tumors in children under 15 years of age in Curitiba, Brazil. Pediatr Blood Cancer 47(1):56–60
12. Ribeiro RC et al (2001) An inherited p53 mutation that contributes in a tissue-specific manner to pediatric adrenal cortical carcinoma. Proc Natl Acad Sci USA 98(16):9330–9335
13. Wajchenberg B et al (2000) Adrenocortical carcinoma: clinical and laboratory observations. Cancer 88(4):711–736
14. Bilimoria KY et al (2008) Adrenocortical carcinoma in the United States: treatment utilization and prognostic factors. Cancer 113(11):3130–3136
15. Fassnacht M, Allolio B (2009) Clinical management of adrenocortical carcinoma. Best Pract Res Clin Endocrinol Metab 23(2):273–289
16. Fassnacht M et al (2009) Limited prognostic value of the 2004 International Union Against Cancer staging classification for adrenocortical carcinoma: proposal for a revised TNM classification. Cancer 115(2):243–250
17. Icard P et al (2001) Adrenocortical carcinomas: surgical trends and results of a 253-patient series from the French Association of Endocrine Surgeons study group. World J Surg 25(7):891–897
18. Koschker AC et al (2006) Adrenocortical carcinoma – improving patient care by establishing new structures. Exp Clin Endocrinol Diabetes 114(2):45–51
19. Luton JP et al (1990) Clinical features of adrenocortical carcinoma, prognostic factors, and the effect of mitotane therapy. N Engl J Med 322(17):1195–1201
20. Icard P et al (1992) Survival rates and prognostic factors in adrenocortical carcinoma. World J Surg 16(4):753–758
21. Wooten MD, King DK (1993) Adrenal cortical carcinoma. Epidemiology and treatment with mitotane and a review of the literature. Cancer 72(11):3145–3155
22. Montanaro D et al (2005) Antiestrogens upregulate estrogen receptor beta expression and inhibit adrenocortical H295R cell proliferation. J Mol Endocrinol 35(2): 245–256
23. Somjen D et al (2003) Carboxy derivatives of isoflavones as affinity carriers for cytotoxic drug targeting in adrenocortical H295R carcinoma cells. J Endocrinol 179(3): 395–403
24. Hsing AW et al (1996) Risk factors for adrenal cancer: an exploratory study. Int J Cancer 65(4):432–436
25. Chow WH et al (1996) Smoking and adrenal cancer mortality among United States veterans. Cancer Epidemiol Biomarkers Prev 5(2):79–80
26. Dalbey WE et al (1980) Chronic inhalation of cigarette smoke by F344 rats. J Natl Cancer Inst 64(2):383–390
27. Kuper H et al (2002) Tobacco use and cancer causation: association by tumour type. J Intern Med 252(3):206–224
28. Hutter AM, Jr, Kayhoe DE (1966) Adrenal cortical carcinoma. Clinical features of 138 patients. Am J Med 41(4):572–580
29. Allolio B (2001) Adrenal incidentalomas. In: Margioris AN, Chrousos GP (eds) Adrenal disorders. Humana, Totawa, NJ, pp 249–261
30. Hamwi GJ et al (1957) Does adrenocortical hyperplasia result in adrenocortical carcinoma. N Engl J Med 257(24):1153–1157

31. Abiven G et al (2006) Clinical and biological features in the prognosis of adrenocortical cancer: poor outcome of cortisol-secreting tumors in a series of 202 consecutive patients. J Clin Endocrinol Metab 91(7):2650–2655
32. Kendrick ML et al (2001) Adrenocortical carcinoma: surgical progress or status quo? Arch Surg 136(5):543–549
33. Schulick RD, Brennan MF (1999) Adrenocortical carcinoma. World J Urol 17(1):26–34
34. Durusu M et al (2002) Adrenal cortical carcinoma presenting initially with radius metastasis. Clin Oncol (R Coll Radiol) 14(1):83–84
35. Solans R et al (2001) Bone metastases as presentation of adrenocortical carcinoma. Med Clin (Barc) 116(2):76–77
36. Bellantone R et al (1997) Role of reoperation in recurrence of adrenal cortical carcinoma: results from 188 cases collected in the Italian National Registry for Adrenal Cortical Carcinoma. Surgery 122(6):1212–1218
37. Haak HR et al (1994) Optimal treatment of adrenocortical carcinoma with mitotane: results in a consecutive series of 96 patients. Br J Cancer 69(5):947–951
38. Pommier RF, Brennan MF (1992) An eleven-year experience with adrenocortical carcinoma. Surgery 112(6):963–970; discussion 970–971
39. Soreide JA et al (1992) Adrenal cortical carcinoma in Norway, 1970–1984. World J Surg 16(4):663–667; discussion 668
40. Venkatesh S et al (1989) Adrenal cortical carcinoma. Cancer 64(3):765–769

Chapter 4
Clinical Presentation and Initial Diagnosis

Bruno Allolio and Martin Fassnacht

4.1 Clinical Presentation

The initial clinical presentation of adrenocortical carcinoma (ACC) consists of signs and symptoms of hormone excess, local or regional manifestations of tumor growth, complications of metastatic disease, or more general manifestations of malignancy such as weight loss, fever, and malaise. Currently, an increasing number of patients is detected incidentally by modern imaging.

4.1.1 Hormone Excess

Clinically apparent hormone excess is the most frequent manifestation of ACC and is the reason to seek medical advice in 45–60% of cases [1–8]. In an extensive older review of all available series published in 1993 and reporting on a total of 1891 cases, 59.3% of tumors were classified as functional [8]. In a recently published series from France collecting 202 consecutive patients beginning in 1963, the disease was revealed in 54% by endocrine features [1]. Similarly, in the German ACC Registry, about 50% of patients showed clinical signs and symptoms of hormone excess at presentation (Fig. 4.1). However, not in all of these cases evidence of hormone excess was the main reason to seek medical advice. Furthermore, while in older series most patients were diagnosed with advanced disease (stage IV), today patients in stage IV comprise less than 35% of patients at the time of presentation [9]. Obviously, earlier detection of disease will be associated with less severe clinical signs and symptoms of hormone excess. Another aspect that may influence the variable percentage of functional tumors in different series is probably related to the center reporting the patients, with a higher percentage of patients presenting with

B. Allolio (✉)
Department of Internal Medicine I, Endocrine and Diabetes Unit, University of Würzburg, Josef-Schneider-Str. 2, 97080 Würzburg, Germany
e-mail: allolio_b@medizin.uni-wuerzburg.de

G.D. Hammer, T. Else (eds.), *Adrenocortical Carcinoma*,
DOI 10.1007/978-0-387-77236-3_4, © Springer Science+Business Media, LLC 2011

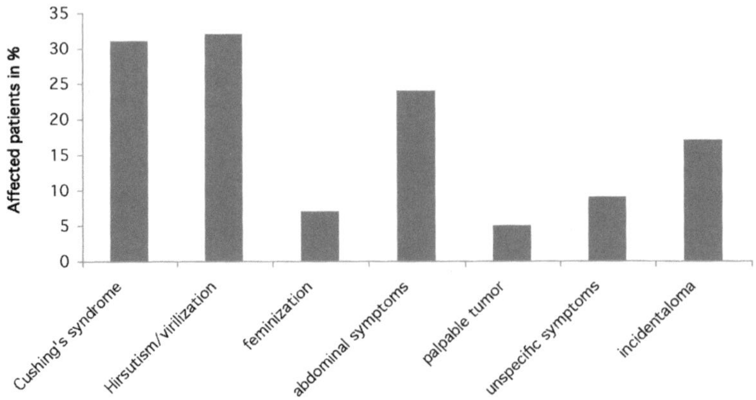

Fig. 4.1 Symptoms at the time of initial diagnosis in 533 patients with ACC. Data from the German ACC Registry. In some patients several symptoms were described. For hirsutism/virilization percentage of women and for feminization percentage of men were calculated

clinical evidence of hormone hypersecretion in series from endocrine departments compared to surgical series.

Cushing's syndrome (CS) is the most frequent presentation in functioning ACC [1, 4, 6, 10–14]. All typical features of CS [15] including central obesity, facial plethora, rounded face, skin atrophy, easy bruising, muscle weakness, supraclavicular fat pads, menstrual irregularity, hypertension, diabetes mellitus, nephrolithiasis, and osteoporosis with fractures may be found at presentation. However, the rapid development of the disease often changes the clinical presentation with less or no weight gain, rapid development of muscle atrophy, profound hypertension, and glucose intolerance as key features. A history of <12 months from the first clinical changes to the detection of CS is highly suspicious of ACC (or ectopic ACTH secretion by a malignant neoplasm). Appearance of psychiatric symptoms like profound depression or acute psychosis warrants immediate attention to avert suicide. Massive hypercortisolism may lead to hypertension and severe hypokalemia, requiring replacement doses of potassium of >120 mmol/day due to excessive renal potassium loss. The pathophysiological basis is incomplete renal inactivation of cortisol by 11-beta-dehydrogenase type II, and hence grossly elevated mineralocorticoid receptor activation [16].

On the other hand, due to the low efficiency in steroid production per cell, clinical abnormalities in functioning ACC may be subtle and often require an astute physician for early recognition of CS. Furthermore, the concomitant secretion of anabolic androgens may mitigate the catabolic activity of excess glucocorticoids on muscle and bone.

A high percentage of female patients present with signs and symptoms of androgen excess (hirsutism, acne, androgenetic effluvium) and virilization with or without concomitant CS (Fig. 4.2). In fact, the combination of hypercortisolism and substantial androgen excess in an adrenal tumor raises the suspicion of ACC significantly.

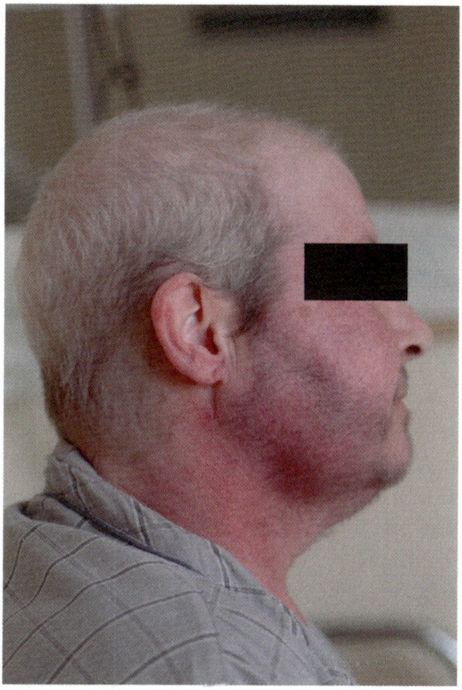

Fig. 4.2 A woman with advanced ACC hypersecreting both cortisol and androgens demonstrating a combination of Cushingoid features and signs of hyperandrogenism

In a series of patients with pure androgen-secreting tumors, women presented with menstrual alterations including amenorrhea and metrorrhagia together with hirsutism [17]. Signs of virilization (clitoral enlargement, deepening of the voice, baldness) were also seen, but only in a minority of women with ACC and androgen excess. Many series do not clearly differentiate between signs of androgen excess like hirsutism, acne, as also seen for example in polycystic ovary syndrome, and clinical virilization with male pattern baldness, deepening of the voice, and changes in clitoral size [4, 14]. Different from other adult disorders of androgen excess in women like late onset congenital adrenal hyperplasia or polycystic ovary syndrome, clinical signs of androgen excess in ACC usually develop rapidly (often <12 months), with no relationship to puberty.

In men, androgen-secreting ACC is usually not associated with clinical changes, as high testicular androgen secretion dominates total androgen activity, and ceiling effects of androgen action obscure additional androgen secretion from an ACC.

In contrast, estrogen-secreting ACC may lead to feminization in males presenting with gynecomastia, loss of libido, and testicular atrophy [18, 19]. In particular, recent onset of bilateral gynecomastia has been repeatedly reported as the first sign of ACC [18, 19]. However, feminizing ACCs are rare, and in the series by Icard [4] only 4 out of 253 patients had evidence of feminization. Based on current data of the German ACC Registry including 533 patients, only 14 out of 195 males showed clinical signs of feminization (7%), supporting the view that gynecomastia is an unusual presentation of ACC. In premenopausal females, estrogen-secreting tumors may lead to disturbance of the menstrual cycle, and in postmenopausal women to reappearance of uterine bleeding [20].

Aldosterone-producing ACC is also rare, probably comprising <2% of patients with ACC [1, 4, 6, 14] (see Chapter 27). Based on a detailed review of 58 cases [21], the median age of the patients ranges between 40 and 50 years, with the vast majority presenting with hypertension and hypokalemia suggestive of Conn's syndrome. However, in rare instances either hypertension or hypokalemia may be the only presenting feature [21]. The mean potassium level is 2.3 ± 0.08 mmol/l and the mean blood pressure $188 \pm 4/111 \pm 2$ mmHg. As outlined above, the combination of hypertension and hypokalemia more often results from massive hypercortisolism due to a glucocorticoid-secreting ACC.

In fact, detailed analysis in hormonally active ACC often reveals hypersecretion of a large spectrum of adrenal steroids, leading to combinations of clinical features like CS plus virilization (Fig. 4.2). Intriguingly, in some cases the clinical pattern may shift from Conn's syndrome to CS, or a previously hormonally active tumor may appear nonfunctioning at recurrence [22, 23]. However, in general, the hormonal pattern of ACC remains stable and allows the use of the hormonal phenotype for monitoring complete tumor removal and recurrence. In addition, hormone precursors are almost invariably detectable in both functional and nonfunctional tumors by sophisticated technology, making the distinction between non-functioning and functioning ACCs somewhat blurred. However, in clinical terms, purely precursor-secreting ACCs appear as hormonally silent tumors.

Some tumors may secrete hormonal products not related to steroidogenesis, which may play a role in the initial clinical manifestation. Tumor-induced hypoglycemia has been reported in ACC, and most likely is related to increased glucose utilization by a large tumor induced by paracrine release of IGF2 and pro-IGF2 acting at the insulin receptor [14, 24, 25]. Occasional ectopic secretion of ADH may present as symptomatic hyponatremia [26]. High secretion of renin by an ACC may contribute to hypertension [27], whereas secretion of erythropoietin may induce erythrocytosis [28], which is reversed after tumor removal. In addition, excessive secretion of inhibin has been described leading to isolated suppression of FSH [29]. Also ectopic calcitonin secretion from an ACC has been reported [30].

4.1.2 Loco-Regional Manifestations

Patients with a nonfunctioning ACC usually present with symptoms related to local mass effects of the tumor like abdominal fullness, pain, indigestion, nausea, and vomiting [14, 20]. These symptoms are related to the large tumor size with a median diameter of >10 cm and a median weight of >500 g in most series [1–6, 8, 12]. In some cases, spontaneous tumor rupture may present as acute abdomen or as retroperitoneal hemorrhage [31, 32]. Tumor invasion into large veins including the inferior vena cava is not uncommon and may influence clinical presentation [33–36] and prognosis [37]. Impaired venous flow may lead to complaints suggestive of deep vein thrombosis [38] and to varicocele [14, 39]. Extension of tumor invasion up to the level of the right atrium has been repeatedly described, leading to shortness of breath and respiratory distress [40]. Furthermore, involvement of hepatic veins has been reported [40] occasionally presenting as acute Budd-Chiari syndrome [41].

4.1.3 Unspecific Symptoms – Metastatic Disease

Nonspecific symptoms of malignancy like fever, weight loss, myalgia, and general malaise only affect a minority of patients with ACC at the time of presentation. In the series from Cochin [1], only 13 of 202 cases were revealed by weakness and weight loss. In fact, in our experience it is a peculiar feature of ACC that it often completely lacks nonspecific symptoms of malignancy even in the presence of extensive tumor burden and progressive disease. However, in rare cases, high expression of *CXC* chemokines by an ACC may lead to a distinct presentation with fever, leukocytosis, and increased acute-phase reactants, probably related to secretion of IL-8 and epithelial neutrophil-activating protein-78 [42].

A substantial fraction of patients with tumors are in stage IV (metastatic disease) at presentation, with lung, liver, and bone being the most frequent sites of metastases [8, 9] (see Fig. 4.3). Bone metastases with local pain or fractures may become the presenting feature of advanced ACC [43, 44]. Other unusual manifestations of advanced ACC are pelvic complaints, paraplegia, urinary obstruction, hematuria [14, 45], and cervical or axillary lymph node enlargement [10].

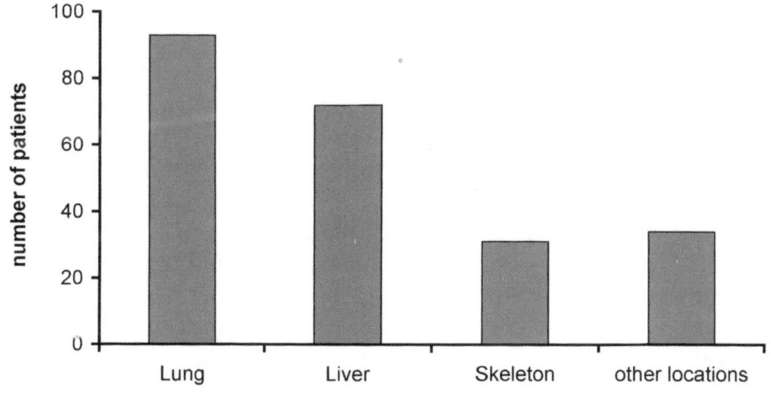

Fig. 4.3 Localization of distant metastases in 160 patients with metastatic ACC (at the time of primary diagnosis). Data from the German ACC Registry (October 2009)

4.1.4 Incidentally Detected Adrenocortical Carcinoma

ACCs discovered incidentally by modern imaging are increasingly frequent in more recent series. In the French series published by Abiven et al. [1] collecting data since 1963, 13% of all patients were investigated for an adrenal incidentaloma, all of them were diagnosed after 1983. Similarly, in the German ACC Registry, 16.7% of 533 patients presented initially as an adrenal incidentaloma. Thus, the widely available modern imaging technologies in affluent countries have a growing impact on the diagnosis of ACC and may contribute to the fact that today ACC is more often detected at an earlier stage.

4.2 Laboratory Work-Up

As discussed above, 45–60% of the patients suffer from clinically evident hormone excess. However, with more sophisticated methodology becoming available, it is evident that only a small proportion of ACCs (if any at all) do not autonomously secrete at least some adrenal steroids. On the other hand, a detailed endocrine assessment is expensive and needs to be justified. Nonetheless, a thorough initial hormonal work-up is important for several reasons. (1) The diagnosis of autonomous steroid hormone excess establishes the adrenocortical origin of the tumor and effectively excludes other diagnoses requiring different therapeutic approaches (e.g., pheochromocytoma or lymphoma). (2) The steroid pattern may indicate, and in some cases even prove, malignancy in an adrenal tumor. An adrenal mass that co-secretes different types of steroids is highly suspicious for an ACC, and co-secretion of glucocorticoids in combination with sex hormones and precursors in our experience establishes the diagnosis and this may influence the surgical approach. In some cases of metastastic disease, evidence of steroid hypersecretion may even obviate the need of a histopathological diagnosis of ACC. In general, low DHEAS suggests a benign adrenocortical tumor, whereas highly elevated DHEAS levels are indicative for ACC [46]. (3) Preoperatively elevated hormones can serve as tumor markers during follow-up. Although imaging methods have improved significantly in the past decades, in some patients disease recurrence may be first detected by an increase of circulating hormones. (4) From a clinical perspective, the probably most relevant reason to search for autonomous hormone secretion is the identification of patients with (subclinical) cortisol excess. If significant cortisol secretion is present and remains undiagnosed, complete resection may lead to life-threatening adrenal insufficiency peri- or postoperatively due to suppression and atrophy of the contralateral adrenal. In this context, the standard 1 mg dexamethasone overnight test is the most sensitive test to screen for glucocorticoid excess. A serum cortisol value <1.8 μg/dl (50 nmol/l) after 1 mg dexamethasone excludes Cushing's syndrome [47, 48]. In all other patients subsequent tests should be performed (e.g., 24-h urinary-free cortisol, midnight salivary or serum cortisol, ACTH, CRH-test). All patients with proven or suspected cortisol excess need perioperative coverage with hydrocortisone.

Aldosterone-secreting ACCs are rare and usually present with severe hypokalemia and high serum aldosterone concentration. In the German ACC Registry, co-secretion of other steroids has been documented in 24 of 37 patients with aldosterone-producing tumors. Therefore, purely aldosterone-secreting adrenal tumors <4 cm are suggestive of a benign adenoma.

Of special importance is the exclusion of a pheochromocytoma. In the past decade, measurement of metanephrines (either as free metanephrine in plasma or as fractionated metanephrines in 24-h urine) has become the method of choice for the exclusion of pheochromocytoma [49–54]. Only in patients with indisputable adrenocortical steroid excess one might skip this analysis.

As discussed above, ACC may rarely produce other hormones like ADH, renin, inhibin, or calcitonin. However, screening for these hormones on a routine basis is not suggested.

In conclusion, the detailed endocrine work-up that was proposed by the ACC Working Group of ENSAT is recommended in all patients with suspected ACC. When applying these tests, only a minority of ACCs are hormonally inactive. Figure 4.4 provides the results of the endocrine work-up in 377 patients in the German ACC Registry. However, in this analysis all patients in whom at least one single adrenocortical hormone had been measured were included. Even with this limitation, almost 80% of tumors were hormonally active. Thus, it is very likely that the percentage of endocrine inactive tumors is largely overestimated. Therefore, in cases in which detailed hormone analyses reveal no autonomous hormone secretion, caution is warranted not to misdiagnose a nonadrenocortical tumor of the adrenal region as an ACC. As demonstrated in other series also, the data from the German Registry confirm that glucocorticoid and androgen excess are by far the most frequent types of hormonal abnormality. In 205 of 354 evaluated patients (54.5%), endocrine work-up demonstrated hypercortisolism and in 172 patients (45.6%) androgen excess (Fig. 4.4).

Preliminary results derived from the analysis of 24-h urinary steroid profiles utilizing gas-chromatography mass-spectrometry (GC-MS) are further supporting the

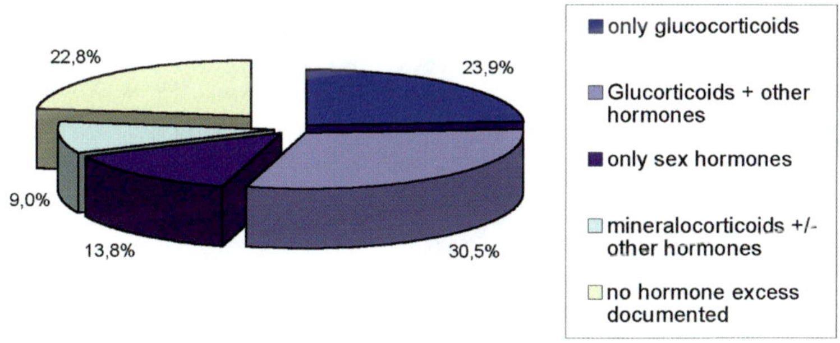

Fig. 4.4 Results of hormonal work-up in 377 patients with adrenocortical carcinoma. Data from the German ACC Registry (October 2009). All patients in which at least one adrenocortical hormone was measured were included in this analysis. Based on this data, it is very likely that the percentage of endocrine-inactive tumors is largely overestimated

Table 4.1 Hormonal work-up in patients with suspected or proven ACC. Recommendations of the ACC Working Group of the European Network for the Study of Adrenal Tumors (ENSAT), May 2005

• Glucocorticoid excess (minimum three out of four tests)	- Dexamethasone suppression test (1 mg, 23:00 h) - Excretion of free urinary cortisol (24-h urine) - Basal cortisol (serum) - Basal ACTH (plasma)
• Sexual steroids and steroid precursors	- DHEAS (serum) - 17-OH-Progesterone (serum) - Androstenedione (serum) - Testosterone (serum) - 17-Beta-estradiol (serum, only in men and postmenopausal women)
• Mineralocorticoid excess	- Potassium (serum) - Aldosterone/renin ratio (only in patients with arterial hypertension and/or hypokalemia)
• Exclusion of a pheochromocytoma	- Catecholamine or metanephrine excretion (24-h urine) - Meta- and normetanephrines (plasma)

concept that virtually all ACCs secret steroids. With this highly accurate method in >95% of all patients with ACC, autonomous secretion of steroids or steroid hormone precursors is detectable [55]. Therefore, this method (when more widely available) may become a corner stone in the diagnosis of adrenal masses.

Although the evidence level for the proposed work-up (Table 4.1) is still low, it provides important guidance in this difficult clinical situation. In a recent analysis in Germany, 16% of patients with ACC had no preoperative hormonal assessment performed, and in less than a quarter of patients the endocrine work-up could be judged as sufficient (Fig. 4.5) [56]. Although comparable data are missing, it is

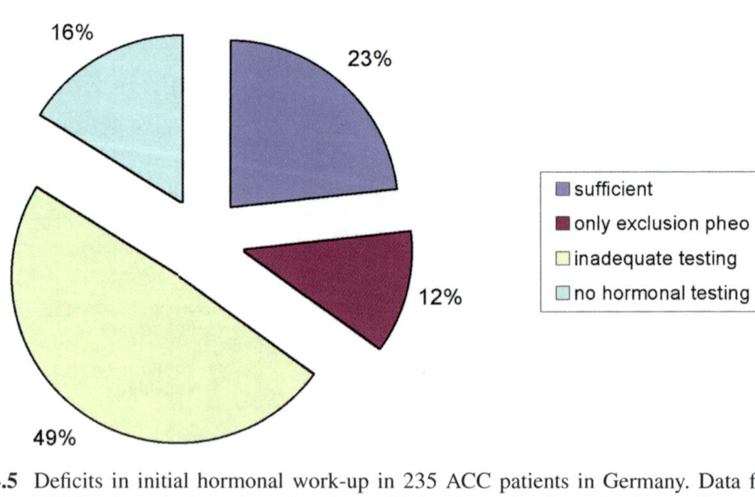

Fig. 4.5 Deficits in initial hormonal work-up in 235 ACC patients in Germany. Data from the German ACC Registry (only patients in whom all data from the time of primary diagnosis were available were analyzed.)

predicted that in other countries the situation is similar. Therefore, major efforts need to be taken to improve the diagnostic work-up in patients with adrenal tumors to avoid putting patients at unnecessary perioperative risks and impairing structured follow-up.

Laboratory parameters other than hormones are of less importance in ACC although blood count, electrolytes, kidney and liver function have to be assessed prior surgical or medical treatment to avoid unexpected toxicity. In addition, serum LDH may serve as a marker of disease progression in aggressive and metastasized disease.

4.3 Imaging at Presentation

Imaging plays a key role in the diagnostic work-up of patients presenting with suspected ACC, and is in more detail discussed in Chapters 6 and 7. Both size and appearance of an adrenal mass are usually well suited to differentiate benign and malignant adrenocortical lesions. In an analysis of the German ACC Registry comprising 489 informative patients, the median tumor diameter at diagnosis was 11.6 ± 4.7 cm (ranging from 3 to 40 cm), making size alone a highly valuable parameter to assess malignancy. Most ACCs are inhomogeneous with areas of necrosis or hemorrhage, with irregular margins, and occasionally with calcifications [57].

Ultrasound. Sonography is an inexpensive and safe method that detects adrenal lesions larger than 2–3 cm. However, it is strongly user-dependent and sonographic evaluations poorly characterize solid adrenal lesions. Using contrast-enhanced sonography, malignant lesions more often show hypervascularization (57% vs. 7% for benign lesions) [58]. In addition, in a series of 12 patients liver metastases were detected in 67% by contrast-enhanced ultrasound compared to only 50% by contrast-enhanced multislice spiral computed tomography [59].

CT. Thin collimation CT is widely used in the diagnosis of ACC and offers high spatial resolution. Detection of invasion into surrounding structures indicates malignancy. Local invasion or tumor extension into the inferior vena cava as well as lymph node or other metastases are regularly demonstrated in advanced ACC at presentation and may greatly influence surgical strategy. Measurement of Hounsfield Units (HU) in unenhanced CT is a helpful tool to differentiate benign adrenal lesions from malignancy. Using a threshold value of 10 HU, sensitivity and specificity for characterizing an adrenal mass as a benign adenoma in unenhanced CT are 71% and 98%, respectively, based on a meta-analysis of ten studies [60]. In cases of a lipid-poor lesion with unenhanced HU values >10, delayed post contrast CT yields high sensitivity and specificity in the diagnosis of ACC [61, 62]. Adrenal lesions with an attenuation value of >10 HU in unenhanced CT and an enhancement washout of <50% and a delayed attenuation of >35 HU are suspicious for malignancy [51, 63–65]. Delayed enhanced CT is also able to characterize some adrenal masses that cannot be characterized by chemical shift MRI [66].

MRI. Similarly effective to CT in characterizing adrenal lesions is MRI with dynamic gadolinium-enhanced and chemical shift technique [63, 64]. Multiplanar MRI is well suited to separate adrenal masses from surrounding structures like liver, pancreas, spleen, and kidneys. MRI may thus be particularly helpful to better define the surgical approach to ACC at the time of diagnosis. ACCs typically present isointense to liver on T1-weighted images and show an increase in intensity in T2-weighted sequences. As with all imaging techniques, heterogeneity due to hemorrhage and necrosis is usually observed. Enhancement after gadolinium is distinct and followed by a slow washout. The sensitivity of MRI for differentiating benign and malignant adrenal lesions has been calculated at 81–89% with a specificity of 92–99% [63, 67]. New developments for MRI imaging include fast low-angle shot, in vivo proton, MR spectroscopy [68, 69], but these methods have not yet entered routine practice.

FDG-PET. In case of uncertainty, [^{18}F]-FDG-PET may be of significant value in patients with suspected ACC. High uptake of [^{18}F]-FDG indicates increased glucose metabolism and is highly suspicious of malignancy, whereas a very low standardized uptake value (SUV) strongly points to a benign lesion. In a prospective study in 77 operated patients, the sensitivity and specificity to distinguish adenomas from ACCs were 1.0 (0.85–1.00) and 0.88 (0.75–0.96) respectively, using a cut-off value above 1.45 for adrenal to liver SUV max ratio [70]. Similarly, in a consecutive sample of 150 patients with documented adrenal lesions and a known malignancy, PET-CT was highly valuable to differentiate benign from malignant adrenal masses. Particularly, all 26 malignant lesions showed qualitative and quantitative signal intensity greater than the liver. By combining unenhanced and qualitative CT data with PET data, the analysis yielded a sensitivity of 100% for the detection of malignancy, a specificity of 99%, a positive predictive value of 93%, and a negative predictive value of 100% [71]. Similar findings using a slightly different cut-off for tumor to liver SUV max ratio were reported in a series from Japan [72]. Thus, in indeterminate cases, FDG-PET may be used to preoperatively better define the malignant potential of an adrenal lesion. In addition, FDG-PET offers a way to detect distant metastases not easily detected by chest CT or abdominal MRI (e.g., bone metastases).

Staging at diagnosis. Prior to undergoing surgery for suspected ACC, careful tumor staging including high-resolution CT of the chest and abdomen for detection of lung and liver metastases is mandatory, as in case of disseminated disease removal of the primary tumor remains of questionable value [57]. FDG-PET cannot substitute for a chest CT, as it has a low sensitivity for small lung lesions (<1 cm) [73, 74]. A bone scan is only required if the patient complains of bone pain and we perform cerebral imaging only in patients with clinical evidence for brain metastases, because bone and brain metastases occur rarely without concomitant metastases in liver or lung (in the German ACC Registry <6% of patients with metastatic ACC).

In the past, various staging systems have been introduced for classification of ACC to assess prognosis and to guide treatment strategies. In 2004, for the first time, a staging system was published by the Union International Contre Cancer (UICC) and the World Health Organization [75]. However, this staging system, which is

Table 4.2 Staging systems for adrenocortical carcinoma proposed by the European Network for the Study of Adrenal Tumors ENSAT 2008 [37]

Stage	ENSAT 2008
I	T1, N0, M0
II	T2, N0, M0
III	T1-2, N1, M0
	T3-4, N0-1, M0
IV	T1-4, N0-1, M1

T1, tumour ≤5 cm; T2, tumour >5 cm; T3, tumour infiltration in surrounding tissue; T4, tumour invasion in adjacent organs or venous tumor thrombus in vena cava/renal vein; N0, no positive lymph nodes; N1, positive lymph node(s); M0, no distant metastases; M1, presence of distant metastasis

largely based on the Macfarlane classification as modified by Sullivan [45, 76], showed limited prognostic power in a recent analysis [37]. Based on this analysis, a revised TNM classification was proposed by ENSAT (see Table 4.2). In this staging system, stage III is defined by tumour infiltration in surrounding tissue or tumour thrombus in vena cava/renal vein or positive lymph nodes, whereas stage IV is defined by the presence of distant metastasis only. The ENSAT staging system provides an important tool for predicting the outcome in patients with ACC (see Fig. 3.4 in Chapter 3).

4.4 Fine-Needle Aspiration/Cut Biopsy

The use of percutaneous needle biopsy of adrenal masses is still a controversial issue. The main reasons are fine-needle aspiration (FNA)-associated morbidity and mortality, and the fact that biopsy often does not alter clinical management and therefore is of questionable utility [77]. Main complications are hemorrhage, pneumothorax, abscess, pancreatitis, tumor rupture, and cardiovascular complications after puncture of an unsuspected pheochromocytoma [78–82]. In older series, the risk of complications ranged between 5 and 12% [79], whereas more recent series reported a complication rate between 0% and 4% [80, 83]. However, in a most recent series, complications due to biopsy occurred in 14% of patients including liver hematoma, biopsy of a paraganglioma complicated by a duodenal hematoma and intravenous nutrition, and hemothorax all requiring hospitalization [77]. Most importantly, occasional needle-track metastases have been described in patients with ACC [84, 85]. This is of particular concern as a major strategy of surgery for ACC aims at keeping the tumor capsule intact to avoid the dissemination of tumor cells. Based on this concept, it makes no sense to biopsy a suspected ACC, at least not in the setting of localized disease potentially amenable to R_0 resection. In contrast, in a metastasized ACC, removal of the primary adrenal mass is frequently of no benefit to the patient. In this case, FNA or cut/core biopsy allowing both cytologic and histologic evaluation may be justified to establish the diagnosis of ACC beyond doubt.

In general, CT or MRI is used to guide biopsy, although due to the large tumor size in ACC ultrasound guidance should be equally effective in most cases. While sensitivity of FNA/cut biopsy is high in adrenal metastases [86–91], the distinction between benign and primary malignant adrenal lesions is often difficult. In a recent analysis of the cytologic features of 20 adrenocortical carcinomas (9 primary tumors and 11 metastases) from 19 patients, a varied morphologic spectrum was found with the potential of diagnostic confusion [92]. As no single specific feature allows a definitive diagnosis of ACC, a combination of cytologic features is required. The typical cytologic features included hypercellularity, necrotic debris, nuclear pleomorphism, mitotic figures, and prominent nucleoli [92]. However, the authors have pointed out that pathological findings need to be combined with clinical information to achieve a proper FNA diagnosis.

At present, the only widely accepted indication for adrenal biopsy is a suspected metastasis from a known primary tumor in a patient in whom the result of the histopathological diagnosis would change the therapeutic approach (e.g., surgery for limited disease vs. chemotherapy for metastatic disease) [46]. In this setting, adrenal biopsy, either as FNA cytology or as adrenal cut biopsy, will give a sensitivity and specificity of more than 80% and an overall accuracy of 90% [79]. Some researchers, however, are more enthusiastic concerning the use of image-guided FNA cytology for the characterization of adrenal masses. In 34 consecutive patients, image-guided FNA cytology using spinal-type narrow gauge needles prior to further procedures was used [93]. Compared to the final pathology in 19 patients and follow-up, the sensitivity, specificity, and positive predictive value for FNA cytology were 83.3%, 100%, and 100% superior to CT or MRI imaging. However, limited information is available on the long-term follow-up of those four ACCs that underwent FNA and the potential risk of local recurrence. In a prospective German and Austrian center trial, an ex vivo approach was used to evaluate the role of adrenal cut biopsy in 220 consecutive patients [94]. The evaluating pathologist was blinded for clinical data and the definite diagnosis was eventually made by histopathology of the complete surgical specimen. Two of 39 malignant lesions were misclassified as benign and two as only possibly malignant, resulting in an overall sensitivity and specificity for malignancy of 94.6% and 95.3%, respectively. While none of the adrenocortical carcinomas was misclassified as benign tumor, 5 out of 22 ACCs were diagnosed as metastases.

Recently, it has been claimed that endoscopic ultrasound-guided FNA biopsy of the adrenal glands might be both safe and useful. In a series from Alabama, 24 biopsy specimens were obtained from adrenal glands and adequate cellularity was noted in all 24 samples. Twenty nine percent were diagnosed as metastatic carcinoma and confirmed on subsequent follow-up [95]. While in this series no significant complications were reported, others have described left adrenal gland hemorrhage as a complication of endoscopic ultrasound-guided FNA [96].

The clinical reality of the role of FNA biopsy in patients with incidentally discovered adrenal masses has been impressively highlighted by Quayle and co-workers

[77]. Of 347 patients evaluated for adrenal masses, 22 had undergone needle biopsy before referral. Clinical presentations were incidentaloma ($n = 15$), suspected metastases ($n = 4$), and symptomatic large mass ($n = 3$). Of the 15 patients with incidentaloma, 80% had nondiagnostic biopsy results and two showed a pheochromocytoma. Biopsies were diagnostic in 50% of patients with suspected metastases and in only one of three patients with a large symptomatic mass. Five of the 22 patients were ultimately diagnosed with pheochromocytoma, none had received biochemical testing for pheochromocytoma prior to biopsy. Most importantly, biopsy results did not alter clinical management in any of the 22 patients in this study. These findings indicate that FNA is still overused in the diagnostic work-up of adrenal masses and poses a significant risk to the patient.

In summary, in suspected ACC FNA/cut biopsy is almost never indicated. Rare exceptions are metastatic nonfunctioning ACC. In this situation, diagnostic biopsy may be justified, as removal of the primary tumor may be of questionable value to the patient. Furthermore, on rare occasions a differential diagnosis between a primary pulmonary tumor with a large adrenal metastasis and a nonfunctioning adrenocortical carcinoma with an isolated large pulmonary metastasis, which is difficult to biopsy, may justify an adrenal FNA/cut biopsy.

References

1. Abiven G et al (2006) Clinical and biological features in the prognosis of adrenocortical cancer: poor outcome of cortisol-secreting tumors in a series of 202 consecutive patients. J Clin Endocrinol Metab 91(7):2650–2655
2. Crucitti F et al (1996) The Italian Registry for Adrenal Cortical Carcinoma: analysis of a multiinstitutional series of 129 patients. The ACC Italian Registry Study Group. Surgery 119(2):161–170
3. Dackiw AP et al (2001) Adrenal cortical carcinoma. World J Surg 25(7):914–926
4. Icard P et al (2001) Adrenocortical carcinomas: surgical trends and results of a 253-patient series from the French Association of Endocrine Surgeons study group. World J Surg 25(7):891–897
5. Kendrick ML et al (2001) Adrenocortical carcinoma: surgical progress or status quo? Arch Surg 136(5):543–549
6. Koschker AC et al (2006) Adrenocortical carcinoma – improving patient care by establishing new structures. Exp Clin Endocrinol Diabetes 114(2):45–51
7. Schulick RD, Brennan MF (1999) Adrenocortical carcinoma. World J Urol 17(1):26–34
8. Wooten MD, King DK (1993) Adrenal cortical carcinoma. Epidemiology and treatment with mitotane and a review of the literature. Cancer 72(11):3145–3155
9. Fassnacht M, Allolio B (2009) Clinical management of adrenocortical carcinoma. Best Pract Res Clin Endocrinol Metab 23(2):273–289
10. Didolkar MS et al (1981) Natural history of adrenal cortical carcinoma: a clinicopathologic study of 42 patients. Cancer 47(9):2153–2161
11. Favia G et al (2001) Adrenocortical carcinoma: is prognosis different in nonfunctioning tumors? Results of surgical treatment in 31 patients. World J Surg 25(6):735–738
12. Pommier RF, Brennan MF (1992) An eleven-year experience with adrenocortical carcinoma. Surgery 112(6):963–970; discussion 970–971
13. Vassilopoulou-Sellin R, Schultz PN (2001) Adrenocortical carcinoma. Clinical outcome at the end of the 20th century. Cancer 92(5):1113–1121

14. Wajchenberg B et al (2000) Adrenocortical carcinoma: clinical and laboratory observations. Cancer 88(4):711–736
15. Newell-Price J et al (2006) Cushing's syndrome. Lancet 367(9522):1605–1617
16. Stewart PM et al (1995) 11 beta-Hydroxysteroid dehydrogenase activity in Cushing's syndrome: explaining the mineralocorticoid excess state of the ectopic adrenocorticotropin syndrome. J Clin Endocrinol Metab 80(12):3617–3620
17. Moreno S et al (2004) Profile and outcome of pure androgen-secreting adrenal tumors in women: experience of 21 cases. Surgery 136(6):1192–1198
18. Gabrilove J et al (1965) Feminizing adrenocortical tumors in the male: a review of 52 cases including a case report. Medicine 44: 37–39
19. Lanigan D et al (1993) A feminizing adrenocortical carcinoma presenting with gynaecomastia. Postgrad Med J 69(812):481–483
20. Allolio B et al (2004) Management of adrenocortical carcinoma. Clin Endocrinol (Oxf) 60:273–287
21. Seccia TM et al (2005) Aldosterone-producing adrenocortical carcinoma: an unusual cause of Conn's syndrome with an ominous clinical course. Endocr Relat Cancer 12(1):149–159
22. Barzon L et al (2005) Shift from Conn's syndrome to Cushing's syndrome in a recurrent adrenocortical carcinoma. Eur J Endocrinol 153(5):629–636
23. Hisamatsu H et al (2002) Adrenocortical carcinoma with primary aldosteronism associated with Cushing syndrome during recurrence. BJU Int 90(9):971–972
24. Hyodo T et al (1977) Adrenocortical carcinoma and hypoglycemia: evidence for production of nonsuppressible insulin-like activity by the tumor. J Clin Endocrinol Metab 44(6): 1175–1184
25. Luton JP et al (1990) Clinical features of adrenocortical carcinoma, prognostic factors, and the effect of mitotane therapy. N Engl J Med 322(17):1195–1201
26. Falchuk KR (1973) Inappropriate antidiuretic hormone-like syndrome associated with an adrenocortical carcinoma. Am J Med Sci 266(5):393–395
27. Yamanaka K et al (2000) A case of renin-producing adrenocortical cancer. Endocr J 47(2):119–125
28. Oka T et al (1996) Erythropoietin-producing adrenocortical carcinoma. Urol Int 56(4): 246–249
29. Fragoso MC et al (2007) An inhibin B and estrogen-secreting adrenocortical carcinoma leading to selective FSH suppression. Horm Res 67(1):7–11
30. Pegoli W Jr. et al (1987) Ectopic calcitonin in adrenocortical carcinoma: a new tumor marker. J Pediatr Surg 22(12):1183–1184
31. Bussani R et al (2003) Chance diagnosis of low stage non-metastasized adrenal cortical carcinoma in a young woman with retroperitoneal hemorrhage. Pathol Res Pract 199(11):761–763
32. Suyama K et al (2007) Spontaneous rupture of adrenocortical carcinoma. Am J Surg 194(1):77–78
33. Chesson JP, Theodorescu D (2002) Adrenal tumor with caval extension – case report and review of the literature. Scand J Urol Nephrol 36(1):71–73
34. Hisham AN et al (2003) Large adrenocortical carcinoma extending into the inferior vena cava and right atrium. Asian J Surg 26(1):40–42
35. Radecka E et al (2003) An unusual case of tumor thrombus in the inferior vena cava. A case report. Acta Radiol 44(2):160–161
36. Yeh MW et al (2006) Virilizing adrenocortical carcinoma with cavoatrial extension. Am J Surg 192(2):209–210
37. Fassnacht M et al (2009) Limited prognostic value of the 2004 International Union Against Cancer staging classification for adrenocortical carcinoma: proposal for a Revised TNM Classification. Cancer 115(2):243–250
38. Bakthavathsalam G et al (2008) Nonfunctioning adrenocorticalcarcinoma. Int Surg 93(2): 81–87
39. Brand TC et al (2001) Adrenal cortical carcinoma presenting as right varicocele. J Urol 165(2):503

40. Wright CB et al (2008) Adrenocortical tumor with left renal vein, vena cava and intrahepatic venous extension. J Cardiovasc Surg (Torino) 49(1):79–81
41. Carbonnel F et al (1988) Acute Budd-Chiari syndrome as first manifestation of adrenocortical carcinoma. J Clin Gastroenterol 10(4):441–444
42. Schteingart DE et al (2001) Overexpression of CXC chemokines by an adrenocortical carcinoma: a novel clinical syndrome. J Clin Endocrinol Metab 86(8):3968–3974
43. Durusu M et al (2002) Adrenal cortical carcinoma presenting initially with radius metastasis. Clin Oncol (R Coll Radiol) 14(1):83–84
44. Solans R et al (2001) [Bone metastases as presentation of adrenocortical carcinoma]. Med Clin (Barc) 116(2):76–77
45. Macfarlane DA (1958) Cancer of the adrenal cortex: the natural history, prognosis and treatment in a study of fifty-five cases. Ann R C Surg Engl 23(3):155–186
46. Fassnacht M et al (2004) Adrenal tumors: how to establish malignancy? J Endocrinol Invest 27(4):387–399
47. Elamin MB et al (2008) Accuracy of Diagnostic Tests for Cushing's Syndrome: a Systematic Review and Metaanalyses. J Clin Endocrinol Metab 93(5):1553–1562
48. Nieman LK et al (2008) The Diagnosis of Cushing's Syndrome: an Endocrine Society Clinical Practice Guideline. J Clin Endocrinol Metab 93(5):1526–1540
49. Boyle JG et al (2007) Comparison of diagnostic accuracy of urinary free metanephrines, vanillyl mandelic acid, and catecholamines and plasma catecholamines for diagnosis of pheochromocytoma. J Clin Endocrinol Metab 92(12):4602–4608
50. Eisenhofer G (2003) Editorial: biochemical diagnosis of pheochromocytoma – is it time to switch to plasma-free metanephrines? J Clin Endocrinol Metab 88(2):550–552
51. Pacak K et al (2007) Pheochromocytoma: recommendations for clinical practice from the First International Symposium. October 2005. Nat Clin Pract Endocrinol Metab 3(2):92 102
52. Perry CG et al (2007) The diagnostic efficacy of urinary fractionated metanephrines measured by tandem mass spectrometry in detection of pheochromocytoma. Clin Endocrinol (Oxf) 66(5):703–708
53. Unger N et al (2006) Diagnostic value of various biochemical parameters for the diagnosis of pheochromocytoma in patients with adrenal mass. Eur J Endocrinol 154(3):409–417
54. Vaclavik J et al (2007) Free plasma metanephrines as a screening test for pheochromocytoma in low-risk patients. J Hypertens 25(7):1427–1431
55. Arlt W et al (2008) Steroid profiling in the diagnosis and monitoring of adrenocortical cancer – results of the EURINE ACC Study of the European Network For The Study Of Adrenal Tumors (ENS@T). Abstracts of the 90th annual meeting of the Endocrine Society (San Francisco): OR40-2
56. Johanssen S, et al (2010) Need for improvement in the clinical management of patients with adrenocortical carcinoma in Germany. Dt Aerzteblatt in press
57. Allolio B, Fassnacht M (2006) Clinical review: adrenocortical carcinoma: clinical update. J Clin Endocrinol Metab 91(6):2027–2037
58. Friedrich-Rust M et al (2008) Contrast-enhanced sonography of adrenal masses: differentiation of adenomas and nonadenomatous lesions. AJR Am J Roentgenol 191(6):1852–1860
59. Bauditz J et al (2008) Improved detection of hepatic metastases of adrenocortical cancer by contrast-enhanced ultrasound. Oncol Rep 19(5):1135–1139
60. Boland GW et al (1998) Characterization of adrenal masses using unenhanced CT: an analysis of the CT literature. AJR Am J Roentgenol 171(1):201–204
61. Caoili EM et al (2002) Adrenal masses: characterization with combined unenhanced and delayed enhanced CT. Radiology 222(3):629–633
62. Hamrahian AH et al (2005) Clinical utility of noncontrast computed tomography attenuation value (Hounsfield units) to differentiate adrenal adenomas/hyperplasias from nonadenomas: cleveland Clinic experience. J Clin Endocrinol Metab 90(2):871–877
63. Heinz-Peer G et al (2007) Imaging of adrenal masses. Curr Opin Urol 17(1):32–38
64. Ilias I et al (2007) The optimal imaging of adrenal tumours: a comparison of different methods. Endocr Relat Cancer 14(3):587–599

65. Szolar DH et al (2005) Adrenocortical carcinomas and adrenal pheochromocytomas: mass and enhancement loss evaluation at delayed contrast-enhanced CT. Radiology 234(2): 479–485
66. Park BK et al (2007) Comparison of delayed enhanced CT and chemical shift MR for evaluating hyperattenuating incidental adrenal masses. Radiology 243(3):760–765
67. Honigschnabl S et al (2002) How accurate is MR imaging in characterisation of adrenal masses: update of a long-term study. Eur J Radiol 41(2):113–122
68. Al-Hawary MM et al (2005) Non-invasive evaluation of the incidentally detected indeterminate adrenal mass. Best Pract Res Clin Endocrinol Metab 19(2):277–292
69. Faria JF et al (2007) Adrenal masses: characterization with in vivo proton MR spectroscopy – initial experience. Radiology 245(3):788–797
70. Groussin L et al (2009) 18F-Fluorodeoxyglucose positron emission tomography for the diagnosis of adrenocortical tumors: a prospective study in 77 operated patients. J Clin Endocrinol Metab 94(5):1713–1722
71. Boland GW et al (2009) PET/CT for the characterization of adrenal masses in patients with cancer: qualitative versus quantitative accuracy in 150 consecutive patients. AJR Am J Roentgenol 192(4):956–962
72. Okada M et al (2009) Adrenal masses: the value of additional fluorodeoxy-glucose-positron emission tomography/computed tomography (FDG-PET/CT) in differentiating between benign and malignant lesions. Ann Nucl Med 23(4):349–354
73. Leboulleux S et al (2006) Diagnostic and prognostic value of 18-fluorodeoxyglucose positron emission tomography in adrenocortical carcinoma: a prospective comparison with computed tomography. J Clin Endocrinol Metab 91(3):920–925
74. Mackie GC et al (2006) Use of [18F]fluorodeoxyglucose positron emission tomography in evaluating locally recurrent and metastatic adrenocortical carcinoma. J Clin Endocrinol Metab 91(7):2665–271
75. DeLellis RA et al (2004) World Health Organization Classification of Tumours. Pathology and genetics of tumours of endocrine organs (IARC), Lyon, France, pp 136
76. Sullivan M et al (1978) Adrenal cortical carcinoma. J Urol 120(6):660–665
77. Quayle FJ et al (2007) Needle biopsy of incidentally discovered adrenal masses is rarely informative and potentially hazardous. Surgery 142(4):497–502; discussion 502–504
78. Casola G et al (1986) Unsuspected pheochromocytoma: risk of blood-pressure alterations during percutaneous adrenal biopsy. Radiology 159(3):733–735
79. Kloos RT et al (1995) Incidentally discovered adrenal masses. Endocr Rev 16(4):460–484
80. Lumachi F et al (2001) Fine-needle aspiration cytology of adrenal masses in noncancer patients: clinicoradiologic and histologic correlations in functioning and nonfunctioning tumors. Cancer 93(5):323–329
81. McCorkell SJ, Niles NL (1985) Fine-needle aspiration of catecholamine-producing adrenal masses: a possibly fatal mistake. AJR Am J Roentgenol 145(1):113–114
82. Yankaskas B et al (1986) Delayed complications from fine-needle biopsies of solid masses of the abdomen. Invest Radiol 21(4):325–328
83. Fassina AS et al (2000) Fine needle aspiration cytology (FNAC) of adrenal masses. Cytopathology 11(5):302–311
84. Habscheid W et al (1990) [Puncture track metastasis after ultrasound-guided fine-needle puncture biopsy. A rare complication?]. Dtsch Med Wochenschr 115(6):212–215
85. Mody MK et al (1995) Percutaneous CT-guided biopsy of adrenal masses: immediate and delayed complications. J Comput Assist Tomogr 19(3):434–439
86. de Agustin P, Lopez-Rios F et al (1999) Fine-needle aspiration biopsy of the adrenal glands: a ten-year experience. Diagn Cytopathol 21(2):92–97
87. Katz RL et al (1984) Fine needle aspiration cytology of the adrenal gland. Acta Cytol 28(3):269–282
88. Silverman SG et al (1993) Predictive value of image-guided adrenal biopsy: analysis of results of 101 biopsies. Radiology 187(3):715–718

89. Wadih G et al (1992) Fine-needle aspiration cytology of the adrenal gland. Fifty biopsies in 48 patients. Arch Pathol Lab Med 116(8):841–846
90. Welch TJ et al (1994) Percutaneous adrenal biopsy: review of a 10-year experience. Radiology 193(2):341–344
91. Wu HH et al (1998) Fine needle aspiration cytology of benign adrenal cortical nodules. A comparison of cytologic findings with those of primary and metastatic adrenal malignancies. Acta Cytol 42(6):1352–1358
92. Ren R et al (2006) Fine-needle aspiration of adrenal cortical carcinoma: cytologic spectrum and diagnostic challenges. Am J Clin Pathol 126(3):389–398
93. Lumachi F et al (2003) CT-scan, MRI and image-guided FNA cytology of incidental adrenal masses. Eur J Surg Oncol 29(8):689–692
94. Saeger W et al (2003) High diagnostic accuracy of adrenal core biopsy: results of the German and Austrian adrenal network multicenter trial in 220 consecutive patients. Hum Pathol 34(2):180–186
95. Jhala NC et al (2004) Endoscopic ultrasound-guided fine-needle aspiration biopsy of the adrenal glands: analysis of 24 patients. Cancer 102(5):308–314
96. Haseganu LE, Diehl DL (2009) Left adrenal gland hemorrhage as a complication of EUS-FNA. Gastrointest Endosc 69(6):e51–52

Chapter 5
Diagnostic Approach to Incidentaloma

Holger S. Willenberg and Stefan R. Bornstein

Adrenal incidentalomas (AI) are masses of the adrenal gland discovered inadvertently during diagnostic imaging for other conditions unrelated to adrenal disease. Incidentally found adrenal tumors were first described more than 25 years ago [1–3]. Improvements in imaging technologies, their increasing availability and use have led to increasing recognition of AI as a public health problem in the aging population [4–6]. Prevalences of AI discovered by CT vary in an age-dependent manner from as low as 0.2% in the young (<30 years) to 6.9% or more in the elderly (50–80 years) [6–9]. AI seems to be more frequent in female subjects [6]. However, they comprise a heterogeneous group of diseases, including primary and secondary tumors, benign and malignant lesions, and endocrine masses with or without clinically relevant autonomous hormone secretion [10]. Patients with an AI have a decreased life expectancy, and evidence-based clinical management is cost-effective [11].

During a process guided by the NIH [12], the information on the AI of initially 5400 and finally over 600 available clinical studies and articles was systematically reviewed [6] and a consensus document was worked out and published by an independent board [5]. As recommended by the panel and other groups, two main questions have to be answered when an adrenal mass was incidentally discovered.

1. Does the adrenal lesion show a biologically benign or malignant behavior?
2. Is the adrenal lesion a source of autonomous hormone hypersecretion?

The answers to these two questions will facilitate decision making as to whether clinical follow-up and observation or surgical removal is the more reasonable approach.

H.S. Willenberg (✉)
Department of Endocrinology, Diabetes and Rheumatology, University Hospital Duesseldorf, Moorenstr. 5, D–40225 Duesseldorf, Germany
e-mail: holger.willenberg@uni-duesseldorf.de

G.D. Hammer, T. Else (eds.), *Adrenocortical Carcinoma*,
DOI 10.1007/978-0-387-77236-3_5,

5.1 Does the Adrenal Lesion Exhibit a Biologically Benign or Malignant Behavior?

5.1.1 Evidence from Epidemiological Studies – Adrenocortical Tumors

Based on studies that report 20 or more individual cases, AI are cortical adenomas in 40%, metastases in 20%, adrenal cortical carcinoma (ACC) in 10%, myelolipoma in 10%, pheochromocytoma in 8%, and other lesions including adrenal cysts [13–22]. Such a distribution was also found in a series of more than 1000 cases, whereby adenomas were a little more and metastasis a little less frequent because patients with known malignancies had been excluded from this study [8] (Fig. 5.1a).

Adrenal adenomas are of benign nature, and there is little evidence that they progress to ACC [12, 17, 23]. However, aberrations in the Wnt signaling pathway have been found in hereditary and spontaneous adrenal cortical tumors, including

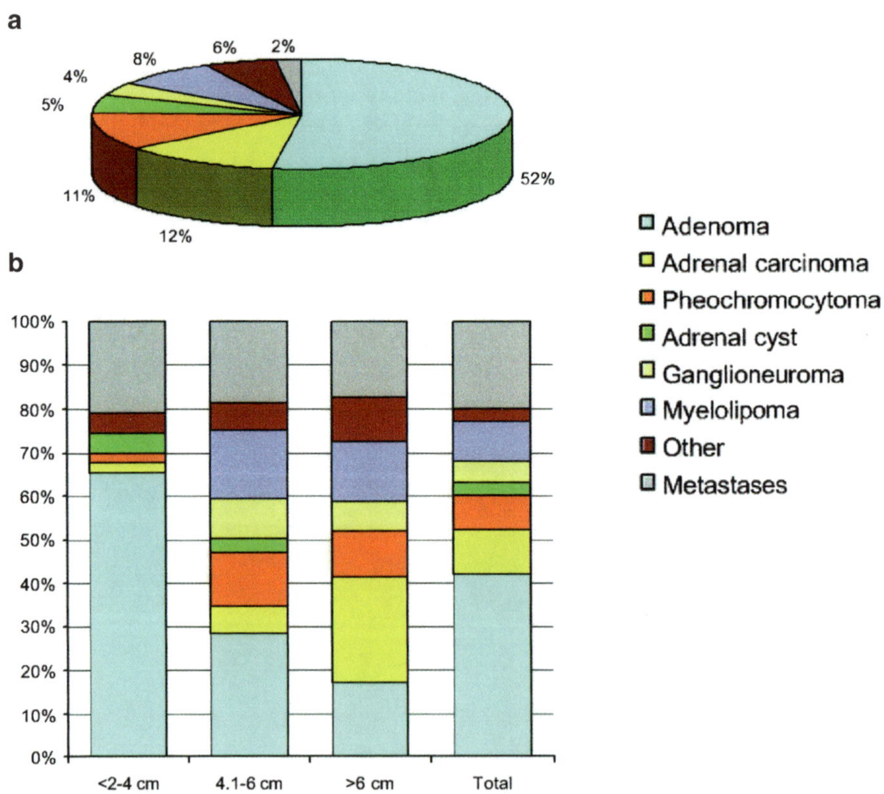

Fig. 5.1 Distribution of pathologic diagnoses of adrenal masses: (**a**) distribution across all sizes of adrenal masses; (**b**) distribution according to size of adrenal mass [6]

adenomas and carcinomas [24, 25]. Also, in a few cases of multiple endocrine neoplasia type 1, the development of rapidly growing ACCs out of slowly growing tumors has been documented. However, in hereditary syndromes, e.g., congenital adrenal hyperplasia, adrenal tumors seem to develop frequently and, usually, even huge benign tumors do not become malignant [26].

The mean size of adrenal adenomas is 3.5 cm, but varies from smaller, almost undetectable masses to 15 cm [8, 27]. The prevalence of adrenal adenomas decreases with the tumor size and is 65% in tumors <4 cm and 18% in tumors >6 cm. This decrease occurs in favor of ACC that represent a minor part of AI if they are less than 4 cm (≈2% of cases) or 4–6 cm (≈6% of cases) in size. However, their prevalence increases substantially, and their portion among adrenal tumors >6 cm is probably up to 25% (see Fig. 5.1b).

5.1.2 Evidence from Epidemiological Studies – Pheochromocytomas

Literature reviews indicate a frequency of 5.1–8.0% for pheochromocytomas among incidentally discovered adrenal masses [6, 9]. In a large autopsy series that had a time span of 50 years, pheochromocytomas were found in 0.13% of cases and 75% of those had not been detected when the patient was alive [28]. Thus, patients with pheochromocytomas found as AI are often normotensive and usually do not display the classic symptoms of catecholamine excess [8, 29, 30]. However, 10% of pheochromocytomas show a malignant behavior and up to 25% grow in the context of hereditary syndromatic disease [31, 32].

5.1.3 Evidence from Epidemiological Studies – Metastasis

The adrenal glands are frequently involved in metastatic disease. Metastasis occurs in about 20% of patients with known malignancies [33]. Nevertheless, if the adrenal tumor is smaller than 6 cm, benign adenomas are still more frequent even in patients with known cancer, including breast, kidney and ovarian cancer, non-small cell lung carcinoma, colorectal cancer, melanoma, lymphomas, and others. However, there is one exception to the rule: in patients with small-cell lung carcinoma the likelihood for metastasis is greater than for an adenoma [6]. Although bilateral tumors in such patients are considered to be an expression of metastatic spread, it may well be a single adenoma in one adrenal and a single metastasis in the other. Pathology studies show that both the adrenal glands are affected by metastasis in more than 50% of cases. However, a quarter of metastatic tumors is smaller than 1 mm and half of them between 1 and 10 mm [33].

5.1.4 Evidence from Epidemiological Studies – Other Adrenal Lesions

Myelolipomas are slowly growing, benign neoplasias of the adrenal cortex, comprising mature fat and hematopoietic tissue. Other rarer entities include ganglioneuromas, hematomas, angiomyelolipomas, epithelial carcinomas, primary adrenal lymphoma, "composite adrenal tumors", hybrid tumors, and neurinomas [10, 18, 33]. Infectious diseases, in particular tuberculosis and histoplasmosis, can appear as an AI.

5.1.5 Evidence from Imaging Studies

AI is discovered in 0.1–0.5% of all patients who underwent routine ultrasound of the abdomen [34, 35]. However, this figure is biased because ultrasound misses a third of lesions smaller than 3 cm as compared with computed tomography (CT) or magnetic resonance imaging (MRI) [6, 36]. Therefore, with the exception of endosonography, ultrasound is a not sensitive enough method for detecting or following AI [37] (Chapter 6).

The mainstay of imaging is currently CT. Here, adrenal adenomas typically appear as homogenous lesions with regular margins that are constant in size during follow-up [38–40]. Calcification, necrosis, or hemorrhage is rare in benign adrenal adenomas. Since adrenocortical adenomas and myelolipomas are lipid-rich tumors, they are characterized by low (<18) Hounsfield units on unenhanced CT [39]. A further diagnostic work-up to assess malignancy can be forgone if Hounsfield units are ≤ 10. However, hemorrhage can interfere with such measurements, in particular in myelolipomas. However, if Hounsfield units are greater, benign adrenocortical adenomas that are poor in lipid content may still be possible in 10–40 % of cases [40]. A further characterization can be achieved in analyzing the washout of contrast material 15 min after its application. The enhancement decreases by more than 50% in benign adenomas. Also, lipid-rich as well as lipid-poor adenomas show similar signal intensities after the application of contrast medium of less than 64–70 Hounsfield units [40, 41].

ACCs are usually heterogeneous tumors with irregularities, calcifications, necrosis, and sometimes indistinct borders [42, 43]. However, ACCs that are less than 6 cm in size may appear as benign adenomas. Metastasis can show cystic areas or necrosis if they are large enough; smaller metastasis may appear as homogenous lesions.

Pheochromocytomas show a density similar to the liver on unenhanced CT [44]. They may also consist of cystic, necrotic, and calcified parts in 10% of cases. Because of its typical vascularization, pheochromocytomas show an intensive enhancement after the application of contrast material. Therefore, the majority of pheochromocytomas can be easily recognized in enhanced MRI studies also. However, characteristics may sometimes overlap with ACC.

On MRI, adrenal malignancies appear brighter than adrenal adenomas on T2-weighed images because they have a higher fluid content [45, 46]. However, the identification of lipid-poor adenomas may become problematic. Metastasis and ACCs appear hypodense on T1-weighed and hyperdense on T2-weighed images in comparison to the liver. After the administration of paramagnetic contrast material, malignant lesions show enhanced signals and a slow washout phase [47, 48]. For further characterization, the "chemical shift" MRI has proven to be a good approach in distinguishing benign adenomas from other lesions. Here, the resonance characteristics of protons in fat and water are studied on T1-weighed "in-phase" and "opposed-phase" images in comparison to other liver or spleen tissue [43, 49].

Other imaging techniques include scintigraphic and positron emission tomography (PET) studies and may serve to identify the kind of tumor, its hormonal activity, or its dignity. While [^{131}I]-6-beta-iodomethyl-norcholesterol, [^{75}Se]-selenomethyl-19-norcholesterol, and, more recently, [^{123}I]-iodometomidate may be employed for the visualization of functioning adrenocortical tumors [50–52], [^{123}I]-metaiodobenzylguanidine (MIBG) and [^{111}In]-octreotide are typical tracers used in adrenal medullary tumors [53–55]. [^{18}F]-2-fluoro-D-deoxyglucose (FDG) can be detected on PET and is a marker of increased metabolism in malignant lesions. An adrenal to liver maximum standardized uptake value below 1.45 is a strong argument to assume a benign lesion [56]. If FDG is linked to DOPA or dopamin, e.g., as [^{18}F]-FDG-DOPA PET/CT, it may be more sensitive than MIBG as a tracer for malignant pheochromocytoma [57–64]. Of note, [^{11}C]-metomidate, metomidate can also be used in PET/CT imaging for visualization of adrenocortical tissue [65].

5.1.6 Evidence from Biopsy Studies

The differentiation of adrenal masses can be achieved by the evaluation of histopathological attributes. To separate benign from malignant adrenocortical lesions, several scoring systems have been evaluated. Of those, the nine criteria proposed by Weiss are generally accepted by reference pathologists [66]. In addition, Ki-67 or PCNA proliferation indices and cellular markers such as, α_1 connexin 43, chromogranin A, synaptophysin, vimentin, nestin, steroidogenic factor-1 inhibits, and class II MHC molecules have been studied in addition to molecular characteristics, e.g., p53 expression, loss of heterozygosity for ACTH receptor, beta-catenin stabilization, and others [6, 67–69]. However, the determination of malignancy or the correct classification of an adrenal mass may still remain difficult in some cases [33].

For example, the differentiation between a benign adrenocortical lesion and a renal cell carcinoma or a small ACC may sometimes become problematic despite the availability of specific antibodies and histologic markers. In addition, despite the existence of a histopathological score of 12 criteria, the only criterion that proves malignancy in pheochromocytoma is the appearance of metastasis [70].

Also, the data on fine-needle biopsies (FNB) is still inconclusive because most studies tested this approach without a reference standard (e.g., histology after operation). Also, data is lacking on the utility of this approach for the diagnosis of ACC. From surgical records, it is suggested to leave the tumor capsules of ACC intact [71]. Also, metastatic spread of cancer along the needle tract has been documented after biopsy of adrenal metastasis [72, 73]. A considerable proportion of biopsies is inconclusive (5–50%) and a benign cytologic diagnosis from FNB does not exclude malignancy. Because of these problems and because of difficulties in the histologic work-up of adrenal lesions, performing CT- or ultrasound-guided fine-needle biopsy is generally discouraged as a routine diagnostic test [6] but is potentially beneficial in the differentiation of metastasis. On the other hand, if the tumors and needles are large enough (tumor >2 cm, needle of 19 gauge or larger), sensitivity and specificity for assessing malignancy are 80% and higher [73, 74]. The occurrence of complications that needed immediate attention is reported to be less than 1%. Therefore, FNB may be an additional helpful tool in the evaluation of patients with malignancy and a suspicious adrenal mass on imaging [74, 75] (see Chapter 4). Importantly, the diagnosis of pheochromocytoma has to be dismissed prior to the biopsy attempt on the basis of endocrine function tests to prevent a potentially life-threatening hypertensive crisis [5, 6, 76].

5.2 Is the Adrenal Lesion a Source of Autonomous Hormone Hypersecretion?

5.2.1 Evidence from Epidemiological Studies

Excess secretion of aldosterone is detected in approximately 1.6–5.5% of patients with an AI and hypertension [8, 77–80]. Hypercortisolism is reported to be more frequent, but definitions of hypercortisolism and, therefore, the percentages vary from 5% to 47% [8, 78, 80–82]. Estrogen- or androgen-producing adenomas are rare.

As stated above, pheochromocytomas are detectable in up to 8% of patients with AI [6, 9]. Despite the often asymptomatic nature of such tumors, they remain a dangerous problem capable of releasing catecholamines in large and life-threatening amounts. All patients with AI should therefore be tested for pheochromocytoma.

However, assay methods and normal values have changed over time. Therefore, all the studies mentioned above are to be interpreted with caution. Adrenocortical adenomas and ACCs may or may not hypersecrete different hormones. Thus, the presence or absence of hormone excess syndromes does not establish malignant or benign biological potential.

In conclusion, screening for hypercortisolism and pheochromocytoma is recommended in every patient with AI. While some argue for the importance to rule out hyperaldosteronism in every AI patient, a more prudent approach might be to screen for primary hyperaldosteronism in patients with AI and hypertension.

5.2.2 Hormone Excess

While adrenal tumors that cause powerful hormone excess syndromes are clinically apparent even to the inexperienced physician, subtle autonomous hormone secretion may not be recognized easily. The simple fact that the adrenal mass is discovered during diagnostic imaging for non-adrenal disease does not necessarily mean that patients do not show signs of excess hormone secretion. In addition, adrenal estrogen hypersecretion in women or adrenal androgen hypersecretion in males may be difficult to detect. Therefore, the term "clinically inapparent adrenal mass" is somewhat relative and may even be misleading. This term may also lead to an underestimation of the value of the case history or the physical examination. While laboratory studies are very useful in measuring hormone levels, they do not necessarily reflect hormone action. Hormone levels do vary and are influenced by multiple factors, including time course and medication. For these reasons, we recommend management of patients with adrenal masses by doctors experienced in the field. In the past 10 years, great advances were made in defining excess hormone secretion. For the detection of primary aldosteronism and hypercortisolism, guidelines of the Endocrine Society have recently been published [83, 84]. During an international conference, a consensus on the diagnosis of pheochromocytoma was reached [32]. Table 5.1 summarizes the diagnostic approach to hypercortisolism, hyperaldosteronism and pheochromocytoma.

5.2.2.1 Hypercortisolism

In brief, for the screening of hypercortisolism, a 1 mg overnight dexamethasone-suppression test (DST) is recommended [5, 6, 9, 84]. When serum cortisol

Table 5.1 This table summarizes the step-wise diagnostic approach to hypercortisolism, hyperaldosteronism and pheochromocytoma. Please see text for detailed information (Sections 5.2.2.1, 5.2.2.2 and 5.2.2.3)

	Hypercortisolism	Hyperaldosteronism	Pheochromocytoma
Screening tests	1-mg overnight dexamethasone suppression test	Aldosterone to renin ratio	Metanephrine and normetanephrine in plasma or in 24-h-urine
Confirmation tests	24-h urinary free cortisol/late night salivary cortisol	Saline infusion test/fludrocortisone suppression test/oral sodium load and 24-h urinary aldosterone	Clonidine suppression test
Additional testing	Basal corticotropin/corticotropin-releasing hormone challenge	Captopril test/upright posture/adrenal venous sampling	[^{123}I]-metaiodobenzylguanidine-scintigraphy

concentrations are below 1.8 μg/dL following overnight suppression with 1 mg of oral dexamethasone, a clinically relevant cortisol excess can be excluded, while values >5.0 μ/dL are evidence of hypercortisolism. Also, the determination of urinary free cortisol (UFC) excretion in two independent samples seems reasonable and can be recommended [84]. In addition, the determination of midnight cortisol has similar good sensitivity and specificity as the DST [84, 85]. However, salivary cortisol measures may not be sensitive enough to characterize a probable mild autonomous cortisol secretion in patients with AI [86], as establishing autonomy is difficult in AI and all the tests suggested by the Endocrine Society do not necessarily correlate with each other in each patient [87].

5.2.2.2 Hyperaldosteronism

Patients with AI and hypertension should be investigated for the presence of primary hyperaldosteronism (PHA). As a screening method, the assessment of aldosterone to renin ratio (ARR) is now established. However, different assay methods, calculation models, and study populations resulted in different cut-off recommendations. The pros and cons of the ARR have recently been systematically reviewed [88]. Consensus was reached for an ARR of 30ng/dl per ng/ml × h (57ng/l per ng/l) [83], although other groups found the compromise between sensitivity and specificity more acceptable with values of 33ng/l per ng/l (using the assay by DiaSorin, Italy) [89]. Since autonomous aldosterone secretion can be excluded if values below 50 ng/L are achieved after suppression with 2000 mL saline, infused intravenously over 4 h, or with fludrocortisone, given at doses of 100 μg every 6 h over 4 days, the calculation of the ARR seems not to make sense in patients with aldosterone values below 50 ng/L.

However, if the ARR is elevated and PHA is suspected, a confirmatory test, preferably salt and water loading or fludrocortisone suppression, and subtype differentiation should be performed [83]. This is because evidence of an AI with PHA is not an ultimate proof that the adrenal tumor is the actual source of the aldosterone excess and/or hypertension. Anti-mineralocorticoid agents, including spironolactone, eplerenone, drospirenone, as well as potassium sparing agents such as triamterene, amiloride, have to be withheld for more than 4 weeks. While beta blockers and clonidine tend to falsely elevate the ARR, angiotensin-converting enzyme inhibitors, angiotensin receptor blockers, and diuretics may lead to a false-negative decrease in ARR. Therefore, these antihypertensives should be held for more than a week. The use of alpha_1-receptor blockers and calcium channel blockers is encouraged instead [6, 83]. Limiting to this approach is that the development of hypertension in PHA is dependent on multiple factors, including aldosterone excess, sodium diet, physical activity, kidney function, and others. Therefore, normotensive forms of PHA may remain undiscovered if the screening with ARR is restricted to hypertensive patients with an AI only. A cheap tool to identify mineralocorticoid excess may be to measure serum potassium levels of serum sodium/urinary sodium to serum potassium/urinary potassium ratio (SUSPUP) [89, 90] because normotensive patients with PA may also be hypokalemic [91].

5.2.2.3 Pheochromocytoma

Because of its implications for FNB or surgery and its potential cardiovascular complications, a pheochromocytoma should be ruled out in every case with an AI. This can be achieved with the determination of metanephrine and normatenphrine in plasma using high-pressure liquid chromatography or tandem mass spectrometry. If these methods are not available, urinary excretion rates of metanephrine and normetanephrine can be determined in acidified 24-h-urine samples, [32, 92]. The use of the two different screening tests is still a matter of debate, but in general urinary metanephrine measurements seem to be slightly advantageous due to their low false-positive rate. Depending on the pre-test probability, which is usually low with a simple AI, this approach seems to be preferable. In case of high suspicion (e.g., hypertension or other symptoms of pheochromocytoma), plasma metanephrine and normetanephrine should be measured. Elevations of metanephrine or normetanephrine of more than four times over the upper normal limit is proof of pheochromocytoma. Repeatedly normal values make the presence of a pheochromocytoma unlikely. Intermediate levels of metanephrine and normetanephrine can be followed up and clarified using the clonidine-suppression test that should show a drop in normetanephrine levels by 40% or values within the reference range 3 h after 300 μg oral clonidine [32].

5.2.2.4 Hyperandrogenemia

Routine testing for androgen or estrogen excess is not recommended [5, 6]. If there are clinical signs of androgen or estrogen excess, however, including virilization or feminization or other typical signs of hypogonadism or "hypergonadism", a further endocrine work-up should be performed. Of note, dehydroepiandrostenedione-sulfate levels do not necessarily reflect hyperandrogenemia or involvement of the *zona reticularis* but are also an expression of 17α-hydroxylase activity, e.g., in the context of glucocorticoid secretion and feedback inhibition of corticotropin release.

5.2.2.5 Other Endocrine Functions

For the characterization of hyperandrogenemia, the short-term 250 μg cosyntropin test may be employed. This test is useful for the detection of inherited defects of steroidogenic enzymes causing hyperandrogenemia, including congenital adrenal hyperplasia (CAH). Since patients with CAH may develop adrenal tumors, it was suggested to identify affected individuals with the cosyntropin test

[93]. Exaggerated 17-hydroxyprogesterone responses after corticotropin challenge have been found in 80% of patients with an adrenal tumor [26, 94] and these observations could be reproduced in other studies [95–97]. However, genetic studies later showed that mutations in the 21-hydroxylase gene (*CYP21A2*) are more frequent in patients with adrenal adenomas than in the general population, and that they are by far rarer than suggested by the aforementioned functional studies [98, 99]. However, deficient 11β-hydroxylation or cytochrome P450 oxidoreductase activity may also explain the augmented response in 17-hydroxyprogesterone secretion after corticotropin challenge, but were never studied. Interestingly, the majority of patients with adrenal adenomas who had an abnormal steroid secretion pattern before the operation showed a normal steroid pattern after removal of the tumor. Therefore, defective steroid biosynthesis is rather a functional than an inherited disorder in patients with adrenocortical tumors. However, this phenomenon can be used to define an AI as being an adrenocortical tumor and to differentiate primary adrenocortical from secondary adrenal neoplasms when other diagnostic methods remained inconclusive. The results of this study must be reproduced in prospective setting [97].

5.3 Is Surgical Removal Necessary or Is an Observational Policy a Safe and Reasonable Approach?

While overt hormone excess syndromes are associated with a considerable increase in risk in morbidity and mortality, the case for mild excess hormone secretion is not so clear. Patients with subclinical glucocorticoid hypersecretion seem to be at risk for developing atherosclerosis, the metabolic syndrome, or osteoporosis [100–107]. However, mild excess cortisol secretion progresses to overt Cushing's syndrome in up to 10% of patients [17, 108–111] although a progressive scintigraphic uptake was found in a greater proportion of patients with AI [112]. Also, a still unresolved question is whether or not patients with mild cortisol excess secretion benefit from surgery. Cardiovascular parameters seem to become better after the intervention: weight improves in 55%, hypertension in 74%, and blood glucose levels in 88% of patients subjected to surgery [113–115]. More recent studies, however, could not confirm that indices of an increased cardiovascular risk improve after surgery [17, 105, 109]. Therefore, the decision for a surgical procedure is individual, and a "wait-and-see"-strategy has been proposed for patients with a mild or subclinical hormone hypersecretion [116].

Adrenocortical cancer is a serious differential diagnosis in neoplasms greater than 6 cm. Therefore, such masses should be operated on following staging [5, 6]. If there is suspected malignancy in smaller hormonally inactive tumors or bilateral disease, a work-up for a primary tumor may make sense and the decision to operate will depend on tumor origin and tumor stage. There is no general consensus to remove tumors between 4 and 6 cm [5, 6]. In these cases, additional factors may become more dominant in the decisive process, including the patient's intention and age, functionality of the tumor, comorbidities, etc.

Most AI are benign nonfunctional adenomas, requiring little more than periodic follow-up to assess for increased size. An important proportion, however, are highly malignant adrenocortical carcinomas or functional endocrine tumors, requiring immediate attention. A flowchart summarizes the recommendations made during the NIH consensus process in 2003 [5, 6, 12] (Fig. 5.2).

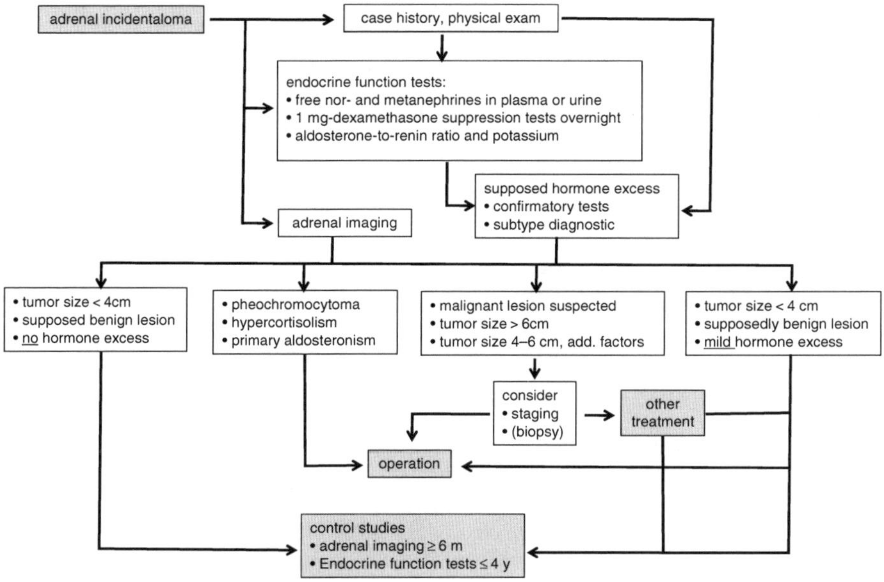

Fig. 5.2 This figure is a flow chart, delineating the diagnostic approach to the incidentally discovered adrenal mass and the consequences for treatment following the suggestions made by and NIH consensus conference [5]

References

1. Copeland PM (1983) The incidentally discovered adrenal mass. Ann Intern Med 98: 940–945
2. Geelhoed GW, Druy EM (1982) Management of the adrenal "incidentaloma". Surgery 92:866–874
3. Prinz RA et al (1982) Incidental asymptomatic adrenal masses detected by computed tomographic scanning. Is operation required? JAMA 248:701–704
4. Aron DC (2001) The adrenal incidentaloma: disease of modern technology and public health problem. Rev Endocr Metab Disord 2:335–342
5. Grumbach MM et al (2003) Management of the clinically inapparent adrenal mass ("incidentaloma"). Ann Intern Med 138:424–429
6. Mansmann G et al (2004) The clinically inapparent adrenal mass: update in diagnosis and management. Endocr Rev 25:309–340
7. Granger P, Genest J (1970) Autopsy study of adrenals in unselected normotensive and hypertensive patients. Can Med Assoc J 103:34–36

8. Mantero F et al (2000) A survey on adrenal incidentaloma in Italy. Study Group on Adrenal Tumors of the Italian Society of Endocrinology. J Clin Endocrinol Metab 85:637–644
9. Young WF Jr (2007) The incidentially discovered adrenal mass. N Eugl J Med 356:601–610
10. Kloos RT et al (1995) Incidentally discovered adrenal masses. Endocr Rev 16:460–484
11. Kievit J, Haak HR (2000) Diagnosis and treatment of adrenal incidentaloma. A cost-effectiveness analysis. Endocrinol Metab Clin North Am 29:69–90
12. Bornstein SR et al (1999) Adrenocortical tumors: recent advances in basic concepts and clinical management. Ann Intern Med 130:759–771
13. Ambrosi B et al (1995) Abnormalities of endocrine function in patients with clinically "silent" adrenal masses. Eur J Endocrinol 132:422–428
14. Corsello SM et al (1993) Incidentally discovered adrenal masses: a functional and morphological study. Exp Clin Endocrinol 101:131–137
15. Gaboardi F et al (1991) Adrenal incidentalomas: what is the role of fine needle biopsy? Int Urol Nephrol 23:197–207
16. Guerrero LA (1985) Diagnostic and therapeutic approach to incidental adrenal mass. Urology 26:435–440
17. Kasperlik-Załuska AA et al (2008) Incidentally discovered adrenal tumors: a lesson from observation of 1444 patients. Horm Metab Res 40:338–341
18. Latronico AC, Chrousos GP (1997) Extensive personal experience: adrenocortical tumors. J Clin Endocrinol Metab 82:1317–1324
19. Osella G et al (1994) Endocrine evaluation of incidentally discovered adrenal masses (incidentalomas). J Clin Endocrinol Metab 79:1532–1539
20. Terzolo M et al (1995) Adrenal incidentaloma, a five year experience. Minerva Endocrinol 20:69–78
21. Schteingart DE (2000) Management approaches to adrenal incidentalomas. A view from Ann Arbor, Michigan. Endocrinol Metab Clin North Am 29:127–139
22. Virkkala A et al (1989) Endocrine abnormalities in patients with adrenal tumours incidentally discovered on computed tomography. Acta Endocrinol (Copenh) 121:67–72
23. Kjellman M et al (2001) Genetic background of adrenocortical tumor development. World J Surg 25:948–956
24. Tadjine M et al (2008) Frequent mutations of beta-catenin gene in sporadic secreting adrenocortical adenomas. Clin. Endocrinol 68:264–270
25. Tissier F et al (2005) Mutations of beta-catenin in adrenocortical tumors: activation of the Wnt signaling pathway is a frequent event in both benign and malignant adrenocortical tumors. Cancer Res 65:7622–7627
26. Jaresch S et al (1992) Adrenal incidentaloma and patients with homozygous or heterozygous congenital adrenal hyperplasia. J Clin Endocrinol Metab 74:685–689
27. Adams JE et al (1983) Computed tomography in adrenal disease. Clin Radiol 34:39–49
28. Sutton MG et al (1981) Prevalence of clinically unsuspected pheochromocytoma. Review of a 50-year autopsy series. Mayo Clin Proc 56:354–360
29. Bernini GP et al (1997) Frequency of pheochromocytoma in adrenal incidentalomas and utility of the glucagon test for the diagnosis. J Endocrinol Invest 20:65–71
30. Mannelli M et al (1999) Pheochromocytoma in Italy: a multicentric retrospective study. Eur J Endocrinol 141:619–624
31. Neumann HP et al (2002) Germ-line mutations in nonsyndromic pheochromocytoma. N Engl J Med 346:1459–1466
32. Pacak K et al (2007) International Symposium on Pheochromocytoma. Pheochromocytoma: recommendations for clinical practice from the First International Symposium. Nat Clin Pract Endocrinol Metab 3:92–102
33. Saeger W et al (1998) Hyperplastic and tumorous lesions of the adrenals in an unselected autopsy series. Endocr Pathol 9:235–239
34. Kluglich M et al (1993) Ultrasound of incidental tumors of the adrenal gland and endocrine hypertension. Bildgebung 60:144–146
35. Masumori N et al (1998) Detection of adrenal and retroperitoneal masses in a general health examination system. Urology 52:572–576

36. Suzuki K et al (1995) Efficacy of an ultrasonic surgical system for laparoscopic adrenalectomy. J Urol 154:484–486
37. Kann P et al (1998) Endosonography of the adrenal glands: normal size--pathological findings. Exp Clin Endocrinol Diabetes 106:123–129
38. Barzon L et al (1999) Risk factors and long-term follow-up of adrenal incidentalomas. J Clin Endocrinol Metab 84:520–526
39. Korobkin M et al (1998) CT time-attenuation washout curves of adrenal adenomas and nonadenomas. AJR Am J Roentgenol 170:747–752
40. Pena CS et al (2000) Characterization of indeterminate (lipid-poor) adrenal masses: use of washout characteristics at contrast-enhanced CT. Radiology 217:798–802
41. Szolar DH, Kammerhuber F (1997) Quantitative CT evaluation of adrenal gland masses: a step forward in the differentiation between adenomas and nonadenomas? Radiology 202:517–521
42. Lee MJ et al (1991) Benign and malignant adrenal masses: CT distinction with attenuation coefficients, size, and observer analysis. Radiology 179:415–418
43. Mayo-Smith WW et al (2001) State-of-the-art adrenal imaging. Radiographics 21:995–1012
44. Francis IR, Korobkin M (1996) Pheochromocytoma. Radiol Clin North Am 34:1101–1112
45. Chezmar JL et al (1988) Adrenal masses: characterization with T1-weighted MR imaging. Radiology 166:357–359
46. Reinig JW et al (1986) MRI of indeterminate adrenal masses. AJR Am J Roentgenol 147:493–496
47. Korobkin M et al (1996) Adrenal adenomas: relationship between histologic lipid and CT and MR findings. Radiology 200:743–747
48. Tsushima Y (1994) Different lipid contents between aldosterone-producing and nonhyperfunctioning adrenocortical adenomas: in vivo measurement using chemical-shift magnetic resonance imaging. J Clin Endocrinol Metab 79:1759–1762
49. Outwater EK et al (1996) Adrenal masses: correlation between CT attenuation value and chemical shift ratio at MR imaging with in-phase and opposed-phase sequences. Radiology 200:749–752
50. Gross MD et al (2002) Is there a future for adrenal scintigraphy? Nucl Med Commun 23:197–202
51. Hahner S et al (2008) [123 I] Iodometomidate for molecular imaging of adrenocortical cytochrome P450 family 11B enzymes. J Clin Endocrinol Metab 93:2358–2365
52. Rubello D et al (2002) Functional scintigraphy of the adrenal gland. Eur J Endocrinol 147:13–28
53. Shapiro B et al (1985) Iodine-131 metaiodobenzylguanidine for the locating of suspected pheochromocytoma: experience in 400 cases. J Nucl Med 26:576–585
54. Tenenbaum F et al (1995) Comparison of radiolabeled octreotide and metaiodobenzylguanidine (MIBG) scintigraphy in malignant pheochromocytoma. J Nucl Med 36:1–6
55. van der Harst E et al (2001) [(123)I]metaiodobenzylguanidine and [(111)In]octreotide uptake in benign and malignant pheochromocytomas. J Clin Endocrinol Metab 86: 685–693
56. Groussin L et al (2009) 18F-FDG PET for the diagnosis of adrenocortical tumors: a prospective study in 77 operated patients. J Clin Endocrinol Metab, PMID: 19190108
57. Boland GW et al (1995) Indeterminate adrenal mass in patients with cancer: evaluation at PET with 2-[^{18}F]-fluoro-2-deoxy-D-glucose. Radiology 194:131–134
58. Hoegerle S et al (2002) Pheochromocytomas: detection with 18F-DOPA whole body PET – initial results. Radiology 222:507–512
59. Ilias I et al (2003) Superiority of 6-[18F]-fluorodopamine positron emission tomography versus [131I]-metaiodobenzylguanidine scintigraphy in the localization of metastatic pheochromocytoma. J Clin Endocrinol Metab 88:4083–4087
60. Pacak K et al (2001) 6-[18F]fluorodopamine positron emission tomographic (PET) scanning for diagnostic localization of pheochromocytoma. Hypertension 38:6–8

61. Pacak K et al (2001) Recent advances in genetics, diagnosis, localization, and treatment of pheochromocytoma. Ann Intern Med 134:315–329
62. Pacak K et al (2004) Functional imaging of endocrine tumors: role of positron emission tomography. Endocr Rev 25:568–580
63. Shulkin BL et al (2006) Current trends in functional imaging of pheochromocytomas and paragangliomas. Ann N Y Acad Sci 1073:374–382
64. Yun M et al (2001) 18F-FDG PET in characterizing adrenal lesions detected on CT or MRI. J Nucl Med 42:1795–1799
65. Bergström M et al (2000) PET imaging of adrenal cortical tumors with the 11 beta-hydroxylase tracer 11C-metomidate. J Nucl Med 41:2752–2782
66. Weiss LM (1984) Comparative histologic study of 43 metastasizing and nonmetastasizing adrenocortical tumors. Am J Surg Pathol 8:163–169
67. Lachenmayer A et al (2009) Nestin as a Marker in the Classification of Adrenocortical Tumors. Horm Metab Res 41:397–401
68. Marx C et al (1996) MHC class II expression – a new tool to assess dignity in adrenocortical tumours. J Clin Endocrinol Metab 81:4488–4491
69. Sasano H et al (1995) Transcription factor adrenal 4 binding protein as a marker of adrenocortical malignancy. Hum Pathol 26:1154–1156
70. Thompson LD (2002) Pheochromocytoma of the adrenal gland scaled score (PASS) to separate benign from malignant neoplasms: a clinicopathologic and immunophenotypic study of 100 cases. Am J Surg Pathol 26:551–566
71. Kopf D et al (2001) Clinical management of malignant adrenal tumors. J Cancer Res Clin Oncol 127:143–155
72. Mody MK et al (1995) Percutaneous CT-guided biopsy of adrenal masses: immediate and delayed complications. J Comput Assist Tomogr 19:434–439
73. Welch TJ et al (1994) Percutaneous adrenal biopsy: review of a 10-year experience. Radiology 193:341–344
74. Harisinghani MG et al (2002) Predictive value of benign percutaneous adrenal biopsies in oncology patients. Clin Radiol 57:898–901
75. Saboorian MH et al (1995) Fine needle aspiration cytology of primary and metastatic lesions of the adrenal gland. A series of 188 biopsies with radiologic correlation. Acta Cytol 39: 843–851
76. Beuschlein F (2007) Adrenal incidentalomas: presentation and clinical work-up. Horm Res 68(Suppl 5):191–194
77. Aso Y, Homma Y (1992) A survey on incidental adrenal tumors in Japan. J Urol 147:147814–147881
78. Bernini G et al (2002) Primary aldosteronism in normokalemic patients with adrenal incidentalomas. Eur J Endocrinol 146:523–529
79. Caplan RH et al (1994) Subclinical hormone secretion by incidentally discovered adrenal masses. Arch Surg 129:291–296
80. Barzon L et al (1998) Incidentally discovered adrenal tumors: endocrine and scintigraphic correlates. J Clin Endocrinol Metab 83:55–62
81. Terzolo M et al (1998) Subclinical Cushing's syndrome in adrenal incidentaloma. Clin Endocrinol (Oxf) 48:89–97
82. Valli N et al (2001) Biochemical screening for subclinical cortisol-secreting adenomas amongst adrenal incidentalomas. Eur J Endocrinol 144:401–408
83. Funder JW et al (2008) Case detection, diagnosis, and treatment of patients with primary aldosteronism: an endocrine society clinical practice guideline. J Clin Endocrinol Metab 93:3266–3281
84. Nieman LK et al (2008) The diagnosis of Cushing's syndrome: an Endocrine Society Clinical Practice Guideline. J Clin Endocrinol Metab 93:1526–1540
85. Reimondo G et al (2005) Evaluation of the effectiveness of midnight serum cortisol in the diagnostic procedures for Cushing's syndrome. Eur J Endocrinol 153:803–809

86. Masserini B et al (2009) The limited role of midnight salivary cortisol levels in the diagnosis of subclinical hypercortisolism in patients with adrenal incidentaloma. Eur J Endocrinol 160:87–92
87. Tanabe A et al (2001) Autonomy of cortisol secretion in clinically silent adrenal incidentaloma. Horm Metab Res 33:444–450
88. Montori VM, Young WF Jr (2002) Use of plasma aldosterone concentration-to-plasma renin activity ratio as a screening test for primary aldosteronism: a systematic review of the literature. Endocrinol. Metab Clin North Am 31:619–632
89. Willenberg HS et al (2009) The serum sodium to urinary sodium to (serum potassium)2 to urinary potassium (SUSPPUP) ratio in patients with primary aldosteronism. Eur J Clin Invest 39:43–50
90. Balaş M et al (2010) Indicators of mineralocorticoid excess in the evaluation of primary aldosteronism. Hypertension Res *Published online*.
91. Médeau V et al (2008) Clinical and Biochemical Characteristics of Normotensive Patients with Primary Aldosteronism: a Comparison with Hypertensive Cases. Clin Endocrinol 69:20–28
92. Lenders JW et al (2002) Biochemical diagnosis of pheochromocytoma: which test is best? JAMA 287:1427–1434
93. Jaresch S et al (1987) Silent adrenal gland tumors in patients with adrenogenital syndrome. Klin Wochenschr 65:627–633
94. Seppel T, Schlaghecke R (1994) Augmented 17a-hydroxy-progesterone response to ACTH stimulation as evidence of decreased 21-hydroxylase activity in patients with incidentally discovered adrenal tumours (incidentalomas). Clin Endocrinol 41:445–451
95. Mantero F et al (1997) Adrenal incidentaloma: an overview of hormonal data from the National Italian Study Group. Horm Res 47:284–289
96. Terzolo M et al (1996) Different patterns of steroid secretion in patients with adrenal incidentaloma. J Clin Endocrinol Metab 81:740–744
97. Willenberg HS et al (2002) The short synacthen test in the evaluation of adrenal masses in patients with malignancies. Endocr Res 4:793–797
98. Beuschlein F et al (1998) Steroid 21-hydroxylase mutations and 21-hydroxylase messenger ribonucleic acid expression in human adrenocortical tumors. J Clin Endocrinol Metab 83:2585–2588
99. Patócs A et al (2002) Hormonal evaluation and mutation screening for steroid 21-hydroxylase deficiency in patients with unilateral and bilateral adrenal incidentalomas. Eur J Endocrinol 147:349–355
100. Francucci CM et al (2002) Bone metabolism and mass in women with Cushing's syndrome and adrenal incidentaloma. Clin Endocrinol 57:587–593
101. Garrapa GG et al (2001) Body composition and metabolic features in women with adrenal incidentaloma or Cushing's syndrome. J Clin Endocrinol Metab 86:5301–5306
102. Midorikawa S et al (2001) The improvement of insulin resistance in patients with adrenal incidentaloma by surgical resection. Clin Endocrinol (Oxf) 54:797–804
103. Osella G et al (2001) The patients with incidentally discovered adrenal adenoma (incidentaloma) are not at increased risk of osteoporosis. J Clin Endocrinol Metab 86:604–607
104. Rossi R et al (2000) Subclinical Cushing's syndrome in patients with adrenal incidentaloma: clinical and biochemical features. J Clin Endocrinol Metab 85:1440–1448
105. Sereg M et al (2009) Atherosclerotic risk factors and complications in patients with non-functioning adrenal adenomas treated with or without adrenalectomy: a long-term follow-up study. Eur J Endocrinol 160:647–655
106. Tauchmanova L et al (2001) Bone loss determined by quantitative ultrasonometry correlates inversely with disease activity in patients with endogenous glucocorticoid excess due to adrenal mass. Eur J Endocrinol 145:241–247

107. Tsagarakis S et al (1998) The low-dose dexamethasone suppression test in patients with adrenal incidentalomas: comparisons with clinically euadrenal subjects and patients with Cushing's syndrome. Clin Endocrinol 48:627–633
108. Barzon L et al (2002) Development of overt Cushing's syndrome in 386 patients with adrenal incidentaloma. Eur J Endocrinol 146:61–66
109. Bülow B et al (2006) Adrenal incidentaloma – follow-up results from a Swedish prospective study. Eur J Endocrinol 154:419–423
110. Charbonnel B et al (1981) Does the corticoadrenal adenoma with "pre-Cushing's syndrome" exist? J Nucl Med 22:1059–1061
111. Terzolo M et al (2002) Adrenal incidentaloma: a new cause of the metabolic syndrome? J Clin Endocrinol Metab 87:998–1003
112. Fagour C et al (2009) Usefulness of adrenal scintigraphy in the follow-up of adrenocortical incidentalomas: a prospective multicenter study. Eur J Endocrinol 160:257–264
113. Reincke M et al (1992) Preclinical Cushing's syndrome in adrenal "incidentalomas": comparison with adrenal Cushing's syndrome. J Clin Endocrinol Metab 75:826–832
114. Sippel RS, Chen H (2004) Subclinical Cushing's syndrome in adrenal incidentalomas. Surg Clin N Am 84:875–885
115. Tauchmanova L et al (2002) Patients with subclinical Cushing's syndrome due to adrenal adenoma have Increased cardiovascular risk. J Clin Endocrinol Metab 87:4872–4878
116. Reincke M (2000) Subclinical Cushing's syndrome. Endocrinol Metab Clin North Am 29:43–56

Part III
Imaging

Chapter 6
Computed Tomography/Magnetic Resonance Imaging of Adrenocortical Carcinoma

Melvyn Korobkin, Anca M. Avram, and Hero K. Hussain

This chapter describes the imaging features of adrenocortical carcinoma (ACC) and their use in detection, staging, and follow-up of the disease. The diagnostic imaging modalities most commonly used for this purpose are computed tomography (CT), magnetic resonance imaging (MRI), and FDG-positron emission tomography (PET).

About half of the cases of ACC present with signs and symptoms of Cushing's syndrome. The other half are not associated with a hypersecretory adrenal syndrome and are often detected as an incidental finding on a CT examination performed for other indications. Specialized techniques have been developed in CT and MRI to help characterize adrenal incidentalomas as adenomas vs. non-adenomas, most of which represent metastases but occasionally are ACCs. First the techniques that usually are applied to nearly all adrenal masses when first discovered will be reviewed. Then a discussion of the features of ACC itself follows. FDG-PET is a radionuclide study that detects hypermetabolic activity within tissues, most commonly seen in neoplastic disease although occasionally also seen in inflammatory conditions. The principles of FDG-PET scanning will be reviewed, and then the role it plays in contemporary imaging of ACC will be described and illustrated.

The role of CT, MRI, and FDG-PET scanning in the detection, diagnosis, staging, and follow-up of ACC in contemporary medicine will be illustrated in several recent cases from our extensive experience with this uncommon disorder.

CT is currently the primary method of imaging the adrenal gland, both for evaluating patients with abnormal adrenal function and for demonstrating adrenal anatomy in patients with incidentally discovered adrenal masses. MRI can also detect the normal and abnormal adrenal gland with accuracy similar to CT, and

M. Korobkin (✉)
Department of Radiology, University of Michigan Health System, University of Michigan, 1500 East Medical Center Drive, Ann Arbor, MI 48105, USA
e-mail: korobkin@umich.edu

Portions of this chapter have been described previously and are reproduced here with permission from Gross M, Korobkin M, Hussain HK et al (2010) Adrenal gland imaging. In: DeGroot LJ, Jameson JL (eds.) Endocrinology, 6th edn. Elsevier, Philadelphia, PA.

G.D. Hammer, T. Else (eds.), *Adrenocortical Carcinoma*,
DOI 10.1007/978-0-387-77236-3_6, © Springer Science+Business Media, LLC 2011

is frequently used to help characterize many incidental adrenal masses as adenomas. Because CT is used much more often to evaluate the abdomen for a variety of known or suspected abnormalities unrelated to the adrenal glands, it is the imaging modality with which most incidental adrenal masses are first detected [1].

With the use of modern CT scanners, the normal adrenals can be visualized in virtually 100% of cases. With the advent of helical CT technology, axial slices of 3–5 mm can be routinely obtained in patients suspected of adrenal pathology. Oral contrast and intravenous contrast are not necessary for the detection of adrenal masses, but are routinely used in abdominal CT.

Recent advances in MRI technology have improved its ability to demonstrate the normal adrenal glands and small adrenal masses. Most notably, the development of breath-hold pulse sequence has dramatically decreased artifacts limiting the utility of adrenal MRI. The traditional advantages of MRI – improved tissue contrast resolution, ability to image in multiple planes, prevention of exposure to radiation, and utility in patients with renal insufficiency and previous idiosyncratic reaction to iodinated contrast material – have always made it a useful alternative to CT. But the image quality of gradient-echo breath-hold scans, use of in-phase and opposed-phrase imaging to detect intracellular lipid in adrenal adenomas, as well as the improved spatial resolution on three-dimensional dynamic imaging with thin slices make MRI a truly competitive method with CT for imaging the normal and pathologic adrenal gland.

The cross-sectional anatomy of the normal adrenal gland is nearly identical on CT and MRI. The right adrenal lies higher in the abdomen than the left adrenal. It is superior to the upper pole of the right kidney, whereas the left adrenal is anteromedial to the upper pole of the left kidney. The basic morphology of the adrenal glands on transverse axial CT and MRI is that of an inverted V or inverted Y. In the inverted Y configuration, the anterior limb is shorter and thicker than the posteromedial and posterolateral limbs, and is sometimes undetectable, thus the inverted V appearance (Fig. 6.1).

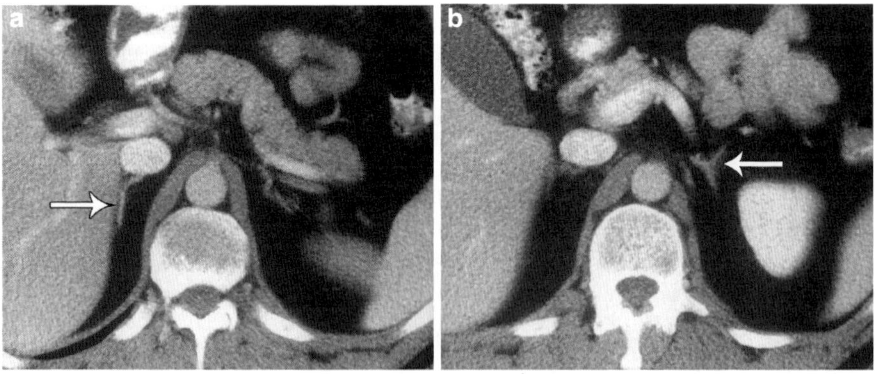

Fig. 6.1 Computed tomography (CT) appearance of normal adrenal glands. (**a**) The cephalad portion of the right adrenal (*arrow*) is seen. (**b**) The three limbs of the left adrenal (*arrow*) are shown at this level. (Reprinted with permission from [59])

6.1 Clinical Utility of CT and MRI

About 30% of cases of Cushing's syndrome are due to an ACTH-independent adrenal cortical neoplasm, about two thirds of these due to adrenal adenomas (ACAs) and the other one third due to ACC. These tumors are easily detectable on both CT and MRI. ACA are nearly always less than 5 cm in diameter, typically 2–2.5 cm, and have a nonspecific morphologic appearance (Fig. 6.2). ACC are typically larger than 5 cm in diameter, often show evidence of necrosis on enhanced CT and MRI scans, and frequently present with spread to adrenal or renal veins or evidence of distant metastatic disease (Fig. 6.3). Carcinomas are usually hypointense relative to liver on T1-weighted images and hyperintense to liver on T2-weighted images.

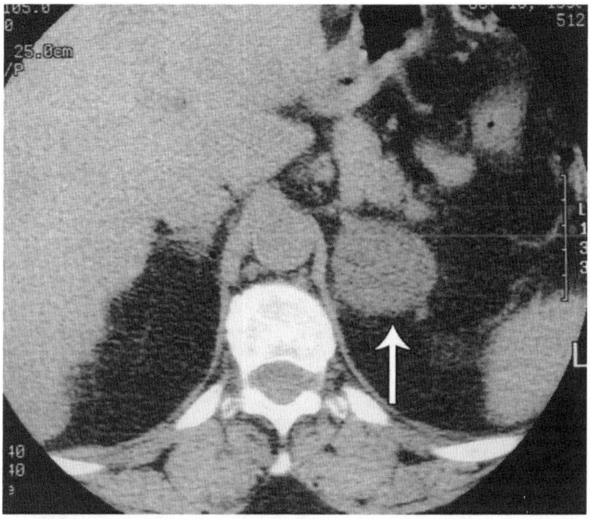

Fig. 6.2 Adrenal adenoma causing Cushing's syndrome. Homogeneous 4-cm left adrenal mass (*arrow*) has a nonspecific computed tomography (CT) appearance. L, left. (Reprinted with permission from [8])

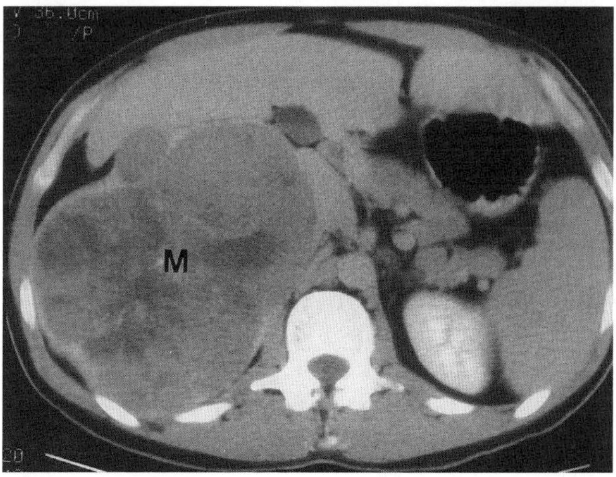

Fig. 6.3 Adrenal carcinoma causing Cushing's syndrome. Computed tomography (CT) scan shows a huge, inhomogeneous, right adrenal mass (M). (Reprinted with permission from [59])

6.2 Pheochromocytoma

Most pheochromocytomas are readily detected on CT, because they typically measure 2–5 cm in diameter. Although some are small and homogeneous in attenuation, many have regions of necrosis or hemorrhage and can have a fluid density on unenhanced CT. For many years, intravenous ionic contrast material was avoided in patients with known or suspected pheochromocytoma because of an effect on catecholamine levels and the fear of inducing a hypertensive crisis [2]. More recently, however, a study using non-ionic IV contrast showed no significant increases in catecholamine levels in either control subjects or patients with pheochromocytomas [3].

Contrast-enhanced CT of adrenal pheochromocytoma shows nonspecific homogeneous or, more commonly, inhomogeneous enhancement of a solid mass, similar to the finding in adrenal metastasis or adrenal cortical carcinoma (Fig. 6.4). Most pheochromocytomas have an unenhanced attenuation greater than 10 Hounsfield units (HU), although a recent report described a single case each of pheochromocytoma (9 HU) and medullary hyperplasia (2 HU) with lipid degeneration [4].

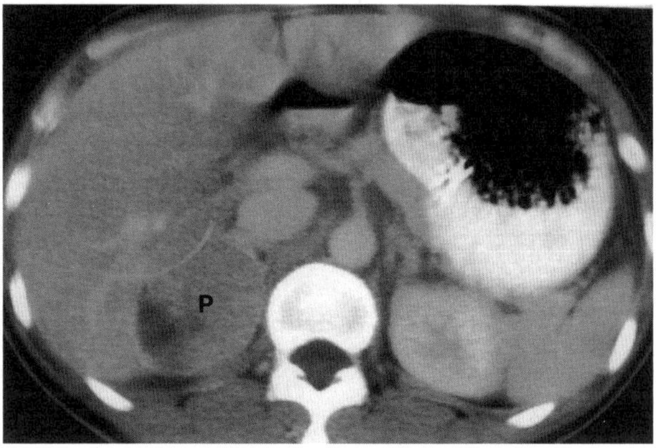

Fig. 6.4 Intravenous contrast-enhanced computed tomography (CT) shows a right adrenal pheochromocytoma (P) with areas of necrosis. (Reprinted with permission from [58])

On MRI, most pheochromocytomas are hypointense on T1-weighted images and markedly hyperintense on T2-weighted images. The cause may be related to necrotic or cystic areas so common within these tumors. MRI angiography is useful to demonstrate the presence or absence of intracaval extension of adrenal pheochromocytoma, and MRI is useful in the search for an extra-adrenal paraganglioma from the neck to the bladder.

6.3 The Incidentally Discovered Adrenal Mass (Incidentaloma)

The more widespread application of high-resolution anatomic imaging to screen the abdomen for diseases or to stage diseases unrelated to the adrenal has identified a growing number of unexpected adrenal masses or "incidentalomas" [5–8].

Given their prevalence ranging from 4 to 10% in patients studied with CT or MRI for indications other than suspected adrenal disease, novel adaptations to imaging have been made to distinguish frequent, nonhypersecretory, benign, adrenal masses from adrenal metastases and ACC [6]. The discovery of an adrenal mass presents a diagnostic and, at times, therapeutic challenge. Since the overwhelming majority of incidentalomas are benign and nonhypersecretory, an aggressive approach to them is not indicated [5–7]. Of course, a solitary adrenal metastasis or incidentally discovered ACC treated earlier would have a more favorable result. Given the uncertainty in the diagnosis of adrenal masses other than cysts and myelolipoma, many diagnostic algorithms and approaches have been offered, making the evaluation of adrenal incidentalomas controversial [5–9]. A thoughtful approach to such patients must include a biochemical evaluation sufficient to exclude both cortical and medullary hyperfunction and an anatomic and/or functional imaging evaluation sufficient to exclude a malignancy [5, 9–11]. The continuing uncertainty about the appropriate clinical and imaging management of adrenal incidentalomas was attested to at a National Institutes of Health Consensus Conference on this subject in February 2002 [12].

6.4 Myelolipoma

A myelolipoma is a benign tumor composed of bone marrow elements. Myelolipomas do not produce hormones and most are detected as incidental findings. Occasionally, large tumors or those undergoing tumor necrosis or spontaneous hemorrhage may cause flank pain. Although most are adrenal in location, extra-adrenal myelolipomas have been reported. Due to large amounts of mature fat, most myelolipomas are easily recognized on CT (Fig. 6.5) [13, 14]. Elements of soft-tissue density are found in varying amounts, and calcification is seen in up to 20% of cases.

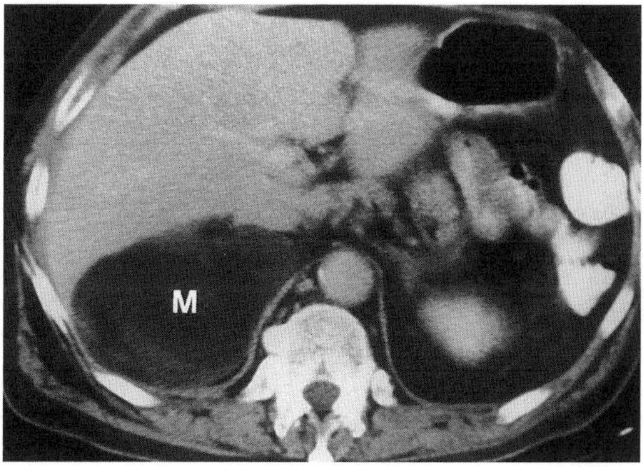

Fig. 6.5 Myelolipoma. Large, fatty right adrenal mass (M) is seen on this contrast-enhanced computed tomography (CT) examination. (Reprinted with permission from [26])

The appearance of a myelolipoma on MRI reflects the portions of fat and bone marrow elements in the tumor. Fat exhibits high-signal intensity on both T1- and T2-weighted sequences. The bone marrow elements have a low-signal intensity on T1-weighted images and moderate signal intensity on T2-weighted scans. Since a confident diagnosis of myelolipoma can usually be made with CT or MRI, the majority is treated conservatively.

6.5 Cyst

Adrenal cysts are uncommon lesions with infrequent reports of their CT appearance. There is a 3:1 female predilection, and there are four types of cysts based on pathologic classification: endothelial, epithelial, parasitic, and posttraumatic pseudocysts. A recent report of 13 new cystic adrenal masses and review of 26 benign adrenal cysts from the literature included one cystic adrenal cortical carcinoma [15]. Of 37 reviewed benign cysts, 19 had mural and 7 had central calcification, 28 were unilocular, and 7 had high attenuation values. Wall thickness was 3 mm or less in 31 lesions. The authors concluded that a CT finding of a nonenhancing mass with or without wall calcification allows differentiation of an adrenal cyst from an adenoma (Fig. 6.6). A small adrenal cyst with near-water attenuation and a thin ($\leq$3 mm) wall is likely to be benign.

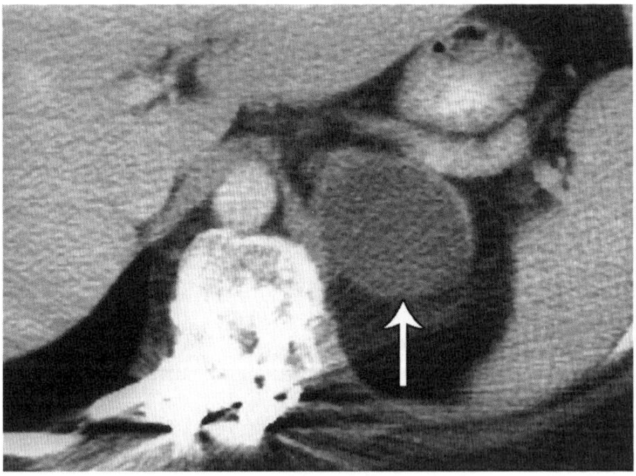

Fig. 6.6 Adrenal pseudocyst. This homogeneous left adrenal mass measured near-water density (8 HU). The wall is thickened, but smooth and less than 3 mm. (Reprinted with permission from [11])

6.6 Hemorrhage

Adrenal hemorrhage can be bilateral or unilateral. When bilateral, the cause is usually associated with anticoagulation therapy or a blood dyscrasia; less commonly, it is associated with the stress of surgery, sepsis, or hypotension, and, rarely, it is caused by trauma [16]. Unilateral adrenal hemorrhage is usually caused by blunt abdominal trauma, and involves the right gland more often than the left [17]. Adrenal vein thrombosis may also cause unilateral adrenal hemorrhage. This may be caused by catheterization to collect blood samples from the adrenal vein in patients with suspected adrenal endocrine disease. In the absence of catheterization or blunt trauma, unilateral adrenal hemorrhage may occur into a preexisting neoplasm, necessitating surgical exploration if follow-up imaging does not show a nearly normal adrenal gland.

Acute or subacute adrenal hemorrhage typically has an unenhanced attenuation value of 55–90 HU (Fig. 6.7). Follow-up studies show diminution in size of the adrenal mass with gradual decrease in attenuation value [18]. The high attenuation value of a recent adrenal hemorrhage is usually readily apparent on unenhanced CT, but is indistinguishable from a solid adrenal neoplasm on contrast-enhanced CT. An adrenal mass detected on contrast-enhanced CT after trauma is usually assumed to be due to a hematoma, but an unrelated adrenal neoplasm can only be excluded by unenhanced CT or serial follow-up CT. Similarly, MRI may indicate hemorrhage by the high-signal intensity on T1-weighted scans, reflecting the presence of methemoglobin [19, 20].

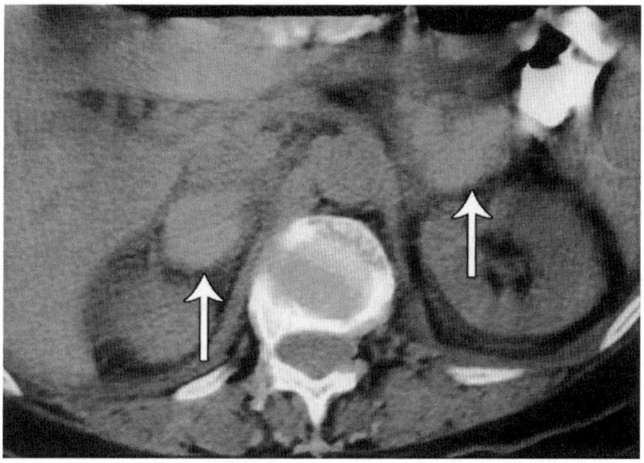

Fig. 6.7 Adrenal hematoma. Bilateral adrenal masses (arrows) are seen in this unenhanced computed tomography (CT) examination. High density of masses suggests hematoma. (Reprinted with permission from [11])

6.7 Adrenocortical Adenoma

A nonfunctioning adenoma is the most common adrenal tumor. It is reported as occurring in 1.4–8.7% of postmortem examinations, depending on the criteria used [21–24]. The incidence is even higher among patients with hypertension or diabetes mellitus [22–24]. Adenomas large enough to be recognized on survey abdominal CT examinations are found in approximately 1% of patients, but may be increasing with improvements in CT technology [25]. On CT, adenomas may have the same density as normal adrenal tissue. Since most adenomas contain large amounts of intracytoplasmic lipid, many have a low density, often near that of water on unenhanced examinations [26] (Fig. 6.8). Calcification is rare. Adenomas enhance significantly after the intravenous administration of iodinated contrast media. Although the degree of enhancement is not significantly different from that of other adrenal tumors, they show more rapid washout of contrast than adrenal metastases [27–29].

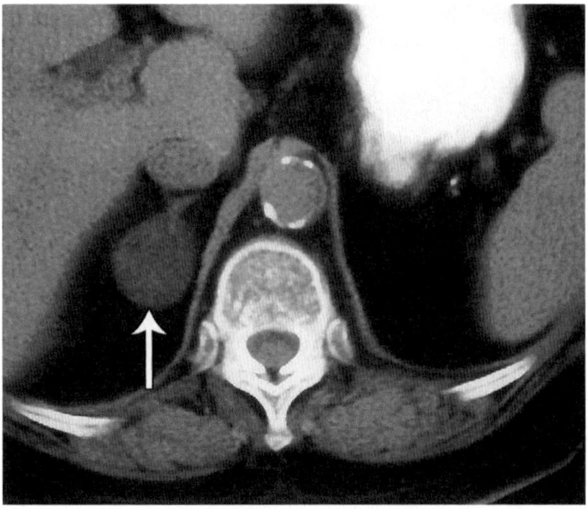

Fig. 6.8 Lipid-rich adenoma. Three cm right adrenal mass (*arrow*) is shown on this unenhanced computed tomography (CT) scan. Attenuation value of –4 HU allows confident diagnosis of benign lesion, either cyst or lipid-rich adenoma. (Reprinted with permission from [11])

The MRI signal characteristics of adenomas are also similar to normal adrenal tissue. Although the signal intensity of an adenoma tends to be low on T2-weighted sequences, this is not a useful way to distinguish adenomas from metastases as there is an overlap of 20–30% with metastases. Chemical shift imaging is used to identify the intracytoplasmic lipid and can distinguish many adenomas from metastases [30, 31] (Fig. 6.9).

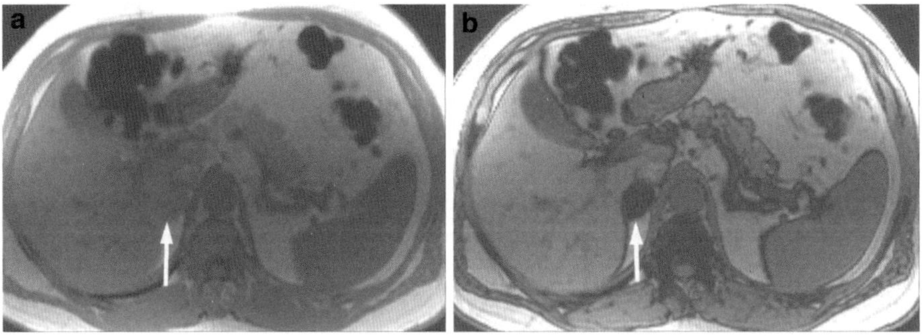

Fig. 6.9 Adrenal adenoma. (**a**) Right adrenal mass (*arrow*) is seen on this in-phase (MRI). (**b**) There is a significant decrease in signal on the out-of-phase MRI

6.8 Adrenocortical Carcinoma

ACC is a rare tumor, with a reported incidence of 1–2 cases per million [32]. Patients may present with abdominal pain, a palpable mass, or Cushing's syndrome, as about 50% of these tumors elaborate unregulated amounts of cortisol. Many of these elaborate insufficient amounts of hormone to produce obvious clinical manifestations. Other endocrine manifestations of ACC include Conn's syndrome, virilization, and feminization, but these are very rare. The tumors tend to be very large at the time of presentation.

The CT appearance of an adrenal carcinoma is a large mass. Central necrosis is common and calcification is seen in 20–30% of cases [33, 34] (Fig. 6.10a). Enhancement is heterogeneous after intravenous contrast administration. Venous extension of tumor into the left renal vein or inferior vena caval is common and can usually be identified on the contrast-enhanced images [33] (Fig. 6.10b). It is important to define precisely the cephalad extent of the intravenous tumor, as this defines the point where the surgeon can gain vascular control of the tumor [35]. Although this can often be done with CT, MRI may be helpful in problem cases [36]. On MRI, carcinomas are usually heterogeneously hyperintense on both T1- and T2-weighted images, reflecting the frequent internal hemorrhage and central necrosis (Fig. 6.11). Enhancement is also heterogeneous, revealing nodular areas of intense enhancement and other areas with no enhancement. Intravenous extension of tumor is typically well seen on MRI due to the multiple planes in which the data sets can be projected [36, 37].

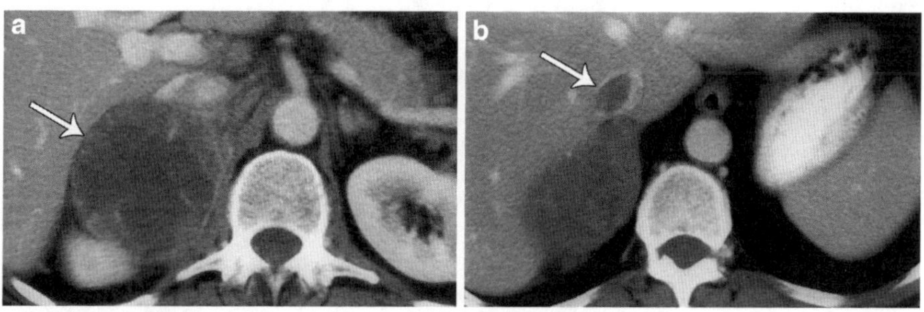

Fig. 6.10 Adrenal cortical carcinoma. (**a**) Contrast-enhanced computed tomography (CT) examination shows 9-cm right adrenal mass. Irregular wall and low-density center indicate necrosis. (**b**) More cephalad image in same examination reveals tumor extension into inferior vena cava (*arrow*). (Reprinted with permission from [11])

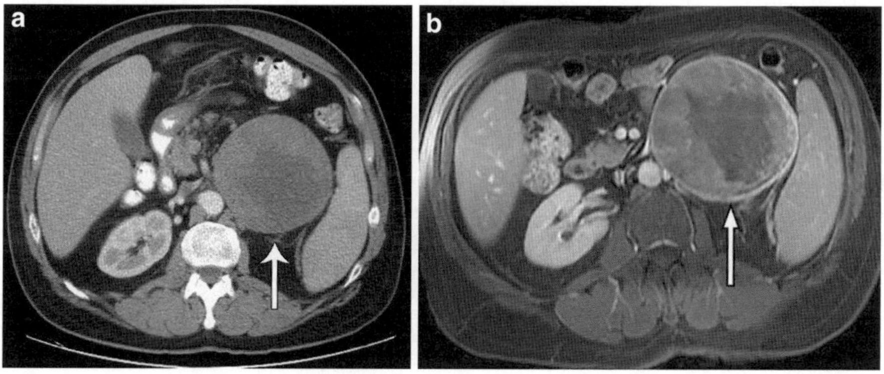

Fig. 6.11 Adrenal cortical carcinoma. (**a**) Contrast-enhanced CT shows a 11 × 16 cm left adrenal mass (*arrow*), with a large central region of low attenuation indicating necrosis and/or hemorhage. (**b**) Gadolinum-enhanced MR shows a similar mass (*arrow*) with central low signal intensity

6.9 Metastasis

The adrenal glands are a common site of metastatic disease, found in about 27% of postmortem examination of patients with malignant neoplasms of epithelial origin [38]. The most common neoplasms with adrenal metastases are carcinomas of the lung and breast and melanoma [38, 39]. Small metastases are often homogeneous on contrast-enhanced CT (Fig. 6.12) or MRI, whereas large metastases often have local regions of heterogenous appearance due to necrosis or hemorrhage or both (Fig. 6.13). Calcification is rare in adrenal metastases.

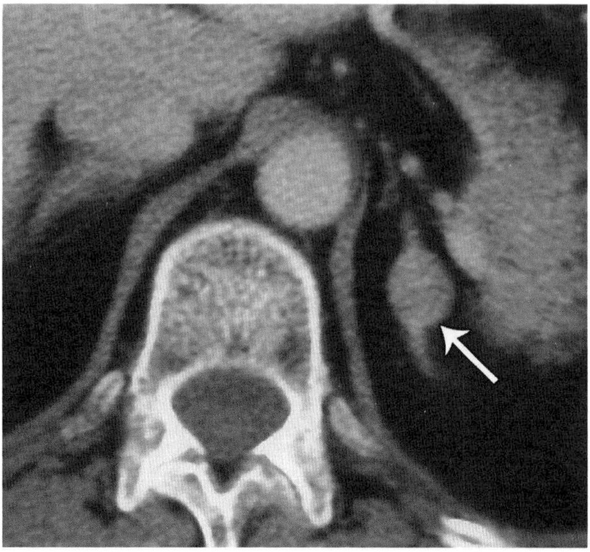

Fig. 6.12 Metastasis from renal carcinoma in a 31-year-old woman. Small, homogeneous left adrenal mass (*arrow*) is seen on this contrast-enhanced computed tomography (CT) examination. (Reprinted with permission from [11])

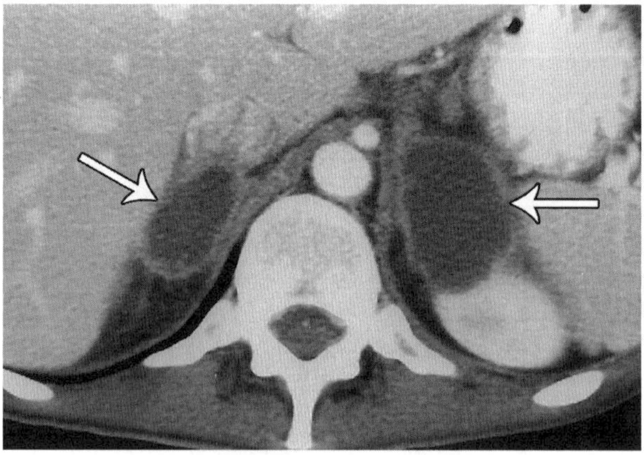

Fig. 6.13 Necrotic metastases from adenocarcinoma of the lung in a 34-year-old woman. Bilateral adrenal masses (*arrow*) with areas of central necrosis are seen on this contrast-enhanced computed tomography (CT) examination. (Reprinted with permission from [11])

6.10 Differential Diagnosis: Adrenocortical Adenoma or Metastasis?

Although this section discusses the different methods of CT and MRI that may be used to differentiate a benign (usually adenoma) from malignant (usually metastasis) adrenal mass, not all lesions or patients require an evaluation. The prevalence of adrenal adenomas is high, and small homogeneous adrenal masses discovered incidentally are likely to be adenomas. If a patient shows evidence of metastases elsewhere and the presence of an adrenal metastasis will not alter therapy, further evaluation is not justified.

Evidence has accumulated that unenhanced CT densitometry can be used to differentiate adrenal adenomas from metastases accurately [40–42]. Most adenomas have unenhanced CT attenuation values lower than metastases, and the scatter plot data from such studies were used to determine a threshold value that resulted in calculation of the optimal combination of sensitivity and specificity for the diagnosis of adenoma. In an oncologic patient with an adrenal mass but no other evidence of distant metastatic disease, the goal of noninvasive diagnostic imaging is to characterize the adrenal mass as an adenoma with high specificity.

Using pooled data from multiple published studies of calculated accuracies and corresponding threshold values of unenhanced attenuation values, it has been shown that the most optimal sensitivity (71%) and specificity (98%) for the diagnosis of adrenal adenoma result from choosing a threshold attenuation value of 10 HU on unenhanced CT [42]. Unlike unenhanced attenuation values, however, intravenous contrast-enhanced CT values show too much overlap between adenomas and metastases to allow an accurate differentiation between them.

Evidence has also accumulated that chemical shift MRI can also be used to differentiate adrenal adenomas from metastases. Taking advantage of the different resonant frequency peaks for the hydrogen atom in water and triglyceride (lipid) molecules, chemical shift MRI results in a decrease in signal intensity of the tissue containing both lipid and water in comparison with the tissue containing no lipid [43]. Using a breath-hold gradient echo technique, signal intensity loss on opposed-phase compared to in-phase images indicates a mixture of lipid and nonlipid tissue that is often present in adrenal adenomas and absent in metastases. Assessment of the chemical shift change can be made using simple visual analysis or by quantitative methods using standard region-of-interest cursor measurements of the mass, and often of an adjacent reference tissue, on in-phase and opposed-phase images. Several different formulas have been proposed to measure the amount of chemical shift change and optimal threshold values, determined by analysis of scatter plot data [44].

Recent observation suggests that quantitative methods may be more sensitive for detecting lipid in an adenoma [44].

Two studies have suggested that unenhanced CT densitometry and chemical shift MRI both detect the presence and amount of lipid within adrenal adenomas. In one study of 47 adrenal masses, which were all imaged with both techniques, there was good inverse linear correlation between the CT attenuation value and the amount of chemical shift change on MRI [45]. In a histologic/radiologic study of a small number of resected adrenal adenomas that had undergone presurgical CT, chemical shift MRI, or both, there was good inverse linear correlation between the estimated number of lipid-rich cells and the unenhanced CT attenuation value and good linear correlation with the relative change in signal intensity on opposed-phase MRI (Figs. 6.14 and 6.15) [26].

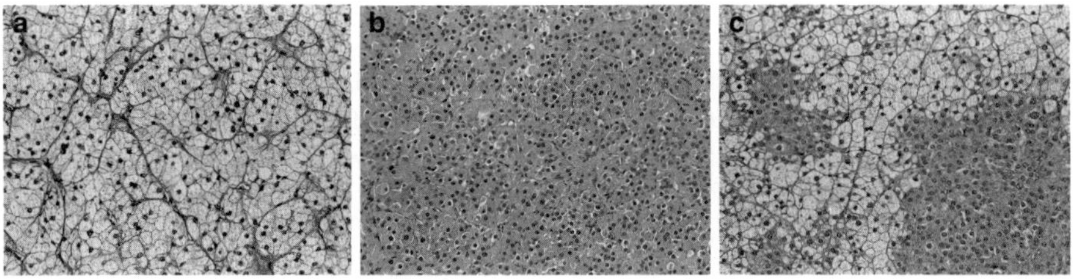

Fig. 6.14 Histologic specimens from resected adrenal adenomas: (**a**) primarily of lipid-rich clear cells; (**b**) primarily of lipid-poor clear cells; and (**c**) of an admixture of clear and compact cortical cells. (Hematoxylin-eosin stain's original magnification, ×200). (Reprinted with permission from [26])

Fig. 6.15 Plot of unenhanced computed tomography (CT) attenuation number vs. the percentage of lipid-rich cells in 13 surgically resected adrenal adenomas. HU, Hounsfield units. (Reprinted with permission from [26])

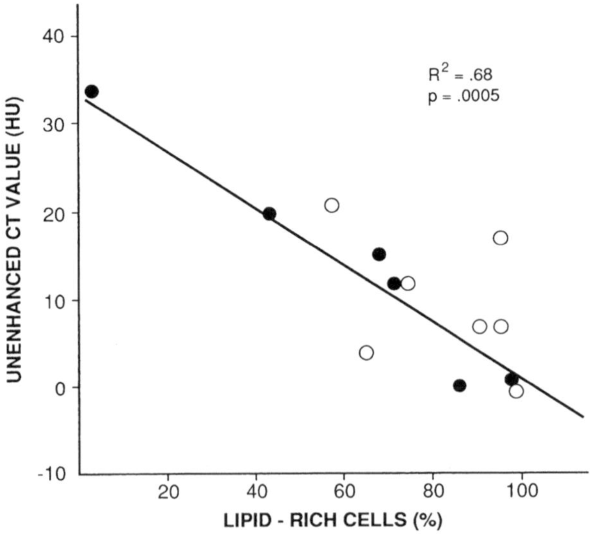

But two more recent publications indicate that chemical shift MRI is more sensitive by detecting sufficient lipid in adenomas with unenhanced CT values between 10 and 30 HU [44, 46].

Standard contrast-enhanced CT images of the adrenal glands are obtained about 60 s after the beginning of bolus intravenous injection of contrast material. Studies suggest this is the only time when the attenuation values of adenomas and metastases are nearly identical. Adenomas have a much more rapid loss of enhancement, as early as 5 min after contrast injection, and attenuation values at 10 or 15 min after contrast administration can be used to differentiate adenomas from other masses [29, 47] (Fig. 6.15). Although the threshold attenuation value for the diagnosis of an adenoma has varied among series, masses with an attenuation value less than 30–40 HU on 15-min delayed contrast-enhanced CT are almost always adenomas (Fig. 6.16).

Prior reports indicated that the more rapid washout of gadolinium enhancement on MRI of adrenal adenomas could also differentiate them from metastases [48]. Subsequent reports could not confirm these results, however, and dynamic gadolinium-enhanced MRI is not widely used for this purpose.

In addition to the delayed CT attenuation value itself, it is also possible to calculate the percentage washout of initial enhancement, which is probably independent of type, amount, and injection rates of contrast administration [29, 49]. The optimal threshold enhancement washout at 15 min is 60%, resulting in a sensitivity of 88% and a specificity of 96% for the diagnosis of adenoma [29]. Of particular interest is the apparent independence of this rapid enhancement washout from the lipid content of an adenoma. Lipid-poor adenomas, those with unenhanced attenuation values greater than 10 HU on unenhanced CT, have enhancement washout features nearly identical to lipid-rich adenomas [50].

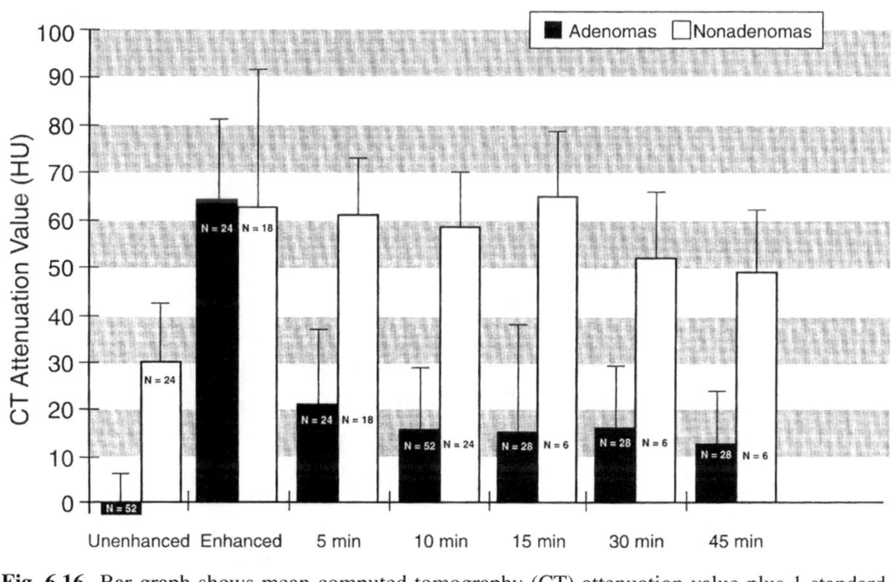

Fig. 6.16 Bar graph shows mean computed tomography (CT) attenuation value plus 1 standard deviation for adrenal adenomas (*black*) and nonadenomas (*white*) on unenhanced, enhanced, and delayed enhanced scans. (Reprinted with permission from [29])

It is easy to calculate the enhancement washout of adrenal masses:

$$\%\ \text{enhancement washout} = [(E - D)/(E - U)] \times 100,$$

where *E* is the enhanced attenuation value, *D* is the delayed enhanced value, and *U* is the unenhanced value. For example, if the unenhanced attenuation is 20 HU, the enhanced attenuation is 100 HU, and the 15-min delayed enhanced attenuation is 40 HU, the percent washout is:

$$[(100 - 40)/(100 - 20)] \times 100 = [60/80] \times 100 = 75\%$$

Using the threshold value of 60%, the mass is likely a lipid-poor adenoma. If there is no unenhanced CT, or the unenhanced attenuation value is unknown, a relative enhancement washout can be calculated as follows:

$$\%\ \text{relative enhancement washout} = [(E - D)]/(E)] \times 100$$

In our department, the optimal threshold value for the relative enhancement washout calculation is 40%, resulting in a sensitivity of 96% and a specificity of 100% for the diagnosis of adenoma. Another study of the accuracy of relative enhancement washout to characterize adrenal masses reported an optimal threshold of 50% [51], resulting in a sensitivity and specificity of 100%.

In the previous example, the calculation for relative enhancement washout is as follows:

$$[(100 - 40)/100] \times 100 = 60\%$$

Using the threshold value for relative enhancement washout of 40%, this calculation again indicates an adenoma.

Assessment of enhancement washout curves of adrenal masses is valid only for lesions with relatively homogeneous attenuation after contrast enhancement. Large regions of low attenuation, probably representing areas of necrosis or hemorrhage, were specifically excluded from evaluation in the papers that described and quantitated the washout curves. The calculations apply only to solid tissue with an intact capillary bed. The diagnosis of adrenal adenoma cannot be made in masses that contain prominent regions of necrosis or hemorrhage.

Combination of the two independent CT properties of adrenal adenomas, rapid contrast enhancement washout and a propensity for intratumoral lipid, leads to a protocol that spares most adenomas from contrast enhancement. It was reported the accuracy of combined unenhanced and delayed enhanced CT densitometry for characterization of adrenal masses [52]. 166 adrenal masses were studied prospectively with unenhanced CT; those with attenuation values greater than 10 HU underwent contrast-enhanced and 15-min delayed enhanced CT. This protocol correctly characterized 160 of the 166 masses (96%). When the five nonadenomas that were not metastases were excluded, the sensitivity and specificity for characterizing a mass as adenoma versus metastasis were 98% (124/127) and 97% (33/34), respectively. Similar results were subsequently reported using a very similar protocol [53].

6.11 Differential Diagnosis: Adrenocortical Adenoma or Carcinoma?

In patients without a primary extra-adrenal neoplasm, an adrenal mass without specific morphologic features is almost always an adenoma, especially if less than 3 cm in diameter. In order to obviate the common practice of serial CT imaging over several years to assure a benign lesion, in order to show stability in size, the imaging techniques described previously are often used to confirm the findings characteristic of an adenoma. If these features are present, a diagnosis of adenoma can be made without the need for follow-up imaging. In a recent study of incidentally detected indeterminate, but benign appearing, adrenal masses with no known primary malignancy, all of the 321 lesions studied were confirmed to be benign. Follow-up imaging appears to have a limited role in this common patient cohort [54].

A unilateral adrenal mass larger than 5 or 6 cm in diameter is considered suspicious for ACC, and many will show evidence of metastatic disease. It is important to remember that a large nonhyperfunctioning pheochromocytoma and a large adrenal metastasis can have a CT and MRI appearance identical to that of a carcinoma. In the absence of metastases, the differential diagnosis is usually ACC versus adenoma. The larger the mass, the greater is the likelihood of carcinoma, although on rare occasion adenomas can be larger than 5 cm and can have large regions of hemorrhage, necrosis, and calcification [55]. The size criteria for resection of adrenal incidentaloma varies widely, but most adrenal masses greater than 6 cm are resected for fear of possible ACC.

Very little is known about chemical shift MRI and CT densitometry of ACC. In one of the reported series of delayed enhanced CT attenuation values and enhancement washout curves, only one included three cases of adrenal carcinomas, but the carcinomas were included in the data set for nonadenomas and their location in the scatter plots of the individual cases was not provided [47]. ACCs greater than 6 cm often have large regions of central necrosis or hemorrhage, invalidating attempts to assess contrast enhancement washout. It is not yet established whether chemical shift MRI, unenhanced CT, or delayed enhanced CT can reliably differentiate ACA from ACC. The answer may depend on the histologic grade of malignancy involved. In one series that included 11 ACCs, the absolute and relative enhancement loss on 10-min delayed imaging of the carcinomas was significantly smaller than for the adenomas, and was similar to that for the metastases and the pheochomocytomas [56]. In another series of seven patients with ACC, delayed enhanced images at approximately 20 min showed a relative percentage of enhancement washout less than 40%, consistent with malignancy [57].

6.12 Imaging and Staging of Adrenocortical Carcinoma

Imaging plays an important role in the diagnosis, differential diagnosis, staging, and follow-up of ACC. If the CT or MR features of a unilateral adrenal mass are typical of a benign entity such as a cyst, myelolipoma, or hemorrhage, further diagnostic evaluation including additional imaging is often not necessary. If the cross-sectional imaging features of these uncommon entities are not present, but the CT densitometry or chemical shift MRI features are highly suggestive of a benign adenoma (especially if the lesion is less than 4 cm in diameter and is not associated with an abnormal adrenal hormone evaluation), often little or no further evaluation is necessary. If there are features that are not typical for a benign adenoma, such as calcifications or heterogeneous appearance on the intravenous contrast-enhanced appearance of a CT or MRI examination, diagnosis of ACC or metastatic lesion must be excluded. If an extra-adrenal primary neoplasm is present and no other sites of metastases are known, image-guided percutaneous biopsy is often used to confirm the diagnosis. In the absence of a known primary extra-adrenal malignancy, ACC is the most likely diagnosis, especially if the adrenal mass is larger than 4 cm.

Imaging is used in staging of ACC before and after initial treatment. Cross-sectional imaging is used to detect both local spread and widespread metastases. FDG PET/CT is used to confirm the likely malignant nature of CT/MR findings or to detect likely metastatic sites not detectable on the anatomic studies. Serial CT or MR findings are sometimes necessary to differentiate residual local tumor or tumor recurrence from post-surgical changes. Metastases are most frequently seen in the lung parenchyma, liver, abdominal and pulmonary lymph nodes, peritoneum and osseous structures. Fig. 6.17 illustrates the correlation of CT findings with FDG-PET imaging (Fig. 6.17).

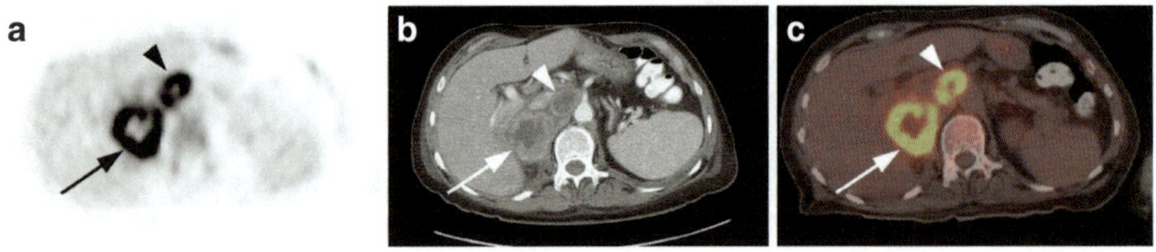

Fig. 6.17 A 61-year-old man without prior history of malignancy presenting with right upper abdominal pain. Transaxial abdominal PET, CT, and PET-CT fused images demonstrate a large right adrenal mass with intense peripheral metabolic activity and central photopenia consistent with aggressive neoplasm with central tumor necrosis (*arrow*). Additionally, there is focal FDG activity in an enlarged right para-aortic mass (*arrowhead*), which is centrally photopenic consistent with regional metastasis with associated intra-tumoral necrosis

References

1. Francis IR et al (1992) Integrated imaging of adrenal disease. Radiology 182:1–13
2. Raisanen J et al (1984) Plasma catecholamines in pheochromocytoma: Effect of urographic contrast media. Am J Roentgenol 143:43–46

3. Mukherjee JJ et al (1997) Pheochromocytoma: Effect of nonionic contrast medium in CT on circulating catecholamine levels. Radiology 202:227–231
4. Blake MA et al (2003) Low-density pheochromocytoma on CT: a mimicker of adrenal adenoma. Am J Roentgenol 181:1663–1668
5. Kloos RT et al (1995) Incidentally discovered adrenal masses. Endocr Rev 16:460–484
6. Barzon L, Boscaro M (2000) Diagnosis and management of adrenal incidentalomas. J Urol 163:398–407
7. Bardet S et al (1996) ^{131}I–6β–Iodomethylnorcholesterol scintigraphy: An assessment of its role in the investigation of adrenocortical incidentalomas. Clin Endocrinol 44:587–596
8. Korobkin M et al (1996) The incidental adrenal mass. Radiol Clin North Am 34: 1037–1054
9. Gross MD, Shapiro B (1993) Clinically silent adrenal masses. J Clin Endocrinol Metab 77:885–888
10. Osella G et al (1994) Endocrine evaluation of incidentally discovered adrenal masses (incidentalomas). J Clin Endocrinol Metab 79:1532–1539
11. Dunnick NR, Korobkin M (2002) Imaging of adrenal incidentalomas: Current status. Am J Roentgenol 179:559–568
12. Incidentally discovered adrenal mass (2002) National Institutes of Health (NIH) Consensus conference, Bethesda, MD, 4–6, February 2002
13. Cyran KM et al (1996) Adrenal myelolipoma. Am J Roentgenol 166:395–400
14. Rao P et al (1997) Imaging and pathologic features of myelolipoma. Radiographics 17: 1373–1385
15. Rozenblit A et al (1996) Cystic adrenal lesions: CT features. Radiology 201:541–548
16. Xarli VP et al (1978) Adrenal hemorrhage in the adult. Medicine 57:211–221
17. Burks DW et al (1992) Acute adrenal injury after blunt abdominal trauma: CT findings. Am J Roentgenol 158:503–507
18. Ling D et al (1983) CT demonstration of bilateral adrenal hemorrhage. Am J Roentgenol 141:307–308
19. Roubidoux MA (1994) MR imaging of hemorrhage and iron deposition in the kidney. Radiographics 14:1033–1044
20. Kawashima A et al (1999) Imaging of nontraumatic hemorrhage of the adrenal gland. Radiographics 19:949–963
21. Commons RR, Callaway CP (1948) Adenomas of the adrenal cortex. Arch Intern Med 81: 37–41
22. Kokko JP et al (1967) Adrenal adenoma and hypertension. Lancet 1:468–470
23. Hedeland H et al (1968) On the prevalence of adrenocortical adenomas in an autopsy material in relation to hypertension and diabetes. Acta Med Scand 184:211–214
24. Russi S et al (1945) Small adenomas of the adrenal cortex in hypertension and diabetes. Arch Intern Med 76:284–291
25. Aso Y, Homma Y (1992) A survey on incidental adrenal tumors in Japan. J Urol 147: 1478–1481
26. Korobkin M FJ et al (1996) Adrenal adenomas: relationship between histologic lipid and CT and MR findings. Radiology 200:743–747
27. Krestin GP et al (1991) Evaluation of adrenal masses in oncologic patients: dynamic contrast-enhanced MR vs CT. J Comput Assist Tomogr 15:104–110
28. Dunnick NR et al (1996) Adrenal radiology: distinguishing benign from malignant adrenal masses. Am J Roentgenol 167:861–867
29. Korobkin M et al (1998) CT time-attenuation washout curves of adrenal adenomas and nonadenomas. Am J Roentgenol 170:747–752
30. Reinig JW et al (1986) Adrenal masses differentiated by MR. Radiology 158:81–84
31. Outwater EK et al (1995) Distinction between benign and malignant adrenal masses: value of T1-weighted chemical-shift MR imaging. Am J Roentgenol 165:579–583
32. Hedican SP, Marshall FF (1997) Adrenocortical carcinoma with intracaval extension. J Urol 158:2056–2061

33. Dunnick NR et al (1982) CT appearance of adrenal cortical carcinoma. J Comput Assist Tomogr 6:978–982
34. Fishman EK et al (1987) Primary adrenocortical carcinoma: CT evaluation with clinical correlation. Am J Roentgenol 148:531–535
35. Dunnick NR et al (1980) Intravenous extension of endocrine tumors. Am J Roentgenol 135:471–476
36. Lee MJ et al (1994) State-of-the-art MR imaging of the adrenal gland. Radiographics 14:1015–1029, 1994
37. Schlund JF et al (1995) Adrenocortical carcinoma: MR imaging appearance with current techniques. J Magn Reson Imaging 5:171–174
38. Abrams HL et al (1950) Metastases in carcinoma: analysis of 1000 autopsied cases. Cancer 3:74–85
39. Zornoza J et al (1976) Radiologic features of adrensal metastases. Urology 8:295–299
40. Lee MJ et al (1991) Benign and malignant adrenal masses: CT distinction with attenuation coefficients, size, and observer analysis. Radiology 179:415–418
41. Korobkin M et al (1996) Differentiation of adrenal adenomas from nonadenomas using CT attenuation values. Am J Roentgenol 166:531–536
42. Boland GW et al (1998) Characterization of adrenal masses using unenhanced CT: an analysis of the CT literature. Am J Roentgenol 171:201–204
43. Mitchell DG et al (1992) Benign adrenocortical masses: diagnosis with chemical shift MR imaging. Radiology 185:345–351
44. Israel GM et al (2004) Comparison of unenhanced CT and chemical shift MR imaging in evaluating lipid rich adrenal adenomas. Am J Roentgenol183:215–219
45. Outwater EK et al (1996) Adrenal masses: correlation between CT attenuation value and chemical shift ratio at MR imaging with in-phase and opposed-phase sequences. Radiology 200:749–752
46. Haider MA et al (2004) Chemical shift MR imaging of hyperattenuating (>10 HU) adrenal masses: does it still have a role? Radiology 231:711–716
47. Szolar DH, Kammerhuber F (1997) Quantitative CT evaluation of adrenal gland masses: a step forward in the differentiation between adenomas and nonadenomas? Radiology 202: 517–521
48. Krestin GP et al (1989) Adrenal masses: evaluation with fast gradient-echo MR imaging and Gd-DTPA-enhanced dynamic studies. Radiology 171:675–680
49. Szolar DH, Kammerhuber FH (1998) Adrenal adenomas and nonadenomas: assessment of washout at delayed contrast-enhanced CT. Radiology 207:369–375
50. Caoili EM et al (2000) Delayed enhanced CT of lipid-poor adrenal adenomas. Am J Roentgenol 175:1411–1415
51. Peña CS et al (2000) Characterization of indeterminate (lipid-poor) adrenal masses: use of washout characteristics at contrast-enhanced CT. Radiology 217:798–802
52. Caoili EM et al (2002) Combined unenhanced and delayed enhanced CT for characterization of adrenal masses. Radiology 222:629–633
53. Blake MA et al (2006) Distinguishing benig from maligant adrenal masses: multidetector row CT protocal with 10 minutes delay. Radiology 238: 578–585
54. Song JH et al (2007) The incidental indeterminate adrenal mass on CT (>10 HU) in patients without cancer. Is futher imaging necessary: follow up of 321 consecutive indeterminate adrenal masses. Am J Roentgenol 189:1119–1123
55. Newhouse JH et al (1999) Large degenerated adrenal adenomas: radiologic-pathologic correlation. Radiology 210:385–391
56. Szolar DH et al (2005) Adrenocortical carconomas and adrenal pheochromocytomas: Mass and enhancement loss evaluation at delayed contrast-enhanced CT. Radiology 234:479–485
57. Slattery JM et al (2006) Adrenocortical carcinoma: contrast washout characteristics on CT. Am J. Roetgenol 187: W21–W24
58. Korobkin M, Francis IR (1997) Imaging of adrenal masses. Urol Clin North Am 24:603–622
59. Korobkin M, Francis IR (1995) Adrenal imaging. Semin Ultrasound CT MR 16:317–330

Chapter 7
Functional Imaging of Adrenocortical Carcinoma

Anca M. Avram and Stephanie Hahner

7.1 $[^{18}F]$-FDG-PET-CT in Adrenocortical Carcinoma

Increased glucose metabolism through the activation of aerobic glycolysis is a central feature of malignant transformation and progression (the Warburg effect) [1]. Malignant tumors can be detected with high sensitivity and specificity by imaging their increased metabolic rate for glucose; and positron emission tomography (PET) using the glucose analog fluorine-18 labeled fluoro-deoxyglucose ($[^{18}F]$-FDG) has become a routine clinical imaging strategy for staging and restaging most solid tumors. In recent years, metabolic imaging has been increasingly combined with computed tomography (CT) imaging for precise anatomic localization resulting in fusion PET-CT. After intravenous injection $[^{18}F]$-FDG is transported across cell membrane by sodium-independent, facilitative glucose transporters (GLUTs), and in most malignant tumors GLUT1 is frequently highly expressed. Intracellularly, $[^{18}F]$-FDG is phosphorylated by hexokinase to $[^{18}F]$-FDG-6 phosphate, which cannot be further metabolized in the glycolytic pathway and becomes trapped within the cell steadily accumulating in metabolically active cells [2]. This process has enabled accurate metabolic imaging of malignant tumors based on their increased rate of metabolism and glucose utilization as compared to surrounding normal tissues.

Early clinical studies assessed the ability of $[^{18}F]$-FDG-PET to accurately characterize the nature of adrenal masses in patients with cancer and differentiate between benign incidental adrenal lesions and adrenal metastases. Incidentally detected adrenal masses are common, with 2–9% of the general population harboring benign adrenal adenomas detected at autopsy [3]; however, an adrenal mass detected in a patient with cancer has a 27–36% chance of being malignant [4]. Several studies have shown the utility of FDG PET for non-invasive characterization of metastatic adrenal lesions in patients with extra-adrenal malignancies, with focally increased FDG uptake in malignant lesions vs. benign adrenal lesions. In

A.M. Avram (✉)
Division of Nuclear Medicine/Radiology, University of Michigan Health System, University of Michigan, 1500 East Medical Center Drive, Ann Arbor, MI 48105, USA
e-mail: ancaa@umich.edu

G.D. Hammer, T. Else (eds.), *Adrenocortical Carcinoma*,
DOI 10.1007/978-0-387-77236-3_7,

a series of 20 patients, Boland et al. demonstrated a statistically significant difference between mean tumor-to-background ratios for malignant (mean, 7.4; range, 2.9–16.6; median, 6.9) vs. benign (mean, 0.8; range, 0.2–1.2; median, 0.6) adrenal lesions [5]. Similarly, in a group of 94 patients with lung cancer [^{18}F]-FDG-PET demonstrated a sensitivity, specificity, and accuracy for detecting metastatic disease of 93%, 90%, and 92%, respectively; however, false-negative results were encountered with adrenal metastases with large necrotic core, with central hemorrhaging, and in small, <11 mm metastatic lesions [6]. FDG-PET was most useful for the characterization of adrenal lesions that were considered indeterminate on anatomic imaging with CT in a group of 92 patients with non-ACC, and qualitative visual evaluation (adrenal uptake exceeding liver uptake) being considered as accurate as quantitative evaluation with standardized uptake value (SUV). PET was 93% sensitive and 96% specific for metastases; a SUV(max) of 3.4 providing 95% sensitivity and 86% specificity [7]. PET/CT proved superior to PET alone in differentiating benign from malignant adrenal lesions in cancer patients, demonstrating sensitivity, specificity, positive predictive value (PPV), and negative predictive value (NPV) of 100%, 98%, 97%, and 100% respectively; when a cut-off SUV of 3.1 was used [^{18}F]-FDG-PET/CT correctly classified all lesions [8]. Algorithms for pre-operative evaluation of adrenal lesions based on anatomic (CT, MRI) and functional imaging (PET/CT) were developed in patients with lung cancer [9, 10]: while a mean CT attenuation of less than 10 Hounsfield units (HU) in an adrenal nodule is highly specific for benign lesions [11], adrenal lesions with mean CT attenuation greater than 10 HU are considered indeterminate and require evaluation with PET/CT or MRI; for adrenal lesions that remain indeterminate after performing these imaging studies, further histopathologic confirmation is required [9].

Assessing the adrenal lesion–liver activity ratio has been proven a useful method for the detection of malignant adrenal lesions which exhibit a high ratio (mean 4, range 1.53–17.08) in contrast to benign adrenal lesions that display activity less than that of the liver (mean ratio 0.66, range 0.22–0.94) [12]. An SUV ratio (adrenal nodule SUV_{max}/liver SUV_{avg}) cut-off of greater than 2.5 has been proposed for definitive identification of adrenal metastases with a specificity of 100%, sensitivity of 59.5%, and accuracy of 84.2% [10].

Benign adrenal lesions with moderate to high FDG uptake leading to false-positive PET results have been reported in several studies [12–15]. It is not fully understood why some benign adrenal nodules demonstrate increased FDG uptake, but the functional status of the nodule is presumed to be a factor, with increased uptake in functioning adenomas [14]. In addition, pheochromocytomas have been reported to show increased FDG uptake on PET [16, 17]. Shulkin et al. demonstrated that most pheochromocytomas, either benign or malignant, are metabolically active, although focal FDG uptake is found in greater percentage of malignant than in benign pheochromocytomas [18]. Other benign adrenal lesions reported to demonstrate increased FDG uptake are adrenal nodular cortical hyperplasia, adrenal endothelial cysts, and inflammatory/infectious adrenal lesions [19]. In a series by Caoili et al., 5 of 47 adrenal adenomas (10%) demonstrated FDG activity greater than liver [20], and in a study of 112 adrenal nodules Vikram et al. found that

12 of 82 (15%) benign adrenal nodules were considered PET-positive (false-positive PET results), demonstrating focal FDG activity greater than liver (adrenal/liver SUV ratio of 1.32) [21]. Moreover, the coexistence of an adrenal adenoma and a metastasis resulting in a collision adrenal tumor has been reported, leading to apparently increased FDG activity in a benign lesion; careful co-registration of PET and CT data and meticulous analysis of anatomic details on CT are essential for accurate diagnosis of two different pathologic processes within the adrenal gland [22].

Malignant adrenal lesions that may produce false-negative PET results have been reported in patients with adrenal metastases secondary to pulmonary carcinoid [7] and bronchioloalveolar lung carcinoma [19]. Hemorrhage and necrosis within a metastatic adrenal lesion and small metastatic lesions ($\leq$10 mm) have been shown to be other common causes of false-negative PET results [6–8, 19].

PET-CT image analysis using a combination of CT densitometry information (unenhanced adrenal attenuation > 10 HU for malignant lesions) and PET data (qualitative signal intensity greater than the liver for malignant lesions) resulted in improved characterization of adrenal masses in patients with cancer: (sensitivity of 100%, specificity of 99%, positive predictive value (PPV) of 93%, negative predictive value (NPV) of 100%, and an accuracy of 99% for the detection of malignancy). Conversely, for the detection of benignity, the sensitivity, specificity, PPV, NPV, and accuracy were 99%, 100%, 100%, 93%, and 99%, respectively [23].

Adrenal masses discovered in patients without a history of malignancy pose a particular diagnostic challenge, and differentiation between a benign process vs. a malignant lesion is fundamental for the patient's clinical management. The prevalence of incidentally discovered adrenal masses on CT examinations has been reported to be 0.35–5.0% [24, 25]. Biochemical testing of secretory function (screening for mineralocorticoid, glucocorticoid, and catecholamine secretion) is necessary to distinguish between functional vs. nonfunctional adrenal masses, and dedicated anatomic and metabolic imaging are required to differentiate between benign and malignant adrenal lesions. In a series of 105 patients with incidental adrenal masses, 49 lesions were characterized as primary adrenal tumors, of which 8 were malignant lesions (3 ACCs (ACC) and 5 neuroblastomas) and 41 were benign lesions: 34 benign tumors were PET negative, and 7 benign tumors were PET positive. Functional benign adrenal nodules demonstrated variable FDG activity, with 2 of 4 (50%) aldosterone-secreting adenomas, and 2 of 3 (66%) of pheochromocytomas being PET positive. Of malignant primary adrenal tumors, the 3 ACCs demonstrated large (8–13 cm) heterogenous masses on CT and high FDG uptake, while 3 of 5 (60%) neuroblastomas demonstrated focal FDG uptake [26]. Tessonier et al. prospectively assessed with PET/CT 37 patients with 41 adrenal masses incidentally discovered and considered indeterminate on cross-sectional anatomic imaging and without biochemical evidence of hormonal hypersecretion: of 29 benign lesions, 4 (14%) nodules demonstrated elevated FDG uptake (false-positive findings); of 12 malignant lesions included in this group, there were 3 ACCs and 9 adrenal metastases (secondary to lung neoplasm, lymphoma, poorly differentiated carcinoma of unknown origin), and all demonstrated focally increased FDG activity (there were no false-negative results); the authors concluded that a negative

FDG PET-CT appears to be a valid predictor of benign behavior, and that visual qualitative interpretation (adrenal lesion activity > liver activity) was more accurate than SUV_{max} alone, resulting in a sensitivity of 100%, a specificity of 86%, and a negative predictive value of 100% [27].

ACC has been consistently demonstrated to display high metabolic activity on [^{18}F]-FDG PET imaging [26–29]. Due to the poor prognosis of ACC, marked by high incidence of disseminated disease (in 50% of patients) at presentation [30], and the high rate of recurrence after initial complete resection (73–86% at 2 years) [31–34], the patients undergo extensive and serial imaging evaluation for staging and re-staging of disease (Fig. 7.1) [35].

Thorax–abdomen–pelvis CT, abdominal MR, and bone scans are routinely used, and accumulating clinical evidence demonstrates that [^{18}F]-FDG PET and PET/CT play an important role in the initial staging and subsequent follow-up for ACC.

Becherer et al. reported an initial series of ten ACC patients studied with FDG-PET (two patients at primary staging and eight patients during follow-up) and showed that all known sites of ACC demonstrated markedly increased FDG uptake; in addition, PET identified pulmonary, abdominal, and multiple skeletal lesions not seen on conventional CT imaging (sensitivity and specificity for PET were 100% and 95%, respectively; for CT were 89% and 100%, respectively). This study also demonstrated that mitotane treatment did not influence FDG uptake in the tumors in a negative manner, as all eight patients undergoing follow-up imaging received the drug and no false-negative results were observed [36].

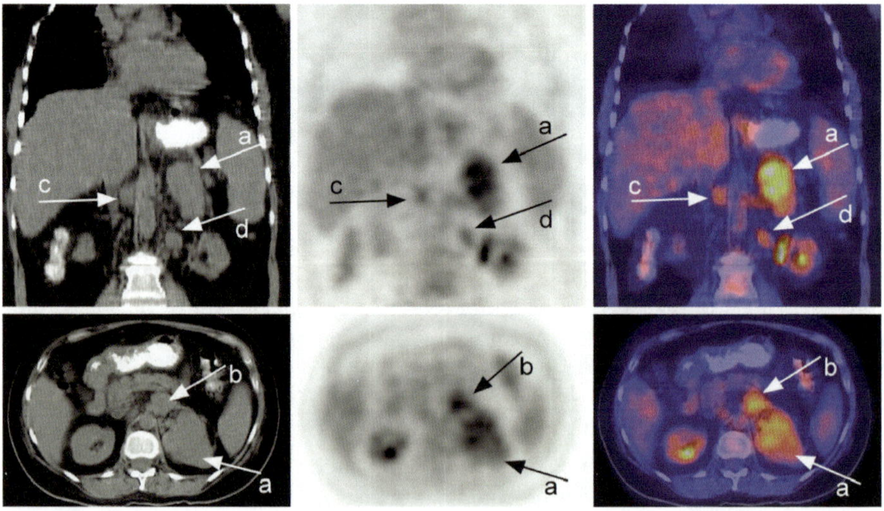

Fig. 7.1 A 51-year-old woman presenting with Cushing's syndrome and large, multilobulated left adrenal mass. Staging [^{18}F]-FDG-PET-CT scan reveals intense and heterogenous FDG activity in 8.2 cm left adrenal mass (**a**) consistent with ACC and retroperitoneal metastatic lymphadenopathy in one aortocaval (**c**) and two left para-aortic lymph nodes (**b**, **d**) (Reprinted with permission from [35])

In a series of 28 consecutive patients with ACC (19 patients with known metastatic disease and 9 patients considered in complete remission; 269 lesions were evaluated), Leboulleaux et al. demonstrated superior diagnostic performance for PET-CT as compared to CT: the sensitivity for the detection of distinct lesions was 90% for PET/CT, and 88% for CT; the sensitivity for the diagnosis of a metastatic organ was 93% for PET/CT, and 82% for CT; 38% of the local relapses were seen only with PET/CT; however, PET/CT depicted three false-positive lesions (axillary lymph node, thyroid, and pancreas). PET/CT is complementary to CT surveillance with 12% percent of the lesions seen on PET/CT only and 10% on CT only. 18% of the metastatic organs were diagnosed with PET/CT only, and 7% with CT only. Morphologic and histopathologic correlation showed that tumor size and mitotic rate were significantly associated with FDG uptake. The intensity of FDG uptake (maximum standardized uptake value >10) and the volume of FDG uptake (>150 ml) were significant prognostic factors for survival [37].

Similarly, in a series of 12 patients studied with FDG PET/CT for the evaluation of locally recurrent and metastatic ACC, Mackie et al. demonstrated that most ACC lesions accumulate and retain FDG and thus can be visualized by PET; however, false-negative results are encountered, especially with small metastatic lesions [38].

A recently published series of 77 patients who underwent surgical resection of incidentally discovered adrenal lesions, comprised 22 ACCs, 43 adrenocortical adenomas and 12 non-adrenocortical lesions, demonstrated that using an adrenal/liver SUV_{max} ratio of 1.45, FDG PET differentiated ACC from benign adrenal adenomas with a sensitivity of 100% and specificity of 88% [39]. FDG PET has been used for staging and restaging of ACC in children, consistently demonstrating focal metabolic activity in primary and metastatic lesions [40, 41].

Based on the current clinical evidence [^{18}F]-FDG-PET and PET/CT have become, in conjunction with classic anatomic cross-sectional imaging, an essential imaging modality for the initial evaluation and follow-up evaluation of patients with ACC.

7.2 Molecular Imaging with Specific Adrenocortical Tracers

Patients that harbor an adrenal mass which cannot be adequately characterized by conventional imaging like CT or MRI may be further evaluated by functional imaging modalities, based on physiological or pathophysiological processes (Fig. 7.2). Imaging modalities include planar scintigraphy or single photon emission computed tomography (SPECT) and positron emission tomography (PET). PET imaging has a higher spatial resolution than SPECT. Whereas [^{18}F]-FDG has been demonstrated to be of great value for establishing malignancy of adrenal lesions and for the detection of metastatic lesions also in ACC, the physiological principal of tracer accumulation is too universal to allow tissue-specific imaging and further differential diagnosis of adrenal tumors. For more tissue-specific imaging and with the aim to also depict target tissue endocrine function,

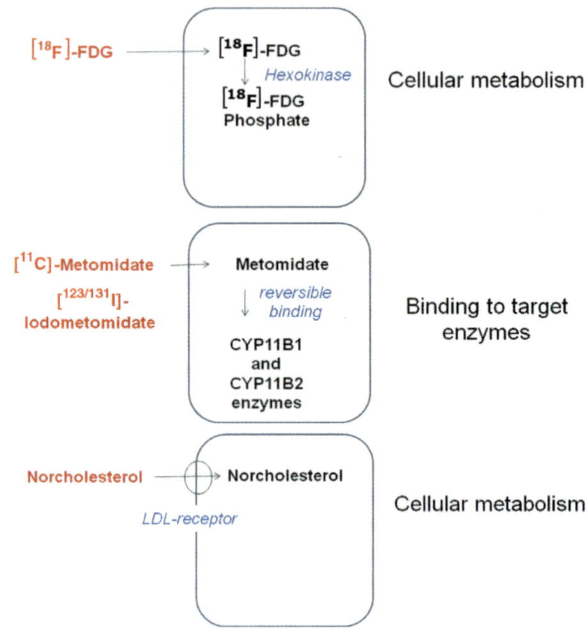

Fig. 7.2 Mechanisms of tissue specific radiotracer accumulation

radiolabeled norcholesterol derivatives have been used for about 40 years for noninvasive imaging of the adrenal glands. Recently, radiotracers using enzyme binding for specific targeting have been introduced in clinical practice as an alternative principle.

7.2.1 Norcholesterol Scintigraphy

The most extensive experience with functional scintigraphic imaging exists with radiocholesterol imaging, which has been available since the early 1970s [42–45]. Radiocholesterol analogues are incorporated into serum LDL particles and accumulated by adrenocortical cells mainly via the LDL receptor under the control of adrenocorticotropic hormone (ACTH) or renin, respectively [46, 47]. High lipoprotein levels and several drugs (e.g., oral contraceptives, mitotane, cholesterol-lowering agents, or glucocorticoids) may interfere with tracer uptake [46–49]. The tracer is esterified within the cell. Further metabolization is negligible [50, 51]. Radiocholesterol underlies an enterohepatic circulation which sometimes increases background activity in the colon [52, 53]. Due to biliary excretion, activity in the gall bladder and the colon is often seen which might interfere with visualization of the adrenals [54]. The initially developed [^{131}I]-19-iodo-cholesterol [43] was followed by [^{131}I]-6β-iodomethyl-norcholesterol (NP-59) or [^{75}Se]-6β-selenomethyl-19-norcholesterol (Scintadren®) that showed slightly higher uptake in the adrenal cortex and improved target to background ratios [45]. Usually, 20–40 MBq of NP-59 or alternatively 7.5–15 MBq of Scintadren is used in adults [55]. Image acquisition is performed over up to 7 days (14 days with Scintadren) after tracer injection, with first images usually obtained after 3 days.

Norcholesterol scintigraphy has been proven useful for localization, differentiation, and lateralization of adrenocortical adenomas [56–61]. An uptake differing more than 50% between the adrenals is considered abnormal, suggesting a unilateral adrenal tumor or hyperplasia. [56–62, 63] A concordant pattern of tracer uptake indicates benign adrenal adenoma or unilateral hyperplasia whereas a discordant pattern hints to nonadrenocortical lesions or ACC [53, 64–66]. In primary hyperaldosteronism, baseline CT or MRI imaging has poor sensitivity due to the mostly small tumors. Tracer uptake in nonsuppressed normal tissue of fasciculata and reticularis cells further hinders differential diagnosis in non-pretreated patients. Systemic dexamethasone suppression reduces ACTH-induced radiocholesterol uptake, which is therefore used to suppress unspecific tracer uptake in the evaluation of primary hyperaldosteronism. [67–70] Radiocholesterol uptake correlates with endocrine activity. The level of radiocholesterol accumulation in adrenocortical tissue is an indicator of the magnitude of hormonal dysfunction [62, 71–76], and has been shown to have relevance for the estimation of later occurrence of adrenal hyperfunction in asymptomatic adrenal incidentalomas [77]. Norcholesterol scintigraphy identifies adrenal adenomas with a sensitivity of 60–100%, depending on the size of tumors investigated, and specificity of 71–100%. [74, 78–81] The adenoma-to-contralateral gland ratio was significantly higher in cortisol releasing than in aldosterone-releasing adenomas [78]. NP-59 has been used to differentiate malignant from benign adrenal lesions, as most malignant tumors exhibit no uptake of NP-59 [82]. Bilateral nonvisualization is suggestive of an ACC as many ACCs secrete glucocorticoids, which suppress uptake in the normal adrenocortical tissue and furthermore do not exhibit tracer uptake sufficient for visualization of the tumor. However, uptake of radiocholesterol into ACC has been studied in only a small number of cases, and in some cases of ACC NP-59 or Scintadren uptake has also been observed in the tumor and also in its metastases, reducing its specificity. [83–95] It was first believed that both the degree of functional abnormality and the cellular differentiation are relevant factors in the scintigraphic imaging of ACCs; however, further studies demonstrated uptake also in undifferentiated ACC [85]. Twenty-one patients with ACC (11 nonfunctioning and 10 hormone-secreting) were investigated with Scintadren scintigraphy by Barzon et al. [85]. In 18 cases no radiocholesterol uptake was found in the adrenal masses (11 nonfunctioning and 7 functioning lesions). Three patients with cortisol-producing carcinomas showed radiotracer uptake by the mass. All three tumors were shown to be undifferentiated ACCs exhibiting an aggressive clinical behavior.

Norcholesterol scintigraphy has proven to be useful for adrenal imaging; however, the method is hampered by several factors. An interval of at least 3–7 days is required from tracer injection to image acquisition, making the method inconvenient for both patient and investigator. Due to the very slow metabolization of the radiopharmacon, the tracer needs to be labeled with a longer lived radionuclide like [^{131}I] or [^{75}Se]. Patients are therefore exposed to very high effective doses (NP-59 30 mSv, Scintadren 17 mSv). Therefore, the use of this radiotracer has been increasingly restricted during recent years and production has been stopped in many countries.

Cholesteryl-*p*-[^{18}F]-fluorobenzoate ([^{18}F]-CFB) has been investigated as a cholesterol derivative for adrenal positron emission tomography (PET) imaging. Normal baboon PET imaging with [^{18}F]-CFB showed adrenal localization at 15 min after injection of the tracer, with enhanced adrenal contrast seen at 60–70 min. Clinical data in humans are, however, so far missing [96].

7.2.2 Enzyme Inhibitors

In the light of the disadvantages of radioiodinated norcholesterol tracers, research aimed at the development of new radionuclides with an improved time frame for imaging and decreased radiation dose. First investigations evaluating inhibitors of adrenocortical steroidogenic enzymes date back to the 1970s where metyrapol and its analog [^{131}I]-SKF-12185 were shown to specifically accumulate in adrenocortical tissue [97]. Further adrenostatic agents like aminoglutethimide and other analogs labeled with [^{125}I] or [^{3}H] have been tested and showed comparable uptake in the adrenals compared to radiocholesterol with faster kinetics, but until recently, none of these enzyme inhibitors was further developed for clinical application. [53, 98, 99] The structural properties that are relevant for binding of the recently developed imidazole derivatives to the CYP11B-enzymes have been further clarified. IC50 values obtained by the displacement of specific [^{131}I]-IMTO binding or by enzyme inhibition studies demonstrated that (*R*)-configuration of the methylbenzyl-group and the substituted imidazole ring are essential for enzyme binding of metomidate/etomidate analogs. Structural changes can be carried out at the phenyl ring and the carbonic acid ester without loss of affinity [98]. Also halogenation of the phenyl ring may offer further versatility for labeling with SPECT and PET radionuclides (i.e., ^{123}I, ^{124}I, ^{76}Br, ^{18}F) [98].

7.2.3 Metomidate

Metomidate (MTO), the methyl-ester of etomidate, is in clinical use for about 40 years as an anesthetic drug in different animal species in veterinary medicine. [100–105] The anesthetic properties are mediated via agonism at $GABA_A$ receptors. [106, 107] Both etomidate and metomidate belong to the most potent inhibitors of the two CYP11B enzymes, 11β-hydroxylase (CYP11B1, $P450_{11\beta}$) and aldosterone synthase (CYP11B2, $P450_{aldo}$) that catalyze the last step of cortisol and aldosterone formation, respectively. [108–110] Both enzymes are located at the inner mitochondrial membrane in adrenocortical cells [111]. Etomidate and metomidate also appear to bind to CYP11A1 (P450side chain cleavage) but with far lower binding affinity. [109, 110] Due to its adrenostatic potency, etomidate has also been used for the correction of severe hypercortisolemia. [112–114]

The expression of the target *CYP11B1* and *CYP11B2* is significant in benign and >95% of ACCs and also in its metastases, suggesting that metomidate and analogs are highly suitable to detect both adrenocortical tumors and adrenocortical metastatic lesions [110, 115] (Hahner et al. unpublished data). In preclinical studies [^{11}C]-etomidate ((*R*)-[*O*-ethyl-1-^{11}C]-etomidate) and [^{11}C]-metomidate ((*R*)-[*O*-methyl-^{11}C]-metomidate) showed very high binding to adrenocortical tissue using frozen section autoradiography of different tissues from rat, pig, and humans [116]. The binding in the adrenal tissue samples correlated with immunostaining for CYP11B1. In addition, in vitro studies using metomidate and different analogs demonstrated high correlation of binding to rat adrenal membranes in displacement experiments with inhibition of cortisol synthesis [98]. (*R*)-configuration appears to be essential for high-affinity binding of metomidate and analogs. In vivo, both [^{11}C]-etomidate and [^{11}C]-metomidate demonstrated high uptake in the adrenal in PET studies in monkeys. Due to its more favorable synthetic characteristics, [^{11}C]-metomidate was selected for further use in clinical studies [116] and preparation methods have been optimized in the meantime resulting in better purification yields [115]. In the first published clinical evaluation of [^{11}C]-metomidate, 15 patients with an adrenal incidentaloma received between 294 and 938 MBq [^{11}C]-metomidate and imaging studies were performed over a time frame of about 45 min. [117, 118] A very high tracer uptake was observed in all tumors of adrenocortical origin, whereas all other adrenal lesions were negative in [^{11}C]-metomidate PET. This was confirmed in several consecutive studies. [119–122] In these studies high uptake was also seen in normal adrenal glands and in the stomach. The uptake was intermediate in the liver and low in other abdominal organs.

As metomidate uptake is mediated by binding to the target enzymes CYP11B1 and CYP11B2, tracer uptake is primarily dependent on the presence and abundance of these targets. Detection limit for tumor size was 1 cm. The sensitivity for proving the adrenocortical origin of a lesion was calculated to be 0.89, with a specificity of 0.96 [122]. False-negative results were mainly due to necrotic or very small tumors.

The values for differential diagnosis between the different adrenocortical tumor entities and for estimation of endocrine activity have also been subsequently analyzed. Among the different adrenocortical tumor lesions investigated, high tracer uptake was observed in several aldosterone-producing adenomas and also in several ACCs, but due to a great variation and overlap in SUVs no significant difference could be demonstrated [120–122] (Table 7.1).

Few patients with ACC have so far been investigated with [^{11}C]-metomidate PET in different trials. Due to the rarity of this disease the number of included ACC is limited (Results of clinical trials involving patients with ACC are summarized in Table 7.2). Khan et al. systematically evaluated 11 patients with ACC (4 with primary tumor, 7 with relapse of a previously histopathologically proven ACC) [119]. In this trial 11 of 16 tumor lesions (primary tumor, local recurrences or distant metastases) that were detected by CT could also be visualized by

Table 7.1 Mean [^{11}C]-metomidate SUV in different adrenocortical tumor entities

	NPA mean SUV	APA mean SUV	CPA mean SUV	ACC mean SUV	normal AG mean SUV
Hennings et al. [122]	18.4 n=7	30.7 n=6	20.3 n=4	15.7 n=10	12.5 n=13
Zettinig et al. [121]	24.0 n=5	19.6 n=5	17.6 n=4	14.3 n=1	17.7 n=13
Minn et al. [120]	14.3 n=5	–	15.3 n=7	28.0 n=1	11.3 n=1

[^{11}C]-metomidate PET with high tracer uptake compared to most organs despite stomach and liver. The lesions that could not be detected by [^{11}C]-metomidate revealed to be necrotic in three cases at histopathological examination. In contrast, two additional lesions were only detected by [^{11}C]-metomidate PET but not by CT, demonstrating that [^{11}C]-metomidate PET not only helps to distinguish between tumors of adrenocortical and nonadrenocortical origin but also adds further information regarding metastatic lesions complementary to CT findings. Tumor lesions showed a more rapid and higher tracer uptake compared to normal adrenals, which was also demonstrated in other studies [120]. But also the liver again exhibited a high tracer uptake that was slightly lower than the uptake in the normal adrenals, limiting the value in identifying hepatic metastases. Treatment with mitotane or with adrenostatic agents like ketoconazole or metyrapone that are frequently used in patients with ACC interferes with tracer uptake, which was demonstrated in the study of Khan et al. [119]. Patients under treatment with those agents exhibited significantly lower tracer uptake compared with patients which were free of treatment.

To further confine the value of [^{11}C]-metomidate first comparative studies applying both [^{11}C]-metomidate-PET and of [^{18}F]-FDG-PET in ACC patients have been performed. However, so far no larger scale studies are available. In smaller cohorts [^{11}C]-metomidate clearly distinguished lesions of adrenocortical origin from lesions of nonadrenocortical origin, whereas [^{18}F]-FDG-PET better performed in distinguishing benign from malignant lesions [120, 121]. Thus, other than norcholesterol, metomidate does not help to distinguish between benign and malignant adrenocortical lesions. These results are as expected as metomidate binds to enzymes that are expressed in both benign and most of the malignant adrenocortical tissues, whereas usually high metabolic activity resulting in increased [^{18}F]-FDG uptake is characteristic for malignant tumors.

Taken together, the main significance of metomidate and its analogs consist of their ability to specifically and noninvasively distinguish adrenocortical from non-adrenocortical lesions, which is particularly helpful in patients with nonsecreting adrenal masses and inconclusive CT or MRI findings and in patients with ACC to detect and characterize metastatic lesions [122]. Imaging after tracer injection is performed after 45 min, which better fits to clinical demands compared to the imaging procedures performed over several days with norcholesterol.

Table 7.2 Studies evaluating [^{11}C]-metomidate-PET including patients with ACC

	Total no. of patients	Patients with ACC	Main study outcome
Juhlin 1998 [117]	13	1	High uptake in all tumors originating from the adrenal cortex, whereas all other processes were negative.
Bergström 2000 [118]	15	2	All adrenocortiocal lesions including ACC with high uptake, whereas the noncortical lesions showed very low uptake. High uptake also seen in normal adrenal glands and in the stomach.
Khan 2003 [119]	11	11	High tracer uptake in all viable tumors. Two more lesions revealed than seen on CT. Three necrotic tumors detected as false-negative observations. Metomidate uptake increased in tumor lesions as compared with normal tissues. Medication with adrenal steroid inhibitors (mitotane, ketoconazole, metyrapone) and chemotherapy decreased the tracer uptake.
Minn et al. 2004 [120]	21	1	Highest uptake found in ACC, followed by active adenomas, nonsecretory adenomas, and noncortical tumors. Patients with adenomas had significantly higher tumor-to-normal-adrenal [^{11}C]-metomidate SUV ratios than patients with noncortical tumors.
Zettinig et al. 2004 [121]	16	1	Sixteen patients investigated using both MTO and [^{18}F]-FDG PET imaging. MTO imaging clearly distinguished cortical from noncortical adrenal masses (median standardized uptake values of 18.6 and 1.9, respectively, $p < 0.01$). MTO uptake slightly, but not significantly, lower in patients with Cushing's syndrome than in those with Conn's syndrome. Uptake was not decreased in the contralateral gland of patients with Conn's syndrome, but in patients with Cushing's syndrome. The single patient with ACC had MTO uptake in the lower range. High [^{18}F]-FDG uptake in malignant lesions.
Hennings et al. 2009 [122]	173 (73 with histological examination)	13	Evaluation of 212 MTO-PET examinations in 173 patients. Sensitivity 0.89, specificity 0.96 for MTO-PET in proving adrenocortical origin of the lesions. Nonadrenocortical lesions were MTO negative. Lesions larger than 1 cm could be differentiated from normal adrenocortical tissue. SUV was higher in aldosterone-hypersecreting adenomas, and the SUV ratio between the tumor and the contralateral gland was significantly higher in all hormonally hypersecreting adenomas as well as in ACC.

Limitations of [^{11}C]-metomidate are the short half-life of [^{11}C] of only 20.3 min, restricting the use to centers with an on-site cyclotron. Moreover, the short half-life also limits its use to the early uptake of the tracer potentially missing the optimum target to background ratio. [^{11}C]-metomidate furthermore shows high uptake into the liver, hampering imaging of the right adrenal gland and also of liver metastases.

In an attempt to improve the tracer, halogenated metomidate analogs have been recently developed that exhibit more favorable adrenal to liver uptake ratios and higher tracer stability in vitro compared to metomidate [123]. This will possibly enable image acquisition at later time points with improved target to nontarget uptake ratios, which has to be proven in in vivo studies.

7.2.4 [^{18}F]-Fluoro-etomidate

As ^{18}F exhibits a longer half-life of 109.7 min compared to ^{11}C, ^{18}F labeled etomidate has been evaluated for adrenal imaging purposes with the aim to possess a better available tracer with more favorable pharmacokinetic properties.

Radiosynthesis of (*R*)-1-(1-phenylethyl)-1*H*-imidazole-5-carboxylic-acid-2-[^{18}F]-fluoroethylester (FETO), a close analog to metomidate and etomidate was established [115]. Binding to CYP11B1 and CYP11B2 is comparable with etomidate and metomidate in in vitro experiments [98, 110]. Binding studies on rat cerebral membranes showed some affinity to the gamma-amino butyric acid (GABA) receptor also [115]. In vivo evaluation in rats demonstrated very high uptake in the adrenal glands, followed by lung, liver, and duodenum [115]. First in vivo evaluation in humans was performed in ten healthy volunteers [124]. Pronounced accumulation of [^{18}F]-FETO was observed in the adrenals, whereas moderate uptake was detected in the liver and only faint uptake in the kidney and bowels. [^{18}F]-FETO also proved to be suitable for imaging of adrenal lesions [125]. In 13 consecutive patients with adrenocortical masses (5 functioning, 8 nonfunctioning adrenal tumors), a high uptake in 12 of the 13 adrenal lesions was observed. The FETO negative lesion revealed to be a rhabdomyosarcoma [125]. So far no data of [^{18}F]-FETO-PET in patients with ACC are available.

Different FETO analogs have recently been described, with 2-[^{18}F]-fluoroethyl 1-[(1*R*)-1-(4-chlorophenyl)ethyl]-1*H*-imidazole-5-carboxylate being a promising alternative as assessed in vitro [126]. Like metomidate, FETO also underlies a rapid metabolization in vivo with a short biological half-life. The metabolic profile showed that FETO kinetics in humans is fast but comparable to metomidate. In vitro experiments demonstrated that FETO stability against esterases is comparable to that of ETO and MTO.

7.2.5 [^{123}I/^{131}I]-Iodo-metomidate

Another approach to receive a longer-lived radionuclide with the potential of a better general availability for adrenocortical imaging [^{123}I]-iodometomidate has been developed for single photon emission computed tomography (SPECT) and planar scintigraphy. Half-life of ^{123}I (13.2 h) and the use of SPECT imaging indicate that [^{123}I]-IMTO is suitable for widespread use as a radiotracer for adrenal tissue. Iodometomidate binds to adrenal membranes with high affinity and inhibits cortisol and aldosterone synthesis via binding to the respective CYP11B enzymes in vitro comparable to metomidate or etomidate. [98, 110, 127] Structural requirements for high-affinity binding are an intact ester group and (*R*)-configuration of the radioligand [127]. Pharmacokinetic studies in rats and mice showed fast and highly specific accumulation in the adrenal glands. [110, 127] Compared to [^{11}C]-metomidate, relatively low uptake appeared within the liver.

Clinical evaluation demonstrated high and specific uptake of [^{123}I]-iodometomidate in adrenocortical tumors and also in distant metastases of ACC [110] (Fig. 7.3). Although ETO, FETO, and MTO have been shown to bind to intracerebral $GABA_A$ receptors, there is only weak tracer uptake in the brain, indicating that binding of IMTO to $GABA_A$ receptors plays no significant role in IMTO imaging. Furthermore, the very low tracer uptake in the testes indicates that binding to side-chain cleavage enzyme (CYP11A1) is not sufficient to lead to relevant tracer uptake in the testes. The effective dose in humans was

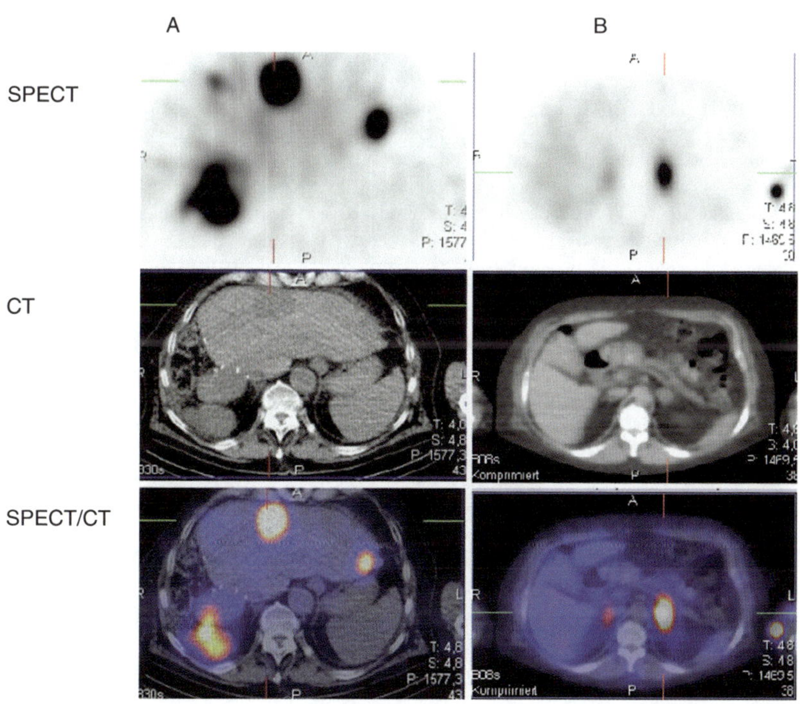

Fig. 7.3 [^{123}I]-Iodometomidate SPECT of a 68-year-old patient with cortisol-producing ACC and liver metastases (**a**) and a 55-year-old patient with nonfunctioning adrenal adenoma at the left side (**b**)

only one tenth compared with norcholesterol scintigraphy [110]. Best visualization of tumor manifestations in humans was observed 4–6 hours after [^{123}I]-IMTO, making IMTO imaging much less time consuming and more convenient than imaging with [^{131}I]-iodomethylnorcholesterol. On the other hand, very low background activity was found after this time and even after 24 h at a time when [^{11}C]-MTO PET imaging is no longer feasible due to the short half-life of C-11 with 20 min. PET imaging has, however, a higher spatial resolution than SPECT, and further studies are needed to define the size of adrenal or metastatic lesions detectable by [^{123}I]-IMTO-SPECT. Similar to [^{11}C]-MTO-PET, [^{123}I]-IMTO-SPECT is unlikely to differentiate benign from malignant adrenocortical lesions.

The use of radioiodine and the very high expression of CYP11B enzymes in some cases of ACC also may hold potential for the treatment of patients with [^{131}I]-IMTO. Preliminary data are available from a small number of patients with ACC so far receiving up to 20 GBq [^{131}I]-iodometomidate. Decrease of tumor lesions could be observed in a substantial percentage of treated patients. Main side effects were transient thrombocytopenia and leucopenia that occurred in most patients. Elimination of [^{131}I]-IMTO from whole body showed a half-life of 20 h. In all patients treatment was well tolerated [128].

References

1. Gillies RJ et al (2008) Causes and consequences of increased glucose metabolism of cancers. J Nucl Med 49(Suppl 2):24S–42S
2. Plathow C, Weber WA (2008) Tumor cell metabolism imaging. J Nucl Med 49 (Suppl 2):43S–63S
3. Hedeland H et al (1968) On the prevalence of adrenocortical adenomas in an autopsy material in relation to hypertension and diabetes. Acta Med Scand 184:211–214
4. Abrams HL et al (1950) Metastases in carcinoma: analysis of 1000 autopsied cases. Cancer 3:74–85
5. Boland GW et al (1995) Indeterminate adrenal mass in patients with cancer: evaluation at PET with 2-[F-18]-fluoro-2-deoxy-D-glucose. Radiology. 194(1):131–134.
6. Kumar R et al (2004) 18F-FDG PET in evaluation of adrenal lesions in patients with lung cancer. J Nucl Med 45(12):2058–2062
7. Jana S et al (2006) FDG-PET and CT characterization of adrenal lesions in cancer patients. Eur J Nucl Med Mol Imaging 33(1):29–35
8. Metser U et al (2006) 18F-FDG PET/CT in the evaluation of adrenal masses. J Nucl Med 47(1):32–37
9. Kim HK et al (2007) Preoperative evaluation of adrenal lesions based on imaging studies and laparoscopic adrenalectomy in patients with otherwise operable lung cancer. Lung Cancer 58(3):342–347
10. Brady MJ et al (2009) Adrenal nodules at FDG PET/CT in patients known to have or suspected of having lung cancer: a proposal for an efficient diagnostic algorithm. Radiology 250(2):523–530
11. Boland GW et al (1998) Characterization of adrenal masses using unenhanced CT: an analysis of the CT literature. AJR Am J Roentgenol 171:201–204
12. Blake MA et al (2006) Adrenal lesions: characterization with fused PET/CT image in patients with proved or suspected malignancy – initial experience. Radiology 238(3): 970–977

13. Han SJ et al (2007) Analysis of adrenal masses by 18F-FDG positron emission tomography scanning. Int J Clin Pract 61(5):802–809
14. Shimizu A et al (2003) High [18F] 2-fluoro-2-deoxy-D-glucose (FDG) uptake of adrenocortical adenoma showing subclinical Cushing's syndrome. Ann Nucl Med 17(5): 403–406
15. Rao SK et al (2004) F-18 fluorodeoxyglucose positron emission tomography-positive benign adrenal cortical adenoma: imaging features and pathologic correlation. Clin Nucl Med 29(5):300–302
16. Yun M et al (2001) 18F-FDG PET in characterizing adrenal lesions detected on CT or MRI. J Nucl Med 42(12):1795–1799
17. Maurea S et al (1999) Imaging of adrenal tumors using FDG PET: comparison of benign and malignant lesions. AJR Am J Roentgenol.173(1):25–29
18. Shulkin BL et al (1999) Pheochromocytomas: imaging with 2-[fluorine-18]fluoro-2-deoxy-D-glucose PET. Radiology. 212:35–41
19. Chong S et al (2006) Integrated PET-CT for the characterization of adrenal gland lesions in cancer patients: diagnostic efficacy and interpretation pitfalls. Radiographics 26(6):1811–1824; discussion 1824–1826
20. Caoili EM et al (2007) Differentiating adrenal adenomas from nonadenomas using (18)F-FDG PET/CT: quantitative and qualitative evaluation. Acad Radiol 14(4):468–475
21. Vikram R et al (2008) Utility of PET/CT in differentiating benign from malignant adrenal nodules in patients with cancer. AJR Am J Roentgenol 191(5):1545–1551
22. Blake MA et al (2004) Collision adrenal tumors on PET/CT. AJR Am J Roentgenol 183(3):864–865
23. Boland GW et al (2009) PET/CT for the characterization of adrenal masses in patients with cancer: qualitative versus quantitative accuracy in 150 consecutive patients. AJR Am J Roentgenol 192(4):956–962
24. Cook DM, Loriaux LD (1996) The incidental adrenal mass. Am J Med 101:88–94
25. Herrera MF et al (1991) Incidentally discovered adrenal tumors: an institutional perspective. Surgery 110:1014–1021
26. Han SJ et al (2007) Analysis of adrenal masses by 18F-FDG positron emission tomography scanning. Int J Clin Pract 61(5):802–809
27. Tessonnier L et al (2008) Does 18FFDG PET/CT add diagnostic accuracy in incidentally identified non-secreting adrenal tumours? Eur J Nucl Med Mol Imaging 35(11):2018–2025
28. Tenenbaum F et al (2004) 18F-fluorodeoxyglucose Adrenocortical tumours? Preliminary results in 13 consecutive patients. Eur J Endocrinol 150:789–792
29. Zettinig G et al (2004) Positron emission tomography imaging of adrenal masses: (18)F-fluorodeoxyglucose and the 11_-hydroxylase tracer (11)C-metomidate. Eur J Nucl Med Mol Imaging 31:1224–1230
30. Luton JP et al (1990) Clinical features of ACC, prognostic factors, and the effect of mitotane therapy. N Engl J Med 322:1195
31. Icard P et al (2001) ACCs: surgical trends and results of a 253-patient series from the French Association of Endocrine Surgeons Study Group. World J Surg 25:891–897
32. Kendrick ML et al (2001) ACC: surgical progress or status quo? Arch Surg 136:543–549
33. Schulick RD, Brennan MF (1999) Long-term survival after complete resection and repeat resection in patients with ACC. Ann Surg Oncol 6:719–726
34. Weiss LM et al (1989) Pathologic features of prognostic significance in ACC. Am J Surg Pathol 13:202–206
35. Gross MD et al (2007) PET in the diagnostic evaluation of adrenal tumors. Q J Nucl Med Mol Imaging 51:272–283
36. Becherer A et al (2001) FDG-PET in ACC. Cancer Biother Radiopharm 16(4): 289–295
37. Leboulleux S et al (2006) Diagnostic and prognostic value of 18-fluorodeoxyglucose positron emission tomography in ACC: a prospective comparison with computed tomography. J Clin Endocrinol Metab 91(3):920–925

38. Mackie GC et al (2006) Use of [18F]fluorodeoxyglucose positron emission tomography in evaluating locally recurrent and metastatic ACC. J Clin Endocrinol Metab 91(7):2665–2671. Epub 2006 Apr 18. PubMed PMID: 16621901
39. Groussin L et al (2009) 18F-Fluorodeoxyglucose positron emission tomography for the diagnosis of Adrenocortical tumors: a prospective study in 77 operated patients. J Clin Endocrinol Metab 94(5):1713–1722
40. Kreissig R et al (2000) The use of FDG-PET and CT for the staging of ACC in children. Pediatr Radiol 30(5):306
41. Binkovitz I et al (2008) Early detection of recurrent pediatric adrenal cortical carcinoma using FDG-PET. Clin Nucl Med 33(3):186–188
42. Lieberman LM et al (1971) Diagnosis of adrenal disease by visualization of human adrenal glands with 131 I-19-iodocholesterol. N Engl J Med 285:1387–1393
43. Beierwaltes WH et al (1971) Visualization of human adrenal glands in vivo by scintillation scanning. JAMA 216:275–277
44. Sarkar SD et al (1975) A new and superior adrenal scanning agent, NP-59. J Nucl Med 16:1038–1042
45. Sarkar SD et al (1977) A new and superior adrenal imaging agent, 131I-6beta-iodomethyl-19-nor-cholesterol (NP-59): evaluation in humans. J Clin Endocrinol Metab 45:353–362
46. Rizza RA et al (1978) Visualization of nonfunctioning adrenal adenomas with iodocholesterol: possible relationship to subcellular distribution of tracer. J Nucl Med 19:458–463
47. Gross MD et al (1981) The role of pharmacologic manipulation in adrenal cortical scintigraphy. Semin Nucl Med 11:128–148
48. Gordon L et al (1980) Failure to visualize adrenal glands in a patient with bilateral adrenal hyperplasia. J Nucl Med 21:49–51
49. Lynn MD et al (1986) The influence of hypercholesterolaemia on the adrenal uptake and metabolic handling of 131I-6 beta-iodomethyl-19-norcholesterol (NP-59). Nucl Med Commun 7:631–637
50. Counsell RE et al (1980) Tissue distribution of high-density lipoprotein labeled with radioiodinated cholesterol. J Nucl Med 21:852–858
51. Nordblom GD et al (1980) A comparison of cholesteryl oleate and 19-iodocholesteryl oleate as substrates for adrenal cholesterol esterase. J Steroid Biochem 13:463–466
52. Lynn MD et al (1986) Enterohepatic circulation and distribution of 131I-6 beta-iodomethyl-19-norcholesterol (NP-59). Nucl Med Commun 7:625–630
53. Rubello D et al (2002) Functional scintigraphy of the adrenal gland. Eur J Endocrinol 147:13–28
54. Shapiro B et al (1983) Value of bowel preparation in adrenocortical scintigraphy with NP-59. J Nucl Med 24:732–734
55. Kampen WU (2003) Significance of 131I-Norvholesterol Scintigraphy for Diagnosis of Adrenal Dysfunction. Der Nuklearmediziner 26:21–24
56. Gross MD et al (1984) Scintigraphic localization of adrenal lesions in primary aldosteronism. Am J Med 77:839–844
57. Yen RF et al (2009) 131I-6beta-iodomethyl-19-norcholesterol SPECT/CT for primary aldosteronism patients with inconclusive adrenal venous sampling and CT results. J Nucl Med 50:1631–1637
58. Avram AM et al (2006) Adrenal gland scintigraphy. Semin Nucl Med 36:212–227
59. Gross MD et al (1987) Functional and scintigraphic evaluation of the silent adrenal mass. J Nucl Med 28:1401–1407
60. Kazerooni EA et al (1990) Diagnostic accuracy and pitfalls of [iodine-131]6-beta-iodomethyl-19-norcholesterol (NP-59) imaging. J Nucl Med 31:526–534
61. Maurea S et al (2001) The diagnostic role of radionuclide imaging in evaluation of patients with nonhypersecreting adrenal masses. J Nucl Med 42:884–892

62. Gross MD et al (1984) The relationship of I-131 6 beta-iodomethyl-619-norcholesterol (NP-59) adrenal cortical uptake to indices of androgen secretion in women with hyperandrogenism. Clin Nucl Med 9:264–270
63. Gross MD et al (1999) Radionuclide imaging of the adrenal cortex. Q J Nucl Med 43: 224–232
64. Kloos RT et al (1995) Incidentally discovered adrenal masses. Endocr Rev 16:460–484
65. Thompson GB, Young WF Jr. (2003) Adrenal incidentaloma. Curr Opin Oncol 15:84–90
66. Kloos RT et al (1997) Diagnostic dilemma of small incidentally discovered adrenal masses: role for 131I-6beta-iodomethyl-norcholesterol scintigraphy. World J Surg 21:36–40
67. Rifai A et al (1978) Adrenal scintigraphy in low renin essential hypertension. Clin Nucl Med 3:282–286
68. Chen YC et al (2009) Seeking the invisible: I-131 NP-59 SPECT/CT for primary hyperaldosteronism. Kidney Int 75:663
69. Volpe C et al (2008) The role of adrenal scintigraphy in the preoperative management of primary aldosteronism. Scand J Surg 97:248–253
70. Simon DR. Palese MA (2008) Noninvasive adrenal imaging in hyperaldosteronism. Curr Urol Rep 9:80–87
71. Moses DC et al (1974) Efficacy of radiocholesterol imaging of the adrenal glands in Cushing's syndrome. Surg Gynecol Obstet 139:201–204
72. Gross MD et al (1983) The relationship of adrenal gland iodomethylnorcholesterol uptake to zona glomerulosa function in primary aldosteronism. J Clin Endocrinol Metab 57:477–481
73. Barzon L et al (1998) Incidentally discovered adrenal tumors: endocrine and scintigraphic correlates. J Clin Endocrinol Metab 83:55–62
74. La Cava G et al (2003) SPECT semiquantitative analysis of adrenocortical (131)I-6 beta iodomethyl-norcholesterol uptake to discriminate subclinical and preclinical functioning adrenal incidentaloma. J Nucl Med 44:1057–1064
75. Donadio F et al (2009) Role of adrenal gland scintigraphy in patients with subclinical hypercortisolism and incidentally discovered adrenal mass. J Endocrinol Invest 32:576–580
76. Barzon L et al (2001) Overnight dexamethasone suppression of cortisol is associated with radiocholesterol uptake patterns in adrenal incidentalomas. Eur J Endocrinol 145:223–224
77. Barzon L et al (1999) Risk factors and long-term follow-up of adrenal incidentalomas. J Clin Endocrinol Metab 84:520–526
78. Yoh T et al (2008) Quantitative evaluation of norcholesterol scintigraphy, CT attenuation value, and chemical-shift MR imaging for characterizing adrenal adenomas. Ann Nucl Med 22:513–519
79. Maurea S et al (2002) Diagnostic accuracy of radionuclide imaging using 131I nor-cholesterol or meta-iodobenzylguanidine in patients with hypersecreting or non-hypersecreting adrenal tumours. Nucl Med Commun 23:951–960
80. Lumachi F et al (2003) Non-invasive adrenal imaging in primary aldosteronism. Sensitivity and positive predictive value of radiocholesterol scintigraphy, CT scan and MRI. Nucl Med Commun 24:683–688
81. Lumachi F et al (2002) Usefulness of CT scan, MRI and radiocholesterol scintigraphy for adrenal imaging in Cushing's syndrome. Nucl Med Commun 23:469–473
82. Maurea S et al (2004) Imaging characterization of non-hypersecreting adrenal masses. Comparison between MR and radionuclide techniques. Q J Nucl Med Mol Imaging 48:188–197
83. Reschini E et al (1984) Uptake of 75Se-selenomethylcholesterol by a nonfunctioning adrenocortical adenoma. J Nucl Med Allied Sci 28:221–224
84. Fig LM et al (1988) Adrenal localization in the adrenocorticotropic hormone-independent Cushing syndrome. Ann Intern Med 109:547–553
85. Barzon L et al (2001) Scintigraphic patterns of ACC: morpho-functional correlates. Eur J Endocrinol 145:743–748
86. Schteingart DE et al (1981) Iodocholesterol adrenal tissue uptake and imaging adrenal neoplasms. J Clin Endocrinol Metab 52:1156–1161

87. Drane WE et al (1983) Imaging of an adrenal cortical carcinoma and its skeletal metastasis. J Nucl Med 24:710–712
88. Chatal JF et al (1976) Uptake of 131I-19-iodocholesterol by an adrenal cortical carcinoma and its metastases. J Clin Endocrinol Metab 43:248–251
89. Pasieka JL et al (1992) Adrenal scintigraphy of well-differentiated (functioning) ACCs: potential surgical pitfalls. Surgery 112:884–890
90. Greathouse DJ et al (1984) Pure primary hyperaldosteronism due to adrenal cortical carcinoma. Am J Med 76:1132–1136
91. Sakashita S et al (1984) Primary aldosteronism due to adrenal cortical carcinoma. J Urol 132:959–961
92. Shenker Y et al (1986) The scintigraphic localization of mineralocorticoid-producing ACC. J Endocrinol Invest 9:115–120
93. Scott HW Jr. et al (1986) Primary hyperaldosteronism caused by ACC. World J Surg 10: 646–653
94. Bossuyt A, Somers G (1975) 131I-19-iodocholesterol visualization of an ACC without clinical manifestations. J Nucl Biol Med 19:225–227
95. Wang FF et al (2006) Unusual visualization of an ACC on NP-59 scintiscan. J Formos Med Assoc 105:340–345
96. Jonson SD, Welch MJ (1999) Synthesis, biological evaluation, and baboon PET imaging of the potential adrenal imaging agent cholesteryl-p-[18F]fluorobenzoate. Nucl Med Biol 26:131–138
97. Beierwaltes WH et al (1978) Imaging the adrenal glands with radiolabeled inhibitors of enzymes: concise communication. J Nucl Med 19:200–203
98. Zolle IM et al (2008) New selective inhibitors of steroid 11beta-hydroxylation in the adrenal cortex. Synthesis and structure-activity relationship of potent etomidate analogues. J Med Chem 51:2244–2253
99. Beierwaltes WH et al (1976) Localization of radiolabeled enzyme inhibitors in the adrenal gland. J Nucl Med 17:998–1002
100. Hillidge CJ et al (1973) Investigations of azaperone-metomidate anaesthesia in the horse. Vet Rec 93:307–311
101. Ryder-Davies P (1973) The use of Metomidate, and intramuscular narcotic for birds. Vet Rec 92:507–509
102. Biver A et al (1976) Combined azaperone and metomidate anaesthesia in liver transplantation in the pig. Eur Surg Res 8:81–88
103. Cadle DR, Martin GR (1976) Metomidate as sole anaesthetic agent in tawny owls. Vet Rec 98:91–92
104. Green CJ et al (1981) Metomidate etomidate and fentanyl as injectable anaesthetic agents in mice. Lab Anim 15:171–175
105. Hansen MK et al (2003) Pharmacokinetic and pharmacodynamic properties of metomidate in turbot (*Scophthalmus maximus*) and halibut (*Hippoglossus hippoglossus*). J Vet Pharmacol Ther 26:95–103
106. Atucha E et al (2009) Structure-activity relationship of etomidate derivatives at the GABA(A) receptor: Comparison with binding to 11beta-hydroxylase. Bioorg Med Chem Lett 19:4284–4287
107. Evans RH, Hill RG (1977) The GABA-mimetic action of etomidate [proceedings]. Br J Pharmacol 61:484P
108. Weber MM et al (1993) Different inhibitory effect of etomidate and ketoconazole on the human adrenal steroid biosynthesis. Clin Investig 71:933–938
109. Fassnacht M (2000) New mechanisms of adrenostatic compounds in a human adrenocortical cancer cell line. Eur J Clin Invest 30(Suppl 3):76–82
110. Hahner S et al (2008) [123 I]Iodometomidate for molecular imaging of adrenocortical cytochrome P450 family 11B enzymes. J Clin Endocrinol Metab 93: 2358–2365

111. Ishimura K, Fujita H (1997) Light and electron microscopic immunohistochemistry of the localization of adrenal steroidogenic enzymes. Microsc Res Tech 36:445–453
112. Allolio B et al (1988) Nonhypnotic low-dose etomidate for rapid correction of hypercortisolaemia in Cushing's syndrome. Klin Wochenschr 66:361–364
113. Schulte HM et al (1990) Infusion of low dose etomidate: correction of hypercortisolemia in patients with Cushing's syndrome and dose-response relationship in normal subjects. J Clin Endocrinol Metab 70:1426–1430
114. Engelhardt D (1994) Steroid biosynthesis inhibitors in Cushing's syndrome. Clin Investig 72:481–488
115. Mitterhauser M et al (2003) *In vivo* and *in vitro* evaluation of [18F]FETO with respect to the adrenocortical and GABAergic system in rats. Eur J Nucl Med Mol Imaging 30:1398–1401
116. Bergstrom M et al (1998) *In vitro* and *in vivo* primate evaluation of carbon-11-etomidate and carbon-11-metomidate as potential tracers for PET imaging of the adrenal cortex and its tumors. J Nucl Med 39:982–989
117. Juhlin C et al (1998) [Differential diagnosis in adrenal gland tumors using PET and [11C]-metomidate]. Nord Med 113:306–307
118. Bergstrom M et al (2000) PET imaging of adrenal cortical tumors with the 11beta-hydroxylase tracer [11C]-metomidate. J Nucl Med 41:275–282
119. Khan TS et al (2003) [11C]-metomidate PET imaging of adrenocortical cancer. Eur J Nucl Med Mol Imaging 30:403–410
120. Minn H et al (2004) Imaging of adrenal incidentalomas with PET using (11)C-metomidate and (18)F-FDG. J Nucl Med 45:972–979
121. Zettinig G et al (2004) Positron emission tomography imaging of adrenal masses: (18)F-fluorodeoxyglucose and the 11beta-hydroxylase tracer (11)C-metomidate. Eur J Nucl Med Mol Imaging 31:1224–1230
122. Hennings J et al (2009) Computed tomography, magnetic resonance imaging and [11C]-metomidate positron emission tomography for evaluation of adrenal incidentalomas. Eur J Radiol 69:314–323
123. Karimi F et al (2008) Synthesis of 11C-labelled metomidate analogues as adrenocortical imaging agents. J Label Compd Radiopharm 51:273–276
124. Wadsak W et al (2006) [18F]FETO for adrenocortical PET imaging: a pilot study in healthy volunteers. Eur J Nucl Med Mol Imaging 33:669–672
125. Rendl G et al (2006) Usefulness of the 11 beta-hydroxylase inhibitor 18F FETO in positron emission tomography imaging of adrenal masses. Nuklearmedizin, Abstract Band of the International Symposium of Nuclear Medicine 2006, Bad Gastein 2006 No 17
126. Erlandsson M et al (2009) (18)F-labelled metomidate analogues as adrenocortical imaging agents. Nucl Med Biol 36:435–445
127. Schirbel A et al (2004) 4-[123/131I]Iodometomidate as a radioligand for functional diagnosis of adrenal disease: synthesis, structural requirements and biodistribution. Radiochim Acta 92:297–303
128. Hahner S et al (2009) 131I-Iodometomidate radiotherapy for metastatic ACC – first clinical experience. Presented at European Congress of Endocrinology, ECE 2009, Istanbul, Turkey. *Endocrine Abstracts* (2009) 20 OC1.3

Part IV
Pathology

Chapter 8
Classical Histopathology and Immunohistochemistry

Wolfgang Saeger

The histopathological diagnosis of adrenocortical carcinoma (ACC) and its differentiation from adrenal adenomas based on nine criteria: nuclear structures, mitotic rate, atypical mitoses, less than 26% clear cells, diffuse architecture, invasion of intratumorous sinusoidal structures, invasion of veins, invasion of capsule, and necroses. If three or more criteria are present and a metastasis of an extra-adrenal tumor or a primary medullary tumor are excluded by structural characteristics or immunohistochemical stainings, an ACC can be diagnosed. Its weight should exceed 100 g, its size should be larger than 5 cm. The typical immunohistochemical marker profile comprehends negativity for chromogranin A and (mostly) for keratin and an expression of inhibin, melan A, calretinin, and (mostly) synaptophysin. The Ki-67 index should exceed 3%. The differential diagnosis to medullary tumors, metastases, and other tumors are presented. The TNM-system for staging is discussed.

ACCs are defined by the WHO [1] as malignant tumors arising from adrenocortical cells. They may or may not be functionally active as evidenced by a clinically recognizable endocrine syndrome or by biochemical abnormalities that indicate a hypercortisolism.

The main problem and challenge for histopathologists is the differentiation of this tumor entity from adrenocortical adenomas (ACAs), medullary tumors, and metastases from other malignancies to the adrenal gland. Therefore, in most cases hematoxylin–eosin stainings have to be complemented by immunohistochemistry.

8.1 Gross Findings

The weight of the tumor is an important parameter [2] as most tumors weighing less than 50 g are benign although exceptional tumors with low weight have been shown

W. Saeger (✉)
Institute of Pathology of the Marienkrankenhaus, Alfredstraße 9, 22087 Hamburg, Germany
e-mail: saeger.patho@marienkrankenhaus.org

G.D. Hammer, T. Else (eds.), *Adrenocortical Carcinoma*,
DOI 10.1007/978-0-387-77236-3_8,

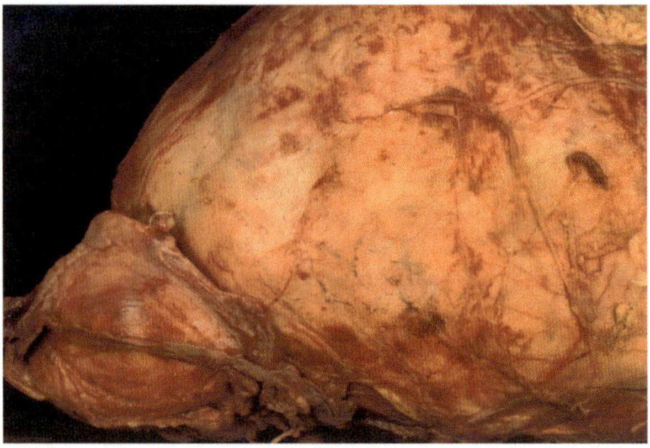

Fig. 8.1 Adrenal cancer: gross findings showing a tumor surrounded by a small rim of retroperitoneal adipose tissue

to be malignant due to demonstration of metastases [3, 4]. The average weight ranges from 500 to 1200 g. Some weigh as much as 5 kg [5]. The average size ranged from 12 to 16 cm, with a minimum of 3 cm [6] and a maximum of 40 cm [2].

The tumors are mostly soft with indistinct capsules (Fig. 8.1) and surrounded by adipose tissue. Cross sections show nodular cut surfaces (Fig. 8.2), irregular areas of necroses (Fig. 8.3) and hemorrhages, and intersecting broad fibrous bands. Necrotic zones appear yellow-white or tan. Cystic degenerations may be seen, but they are not sharply demarcated. The adjacent tumor-free adrenal is often not demonstrable or appears as a very small rim surrounding parts of the tumor.

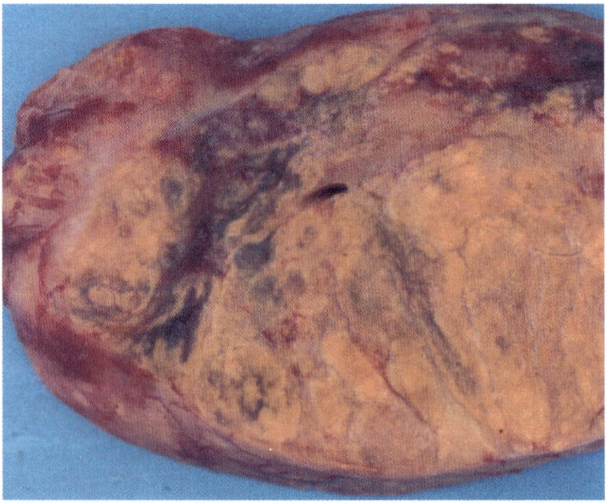

Fig. 8.2 Adrenal cancer: cut surface with nodal structure, lipid-rich areas (*yellow*), bleedings, fibroses (*gray*), no necroses, intact capsule, very small rim of adjacent tumor-free adrenal

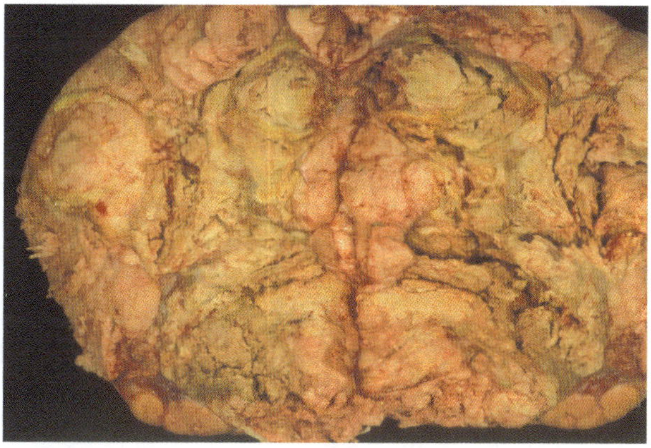

Fig. 8.3 Adrenal cancer: cut surface with extensive necroses, irregular border, invasion of capsule

8.2 Histopathology

Histopathologically, six main parameters have to be evaluated in ACC: growth pattern/architecture, vascularity, invasion, regressive changes, cell structures, and mitoses [7] (Table 8.1).

The *architecture* can be broadly categorized as diffuse (Fig. 8.4), trabecular, or alveolar. The most characteristic feature is the diffuse pattern without distinct partitions. The trabecular pattern shows broad anastomosing cords of tumor cells surrounded by slit-like vascular spaces. The alveolar architecture is characterized by round zellballen separated by net-like connective tissue.

The *vascularity* shows sinusoidal channels with thin endothelia but without distinct muscular fibers or small or medium-sized capillaries. Venous channels are mostly present in the periphery or in the immediate vicinity, showing dilated or collapsed lumina and mostly thin walls.

Invasion affects mostly the differently thick, sometimes very thin capsule, the surrounding connective tissue, rarely the adjacent adrenal gland, and very often the venous channels (Fig. 8.5) at the periphery and the sinusoidal channels in the center of the tumor. In those cases tumor cell nests are found within the lumina of veins or sinusoids whereas the endothelia of the sinusoids are interrupted or damaged. Rarely, thromboses may be found in the sinusoidal lumina (Fig. 8.6).

Regressive changes such as necroses and hemorrhages (Fig. 8.7) are found in different extents and stages whereas single-cell necroses are less significant. From these changes, broad band-like fibroses and larger areas of scars (Fig. 8.8) develop.

The *cell structures* are mostly characterized by eosinophilic or bubbly clear cytoplasm. In highly differentiated tumors, clear cells very similar to normal adrenocortical cells can be found, but also compact cells of normal adrenocortical type with strongly eosinophilic cytoplasm may be demonstrable in more mature carcinomas.

Table 8.1 Pathological features of ACCs [7]

Feature	Number of cases	Percentage
Nuclear grade [8]		
I	0/42	0
II	5/42	12
III	18/42	38
IV	21/42	50
Mitotic rate (per 50 high-power fields)		
0–5	10/42	24
60–20	11/42	26
21–50	16/42	38
>50	5/42	12
Atypical mitoses		
Absent	13/42	30
Present	29/42	70
Cytoplasm		
26–100% clear cells	4/42	10
0–25% clear cells	38/42	90
Architecture of tumor		
Non-diffuse	12/42	29
Diffuse	30/42	71
Necroses		
Absent	21/42	10
Present	38/42	90
Invasion of venous structures		
Absent	21/42	50
Present	21/42	50
Invasion of sinusoidal structures		
Absent	18/42	43
Present	24/42	57
Invasion of capsule		
Absent	18/42	43
Present	24/42	57
Weight (g)		
0–100	2/29	7
101–250	7/29	24
251–1,000	13/29	45
>1,000	7/29	24
Size (cm)		
0–5	2/38	5
6–10	11/38	29
11–20	21/38	55
>20	4/38	11

Myxoid changes in adrenocortical tumors evidenced by Alcian blue staining foci can be found in some carcinomas. Myxoid structures as the main architecture are very rare. In a collection of eight carcinomas, three of these cancers had myxoid

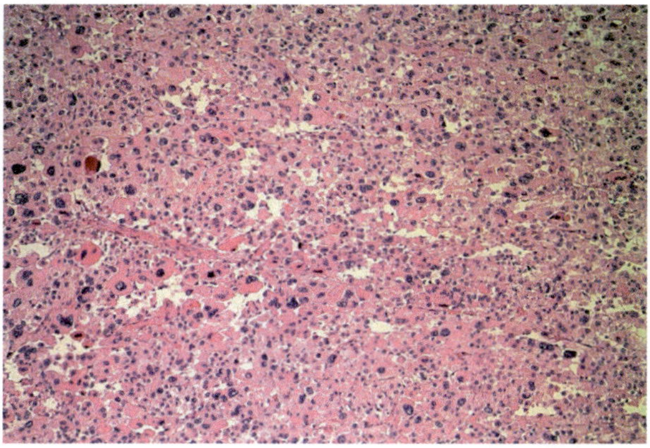

Fig. 8.4 Adrenal cancer: diffuse pattern, high cellularity, pleomorphic giant cells. Haematoxylin–eosin staining

changes in more than 50% of the tumor volume [9]. Additional special subtypes are the oncocytic variant and the sarcomatoid subtype. The *oncocytic carcinoma* [10] shows an intensively eosinophilic, fine granular broad cytoplasm and nuclei with coarsely clumped chromatin and prominent nucleoli. The ultrastructure (see below) is characterized by strongly increased mitochondria that may contain crystalline inclusions or round, homogenously dense bodies [10]. One case of *carcinosarcoma* was reported [11], which consisted of large areas of a typical adrenocortical carcinoma that was interspersed with multiple foci of sarcoma with rhabdomyosarcomatous elements which could be identified both immunohistochemically and ultrastructurally.

Nuclear atypia varies from non-existent to highly pleomorphic (Figs. 8.4 and 8.9) and bi- or multinucleated giant cells can be identified. The chromatin is loosely arranged in the more differentiated tumors or increased and condensed in the more undifferentiated ones. The nucleoli are mostly medium-sized but can also be very large and irregular (Fig. 8.9).

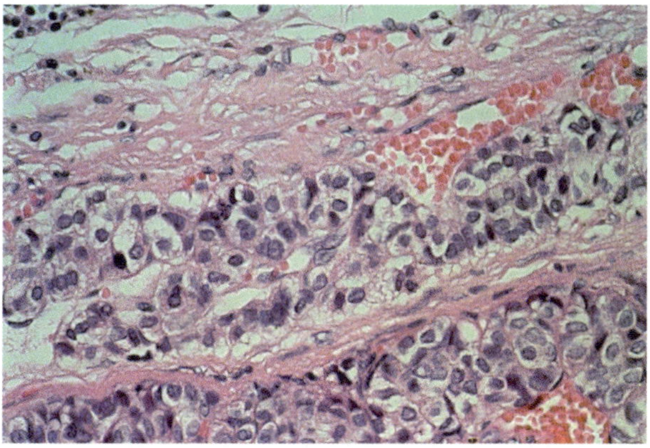

Fig. 8.5 Adrenal cancer: invasion of veins at the tumor periphery. Haematoxylin–eosin staining

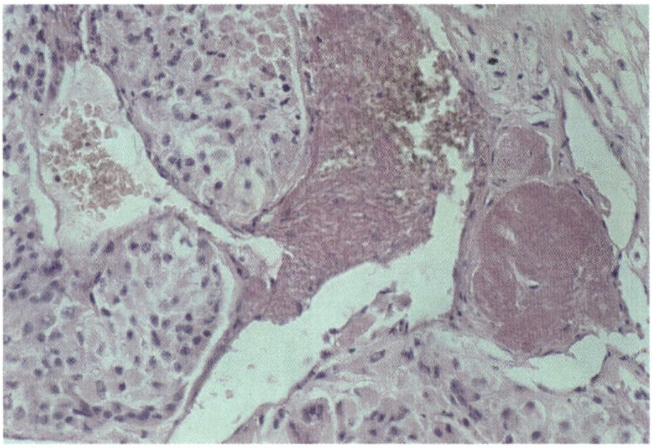

Fig. 8.6 Adrenal cancer: thrombosis due to invasion of sinusoidal channels. Haematoxylin–eosin staining

Mitoses should be counted per high-power field. Minimally 20 high-power fields should be screened. The number varies considerably. Whereas some carcinomas show mitoses very rarely, others contain ten or more per high-power field. Atypical mitoses may be present.

8.3 Scoring Systems

Definitive criteria for malignancy are distant metastases or distinct local invasion [12]. Local recurrences are retrospective evidence of malignancy in many cases [13]. Multiparametric systems have been developed for delineating malignancy using the existence of metastases, distinct invasion, or local recurrence after surgery in retrospective comparison with those tumors that do not show metastases or recurrences.

Three such scoring systems have been developed [7, 13–15] to differentiate ACCs from ACAs. The first system was published by Hough [14] (Table 8.2). They

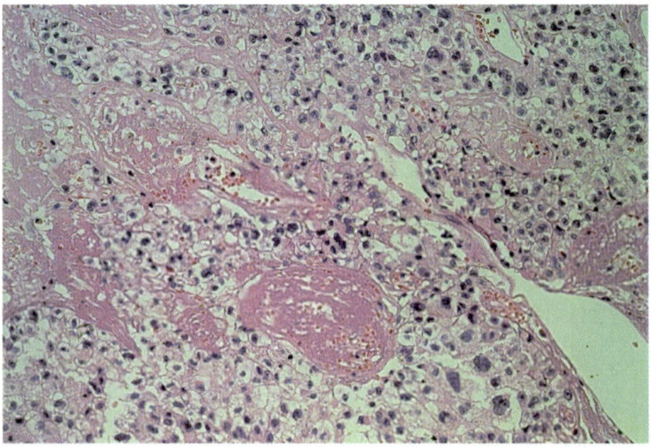

Fig. 8.7 Adrenal cancer: necroses due to thrombosis of sinusoidal channels. Strong pleomorphism of tumor cell nuclei. Haematoxylin–eosin staining

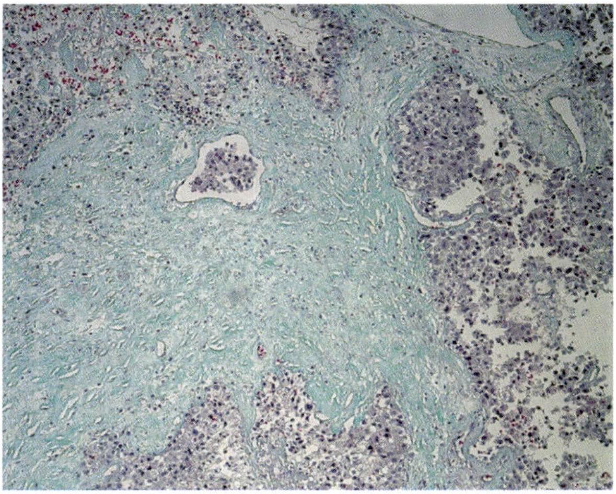

Fig. 8.8 Adrenal cancer: fibroses and scar following necroses. Trichrom staining

combined histological with macroscopical and clinical data. Weight loss and tumor weight of more than 100 g result in high values. The histological criteria underscore broad fibrous bands, the diffuse growth pattern, and the vascular invasion with highest results. The second system was presented by Weiss [13] (Table 8.3). The nine criteria were based on exact definitions and are, therefore, well feasible. All criteria have the same value, and the presence of four or more criteria lead to the diagnosis of adrenocortical cancer. The threshold of malignancy was lowered to three or more by the authors [7] in 1989 since one patient with three criteria in their series of 42 cases turned out to be a cancer. The third system was developed by van Slooten [15] (Table 8.4). Its seven criteria are differently weighted. Highest values are given to the mitotic activity (two or more mitoses per 10 high-power fields) and the regressive changes as necroses, hemorrhages, fibroses, or calcifications. A high mitotic activity alone leads with a value of 9.0 to the diagnosis of cancer as the threshold value is over 8.

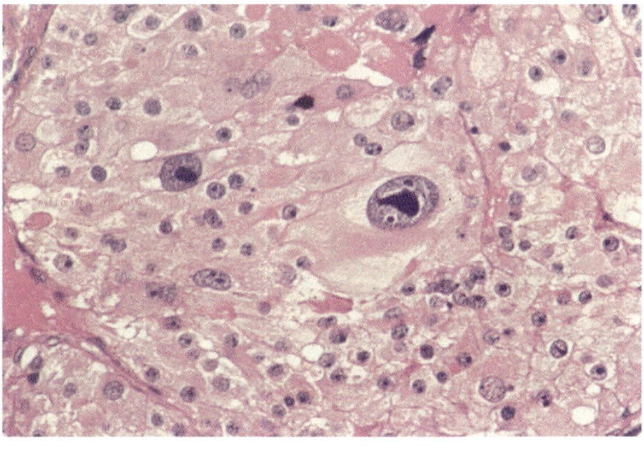

Fig. 8.9 Adrenal cancer: some pleomorphic mononuclear cells with increased chromatin and enlarged irregular nucleoli. Haematoxylin–eosin staining

Table 8.2 The system of Hough [14] for differentiating benign from malignant adrenocortical tumors

	Criterion	Value
Histologic criteria		
1	Diffuse growth pattern	0.92
2	Vascular invasion	0.92
3	Tumor cell necrosis	0.69
4	Broad fibrous bands	1.00
5	Capsular invasion	0.37
6	Mitotic index (1 per 10 high-power field)	0.60
7	Pleomorphism (moderate or marked)	0.39
Nonhistologic criteria		
1	Tumor mass >100 g	0.60
2	Urinary 17-ketosteroids (10 mg/g creatinine/24 h)	
3	Response to ACTH (17-hydroxysteroids increased two times after 50 mg ACTH iv)	0.42
4	Cushing's syndrome with virilism, virilism alone, or no clinical manifestations	0.42
5	Weight loss (10 lb/3 months)	2.00

The mean histologic index of malignant tumors was 2.91, indeterminate tumors 1.00, and benign tumors 0.17

Aubert et al [16] modified the Weiss system (Table 8.5). They reduced the criteria from nine to five and elevated the value for the mitoses and for the low number of clear cells from one to two and defined the threshold value as more than 3. The data were supported by the proliferation marker Ki-67 resp. MiB-1 with an index of more than 3%.

An additional study of a collection of 190 ACCs [17], compared the three different scoring systems using a threshold value of >2.0 for the Hough et al. system, of >3 for the Weiss system, and of >8 for the van Slooten system. Eleven cancers (5.8%) showed a Weiss index lower than 4, but a Hough index of more than 2.01 in six cases. Of the remaining five cases, three had a van Slooten index higher 8. The

Table 8.3 The system of Weiss [7, 13] for differentiating benign from malignant adrenocortical tumors

	Histologic criteria
1	High nuclear grade (Fuhrman criteria [8])
2	More than 5 mitoses per 50 high-power fields
3	Atypical mitotic figures (showing an abnormal distribution of chromosomes or an excessive number of mitotic spindles)
4	Less than 25% of tumor cells are clear cells (resembling the normal zona fasciculata)
5	Diffuse architecture (more than one third of the tumor forming patternless sheets of cells)
6	Necroses (when occurring in at least confluent nests of cells)
7	Venous invasion (smooth muscle as a component of the wall)
8	Sinusoidal invasion (endothelial lined vessel with little supportive tissues)
9	Capsular invasion (present when nests or cords of tumor cells extend into or through the capsule with a corresponding stroma reaction)

The presence of three or more criteria highly correlates with subsequent malignant behavior [7]

Table 8.4 The system of van Slooten [15] for differentiating benign from malignant adrenocortical tumors

	Histologic criteria	Weighted value
1	Extensive regressive changes (necroses, hemorrhages, fibroses, calcifications)	5.7
2	Loss of normal structure	1.6
3	Nuclear atypia (moderate/marked)	2.1
4	Nuclear hyperchromasia (moderate/marked)	2.6
5	Abnormal nuclei	4.1
6	Mitotic activity (≥ 2 per 10 high-power fields)	9.0
7	Vascular or capsular invasion	3.3

Histologic index >8 correlates with subsequent malignant behavior

179 tumors with a Weiss score >3 showed a Hough score <2.0 in 23 tumors and a van Slooten score <8 in nine tumors. In two tumors with nonmalignant indices, the carcinoma diagnosis was based on a high MiB-1 index (>20%; critical index 3%). We found a reliability of 94.2% for the Weiss score, of 85.3% for the Hough score, and of 93.7% for the van Slooten score. The three systems together with the immunostaining for MiB-1 enabled us to differentiate all ACCs from ACAs.

Table 8.5 The system of Weiss [13] for differentiating benign from malignant adrenocortical tumors, revisited and modified by Aubert [16]

	Histologic criteria	Weighted value
1	More than 5 mitoses per 50 high-power fields	2
2	Less than 25% of tumor cells are clear cells	2
3	Abnormal mitoses	1
4	Necroses	1
5	Capsular invasion	1

Threshold value for malignancy ≥3
MiB-1 index ≥ 4%

The most important gross findings and histological criteria including the MiB-1 labeling index are summarized by Aubert [16] (Table 8.6). They found a threshold for the mitotic rate of 5 in 50 high-power fields with a specificity of 100% and for the Weiss score of 3 with a specificity of 96%.

Table 8.6 Thresholds for malignancy according to Aubert [16]

Criterion	Threshold[a]	Specificity (%)	Sensitivity (%)
Tumor weight (g)	50 g	90.9	100
Tumor size (cm)	6.5	91.7	100
Weiss score [13]	3	96	100
Mitotic rate (for 50 high-power fields)	5	100	96
MiB-1 labeling index (%)	4	91.7	95.7

[a]Equal or higher

8.4 Immunocytochemistry

Immunostainings should be used in adrenal pathology for differentiation of cortical tumors from medullary tumors. Proliferation marker MiB-1 may confirm ACC diagnosis by an index of more than 3% (Fig. 8.10). The expression of antigens in the cortex is totally different from that in the medulla, and the same is true for tumors arising from these tissues.

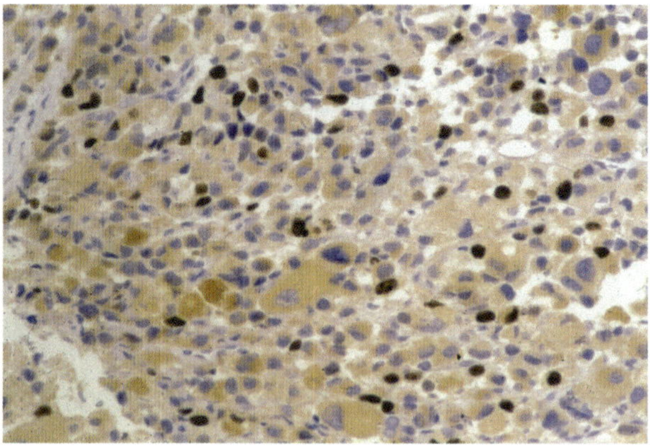

Fig. 8.10 Adrenal cancer: about 20% Ki-67 positive nuclei. Ki-67 (MiB-1) immunostaining

The diagnosis of an ACC should base on the structure in combination with a small panel of immunostainings (Table 8.7). From our experiences, an ACC has to be negative for chromogranin A [18] and epithelial membrane antigen (EMA) [18] although a weak cytoplasmic, not membranous, reaction may be found. Cytokeratin

Table 8.7 Immunostainings for adrenal cancers

Antigen	Reaction in adrenal carcinomas (%)
Cytokeratins	40–50% [18], 50% [19]
Epithelial membrane antigen	– [18]
Chromogranin A	– [18]
Synaptophysin	+ [18]
Neuron specific enolase	30% [20]
Neurofilament	50% [80]
Polysia-NCAM	30% [20]
Vimentin	80–100% [18]
Melan A	+ [18], 21/21 [21]
HMB45	– [18]
Nuclear protein adrenal 4 binding protein	+ [18]
Inhibin	6/6 [22]
Bcl-2	15/16 [23]
Insulin-like growth factor 2	64/69 [24], 4/4 [25]
Calretinin	11/12 [26]
Ki-67 (MiB-1) index	5.8% (+/– 1.3%) [27], 13.7% (+/– 3.1%) [23], 20.8% [28]
P53 index	10–50% in 62.5% of cancers [22], 9/20 [28]
Topoisomerase IIa	6.1% (+/– 1.6%) [27]

should be negative. Although a weak reaction is compatible with an ACC [18, 19], a very strong reaction is a significant argument against an ACC. In far most cases inhibin, melan A (Fig. 8.11) [18, 21], calretinin (Fig. 8.12) [26], and synaptophysin (Fig. 8.13) [18] are positive. The proliferation marker Ki-67 (MiB-1) is positive in

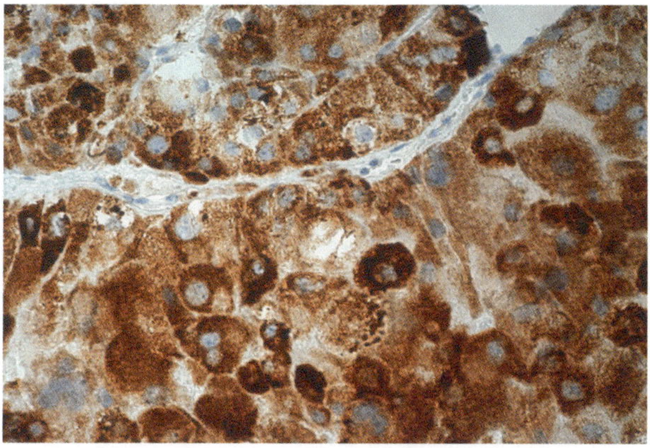

Fig. 8.11 Adrenal cancer: strong cytoplasmic Melan A expression. Melan A immunostaining

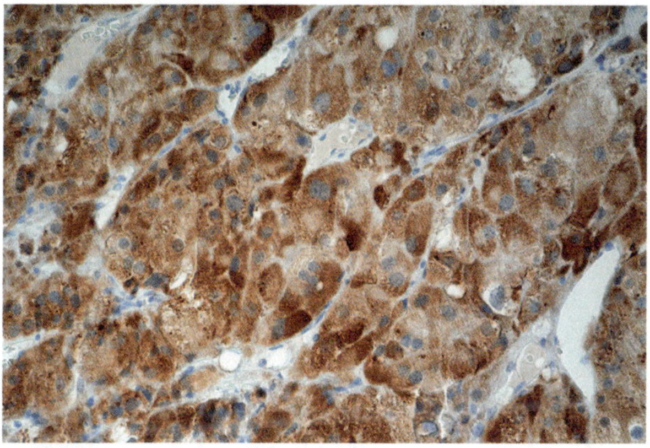

Fig. 8.12 Adrenal cancer: moderate to strong cytoplasmic calretinin expression. Calretinin immunostaining

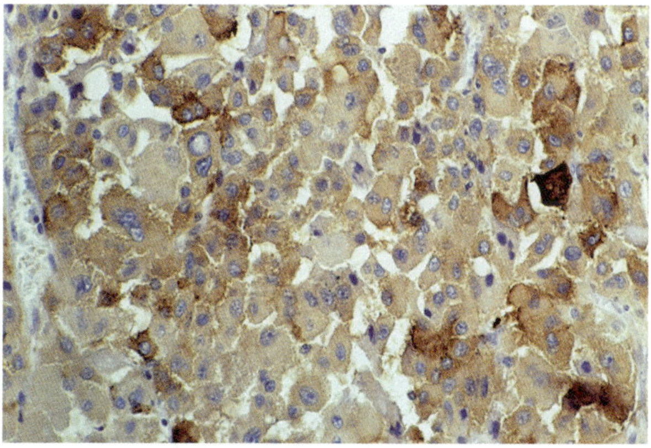

Fig. 8.13 Adrenal cancer: different cytoplasmic expression of synaptophysin. Synaptophysin immunostaining

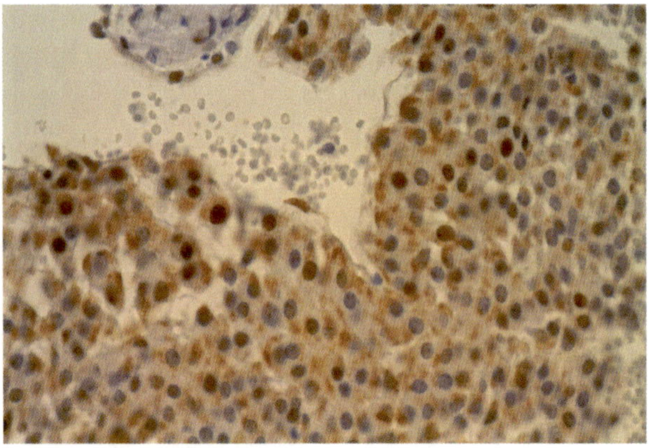

Fig. 8.14 Adrenal cancer: about 20% p53 protein positive nuclei of different intensity. P53 protein immunostaining

more than 3% of nuclei in most cases of ACC (mean 5.8–20%) (Fig. 8.10) [23, 27, 28]. P53 protein is demonstrable in less than one third to two third of ACC samples (Fig. 8.14). [28, 29].

8.5 Ultrastructure

The significance of ultrastructural studies has decreased with the development and progress in immunohistochemistry and molecular pathology. Nevertheless, many interesting structural details can be demonstrated by electron microscopy. Features associated with steroid hormone synthesis are liposomes, smooth endoplasmic reticulum, well-developed Golgi apparatus, and mitochondria [30]. The three zones of the normal adrenal cortex show different organelle structures [31]. Many ACAs are similar to one or occasionally two zones of the normal cortex [30]. Some ACCs may show structures of the normal cortex, as well, but in one study only one third of ACCs show convincing evidence of steroid cell differentiation [32].

The main cell type in ACC is not represented in the normal adrenal gland, but resembles a compact more than the spongiform normal cell type since lipid vacuoles in the cancer cytoplasm are very rare. The nuclei are often the dominant features presenting chromatin dispersed on the nuclear membrane or densely clumped [2] (Figs. 8.15 and 8.16). The nucleoli are mostly enlarged. At the cell membrane microvillous projections can be found. They are not as well developed as those in adenomas. Mitochondria (Fig. 8.17) are pleomorphic, but often small and round to oval. The cristae may show primitive structures or can be tubular, vesicular, or lamellar. A granular matrix may be found within some mitochondria. The amount of rough endoplasmic reticulum is relatively high, but also the smooth endoplasmic reticulum can be strongly developed (Fig. 8.16). Liposomes vary widely in number, size, and arrangement [30].

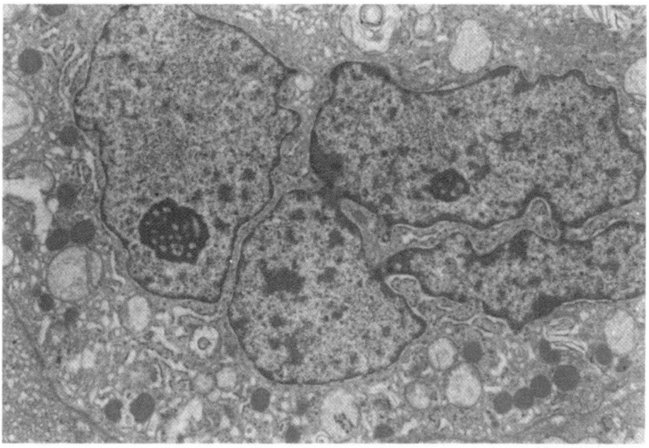

Fig. 8.15 Ultrastructure of adrenal cancer: lobated irregular nucleus with distinct nucleolus, increased rough and smooth endoplasmic reticulum. Uranyl acetate – lead citrate

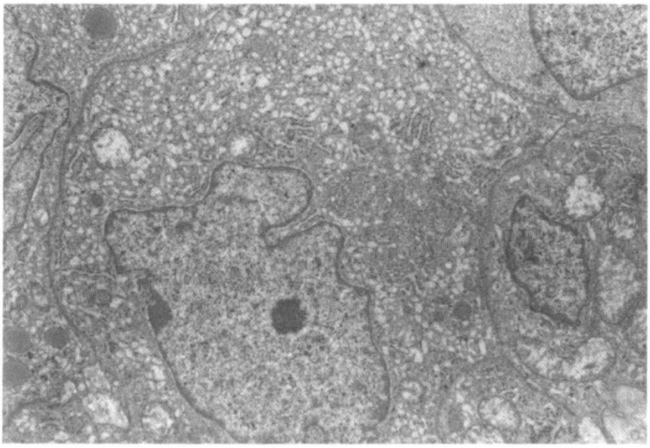

Fig. 8.16 Ultrastructure of adrenal cancer: lobated nucleus, increased smooth endoplasmic reticulum. Uranyl acetate – lead citrate

Morphometric analyses comparing endocrine active and inactive carcinomas as been performed for the adenomas [33] are not known. For androgen- or estrogen-secreting carcinomas, intramitochondrial dense granules are typical (Fig. 8.18) [34, 35].

8.6 Grading

The relationship between cancer morphology and clinical behavior has been known for more than a century and has provided the basis for any tumor grading system. Such a system should ideally have not only prognostic or predictive value but also add significant impact on choosing the optimal treatment [36] as is well established in prostatic [37], urothelial [37], and breast [38] cancer.

In cancers of the endocrine system, a grading system was not established until recently [39]. For ACCs, the Weiss scoring system [47] was developed to identify

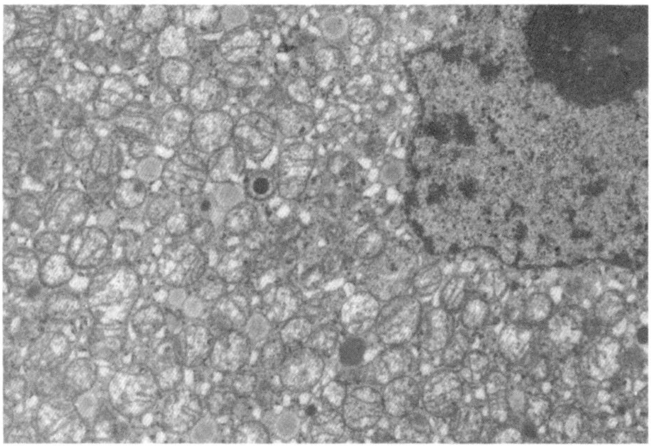

Fig. 8.17 Ultrastructure of adrenal cancer: increased and slightly irregular mitochondria. Uranyl acetate – lead citrate

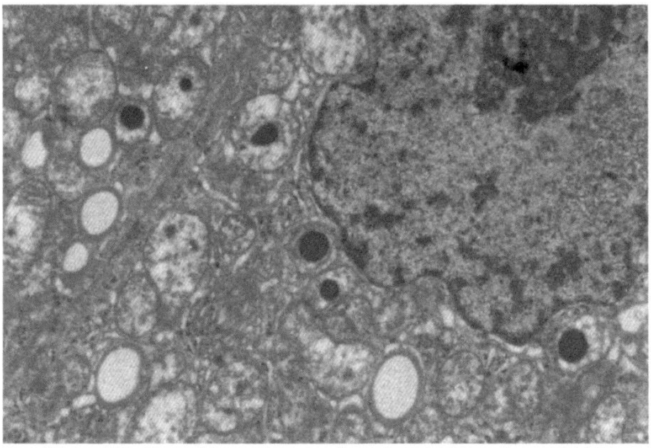

Fig. 8.18 Ultrastructure of adrenal cancer: intramitochondrial granular bodies. Uranyl acetate – lead citrate

the pathologic features of prognostic significance in ACC. Damjanov [36] used the nine criteria of this system to establish a provisional or temporary grading system. Three to four criteria correspond to grading G 1, five to six criteria to G 2, and seven to nine criteria to G 3. A second system to be tested uses the Ki-67 (MiB-1) index. In a provisional data set, an index of 4–5% represents G 1, an index of 6–20% G 2, and an index of more than 20% G 3. This system can be validated after some years of use on a large number of tumors.

8.7 Staging

In 2004, the International Union Against Cancer (UICC) and the World Health Organization (WHO) published the first staging classification for ACCs based on TNM criteria [40] (Table 8.8). Former classification systems were [41, 42] not consensually agreed upon by all. The 2004 classification categorizes localized tumors

Table 8.8 TNM classification and stage grouping of adrenal carcinoma [40]

TNM classification	
T	Primary tumor
Tx	Primary tumor cannot be assessed
T0	No evidence of primary tumor
T1	Tumor 5 cm or less, localized
T2	Tumor more than 5 cm, localized
T3	Tumor any size, locally invasive but not involving adjacent organs
T4	Tumor any size, involving adjacent organs
N	Regional lymph nodes
Nx	Regional lymph nodes cannot be assessed
N0	No regional lymph node metastasis
N1	Regional lymph node metatastasis
M	Distant metastasis
Mx	Distant metastasis cannot be assessed
M0	No distant metastasis
M1	Distant metastasis
Stage grouping	
Stage I	T1, N0, M0
Stage II	T2, N0, M0
Stage III	T1 or T2, N1, M0 or T3, N0, M0
Stage IV	T3, N1, M0 or T4, N0, M0 or any T, any N, M1

up to 5 cm as stage I, localized tumors larger than 5 cm as stage II, locally invasive but not involving adjacent organs as stage III, and tumors involving adjacent organs as stage IV (Table 8.8). The prognostic value of this classification remains to be established. Therefore, it is not incorporated in the recent official TNM classification of the different organ systems [43]. Additionally to the TNM systems, a stage grouping is proposed (Table 8.8) categorizing four stages (stage I – stage IV).

Recently, a proposal of the European Network for the study of Adrenal Tumors Classification [44] was published (see Chapter 4, Table 4.2). The evaluations of this group had shown that patients with stage II disease do not differ considerably in their disease-specific survival from patients with stage III, and patients with stage IV disease with distant metastases have a poorer survival than patients with stage IV disease without distant metastases. Other parameters, especially venous tumor thrombosis, were found to be important. Therefore, the group proposed [44] that stage III should be defined by the presence of positive lymph nodes, infiltration of surrounding tissues, or venous tumor thrombus whereas stage IV should be restricted to patients with distant metatsasis.

8.8 Differential Diagnosis

There are four topics of histological differential diagnosis in ACC: ACAs, medullary tumors, other tumors of the adrenal, and metastases.

Table 8.9 Immunostainings in the differential diagnosis of ACCs (modified from DeLellis and Shin [18])

	Adrenocortical cancer	Pheochromocytoma	Metastasis from renal cell cancer	Metastasis from hepatocellular cancer	Metastasis from other cancers	Sarcomas	Diffuse large B cell lymphomas	Malignnant melanoma
Keratin Kl1	–/+	–	+	+	+	–	–	–
Vimentin	–/+	–/+	+/–	+	–	+	–	–/+
EMA	–	–	–	+	+	–	–	–
S100 prot	–	+ [a]	–	–/+	–	–/+	–	+
Chromogr A	–	+	–	–	–	–	–	–
Synaptophysin	+	+	–	–	–	–	–	–
Neurofilament	+	+	–	–	–	–	–	–
AFP	–	–	–	+	–	–	–	–
Calretinin	+	–	–/+	–/+	–/+	–	–	–
Melan A	+	–	–	–	–	–/+	–	+
Inhibin	+	–	–/+	–/+	–	–	–	–
CEA	–	–	–	+	+/–	–	–	–
RCC	–	–	+	–	–	–	–	–
Heppar-1	–	–	–	+	–	–	–	–
CD 45 (LCA)	–	–	–	–	–	–	+	–
CD 20	–	–	–	–	–	–	+	–

[a]Sustentacular cells only.

EMA Epithelial membrane antigen S100 prot S100 Protein; Chromogr A Chromogranin A; AFP Alpha fetoprotein; CEA Carcinoembryonic antigen; RCC Renal cell carcinoma antigen; HEPPAR-1 Hepatocyte specific antibody; LCA Leukocytic common antigen

Adrenal adenomas have to be differentiated from ACCs by one of the three scoring systems mentioned above [13–15]. The modifications of the Weiss system by Aubert et al. [16] (Table 8.5) are also additionally helpful. If only one of the three systems show values of malignancy, a Ki-67 (MiB-1) index of more than 3% is helpful for the cancer diagnosis. From our experiences, tumors with undetermined malignancy are very rare if the different systems are used uncompromisingly and rigorously.

Medullary tumors, especially pheochromocytomas, can resemble ACCs markedly if the typical zellballen pattern of pheochromocytomas is missed and cells show cytoplasmic vacuoles simulating lipid vacuoles. Those cases have to be clarified by immunostainings (Table 8.9). Pheochromocytomas show a typical marker expression: Chromogranin A positive, keratins negative. A chromogranin A negative or keratin positive tumor cannot be a pheochromocytoma. Sustentacular cells in pheochromocytomas that cannot be found in adrenocortical tumors are demonstrable by S100 protein expression. They are often lacking in malignant pheochromocytomas [45, 46].

Other tumors of the adrenal are soft tissue or germ cell tumors [2], which have to be identified by their typical structures and immunostainings (Table 8.9). Undifferentiated sarcomas may be problematic in the differentiation from adrenocortical cancers. The marker profile of these sarcomas (especially expression of vimentin, smooth muscle antigen for leiomyosarcomas, or endothelial markers for angiosarcomas) are then of critical importance. Diffuse large B cell lymphomas [47–49] should be identified by their cell structures and their marker profile (Table 8.9).

The differentiation from *adrenal metastases* is the most difficult differential diagnosis. Specifically, it can be difficult to differentiate hepatocellular carcinomas, renal cell cancer, or melanomas from a primary adrenocortical tumor. A correct diagnosis in 77% of cases by core biopsy was achieved in our material although clinical data were not transmitted to the pathologist [50]. With distinct clinical data concerning the distribution of the tumor in the body, a demonstration of the metastatic nature of a malignant tumor in the adrenal is easier. Solid or adenoid tumor pattern, keratinizations, or strong PAS reactions and strongly increased connective tissue within the tumor are not compatible with adrenal cancers. If the tumor is strongly positive for keratin and negative for melan A, inhibin, or calretinin (Table 8.9), an adrenocortical cancer should not be diagnosed. Also expression of CEA or a distinct membranous reaction for epithelial membrane antigen are not compatible with an adrenocortical cancer. With distinct structural analyses, a marker panel of six to ten antibodies (Table 8.9), and sufficient clinical data, an exact discrimination of metastasis and adrenal primary tumor is possible in every case.

References

1. Lloyd RV et al (2004) Tumours of the adrenal gland. In: DeLellis RA, Lloyd RV, Heitz PU (eds) Pathology and Genetics. Tumours of endocrine tumours. International Agency for Research and Cancer (IARC), Lyon, pp 135–173

2. Lack EE (2007) Adrenal cortical carcinoma. In Lack, E. E. (Ed) Tumors of the adrenal glands and extraadrenal paraganglia. Armed Forces Institute of Pathology, Washington, DC, pp 131–160
3. Gandour MJ, Grizzle WE (1986) A small ACC with aggressive behavior; an evaluation of criteria for malignancy. Arch Pathol Lab Med 110:1076–1079
4. Saracco S et al (1988) Spontaneously regressing adrenocortical carcinoma in a newborn; a case report with DNA ploidy analysis. Cancer 62:507–511
5. McNicol AM, Laidler P (1996) The adrenal gland and extra-adrenal paraganglia. In: Lewis PD (ed) The endocrine system. Churchill Livingstone, New York, pp 131–186
6. Icard P et al (1992) ACC in surgically treated patients: a retrospective study on 156 cases by the French Association of Endocrine Surgery. Surgery 112:972–979
7. Weiss LM et al (1989) Pathologic features of prognostic significance in adrenal cortical carcinoma. Am J Surg Pathol 13:202–206
8. Fuhrman SA et al (1982) Prognostic significance of morphologic parameters in renal cell carcinoma. The American Journal of Surgical Pathology 6:655–663
9. Brown FM et al (2000) Myxoid neoplasms of the adrenal cortex – A rare histologic variant. Am J Surg Pathol 24:396–401
10. El-Naggar AK et al (1991) Oncocytic adrenal cortical carcinoma. Ultrastruct Pathol 15: 549–556
11. Fischler DF et al (1992) Adrenal carcinosarcoma presenting in a woman with clinical signs of virilization – a case-report with immunohistochemical and ultrastructural findings. Am J Surg Pathol 16:626–631
12. Lewinsky BS et al (1974) Clinical and Pathologic Features of Non-Hormonal Adrenocortical Tumors – Report of 20 New Cases and Review of Literature. Cancer 33: 778–790
13. Weiss LM (1984) Comparative histologic study of 43 metastasizing and non-metastasizing adrenocortical tumors. Am J Surg Pathol 8:163–169
14. Hough AJ et al (1979) Prognostic factors in adrenal cortical tumours. Am J Clin Pathol 72:390–399
15. van Slooten H et al (1985) Morphologic characteristics of benign and malignant adrenocortical tumors. Cancer 55:766–773
16. Aubert S et al (2002) Weiss system revisited – A clinicopathologic and immunohistochemical study of 49 adrenocortical tumors. American J Surg Pathol 26:1612–1619
17. Saeger W, Buurman H (2007) Adrenal carcinomas: comparison of three different scoring-systems for diagnosis in a series of 190 tumors. Pathol Rese Pract 203:382–383
18. DeLellis RA, Shin SJ (2003) Immunohistochemical characteristics of ACC: an overview. Acta Histochem et Cytochem 36:293–298
19. Hiraki H et al (1997) Regular immunohistochemical localization of endothelin-1 and endothelin-B receptor in normal, hyperplastic and neoplastic human adrenocortical cells. Pathol Int 47:117–125
20. Saeger W et al (2001) Pathologie wichtiger Erkrankrungen endokriner Organe (Schilddrüse ausgenommen). Der Pathologe 22:296–309
21. Loy TS et al (2002) A103 immunostaining in the diagnosis of adrenal cortical tumors – An immunohistochemical study of 316 cases. Arch Pathol Lab Med 126:170–172
22. Cho EY, Ahn GH (2001) Immunoexpression of inhibin alpha-subunit in adrenal neoplasms. Appl Immunohistochem Mol Morphol 9:222–228
23. Bernini GP et al (2002) Apoptosis control and proliferation marker in human normal and neoplastic adrenocortical tissues. British Journal of Cancer 86:1561–1565
24. Erickson LA et al (2001) Pathologic features and expression of insulin-like growth factor-2 in adrenocortical neoplasms. Endocr Pathol 12:429–435
25. Ilvesmaki V et al (1993) Insulin-like growth factors (IGFs) and their receptors in adrenal tumors: high IGF-II expression in functional ACCs. J Clin Endocrinol Metab 77: 852–858

26. Zhang PJ et al (2003) The role of calretinin, inhibin, melan-A, BCL-2, and C-kit in differentiating adrenal cortical and medullary tumors: an immunohistochemical study. Mod Pathol 16:591–597
27. Iino K et al (1997) DNA topoisomerase II alpha and Ki-67 in human adrenocortical neoplasms: a possible marker of differentiation between adenomas and carcinomas. Mod Pathol 10:901–907
28. Vargas MP et al (1997) Adrenocortical neoplasms: role of prognostic markers MIB-1, P53, and RB. Am.J Surg Pathol 21:556–562
29. Leung G et al (2002) The effect of flutamide and tamoxifen on sex hormone-induced mammary carcinogenesis and pituitary adenoma. Breast Cancer Res Treat 72: 153–162
30. Saeger W (1990) Tumours of the adrenal gland. In: Beck L, Grundmann E, Ackermann R, Röher HD (eds) Hormone-related malignant tumors. Recent results in cancer research, vol118. Springer, New York. pp 79–96
31. Neville AM, O'Hare MJ (1979) The human adrenal gland. Aspects of structure, function and pathology. In: James VHT (ed) The adrenal gland. Raven, New York, pp. 1–66
32. Mackay B et al (1994) Ultrastructure of adrenal cortical carcinoma. Ultrastruct Pathol 18:181–190
33. Saeger W et al (1979) Ultrastructural and morphometrical study of endocrinologically active and of non-functioning adenomas of the human adrenal cortex. 24. Symposium der Deutschen Gesellschaft für Endokrinologie. Acta endocrinologica (Kopenhagen) 90(Suppl 225):55
34. Mitschke H et al (1978) Feminizing adrenocortical tumor. Histological and ultrastructural study. Virchows Archiv 377:301–309
35. Saeger W, Mitschke H (1989) Androgenbildende Prozesse der Nebennierenrinde. Aktuelle Endokrinologie und Stoffwechselkrankheiten 10:162–169
36. Damjanov I (2007a) History and general aspects of tumor grading. In: Damjanov I, Fan F (eds) Cancer Gradig manual. Springer, New York, pp 1–5
37. Damjanov I, Mikuz G (2007) Tumors of the kidney and the male urogenital system. In: Damjanov, I, Fan F (eds) Cancer Gradig manual. Springer, New York, pp 55–63
38. Fan F, Thomas PA (2007) Tumors of the breast. In: Damjanov I, Fan F (eds) Cancer Gradig manual. Springer, New York, pp 75–81
39. Damjanov I (2007b) Tumors of the endocrine system. In: Damjanov I, Fan F (eds) Cancer Gradig manual. Springer, New York, pp 47–54
40. DeLellis RA et al (2004) Pathology and genetics: tumours of endocrine organs (World Health Organization classification of tumours). International Agency for Research and Cancer (IARC), Lyon
41. Macfarlane DA (1958) Cancer of the adrenal cortex; the natural history, prognosis and treatment in a study of fifty-five cases. Ann R Coll Surg Engl 23:155–186
42. Sullivan M et al (1978) Adrenal cortical carcinoma. J Urol 120:660–665
43. Wittekind C et al (2005) TNM-Atlas. Illustierter Leitfaden zur TNM/pTNM-Klassifikation maligner Tumoren. Springer, New York
44. Fassnacht M et al (2009) Limited prognostic value of the 2004 International Union Against Cancer Staging Classification for ACCs. Cancer 115:243–250
45. Padberg BC et al (1990) Histologie, Immuncytochemie and DNA-Cytophotometrie des adrenalen Phäochromocytoms (PCC) – eine morphologisch-klinische Untersuchung an 64 Tumoren. Verhandlungen der Deutschen Gesellschaft für Pathologie 74:289–294
46. Thompson LDR (2002) Pheochromocytoma of the adrenal gland scaled score (PASS) to separate benign from malignant neoplasms – A clinicopathologic and immunophenotypic study of 100 cases. Am J Surg Pathol 26:551–566
47. Barbaros U et al (2006) Primary adrenal lymphoma presenting as bilateral adrenal masses. The Endocrinol 16:75–76
48. Libe R et al (2006) A primary adrenal non-Hodgkin's lymphoma presenting as an incidental adrenal mass. Exp Clin Endocrinol Diabetes 114:140–144

49. Wang J et al (1998) Clinically silent primary adrenal lymphoma: a case report and review of the literature. Amer J Hematol 58:130–136
50. Saeger W et al (2003) High diagnostic accuracy of adrenal core biopsy: results of the German and Austrian Adrenal Network multicenter trial in 220 consecutive patients. Hum Pathol 34:180–186

Chapter 9
Cellular and Molecular Pathology of Adrenocortical Carcinoma

Tobias Else

Information molecular and genetic alterations as well as about morphological stages of adrenocortical tumorigenesis is sparse in comparison with our understanding of the development of more common neoplasms like those arising in breast or colon tissue. Breast and colon cancer have well-defined pre-cancerous or cancerous precursor lesions, carcinoma in situ, and adenoma, respectively. Stages and related genetic and epigenetic alterations are well defined. In contrast, adrenocortical tumorigenesis is less well defined. It is still a matter of debate whether adrenocortical carcinomas (ACCs) arise from normal tissue via the stages of hyperplasia or adenoma. It is certainly known that some hereditary diseases predispose to the development of ACC and, in fact, some of the alterations caused by these genetic syndromes can also be found in sporadic ACCs (see Chapter 10). The contributions of *p53*, *IGF2*, and WNT/β-catenin signaling pathway to adrenocortical tumorigenesis are discussed in chapters in this book dedicated to hereditary syndromes and their underlying genetic changes. This chapter will focus on the contributions of other known or suggested pathways, genomic and genetic alterations, as well as common principles of carcinogenesis, such as aneuploidy and clonal origin.

Most of the neoplastic changes discussed in this chapter are not unique to tumorigenesis in the adrenal cortex, but have been shown to accompany or cause carcinogenesis of cells of other tissue origin. Therefore, this discussion will in part be about common epiphenomena and the "usual suspects" frequently involved in tumorigenesis in other tissues. Their general role in the pathogenesis of malignant neoplasms will be described only as deemed necessary to understand their contribution to the development of ACC in particular.

Overall, it is remarkable that evolution has provided numerous mechanisms to prevent malignant transformation. As discussed in Chapter 13, this is

T. Else (✉)
Department of Internal Medicine – Division of Metabolism, Endocrinology & Diabetes, University of Michigan Health System, University of Michigan, Domino's Farms, Lobby C, Suite 1300, 24 Frank Lloyd Wright Drive, PO Box 451, Ann Arbor, MI 48106, USA
e-mail: telse@med.umich.edu

G.D. Hammer, T. Else (eds.), *Adrenocortical Carcinoma*,
DOI 10.1007/978-0-387-77236-3_9,

particularly relevant for telomere dysfunction, which can lead to senescence or crisis, both of which result in terminal non-proliferative states and thereby prevent the emergence of cellular progeny with oncogenic mutations that potentially give rise to cancer. Senescence can also be induced by oncogenes, such as oncogenic *RAS* or oncogenic *BRAF* (oncogene-induced senescence). Other mechanisms such as mitotic checkpoints prevent the generation and replication of aneuploid cells. Therefore, as a general scheme the road of oncogenesis can be seen as an interplay between stimulatory forces, such as genomic rearrangements, oncogenic mutations, or supraphysiologic stimulation with extracellular growth factors, and inhibitory forces represented by several checkpoints that when activated, stall the cell cycle until it can safely be resumed (e.g., after DNA repair occurred) or once and forever guide the cell towards a terminal state (senescence or crisis) or cell death (e.g., apoptosis). While mutations in proto-oncogenes play a crucial role in the transformation of normal cells, the action of tumor suppressor genes serves to prevent oncogenesis.

9.1 Clonality

In general, it is assumed that during carcinogenesis tumor-initiating genetic changes occur on the somatic level, followed by tumor-promoting changes. Once a clone has acquired the prerequisites to expand indefinitely, it gives rise to a genetically uniform population of cancer cells. Classically, it has been widely regarded that the origin of a malignant tumor is a single cell and that post-initiation genomic changes are rather rare events in comparison to the initial events leading to the original oncogenic clone[1]. Therefore, most, if not all, malignant neoplasms arise as a uniform monoclonal cell population. Monoclonality can be assessed by several surrogate parameters, such as X chromosome inactivation in female tumors. Somatic female cells maintain an "active" gene dosage of only one X chromosome. According to the Lyon's hypothesis, one X chromosome is epigenetically silenced early in embryogenesis, giving rise to a fixed pattern of X chromosomal expression [2]. This pattern is somatically inherited by the cell progeny, and therefore all cells of a tumor that arose from a single cell clone will have the same X chromosome silenced.

Several studies have analyzed tissues of adrenocortical hyperplasias (ACH), adrenocortical adenomas (ACA), and ACCs. An initial study analyzed three different markers on the X chromosome by methylation-sensitive digestion and found a monoclonal pattern in all informative ACCs (4/4) and in the majority of ACAs (8/14) and ACHs (5/7) [3]. A second study analyzed ACH, ACA, and ACC using two different polymorphic markers on the X chromosome, confirming a polyclonal pattern of the ACH in patients with ACTH-dependent Cushing's disease (5/5) and a predominantly monoclonal pattern in ACAs (7/8) and ACCs (3/3) [4]. A different study analyzing the CAG repeat polymorphic marker within the *AR* gene (Androgen receptor, *NR3C4, Xq11-q12*) compared ACH, ACA, and ACC and found a monoclonal pattern in 4 of 18 ACHs, 19 of 22 ACAs, and 9 of 9 ACCs [5]. Another recent study detected a monoclonal pattern in 14 of 62 ACHs, 49 of 56 ACAs, and 21 of 21

ACCs [6]. Taken together these studies show that the majority of benign ACAs are of monoclonal composition and that most, if not all, ACCs consist of monoclonal cell clones.

9.2 Genomic and Genetic Abnormalities

With the advent of more sophisticated analytic methods to evaluate genomic aberrations, genome resolution has become significantly higher over the recent decade. While earlier studies were able to estimate differences in overall DNA content (e.g., by morphometry or flow cytometry), metaphase analysis and classical comparative genomic hybridization studies were able to identify more precisely the "macroscopic" gains and losses of genomic loci. Until recently, a more detailed analysis had been restricted to certain loci, either through mutation analyses, using direct sequencing, or through loss of heterozygosity (LOH) analyses, using polymorphic markers. However, tiled arrays and whole genome sequencing have made genome analyses far less time consuming and less costly. These methods give accurate high-resolution results, some of them even to the nucleotide level. In the following paragraphs, results from genomic analyses of ACCs, in most cases in comparison to ACAs, will be presented, summarizing first earlier low-resolution techniques followed by modern high resolution techniques.

Since an increasing number of transcriptome analyses are available, they are discussed in a separate chapter dedicated to mRNA/cDNA microarray analyses (see Chapter 29). It should be noted that interpretation and comparison of the different studies of ACC are difficult, due to both several differences in important criteria defining malignancy and the great variation in available clinical data. Most studies do not define malignancy in biologic terms as the presence of distant metastases or tumor invasion. The availability of these data is dependent on the length of clinical follow-up and may not even be possible in the event of surgical cure of small stage I or II ACCs, which could have malignant potential but have not metastasized. Instead, most studies use surrogate parameters, such as the Weiss score, which is usually regarded to determine malignancy if it is greater than 3, or greater than 4, depending on the time studies were conducted (see Chapter 8).

9.2.1 Ploidy and DNA Content of Adrenocortical Tumors

The observation of aberrant mitosis leading to aneuploidy as a basis of malignant transformation is over a 100 years old [7]. Hansemann was the first to give detailed descriptions of unequal distribution of chromatin material in epithelial cancers. A few years later in 1914 Boveri made the same observation and concluded that aberrant mitosis leads to unequal distribution of chromosomes [8]. He hypothesized that in the majority of cases the originating cells will die, but occasionally will give rise to a cell clone that acquired the ability of unlimited malignant cell growth. He also postulated that tumors arise from one malignant cell clone that will pass the malignant characteristics on to its progeny. Over the course of the 20th century and through the work of numerous medical and biological researchers, his hypothesis was proven right [9, 10].

Aneuploidy describes a numeric chromosome anomaly (e.g., $<$ or $>$ 46 chromosomes per cell). Hyperploidy defines the state wherein multiples of a full chromosome set (3n, 4n, 5n, etc.) are present in one nucleus. Both, aneuploidy and hyperploidy have well been described in adrenocortical neoplasms. Several studies in the 1980s analyzed DNA content by morphometry and flow cytometry. An initial analysis found hypotriploid aneuploidy in 4 of 4 ACCs, but not in 4 normal adrenocortical tissue samples or 2 ACAs [11]. In a study of 22 adrenal neoplasms all 16 ACAs were diploid as opposed to 5 of 6 ACCs, which were aneuploid with 4 near triploid ACCs and 1 near tetraploid ACC [12]. Another large study of 39 neoplastic adrenal glands, with follow-up data available for 36 neoplasms, found aneuploidy in 4 of 5 ACC (1 hypotriploid and 3 hypertriploid) but in only 3 of 31 benign lesions (all hypotriploid). Aneuploidy correlated well with histopathologic criteria (Weiss score); 7 of 9 neoplasms that were found to be aneuploid had histopathologic features with a Weiss score $>$ 3 [13]. This correlation was confirmed by another study that found aneuploidy in 9 of 13 ACCs and 6 of 30 ACAs. Interestingly, this study failed to show a significant difference in survival between patients with aneuploid and diploid neoplasms [14]. Later, the finding of aneuploidy predominantly in ACC and only occasionally in ACA was confirmed by several other studies [12, 15]. In general, aneuploidy is a frequent characteristic of ACCs (summary in Table 9.1).

Table 9.1 Studies of aneuploidy in ACC. Several studies have reported aneuploidy in ACC. Aneuploidy is a common feature of malignant tumors that is shared by the majority of ACCs

Study	ACC (aneuploid/total)	ACA (aneuploid/total)
Klein et al. [11]	4/4	0/2
Bowlby et al. [12]	5/6	0/22
Amberson et al. [13]	4/5	3/31
Cibas et al. [14]	9/13	6/30
Takehara et al. [15]	2/3	3/21
Kjellman et al. [16]	8/8	0/14
Total	32/39 (82%)	12/120 (10%)

9.2.2 Genomic Aberrations in Adrenocortical Carcinoma: Analysis by Comparative Genomic Hybridization (CGH)

Consistent with observations from studies of total nuclear DNA content, studies focusing on the chromosome level by simple metaphase analysis defined partial or total chromosome gains or losses. However, these studies, which consisted primarily of case reports or small series of cases, did not reveal a conclusive alteration typical for ACC. Several later studies analyzed ACCs for genomic alterations by CGH. In this method, fluorescent-labeled tumor DNA is hybridized either to "normal" DNA, ideally of the same individual, or to DNA of a standardized cell line with a normal human genome. If no genomic differences exist, the fluorescence intensity will be evenly distributed over the whole metaphase. Loss of a genomic region will be reflected in a lack of fluorescence, while gains will have an increased fluorescence signal, greater than the background hybridization signal. Unfortunately, these studies were conducted before the requirement to submit data sets to a public repository, making combined analysis very difficult.

The first study of CGH on adrenocortical tumors evaluated 22 samples, including 14 ACAs and 8 ACCs [16]. These authors defined malignancy by histopathological features, size, urinary steroid profile, and clinical data (follow-up time 0.3–8.8 years, mean 4 years). 2 of 14 ACAs had a maximum of only two genetic aberrations, while 7 of 8 ACCs had multiple genetic aberrations with a mean of ten gains or losses. Gains were most commonly located on chromosome 4q, 5p, and 5q, and losses observed on chromosome 2, 11q, and 17p (>50% of ACCs). In a later study, the same authors employed LOH analysis using several polymorphic markers and confirmed some of the losses observed by CGH [17]. Most commonly affected in ACCs were 2q(50%), 4p(44%), 11p(60%), 11q(47%), and 18p(57%). Another study reports CGH analysis of 12 ACCs, 23 ACAs, and 6 ACHs [18]. A disadvantage of this study is the relatively short time of follow-up for the majority of patients and the complete absence of follow-up data in others. This study detected a much higher number of aberrations, which affected all ACCs (12/12) and the majority of ACAs (15/23). More than 40% of ACCs showed gains at 20q, 5q12–13, 5q22-ter, 9q32-qter, 12q13–14, and 12q24 and losses at 1p21–31, 9p, 3p, 2q, 3q, 6q, and 11q14-qter. Genomic aberrations in ACAs included gains at 17q11.2–21 and 17q24–25, 17p, and 9q32. A third study classified neoplasms as benign or malignant by histopathological criteria, which unfortunately were different from the classical Weiss score. These authors found genomic aberrations in 13 of 13 ACCs and 11 of 18 ACAs [19]. The mean number of changes was higher in malignant neoplasms (7.6, range 1–15) than in benign neoplasms (1.1, range 0–4). Gains and losses showed an equal distribution. Main changes in ACCs (>30%) were gains at chromosomes 5p, 5q, 12p, 12q, 19, and 4 and losses at 1p, 17p, 22, 2q, 11q. In the group of ACAs gains were observed at chromosome 4q (22%), 5 (11%) and losses at chromosome 3q (11%). A fourth study analyzed 25 adrenocortical tumor samples, including 14 ACCs, 8 ACAs, and the NCI-H295 and SW13 cell lines [20]. The authors found more gains than losses and the number of aberrations is found to correlate with tumor size. Gains in ACCs were most prevalent on chromosome 5, 7, 12, 16. Moreover, this study identified multiple loci of high-level amplification, which were not reported in other studies. These were rarely present in more than one sample, with the exception of 19p13.3 and 19q13.4, which were present in five, and three samples, respectively (of 14 ACC samples).

Overall, the conclusion from these studies is that ACCs are genetically diverse and display heterogeneity regarding genomic gains and losses. While no common "signature" can be derived from the available data, though some chromosomes seem to be affected more often (e.g., gains on chromosome 5 and 12).

A clear disadvantage of conventional CGH is the low resolution of genomic alterations and the inability to reliably differentiate high amplification areas from low amplification areas or to even estimate copy number variation. Most of these obstacles can be overcome using the more recently available technique of hybridization to tiled microarrays. Only one study has so far employed this method and reports gains on chromosomes 5, 6q, 7, 8q, 12, 16q, and 20 and losses on chromosomes 1, 2q, 3, 6p, 7p, 8p, 9, 10, 11, 13q, 14q, 15q, 16, 17, 19q, and 22q [21]. These authors also identified specific genomic alterations that were correlated with a poorer clinical outcome. With more studies this method should allow for the genetic subclassification of ACCs and analysis of clinical characteristics such as treatment response and prognosis. In the future, microarray CGH analysis in conjunction with other array analyses (e.g., mRNA/cDNA microarrays) may lead to a personalized treatment approach (see Chapter 29).

9.2.3 LOH and Mutation Analysis of Genomic Loci and Genes

As detailed above, classical CGH analysis provides a low-resolution picture of genomic alteration. It can not identify small losses or gains let alone detect point mutations in a gene. A more detailed method to identify genomic losses is allele typing using polymorphic microsatellite markers. Point mutations can be identified by gene amplification and direct gene sequencing or by single-strand conformation polymorphisms analysis utilizing pulse field gel electrophoresis. In contrast to full genome analysis, such as CGH, classical LOH studies and sequencing studies focus on a particular target gene or target locus within the genome. Most of the LOH analyses have investigated sporadic ACCs for the losses of genes known to be associated with hereditary ACC, such as *TP53*, *MEN1*, *IGF2*, *IGF2R*. But other loci such as *p16/INK4A* (*CDKN2A*) have also been analyzed. The results are summarized in Tables 9.2 and 9.3. Low frequency of LOH was found at *CDKN2A1* (9p21). The loci containing *MEN1* (11q13), *TP53* (17p13), and *IGF2* (11p15) were affected more commonly.

To date *TP53*, located on 17p13, is the most commonly mutated gene in ACC, with *TP53* mutations found in about one third of ACCs [22–26]. An initial study found *TP53* mutations even in a high percentage of benign ACA (73%, 11/15) [27]. However, this was not confirmed in subsequent studies, where *TP53* mutations were exclusively found in malignant adrenocortical neoplasms. Gicquel et al. showed that LOH at 17p13 was present in 11 of 13 ACC and 23 of 76 ACA [28]. In a follow-up study LOH of *TP53* and mutations in the *TP53* gene were analyzed in more detail only in those tumors (ACAs and ACCs) that had proven LOH at 17p13 [29]. About 12 of 36 tumors had *TP53* point mutations and 16 of 35 informative tumors had LOH of a polymorphic marker within *TP53*. Interestingly, there was no significant overlap of LOH and mutations in the same tumors as one would expect for the classical LOH

Table 9.2 Gene mutations in ACC. This table compiles the majority of studies analyzing mutations of specific genes in ACC. Only studies that incorporated ACCs were used for this table. ACA numbers refer to the ACA samples analyzed in the same studies

Gene	Locus	Function	ACC	ACA	Analysis	Study
KRAS	12p12.1	Small GTPase of the RAS family	1/35		Exon 1,2	Kotoula et al. [54]
			0/24	0/32	Codon 12, 13, 61	Yashiro et al. [57]
			0/15	0/18	Codon 12, 13, 61	Ohgaki et al. [23]
				6/17	Exon 1,2	Lin et al. [56]
HRAS	11p15.5	Small GTPase of the RAS family	0/24	0/32	Codon 12, 13, 61	Yashiro et al. [57]
			0/15	0/18	Codon 12, 13, 61	Ogaki et al. [23]
				0/17	Exon 1,2	Lin et al. [56]
NRAS	1p13.2	Small GTPase of the RAS family	1/35		Exon 1,2	Kotoula et al. [54]
			3/24	4/32	Codon 12, 13, 61	Yashiro et al. [57]
			0/15	0/18	Codon 12, 13, 61	Ohgaki et al. [23]
BRAF	7q34	MAP3K	0/18		Exon 15	Ameur et al. [55]
			2/35		Exon 11, 15	Kotoula et al. [54]
			1/15	0/41	Exon 15	Masi et al. [66]
EGFR	7p12.3-p12.1	EGF-receptor, receptor tyrosine kinase	0/18		Exon 18, 19, 21	Ameur et al. [55]
			4/35		Exon 18–21	Kotoula et al. [54]
PIK3CA	3q26.3	Phosphatidylinositol 3-kinase	0/18		Exon 9, 20	Ameur et al. [55]
JAK2	9p24	Tyrosine kinase	0/18		Exon 12	Ameur et al. [55]
GNAI2	3p21	Guanine nucleotide-binding protein	0/24	0/32	Codon 179, 205	Yashiro et al. [57]
CTNNB1	3p22-p21.3	β-catenin, transcription co-factor	3/15	8/41	Exon 3	Masi et al. [66]
			0/4	5/33	Exon 3	Tadjine et al. [112]
			4/13	7/26	Exon 3	Tissier et al. [113]

Table 9.2 (continued)

Gene	Locus	Function	ACC	ACA	Analysis	Study
TP53	17p13.1	Tumor suppressor, transcription factor	5/20		Exon 2–11	Sidhu et al. [26]
			8/14		PCR/SSCP	Barzon et al. [22]
			0/2	0/25	Exon 4	Reincke et al. [25]
			3/11	0/8	Exon 5–8	Reincke et al. [24]
			3/15	0/8	Exon 5–8	Ohgaki et al. [23]
CDKN1C	11p15.5	CDK-inhibitor	0/14	0/41	Exon 3, 4	Barzon et al. [22]
MENIN	11q13	Unclear function	2/17		Complete coding region	Schulte et al. [33]
			0/11	0/2	Complete coding region	Kjellman et al. [17]
			0/7	0/24	Complete coding region	Heppner et al. [31]
			0/10	1/19	Complete coding region	Gortz et al. [32]
RET	10q11.2			3/21		Lin et al. [44]

Table 9.3 LOH analysis of ACC. Several studies have analyzed specific genetic loci for LOH, a compilation of these studies is shown in this table

Gene	Locus	ACC	ACA	Analysis	Study
TP53	17p13	17/23	2/14		Soon et al. [114]
		11/13	23/76		Gicquel et al. [115], subanalysis 16/35 LOH at VNTR [29]
		5/5	1/23		Wachenfeld et al. [30]
CDKN2A	9p21	3/7	1/7		Pilon et al. [37]
IGF2R	6q26	11/19	2/22		Leboulleux et al. [36]
IGF2	11p15	15/18	32/94		Gicquel et al. [34]
MENIN	11q13	6/8	5/26		Wachenfeld et al. [30]
		8/8	2/13		Kjellman et al. [17]
		5/5	2/21		Heppner et al. [31]
		6/10	1/14		Gortz et al. [32]
		5/5			Schulte et al. [33]

mechanism of a tumor suppressor gene. There are several scenarios that may explain this finding. (1) *TP53* mutated alleles may give rise to a TP53 protein that displays a dominant negative effect on the wild-type TP53 protein function. This, indeed, has been shown for several TP53 variants (see Chapters 11 and 12). (2) Alternative mechanisms, such as promoter methylation, may silence *TP53* in those tumors that lack *TP53* LOH. However, a separate study failed to detect methylation of this region. (3) The 17p13 locus may harbor another oncogene different from *TP53*. This has been suggested in the literature, but to date no clear candidate genes have been identified, and given the known role of TP53 inactivation in the majority of human tumors, it seems to be unlikely that a different unidentified oncogene is located at the 17p13 locus. There is also a possibility that a site important for regulating *TP53* expression may be affected. Future research will be needed to elucidate the mechanisms of allelic inactivation. To this extent, it is worthwhile mentioning that the adrenocortical tumors with *TP53* mutation, but no LOH at the *TP53* locus, have been shown to express exclusively the mutant allele. Other mechanisms, such as increased *MDM2* expression that may affect TP53 activity, have also been largely unexplored in ACC.

The 11q13 locus, which harbors the *MEN1* (*MENIN*) gene, has also been found to undergo LOH in many ACCs [30–33]. However, as in the case of *TP53* this does not seem to follow the general mechanism of LOH, as the remaining allele is usually intact and unaffected by any kind of mutations. LOH is evident in ~83% of 30 ACCs reported in the literature (see Table 9.3). Only one study found two mutations (one nonsense mutation, one premature stop mutation) [33]. Unfortunately, for neither of these two tumors was leukocyte DNA available for LOH analysis. In addition, one of the two patients may represent a classical MEN1 patient with a germline (or mosaic) *MEN1* mutation, as the patient had other symptoms of the MEN1 syndrome. There has been extensive speculation in the literature regarding a different oncogene at the

11q13 locus, but to date no candidate gene has been identified. Alternatively, the observations may be explained by epigenetic factors that downregulate expression of the wild-type allele. However, data supporting this hypothesis are absent. One study that specifically focused on *MEN1* mRNA expression in tumors with proven LOH of 11q13 did not find any alteration in the expression of wild-type *MEN1* mRNA.

Several components of the IGF2 signaling pathway and the *IGF2* locus are regularly affected by LOH. The *IGF2* locus is localized at 11p15 and also harbors the genes for *CDKN1C* (*p57/KIP2*) and *H19*, a noncoding RNA (see Chapter 15). Gicquel et al. found LOH at 11p15 in 15 of 18 ACCs and in 32 of 94 ACAs, suggesting an involvement of this locus in tumorigenesis of sporadic ACC and ACA [34, 35]. Another study focused on point mutations of *CDKN1C*, which is mutated in the monogenetic variant of hereditary BWS, but did not find any mutations in a cohort of 14 ACCs and 41 ACAs [22]. LOH has also been observed at the locus for the *IGF2R*, one study showing LOH in 11 of 19 ACCs and 2 of 22 ACAs [36].

Another locus that has been investigated for LOH contains the *CDKN2A* gene *(p16/INK4A)* [37]. Hereditary mutations in this gene are known to predispose for malignant melanoma and LOH has been observed in several human cancers [38]. About 3 of 7 ACCs showed LOH at this site [37]. In contrast, only 1 of 7 ACAs was positive for LOH. Analyses for mutations in *CDKN2A* in ACC patients have not been conducted.

There are several analyses that have focused exclusively on benign lesions (ACAs and ACHs), which will not be mentioned in detail here. These studies have analyzed mutations, expression, and LOH of *ATR1*, *MC2R* (*ACTHR*), and *GNAS1*, which is mutated in McCune-Albright hereditary osteodystrophy [39–43]. One study is worthwhile mentioning which found *RET* mutations in 23 adrenocortical tumors, which were not further described regarding their clinical or histological features, but most likely are benign ACAs [44]. About 3 of 23 tumors analyzed displayed alterations of the *RET* genes, including 1 point mutation and 2 rearrangement of RET forming the *RET/PTC1* fusion gene. *RET* mutations are the molecular basis of MEN2, which is not associated with adrenocortical neoplasms. Rearrangements entailing the *RET* gene as well as *RET* mutations are found regularly in papillary thyroid cancers. Depending on the study series, 3–60% of sporadic papillary thyroid cancers have rearrangements involving the *RET* gene [45, 46]. *RET/PTC1* is a common rearrangement found in papillary thyroid cancer.

In summary, LOH and point mutations of the above mentioned genes and loci can be found in many ACCs and to a lesser extent in ACAs. It is still a conundrum why most of these genes do not follow the classical mechanism of LOH. According to Knudson's hypothesis, one would expect LOH in exactly those tumors that have a dysfunctional allele. However, studies of ACCs find that the remaining allele is usually intact and there is discordance, as within study series different tumors display LOH or point mutations of the same gene/loci. While the reason for this puzzling finding is unclear, at least three scenarios seem worthy of further inquiry: (1) occurrence of dominant negative alleles; (2) true haploinsufficiency with respect to preventing adrenocortical tumorigenesis; (3) other epigenetic mechanisms serve to silence alleles, either the remaining wild-type allele that has not undergone LOH or the non-mutated allele in case of tumors with gene mutations.

9.3 The RAS-Associated Signaling Networks in Adrenocortical Carcinoma

RAS, BRAF, PI3K, AKT, and mTOR are integral parts of intracellular signaling networks that are activated by binding of extracellular growth factors to their respective receptors (e.g., IGF2R, insulin receptor, PDGFR, EGFR) [47]. Research over the past decades has revealed complicated networks that consist of diversions, alternate signaling routes, and parallel signaling mechanisms. This means that the above mentioned factors are parts of a highly integrated shared signaling network. The following paragraphs will highlight those parts of the RAS-associated signaling network that have been implicated in adrenocortical tumorigenesis (see Fig. 9.1).

Ras oncogenes were first cloned from Harvey and Kirsten rat sarcoma viruses, which had been shown to cause murine tumors [48, 49]. These viruses acted

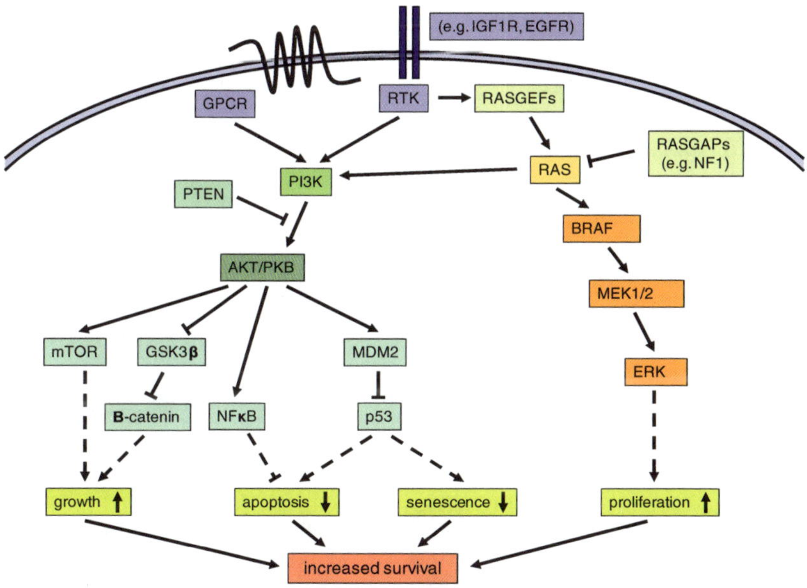

Fig. 9.1 Receptor tyrosine kinase signaling in ACC. Overview of signaling events induced by ligand binding to RTK-coupled receptors and GPCR. This is a very simplified scheme and only highlights of this signaling network are shown as it is important for ACCs. Right side – RAS signaling network. Several of these components are known to be mutated in a subset of ACCs (EGFR, RAS, and BRAF mutations described in ACC). Left side – PI3K signaling network. Activation of PI3K links signaling to Wnt-signaling and p53 inhibition. Several of these components have been shown to be activated in ACC, e.g., AKT. Signaling pathways finally lead to increased proliferation and growth and less senescence or apoptosis, ensuring increased survival of malignant cells

analogous to the Rous sarcoma virus, an avian retrovirus that was identified as early as 1916 as a cause of tumors in chicken [47]. In the 1980s, the first cellular homologs of viral Ras transforming oncogenes were cloned and termed *HRAS* and *KRAS*. Soon thereafter, another homologous proto-oncogene was identified in neuroblastomas and termed *NRAS* [50]. Through further structural and genomic analysis, the universe of *RAS*-related genes expanded to a total of 36 genes in the human genome [47]. It is now known that different members of the RAS family of proteins regulate a magnitude of cellular processes and serve as relays of multiple signaling pathways. They function as small GTPases, acting as binary switches in signaling pathways, with the GTP-bound form being active and the GDP-bound form being inactive. Two classes of factors regulate the RAS switch: GTPase-activating proteins (RASGAPs) turning it "off" and RAS guanine nucleotide-exchange factors (RASGEFs) turning it "on". As true for *RAS* oncogenes themselves, several members of RASGEFs and RASGEPs are known to date. Of interest, *NF1*, the gene mutated in neurofibromatosis type 1, encodes a RASGAP [51]. Mutant forms of this protein fail to activate the RAS GTPase activity, thereby increasing RAS activity. Upstream regulators of RASGAPs and RASGEFs are several tyrosine kinase-associated growth factor receptors (RTKs), such as PDGFR and EGFR [52, 53]. Mutations in the *EGFR* have been found in 11.4% tumors in a series of 34 ACCs [54]. Another study did not find any mutations analyzing 18 ACCs [55]. Adrenal tumors have also been analyzed for *RAS* proto-oncogene mutations in several studies. Mutations in *KRAS* and *NRAS* have been found in ~7% of ACCs and ~20% of all human neoplasms [23, 47, 54, 56, 57]. Interestingly, activating mutations were also found in a high percentage (14%) of ACAs (*KRAS* and *NRAS*), which is evidence for the fact that *RAS* mutations alone are not sufficient for malignant transformation [56, 57]. Interestingly, *RAS* oncogenes introduced into fibroblasts can lead to transformation or oncogene-induced cellular senescence [58, 59]. The process to either transformation or senescence is influenced by the concurrent activation of other cellular pathways, such as the p53/p21 and p16/Rb pathways [60].

Downstream events of GTP-bound RAS include the activation of mitogen-activated protein kinase (MAPK) cascades, which comprise a MAPK kinase kinase (MAP3K), such as BRAF, a MAPK kinase (MAP2K), such as MEK1/2, and the terminal MAPKs, such as ERK1/2, which in turn activates several transcription factors involved in cell proliferation and survival. To date the best described kinase pathway is the RAF-MEK-ERK pathway. Activated RAS interacts with a MAPK of the RAF family of serine/threonine kinase (BRAF, RAF1, ARAF1), which in turn signal through the MEK-ERK pathway [61]. *BRAF* mutations have been found in a variety of tumors. *BRAF* V600E is found in a majority of melanomas and papillary thyroid carcinoma [62, 63]. The *BRAF* V600E mutated allele is able to transform NIH3T3 cells. Interestingly, the *BRAF* V600E mutation is not only found in malignant melanomas but also in melanocytic nevi, where its activity has lead to oncogene-induced senescence, preventing further progression to full malignant transformation [64, 65]. BRAF mutations can be found in ~7% of all cancers and ~4% of ACCs, but have not been reported in adenomas [54, 55, 62, 66]. It has been reported that *NRAS* mutations and *BRAF* mutations are mutually exclusive in malignant tumors, suggesting that they directly act in the same pathway and therefore mutations in both genes would be redundant in view of pathway activation [67, 68].

RAS-mediated activation of the MAPK cascade leads to the activation of the terminal MAPKs. These MAPKs in turn activate several transcription factors (e.g., immediate early genes, such as ETS and AP1 family of transcription factors). Activation of this pathway has been shown to induce proliferation, increase survival, and lead to the acquisition of several malignant characteristics, such as increased motility and ability of tissue invasion. The role and activation of MAPKs downstream of BRAF have not been thoroughly investigated in human ACC. However, in human NCI-H295 cells it has been shown that IGF2 as well as N-POMC 1-24, a peptide that is derived from the same POMC peptide precursor as ACTH, induce phosphorylation of ERK 1/2 [69].

RAS signaling also activates the PI3K/AKT signaling cascade. PI3Ks are major downstream effectors of receptor tyrosine kinases (RTKs) and G-protein-coupled receptors (GPCRs) [70]. These enzymes relay signaling via the production of phospholipids, which in turn activate downstream kinases, such as AKT. PI3Ks exist in several classes and usually consist of a regulatory and catalytic subunit. A heterodimer of these subunits is activated either directly by an RTK or via an adaptor molecule, such as RAS or IRS1. Following activation, PI3K catalyzes the reaction of PIP2 to PIP3, which recruits AKT and leads to conformational changes necessary for full AKT activation. PIP3 generation is counteracted by PTEN, which generates PIP2 by dephosphorylation of PIP3, thus antagonizing PI3K signaling. AKT activation leads to the activation of multiple downstream signaling events, which include, but are not limited to, mTOR activation, NFkB activation, and MDM2 activation (which in turn inhibits p53 activation). Other factors such as FOXO1 or GSK3β are negatively regulated by PI3K. These actions link PI3K signaling to several other pathways, such as p53 inhibition (via MDM2 activation) and activation of WNT signaling (via GSK3beta inhibition). Several components of the PI3K/AKT pathway have been found to be activated or affected by mutations in multiple kinds of cancers. Data supporting abnormal activation of the PI3K/AKT pathway in ACC are sparse. A recent mutational analysis failed to reveal any mutations in *PIK3CA*, a gene encoding one of the main PI3Ks. Immunostaining of ACC tissues detects foci of phosphorylated AKT [71]. In NCI-H295 cells, AKT seems to be constitutively phosphorylated at a baseline level. This level is increased with IGF1R stimulation and can be reduced to levels below baseline using an IGF1R antagonist [72]. The crucial involvement of the PI3/AKT pathway in RTK signaling, specifically signaling of the IGF1R, makes it an important pathway to analyze in ACC.

9.4 Angiogenesis in Adrenocortical Carcinoma

Angiogenesis is thought to be crucial to ensure the nutrient and oxygen supply to the often large ACCs. However, reports regarding vascularization and angiogenesis in ACC are conflicting in the literature. An initial study carefully examined vessel number, vascular area, and endothelial area in adrenocortical neoplasms

[73]. While the latter two parameters were significantly higher in ACCs vs. ACAs, no difference was found regarding vessel number. A second study, which investigated the microvessel density together with clonality [74], detected no difference between microvessel area in monoclonal vs. polyclonal lesions. Vessel area and vessel perimeter were increased in ACC when compared to ACA or ACH, but again no difference was found in the actual vessel density. Another study focused on blood vessels per area in conjunction with angiogenic markers and found that the vessel number was significantly lower in malignant lesions than in normal adrenocortical tissue or ACAs [75]. ACCs had less than one third of the number of blood vessels observed in normal adrenocortical tissue. On the contrary, *VEGF* expression was about twofold higher in ACCs vs. normal adrenocortical tissues and ACAs. Most recently, gene expression array studies found that there is a highly significant correlation between *IGF2* expression, which can be regarded as an almost pathognomonic feature of ACCs, and *VEGF* expression [76]. This observation confirmed prior studies that detected higher mean expression of *VEGF* in ACCs [77]. Results of several studies that examined VEGF as a possible marker of malignancy in ACC indicate that, while serum VEGF levels tend to be higher in patients with malignant adrenocortical neoplasms, absolute levels failed to safely differentiate patients with malignant tumors from patients with benign tumors [78, 79]. On the other hand, VEGF levels show a significant decline post surgery for adrenocortical tumors [80].

While it seems to be difficult to integrate the observation of increased expression of pro-angiogenic factors, but a decrease or no change in number of blood vessels, this may be explained by an extent of tumor growth that can not be sufficiently supported by angiogenesis. This theory is also in accordance with the frequently observed necrotic areas in ACC [73].

9.5 Peptide Hormones and Cytokines in Adrenocortical Carcinoma

Peptide hormones have mainly been shown to regulate steroidogenesis and possibly growth in subsets of ACTH-independent macronodular hyperplasia (AIMAH) and ACAs. AIMAH is the best researched entity with respect to ectopic or illicit hormone receptor expression. A whole variety of ectopically expressed G-protein-coupled receptor genes (*GPCRs*) has been identified in patients. Binding of ligands to these GPCRs has been functionally shown to increase steroidogenesis and result in clinically apparent hormone production. These clinical scenarios include, for example, food-dependent Cushing's syndrome (e.g., GIP-receptor expression) or pregnancy and menopause-associated Cushing's syndrome (LH-receptor expression). Other receptors that have been shown to be functionally active in AIMAH include vasopressin receptor, serotonin receptor, beta-adrenergic receptor, and angiotensin 1 receptor. Lacroix et al. developed a clinical work-up protocol to identify possible ectopic receptor expression as the underlying cause of hormone hypersecretory states [81, 82]. This protocol includes hormone (cortisol) measurements in fasting state and fed state, in the supine and upright position, as well as after stimulation with GPCR ligands suspected to be expressed in these diseases. Ectopic *GPCR* expression has also been associated with hormone production by ACAs, but only one study identified the serotonin-7 receptor to regulate steroidogenesis in an ACC and several other studies did not find any ectopic GPCR expression in series of ACCs [81, 83]. Therefore, while ectopic GPCRs may be involved in AIMAH, it is unlikely that their expression represents a major mechanism in the regulation of growth and steroidogenesis in ACC [81].

More recently, several mutations in genes encoding the enzymes involved in regulating cAMP levels and cAMP-induced signal transduction have been reported to result in clinical syndromes of clinically apparent hormone production. These include mutations in *PPKAR1A*, a PKA regulatory subunit, that result in primary pigmented nodular hyperplasia (Carney-complex), *PDE11A* and *PDE8A*, which catalyze cAMP hydrolysis [84–86]. Mutations in these genes seem to play a role in subclasses of primary hypercortisolism, but are rarely mutated in ACC.

Two case reports have suggested a role for cytokine/chemokine signaling in adrenocortical lesions. A first report showed expression of *IL1R* in an ACA and proved in vitro stimulation of cortisol production by interleukin 1 [87]. The other report describes a case of ACC associated with high expression levels of *CXC8* [87, 88].

It is difficult to state whether the described cases of mutations in the cAMP signaling pathway, ectopic expression of *GPCR*s, or cytokines/chemokines represent common principles in pathogenesis or peculiar presentations of a rare disease. While the role of ectopic *GPCR* expression in regulating steroidogenesis in subclasses of AIMAH and ACAs is well established, involvement in ACCs seems to be the exception rather than the rule.

Gonadotropins and the inhibin/activin system have been suggested to play a role in animal models of adrenocortical tumorigenesis. This topic is discussed in Chapter 19. In short, in certain mouse strains gonadectomy and subsequent rise in LH can induce adrenocortical tumors. The same observation can be made in *Inhα/Tag* mice, which carry the SV40 large T antigen under the control of the inhibin promoter in their genome. In these mouse models, tumorigenesis is gonadotropin dependent as evidenced by the prevention of tumorigenesis on a hypogonadotropic mouse strain background or by treatment with GNRH superagonists. To what extent this model applies to human adrenocortical carcinogenesis is unclear. There are only vague parallels that may suggest the same mechanisms. Tumors observed in these mice are very different from usual human ACCs. They rather resemble a gonadal tissue type and only rarely are of a completely malignant phenotype (e.g., absence of tumor invasion and metastasis). Nevertheless, epidemiology may suggest some role of gonadotropins in human adrenocortical carcinogenesis. ACCs exhibit a slight predominance in females, specifically around the age of menopause, which is accompanied by a rise in LH secretion. Additionally, some reports indicate a significant number of ACCs diagnosed during pregnancy, a time in which βHCG acts on LH-receptors [89, 90]. Nonmalignant adrenocortical changes, which are relatively specific for the post-menopausal female population, have also been described.

Specifically, the peculiar change of thecal metaplasia, which has not been well studied, is commonly observed in this population and may represent a tissue change induced by elevated gonadotropins [91, 92].

9.6 Contributions of Physiological Regulators of the HPA-Axis, ACTH, and Steroid Hormones to Adrenocortical Tumorigenesis

Growth and function of endocrine organs are known to depend on the action of peptide hormones, mainly secreted by the pituitary. This fact is probably best evidenced by the pituitary–thyroid axis, wherein TSH secreted by the pituitary stimulates both thyroid growth and thyroid function. Therefore, in the case of TSH-dependent thyroid cancer, such as papillary thyroid cancer, a main goal in treatment is the suppression of pituitary TSH secretion by slightly supraphysiologic thyroid hormone supplementation.

It has been a longstanding debate whether ACTH represents a functional stimulus only or whether it also influences growth. While the functional role leading to an immediate production of glucocorticoids is well accepted, the possible trophic effect of ACTH on adrenocortical cells or on ACC is not well understood. Steroidogenesis is directly regulated by the signaling cascade induced through binding of ACTH to the MC2R. On the contrary, the effect of ACTH on adrenocortical growth seems to be indirect. In terms of stress, ACTH is known to provide the adrenal cortex with an increase in enzyme expression necessary for an increased cortisol production. Prolonged stress leads to an increase in adrenocortical size [93]. However, this effect does not exclusively depend on the effects of ACTH, but also on other POMC gene derivatives, other pituitary factors and non-pituitary derived factors [69, 94].

ACTH-mediated regulation of ACC growth is unlikely, as can be inferred from several lines of evidence. First, the vast majority of ACCs lose their ability to respond to ACTH stimulation; and second, it has been shown that ACTH treatment inhibits growth of transplanted mouse adrenocortical tumor cells [95]. Data regarding ACTH treatment of adrenocortical cancer cells in vitro are conflicting, but it is widely regarded that ACTH itself does not significantly induce proliferation [69]. Therefore, ACTH-suppressing treatment has never been a goal of ACC treatment.

The majority of (if not all) ACCs produce several different steroid hormones. Whether any of these may be involved in tumorigenesis or tumor maintenance remains a matter of speculation. Cortisol-producing ACCs have a slightly worse prognosis, which may be due to other concurrent genetic defects or due to the generally deleterious effects of high cortisol levels, specifically in cancer patients (e.g., one may speculate that tumor-directed immunity in these patients is disturbed) (see Chapter 4). Beyond these effects, recent studies have shown that *GR* (glucocorticoid receptor, *NR3C1*) expression is significantly increased in ACC vs. ACA and that GR immunohistochemical staining is prominent in ACC and absent in ACA [96]. While these studies were completely observational, one may speculate that the GR could be involved in a feed forward loop. Interestingly the initial growth media for adrenocortical NCI-H295 cells include hydrocortisone as one compound [97].

Minor clinical evidences have suggested a relation of adrenocortical tumorigenesis to estrogens (e.g., diagnosis during pregnancy, female predominance) (see Chapter 3). Estrogen receptors have been shown to be expressed in NCI-H295 cells, with *ERβ* being expressed at significantly higher levels than *ERα* [98]. Furthermore, estrogens increase, while anti-estrogens decrease, the proliferation of NCI-H295 [99, 100].

Another nuclear hormone receptor that has been experimentally shown to play a role in NCI-H295 proliferation is SF1 (NR5A1). SF1 is an important regulator of steroidogenic tissues in general and adrenocortical growth and function in particular [101]. Most genes encoding steroidogenic enzymes harbor response elements for SF1, and they are positively regulated by this orphan nuclear receptor. Mice completely lacking SF1 do not develop adrenal cortices and die in the perinatal period, presumably due to adrenal insufficiency [102]. SF1 has also been proven to be important in several postnatal growth paradigms [103]. In adrenocortical cancer cells proliferation is decreased upon treatment with an inverse agonist of SF1 [104]. However, there is conflicting evidence for a role of SF1 in growth and function of ACCs. *SF1* is expressed in most adrenocortical tumors. A recent profiling study of adult adrenocortical tumors found a decreased *SF1* expression in ACCs vs. ACAs and no significant change in ACCs vs. normal adrenocortical tissues [76]. On the contrary, *SF1* transgenic mice develop adrenocortical hyperplasia and occasional tumors [105]. This discrepancy may be explained by a different biology of childhood ACC vs. adult ACC, as a recent publication describes increased *SF1* expression in childhood ACC, but does not find any alteration of SF1 expression in adult ACC [106].

9.7 Timing of the Occurrence of Tumorigenesis-Related Changes

Whether adrenocortical tumorigenesis follows the common theme of a stepwise progression from normal tissue via precancerous lesions to a malignant tumor, as it has been described for other tumor entities, remains unclear. Colon carcinoma is amongst the best researched malignant tumors for which a histopathological stepwise development has been described. Most colon cancers develop from adenomas. As Fearon and Vogelstein described in their seminal work, the process of tumorigenesis is paralleled by a stepwise acquisition of certain common mutations [107]. Rather than a prerequisite for malignant transformation, this model provides a tool for thinking about how tumors develop. Certainly, there are exceptions to this model. Specifically, hereditary nonpolyposis colorectal cancer (HNPCC)-associated tumors do not develop through the adenoma stage, suggesting an alternative pathway or a different rate of mutation acquisition [108, 109]. Other cancers such as cervical cancer or breast cancer also have well-defined premalignant precursor lesions, which in part are the basis for screening programs of these tumor entities [110]. For other malignant tumors, like melanoma, morphological stages of tumor development are less well described. Malignant melanocytic tumors can arise from preexisting benign nevi or from melanocytes that are not associated with benign nevi [111].

With regards to adrenocortical tumorigenesis, there are two main questions persisting: 1) Are there common precancerous lesions, from which ACCs arise? Are the common ACAs actually precursor lesions that may transform into ACC? 2) Is there a common progression of genetic mutations that lead to ACC?

Overall, there is a significant overlap between genetic aberrations within ACAs and those in ACCs. Moreover, ACAs and ACCs share other common features (see Fig. 9.2). Both malignant and benign tumors are most often monoclonal. Aneuploidy is almost invariably present in ACCs, and is observed in a small percentage of ACAs. A subgroup of ACAs also shows chromosomal gains and losses, though to a much lesser extent than ACCs. Several common genetic mutations can be found in almost the same percentage of ACAs and ACCs (e.g., *CTNNB1, or RAS*), while other mutations are almost exclusively found in ACCs (e.g., *TP53*). While this

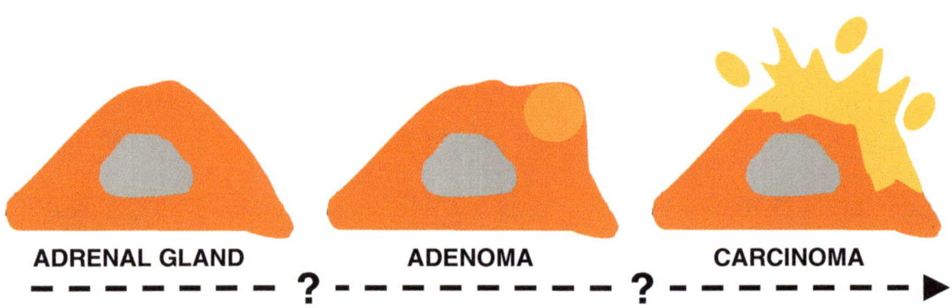

	ADENOMA	CARCINOMA
Monoclonal (%)	83%	100%
Aneuploid (%)	10%	82%
Genomic aberrations	none - moderate	moderate - severe
Mutations (%)		
TP53	0%	30%
CTNNB1	20%	21%
RAS	14%	7%
BRAF	0%	4%
EGFR	0%	11%
LOH		
17p13	23%	80%
6q21	9%	57%
11p15	34%	83%
11q13	13%	83%

Fig. 9.2 Cellular and molecular characteristics of ACA and ACC. Both entities share common characteristics, but there is currently no clear evidence for a progression from benign to malignant lesions

observation may suggest a stepwise acquisition of genetic aberrations, it may also be confounded by the histopathological difficulty of differentiating benign and malignant lesions. Naturally, but unfortunately, most studies use surrogate parameters of malignancy, such as Weiss score and tumor size, rather than true biological evidence of malignancy, such as organ invasion or distant metastasis. Apart from case reports of ACCs that were presumed to have arisen from a more ACA-like portion of the tumor, morphological evidence for an adenoma to carcinoma sequence in adrenocortical tumorigenesis is non-existent. Even evidence from genetic diseases, such as FAP, is not convincing. First, there is no report that suggests morphologically the origin of ACCs from ACAs in these patients. Second, although FAP patients are clearly prone to develop ACAs, an increased frequency of ACCs in these patients has not been proven (see Chapters 10 and 16).

To answer the above mentioned questions it seems safe to conclude that ACAs and ACCs share common genetic aberrations suggesting some similarities in pathogenesis, but current data do not necessarily support a sequential relationship manifesting in an adenoma to carcinoma progression. Moreover, epidemiological data suggest a high prevalence of adenomas (~5% of population), while the incidence of ACCs is very low (~1 per million). Therefore, from these numbers it is evident that even if there is a progression, the frequency is extremely low. Even if there was a true adenoma to carcinoma progression, only 1 in a 50,000 ACAs would progress to an ACC.

References

1. Fialkow PJ (1976) Clonal origin of human tumors. Biochim Biophys Acta 458(3):283–321
2. Lyon MF (1961) Gene action in the X-chromosome of the mouse (Mus musculus L.). Nature 190:372–373
3. Gicquel C (1994) Clonal analysis of human adrenocortical carcinomas and secreting adenomas. Clin Endocrinol (Oxf) 40(4):465–477
4. Beuschlein F (1994) Clonal composition of human adrenocortical neoplasms. Cancer Res54(18):4927–4932
5. Diaz-Cano SJ (2000) Clonality as expression of distinctive cell kinetics patterns in nodular hyperplasias and adenomas of the adrenal cortex. Am J Pathol 156(1):311–319
6. Blanes A, Diaz-Cano SJ (2006) DNA and kinetic heterogeneity during the clonal evolution of adrenocortical proliferative lesions. Hum Pathol 37(10):1295–1303
7. Hansemann DP (1891) Ueber Pathologische Mitosen. Arch Pathol Anat Phys Klin Med 119:299–326
8. Boveri T (1914) Zur Frage der Entstehung maligner Tumoren. Fischer, Jena
9. Hardy PA, Zacharias H (2005) Reappraisal of the Hansemann-Boveri hypothesis on the origin of tumors. Cell Biol Int 29(12):983–992
10. Holland AJ, Cleveland DW (2009) Boveri revisited: chromosomal instability, aneuploidy and tumorigenesis. Nat Rev Mol Cell Biol 10(7):478–487
11. Klein FA (1985) Flow cytometric determinations of ploidy and proliferation patterns of adrenal neoplasms: an adjunct to histological classification. J Urol 134(5):862–826
12. Bowlby LS et al (1986) Flow cytometric analysis of adrenal cortical tumor DNA. Relationship between cellular DNA and histopathologic classification. Cancer 58(7):1499–1505

13. Amberson JB (1987) Flow cytometric analysis of nuclear DNA from adrenocortical neoplasms. A retrospective study using paraffin-embedded tissue. Cancer 59(12): 2091–2095
14. Cibas ES (1990) Cellular DNA profiles of benign and malignant adrenocortical tumors. Am J Surg Pathol 14(10):948–955
15. Takehara K (2005) Proliferative activity and genetic changes in adrenal cortical tumors examined by flow cytometry, fluorescence in situ hybridization and immunohistochemistry. Int J Urol 12(2):121–127
16. Kjellman M (1996) Genetic aberrations in adrenocortical tumors detected using comparative genomic hybridization correlate with tumor size and malignancy. Cancer Res 56(18): 4219–4223
17. Kjellman M (1999) Genotyping of adrenocortical tumors: very frequent deletions of the MEN1 locus in 11q13 and of a 1-centimorgan region in 2p16. J Clin Endocrinol Metab 84(2):730–735
18. Zhao J (1999) Analysis of genomic alterations in sporadic adrenocortical lesions. Gain of chromosome 17 is an early event in adrenocortical tumorigenesis. Am J Pathol 155(4): 1039–1045
19. Sidhu S (2002) Comparative genomic hybridization analysis of adrenocortical tumors. J Clin Endocrinol Metab 87(7):3467–3474
20. Dohna M (2000) Adrenocortical carcinoma is characterized by a high frequency of chromosomal gains and high-level amplifications. Genes Chromosomes Cancer 28(2):145–152
21. Stephan EA (2008) Adrenocortical carcinoma survival rates correlated to genomic copy number variants. Mol Cancer Ther 7(2):425–431
22. Barzon L (2001) Molecular analysis of CDKN1C and TP53 in sporadic adrenal tumors. Eur J Endocrinol 145(2):207–212
23. Ohgaki H et al (1993) p53 mutations in sporadic adrenocortical tumors. Int J Cancer 54(3):408–410
24. Reincke M (1994) p53 mutations in human adrenocortical neoplasms: immunohistochemical and molecular studies. J Clin Endocrinol Metab 78(3):790–794
25. Reincke M (1996) p53 mutations in adrenal tumors: Caucasian patients do not show the exon 4 "hot spot" found in Taiwan. J Clin Endocrinol Metab81(10):3636–3638
26. Sidhu S (2005) Mutation and methylation analysis of TP53 in adrenal carcinogenesis. Eur J Surg Oncol31(5):549–554
27. Lin SR et al (1994) Mutations of the p53 gene in human functional adrenal neoplasms. J Clin Endocrinol Metab78(2):483–491
28. Gicquel C, Le Bouc Y (1997) Molecular markers for malignancy in adrenocortical tumors. Horm Res 47(4–6):269–272
29. Libe R (2007) Somatic TP53 mutations are relatively rare among adrenocortical cancers with the frequent 17p13 loss of heterozygosity. Clin Cancer Res 13(3):844–850
30. Wachenfeld C (2001) Discerning malignancy in adrenocortical tumors: are molecular markers useful? Eur J Endocrinol 145(3):335–341
31. Heppner C (1999) MEN1 gene analysis in sporadic adrenocortical neoplasms. J Clin Endocrinol Metab 84(1):216–219
32. Gortz B (1999) MEN1 gene mutation analysis of sporadic adrenocortical lesions. Int J Cancer 80(3):373–379
33. Schulte KM (1999) MEN I gene mutations in sporadic adrenal adenomas. Hum Genet 105(6):603–610
34. Gicquel C (1994) Rearrangements at the 11p15 locus and overexpression of insulin-like growth factor-II gene in sporadic adrenocortical tumors. J Clin Endocrinol Metab 78(6):1444–1453
35. Gicquel C (1997) Structural and functional abnormalities at 11p15 are associated with the malignant phenotype in sporadic adrenocortical tumors: study on a series of 82 tumors. J Clin Endocrinol Metab 82(8):2559–2565

36. Leboulleux S (2001) Loss of heterozygosity at the mannose 6-phosphate/insulin-like growth factor 2 receptor locus: a frequent but late event in adrenocortical tumorigenesis. Eur J Endocrinol 144(2):163–168
37. Pilon C (1999) Inactivation of the p16 tumor suppressor gene in adrenocortical tumors. J Clin Endocrinol Metab 84(8):2776–2779
38. Hussussian CJ (1994) Germline p16 mutations in familial melanoma. Nat Genet 8(1):15–21
39. Reincke M (1993) No evidence for oncogenic mutations in guanine nucleotide-binding proteins of human adrenocortical neoplasms. J Clin Endocrinol Metab 77(5):1419–1422
40. Yoshimoto K (1993) Rare mutations of the Gs alpha subunit gene in human endocrine tumors. Mutation detection by polymerase chain reaction-primer-introduced restriction analysis. Cancer 72(4):1386–1393
41. Davies E (1997) Somatic mutations of the angiotensin II (AT1) receptor gene are not present in aldosterone-producing adenoma. J Clin Endocrinol Metab, 1997. 82(2):611–615
42. Reincke M (1997) Deletion of the adrenocorticotropin receptor gene in human adrenocortical tumors: implications for tumorigenesis. J Clin Endocrinol Metab 82(9):3054–3058
43. Latronico AC (1995) No evidence for oncogenic mutations in the adrenocorticotropin receptor gene in human adrenocortical neoplasms. J Clin Endocrinol Metab 80(3):875–877
44. Lin SR (1998) Alterations of RET oncogene in human adrenal tumors. Jpn J Cancer Res 89(6):634–640
45. Couto JP (2009) How molecular pathology is changing and will change the therapeutics of patients with follicular cell-derived thyroid cancer. J Clin Pathol 62(5):414–421
46. Sobrinho-Simoes M (2008) Intragenic mutations in thyroid cancer. Endocrinol Metab Clin North Am 37(2):333–362, viii
47. Karnoub AE, Weinberg RA (2008) Ras oncogenes: split personalities. Nat Rev Mol Cell Biol 9(7):517–531
48. DeFeo D (1981) Analysis of two divergent rat genomic clones homologous to the transforming gene of Harvey murine sarcoma virus. Proc Natl Acad Sci U S A 78(6):3328–3332
49. Chang EH (1982) Human genome contains four genes homologous to transforming genes of Harvey and Kirsten murine sarcoma viruses. Proc Natl Acad Sci U S A 79(16):4848–4852
50. Hall A (1983) Identification of transforming gene in two human sarcoma cell lines as a new member of the ras gene family located on chromosome 1. Nature 303(5916):396–400
51. Xu GF (1990) The neurofibromatosis type 1 gene encodes a protein related to GAP. Cell 62(3):599–608
52. Kamata T, Feramisco JR (1984) Epidermal growth factor stimulates guanine nucleotide binding activity and phosphorylation of ras oncogene proteins. Nature 310(5973):147–150
53. Molloy CJ (1989) PDGF induction of tyrosine phosphorylation of GTPase activating protein. Nature 342(6250):711–714
54. Kotoula V (2009) Mutational analysis of the BRAF, RAS and EGFR genes in human adrenocortical carcinomas. Endocr Relat Cancer 16(2):565–572
55. Ameur N (2009) Mutational status of EGFR, BRAF, PI3KCA and JAK2 genes in endocrine tumors. Int J Cancer 124(3):751–753
56. Lin SR (1998) Mutations of K-ras oncogene in human adrenal tumours in Taiwan. Br J Cancer 77(7):1060–1065
57. Yashiro T (1994) Point mutations of ras genes in human adrenal cortical tumors: absence in adrenocortical hyperplasia. World J Surg 18(4):455–60; discussion 460–461
58. Serrano M (1997) Oncogenic ras provokes premature cell senescence associated with accumulation of p53 and p16INK4a. Cell 88(5):593–602
59. Benanti JA, Galloway DA (2004) Normal human fibroblasts are resistant to RAS-induced senescence. Mol Cell Biol 24(7):2842–2852
60. Benanti JA, Galloway DA (2004) The normal response to RAS: senescence or transformation? Cell Cycle 3(6):715–717
61. Montagut C, Settleman J (2009) Targeting the RAF-MEK-ERK pathway in cancer therapy. Cancer Lett 283(2):125–134

62. Davies H (2002) Mutations of the BRAF gene in human cancer. Nature417(6892):949–954
63. Namba H (2003) Clinical implication of hot spot BRAF mutation, V599E, in papillary thyroid cancers. J Clin Endocrinol Metab88(9):4393–4397
64. Michaloglou C (2008) BRAF(E600) in benign and malignant human tumours. Oncogene 27(7):877–895
65. Michaloglou C (2005) BRAFE600-associated senescence-like cell cycle arrest of human naevi. Nature 436(7051):720–724
66. Masi G (2009) Investigation of BRAF and CTNNB1 activating mutations in adrenocortical tumors. J Endocrinol Invest 32(7):597–600
67. Brose MS (2002) BRAF and RAS mutations in human lung cancer and melanoma. Cancer Res 62(23):6997–7000
68. Gorden A (2003) Analysis of BRAF and N-RAS mutations in metastatic melanoma tissues. Cancer Res 63(14):3955–3957
69. Fassnacht, M (2003) N-terminal proopiomelanocortin acts as a mitogen in adrenocortical tumor cells and decreases adrenal steroidogenesis. J Clin Endocrinol Metab 88(5): 2171–2179
70. Liu P (2009) Targeting the phosphoinositide 3-kinase pathway in cancer. Nat Rev Drug Discov 8(8):627–644
71. Fassnacht M (2005) AKT is highly phosphorylated in pheochromocytomas but not in benign adrenocortical tumors. J Clin Endocrinol Metab 90(7):4366–4370
72. Barlaskar FM (2009) Preclinical targeting of the type I insulin-like growth factor receptor in adrenocortical carcinoma. J Clin Endocrinol Metab 94(1):204–212
73. Sasano H (1998) Vascularity in human adrenal cortex. Mod Pathol 11(4):329–333
74. Diaz-Cano SJ (2001) Contribution of the microvessel network to the clonal and kinetic profiles of adrenal cortical proliferative lesions. Hum Pathol 32(11):1232–1239
75. Bernini GP (2002) Angiogenesis in human normal and pathologic adrenal cortex. J Clin Endocrinol Metab 87(11):4961–4965
76. Giordano TJ (2009) Molecular classification and prognostication of adrenocortical tumors by transcriptome profiling. Clin Cancer Res 15(2):668–676
77. de Fraipont F (2000) Expression of the angiogenesis markers vascular endothelial growth factor-A, thrombospondin-1, and platelet-derived endothelial cell growth factor in human sporadic adrenocortical tumors: correlation with genotypic alterations. J Clin Endocrinol Metab 85(12):4734–4741
78. Britvin TA (2005) Vascular endothelium growth factor in the sera of patients with adrenal tumors. Bull Exp Biol Med 140(2):228–230
79. Kolomecki K (2001) Usefulness of VEGF, MMP-2, MMP-3 and TIMP-2 serum level evaluation in patients with adrenal tumours. Endocr Regul 35(1):9–16
80. Jurczynska J (2009) Peripheral blood concentrations of vascular endothelial growth factor and its soluble receptors (R1 and R2) in patients with adrenal cortex tumours treated by surgery. Endokrynol Pol 60(1):9–13
81. Lacroix A (2009) Aberrant G-protein coupled receptor expression in relation to adrenocortical overfunction. Clin Endocrinol (Oxf), Aug 29 epub ahead of print
82. Lacroix A (2001) Ectopic and abnormal hormone receptors in adrenal Cushing's syndrome. Endocr Rev 22(1):75–110
83. Louiset E (2008) Ectopic expression of serotonin7 receptors in an adrenocortical carcinoma co-secreting renin and cortisol. Endocr Relat Cancer 15(4):1025–1034
84. Horvath A (2006) A genome-wide scan identifies mutations in the gene encoding phosphodiesterase 11A4 (PDE11A) in individuals with adrenocortical hyperplasia. Nat Genet 38(7):794–800
85. Horvath A et al (2008) Mutation in PDE8B, a cyclic AMP-specific phosphodiesterase in adrenal hyperplasia. N Engl J Med 358(7):750–752
86. Kirschner LS (2000) Mutations of the gene encoding the protein kinase A type I-alpha regulatory subunit in patients with the Carney complex. Nat Genet 26(1):89–92

87. Willenberg HS (1998) Aberrant interleukin-1 receptors in a cortisol-secreting adrenal adenoma causing Cushing's syndrome. N Engl J Med 339(1):27–31
88. Schteingart DE (2001) Overexpression of CXC chemokines by an adrenocortical carcinoma: a novel clinical syndrome. J Clin Endocrinol Metab 86(8):3968–3974
89. Luton JP (1990) Clinical features of adrenocortical carcinoma, prognostic factors, and the effect of mitotane therapy. N Engl J Med 322(17):1195–1201
90. Icard P (2001) Adrenocortical carcinomas: surgical trends and results of a 253-patient series from the French Association of Endocrine Surgeons study group. World J Surg 25(7): 891–897
91. Fidler WJ (1977) Ovarian thecal metaplasia in adrenal glands. Am J Clin Pathol 67(4): 318–323
92. Wont TW, Warner NE (1971) Ovarian thecal metaplasia in the adrenal gland. Arch Pathol 92(5):319–328
93. Ulrich-Lai YM (2006) Chronic stress induces adrenal hyperplasia and hypertrophy in a subregion-specific manner. Am J Physiol Endocrinol Metab 291(5):E965–973
94. Else T, Hammer GD (2005) Genetic analysis of adrenal absence: agenesis and aplasia. Trends Endocrinol Metab 16(10):458–468
95. Zwermann O (2005) ACTH 1-24 inhibits proliferation of adrenocortical tumors in vivo. Eur J Endocrinol 153(3):435–444
96. Tacon LJ (2009) The glucocorticoid receptor is overexpressed in malignant adrenocortical tumors. J Clin Endocrinol Metab 94(11):4591–4599
97. Gazdar AF (1990) Establishment and characterization of a human adrenocortical carcinoma cell line that expresses multiple pathways of steroid biosynthesis. Cancer Res 50(17): 5488–5496
98. Somjen D (2003) Carboxy derivatives of isoflavones as affinity carriers for cytotoxic drug targeting in adrenocortical H295R carcinoma cells. J Endocrinol 179(3):395–403
99. Barzon L (2008) Expression of aromatase and estrogen receptors in human adrenocortical tumors. Virchows Arch 452(2):181–191
100. Montanaro D (2005) Antiestrogens upregulate estrogen receptor beta expression and inhibit adrenocortical H295R cell proliferation. J Mol Endocrinol 35(2):245–256
101. Parker KL, Schimmer BP (1997) Steroidogenic factor 1: a key determinant of endocrine development and function. Endocr Rev 18(3):361–377
102. Luo X (1999) Steroidogenic factor 1 (SF-1) is essential for endocrine development and function. J Steroid Biochem Mol Biol 69(1–6):13–18
103. Beuschlein F (2002) Steroidogenic factor-1 is essential for compensatory adrenal growth following unilateral adrenalectomy. Endocrinology 143(8):3122–3135
104. Doghman M (2009) Inhibition of adrenocortical carcinoma cell proliferation by steroidogenic factor-1 inverse agonists. J Clin Endocrinol Metab 94(6):2178–2183
105. Doghman M (2007) Increased steroidogenic factor-1 dosage triggers adrenocortical cell proliferation and cancer. Mol Endocrinol 21(12):2968–2987
106. Almeida MQ (2010) Steroidogenic factor 1 overexpression and gene amplification are more frequent in adrenocortical tumors from children than from adults. J Clin Endocrinol Metab 95(3):1458–1462
107. Fearon ER, Vogelstein B (1990) A genetic model for colorectal tumorigenesis. Cell 61(5):759–767
108. Lynch HT (2009) Review of the Lynch syndrome: history, molecular genetics, screening, differential diagnosis, and medicolegal ramifications. Clin Genet 76(1):1–18
109. Imai K, Yamamoto H (2008) Carcinogenesis and microsatellite instability: the interrelationship between genetics and epigenetics. Carcinogenesis 29(4):673–680
110. Allred DC et al (2001) Histological and biological evolution of human premalignant breast disease. Endocr Relat Cancer 8(1):47–61
111. Bevona C (2003) Cutaneous melanomas associated with nevi. Arch Dermatol 139(12):1620–1624; discussion 1624

112. Tadjine M (2008) Frequent mutations of beta-catenin gene in sporadic secreting adrenocortical adenomas. Clin Endocrinol (Oxf) 68(2):264–270
113. Tissier F (2005) Mutations of beta-catenin in adrenocortical tumors: activation of the Wnt signaling pathway is a frequent event in both benign and malignant adrenocortical tumors. Cancer Res 65(17):7622–7627
114. Soon PS (2008) Loss of heterozygosity of 17p13, with possible involvement of ACADVL and ALOX15B, in the pathogenesis of adrenocortical tumors. Ann Surg 247(1):157–164
115. Gicquel C (2001) Molecular markers and long-term recurrences in a large cohort of patients with sporadic adrenocortical tumors. Cancer Res 61(18):6762–6767

Part V
Genetic and Molecular Aspects

Chapter 10
Overview of Genetic Syndromes Associated with Adrenocortical Cancer

Tobias Else

The volume of literature on the association of benign and malignant adrenocortical neoplasms with genetic syndromes is overwhelming. However, inherent problems arise when attempting to determine the specificity of these associations. On one hand, it is difficult to establish a clear link between the common benign adrenocortical adenomas and the rare congenital syndromes, and one must exercise caution when interpreting these observations. An exception, of course, is the case in which a specific phenotype of functional hormone-secreting lesions is observed. For example, diagnosis may be easier with rare syndromes, such as McCune-Albright syndrome, or with a specific diagnostic response to a diagnostic test as in Carney complex (i.e., the paradox of increased cortisol secretion after dexamethasone application).

On the other side, the coincidence of a rare genetic syndrome with adrenocortical carcinoma (ACC), which alone has a very low incidence (less than 2 per million), immediately raises the suspicion of a specific association. This is especially true when individual researchers or clinicians become aware of more than one case or if an increased number of cases are reported in the literature. Such cases raise the possibility that these conditions, ACC and the syndrome, may be either genetically linked or may share the same genetic basis. However, the difficulties in establishing such an association can be illustrated in the following example of ACC and multiple endocrine neoplasia type 1 (MEN1) (Table 10.1). In this example, it is shown that one should not jump to conclusions based on a limited number of case reports. It is estimated that the incidence of ACC is 0.72 per million in the United States – or 216 cases per year [1]. The frequency (=prevalence at birth) of MEN1 is estimated to be 1:5,000 – 1:30,000 [2, 3]. Therefore, assuming no linkage between the *MENIN* gene and another possible gene predisposing to ACC, one would expect a MEN1 patient with ACC roughly every 25–150 years in the United States simply by chance. It

T. Else (✉)
Department of Internal Medicine – Division of Metabolism, Endocrinology & Diabetes, University of Michigan Health System, University of Michigan, Domino's Farms, Lobby C, Suite 1300, 24 Frank Lloyd Wright Drive, PO Box 451, Ann Arbor, MI 48106, USA
e-mail: telse@med.umich.edu

G.D. Hammer, T. Else (eds.), *Adrenocortical Carcinoma*,
DOI 10.1007/978-0-387-77236-3_10, © Springer Science+Business Media, LLC 2011

Table 10.1 Numbers needed for statistical significance of association of ACC with rare syndromes. The numbers in this table serve as an example of numbers needed to reach statistical significance ($p < 0.05$) for an association of MEN1 with ACC, assuming the example total population, time of observation and prevalence as given in this table, which are all crude estimates. For example, to make the conclusion of an estimated prevalence of 1:5000 for MEN1, one would expect four patients with ACC and MEN1 by chance in the European population (estimated at 500,000,000)

		17 years	55 years
Europe			
Population 500,000,000	Expected ACC total	6120	19800
Prevalence 1:5,000	Expected ACC patients with syndrome	1.2	4.0
	Number to reach significance	4	8
Prevalence 1:30,000	Expected ACC patients with syndrome	0.2	0.7
	Number to reach significance	2	3
United States			
Population 300,000,000	Expected ACC total	3672	11880
Prevalence 1:5,000	Expected ACC patients with syndrome	0.7	2.4
	Number to reach significance	2	6
Prevalence 1:30,000	Expected ACC patients with syndrome	0.1	0.4
	Number to reach significance	1	3

is important to note that this assumption not only ignores basic knowledge of population genetics but also is hampered by the fact that we do not know the exact prevalence of MEN1 or the exact incidence of ACC. Of course, incidences can not be derived or even estimated from case report numbers. Furthermore, the threshold to report cases with both entities decreases the more the association becomes established. Interestingly, there are far more reviews mentioning an association of these two entities than actually reports of cases or case series. It also fails to consider the bias produced by the fact that both patient groups (ACC patients and MEN1 patients) are usually cared for by endocrinologists who may more readily diagnose both diseases. In terms of coincidence of ACC and MEN1 as well as other rare syndromes, we rely almost entirely on case reports in which diagnostic criteria and interpretation vary from institution to institution. Furthermore, it is almost impossible to estimate the total reporting population, reporting frequency, and threshold. Nevertheless, as an example, this issue should be approached with the following hypothetical example. In an ideal scenario where every MEN1 and every ACC case were reported, how many cases of patients carrying both conditions would be necessary to find this association convincing? To address this it may be helpful to focus on the aforementioned numbers in more detail. MEN1 serves as a good example to dissect evidences for an association with ACC, but it should be mentioned that this is an arbitrary choice. The following discussion is completely theoretical and does not necessarily need specific disease entities. It should rather guide the reader through the general thought process to determine the significance of the association of a rare complex syndrome with a rare symptom, which can also be observed in the general population (Table 10.1). A total of six cases of MEN1 patients with

ACC have been reported in the literature [4–7]. MEN1 was first described in 1954, 55 years ago, and the first MEN1 patient with an ACC was reported in 1992, 17 years ago [6, 8]. Assuming a MEN1 frequency of 1 in 5000, to attain the accepted $p > 0.05$ statistical significance would require that there be at least six patients in the past 55 years in the United States who display both diseases. An MEN1 frequency of 1 in 30,000 would equate to three patients with MEN1 and ACC in the past 55 years. Thus, the six actual cases reported to date fall well within the significance criteria. However, all 6 patients have been reported from Europe and none have been reported from the United States [4–7]. Therefore, assuming a European population of 500 million people, we would need at least two patients over 17 years, assuming a prevalence of 1:30,000 or eight patients over 55 years for a prevalence of 1:5,000. Therefore, in Europe the reported number almost falls into the expected range for a chance association. Even in this selected population, ACC is still a rare cancer though the risk of ACC development may be slightly increased. It should be mentioned that the association of MEN1 and ACC would be negligible if the United States and Europe together were considered as the reporting population. Again, this calculation does not serve to determine the real association in either the European or US population but rather should serve as an example of an approach to think about the significance of the association of another rare disease with a rare symptom. In conclusion, the evidence for an association between MEN1 and ACC is weak from an epidemiological point of view. This short example may leave the reader better equipped to estimate "real," significant and "non-real," nonsignificant associations.

Perhaps more convincing evidence to persuade the reader that a certain symptom is part of a complex syndrome is experimentally derived evidence. If, for example, the syndrome-causing mutation is known and it is shown in animal models that it leads to comparable phenotypes, we tend to believe the specific association between the symptom and the complex syndrome. It would be also convincing if it were shown that a syndrome-causing mutation impacts a certain signaling pathway and that pathway is also found to be disturbed in sporadic occurrence of a certain cancer – e.g., a germline mutation leads to a genetic syndrome with ACC and a disruption of the same pathway or somatic mutations are found in sporadic cases of ACC.

A third mechanism that influences judgment about an association is personal experience and expert opinion. To this end, communication within a research area is extremely important and beneficial. This mechanism though is of course also challenged by the production of a personal or an expert-derived bias.

Ideally, a clear genetic association together with experimental evidence is the most convincing support for an association. When dealing with a rare disease entity such as ACC, the body of information is relatively sparse compared to other more common cancers. Nevertheless, there are gene mutations that are proven to predispose to ACC development and others for which experimental evidence is convincing. Unfortunately, there are hardly any instances where both types of evidence are available. For example, the connection between Li-Fraumeni syndrome (LFS) and ACC is well established; indeed, the clinical diagnosis is in part based on the diagnosis of ACC in affected families (Tables 10.2 and 10.4). Experimental evidence

Table 10.2 Overview of syndromes reported in the literature to occur with ACC. Summary of clinical, genetic, and epidemiological data of main syndromes, which have either been proven to be associated with ACC or which have been reported to occur with ACC, but for which association of genetics changes

Syndrome	Genes	Locus	Prevalence	clinical features	associated neoplasias
Beckwith-Wiedemann syndrome [17, 20, 32, 33, 35, 38, 74] (OMIM#130650)	*IGF2* *CDKN1C* *H19* *LIT1* *KvLQT1*	*11p15* Mutations or altered methylation	1:13,700 1:76,923	Macroglossia, abdominal wall defects, ear pits, hemangiomas, nevus flammeus, neonatal hypoglycemia, premature birth, cryptorchidism, polyhydramnios, hearing loss, cliteromegaly, hypospadias, adrenocortical cytomegaly	Wilms tumor, hepatoblastoma, ACC, rhabdomyosarcoma, neuroblastoma, others
Isolated hemihyperplasia [18, 76] (OMIM%235000)	*IGF2* *CDKN1C* *H19* *LIT1* *KvLQT1*	*11p15* Mutations or altered methylation	1:86,000	Asymmetric growth involving one or more body parts, isolated, significant overlap with BWS and other overgrowth syndromes	Wilms tumor, hepatoblastoma, ACC, rhabdomyosarcoma, neuroblastoma, others
Li-Fraumeni syndrome [10–16, 37, 41, 43] (OMIM#151623)	*TP53*	*17p13*	1:20,000 or less common	Early age of onset of multiple cancers	*Typical LFS*: soft tissue sarcomas and osteosarcomas, breast cancer, brain tumors, leukemia, and ACC; *Extended LFS:* melanoma, prostate cancer, and pancreatic cancer, others
Familial adenomatous polyposis [49, 50, 78] (OMIM#175100)	*APC*	*5q21-22*	1:7,000–1:8,000	Colon polyps, congenital hypertrophy of the retina, epidermoid cysts, osteoma, desmoid tumor, pigmented epithelium, supernumerary teeth	Colon cancer, thyroid cancer, hepatoblastoma, ACC (?) *Turcot syndrome:* brain tumor

Table 10.2 (continued)

Syndrome	Genes	Locus	Prevalence	clinical features	associated neoplasias
Neurofibromatosis type 1 [75] (OMIM#162200)	*NF1*	*17q11.2*	1:962–1:7,800	Cafe ́au lait patches, skin-fold freckling, cutaneous neurofibromas, plexiform neurofibromas, optic pathway glioma, cerebral gliomas, Lisch nodules, skeletal abnormalities, severe cognitive impairment, learning problems, sphenoid wing dysplasia	Malignant peripheral nerve sheath tumor, malignant CNS tumors, pheochromocytoma, rhabdomyosarcoma, ACC (?)
Multiple endocrine neoplasia type 1 [59] (OMIM+131100)	*MENIN*	*11q13*	1:5,000–1:30,000	Facial angiofibromas, collagenomas, lipomas,	Pituitary adenomas, parathyroid adenomas, foregut carcinoids, pancreatic endocrine tumors (gastrinoma, insulinoma etc.), pheochromocytoma (?), ACC (?)

for a disturbance of p53-dependent pathways in experimental adrenocortical carcinogenesis is less well established. On the other hand, if one considers a possible association between familial adenomatous polyposis coli (FAP) and ACC, defective β-catenin signaling has been observed in sporadic cancers and there is increasing evidence for a role in ACCs in animal models, but the clinical association is less convincing. The details of this genetic and experimental dilemma will not be discussed in this section. Instead, the existing evidence will be outlined followed by clinical recommendations that might be offered based on this evidence. Specific issues regarding FAP, LFS, and Beckwith-Wiedemann syndrome (BWS) will be covered in subsequent chapters that detail the mechanisms involved in syndromes convincingly associated with ACC.

The first careful analysis of childhood ACC was published by Fraumeni et al. in 1967, by the same authors who later described the Li-Fraumeni syndrome, which has become one of the most widely recognized familial syndromes predisposing to cancer [9, 10]. Remarkably, this first publication included cases that, in retrospect, possibly could be identified either as classical LFS, neurofibromatosis type 1 (NF1), or BWS/idiopathic hemihypertrophy (IHH). Therefore, they already covered the two major associations in their descriptions, LFS and BWS/IHH (Tables 10.2 and 10.3). The authors also reported a subgroup with concurrent urogenital malformations, an association that has been well observed in the literature but to date has not been described as a distinct disease entity.

In the setting of genetic syndromes, most ACCs occur early in life, usually within the first decade (Table 10.4). According to the diagnostic criteria for LFS, ACC is a syndrome defining neoplasia and therefore there is a clear association between LFS and ACC (Tables 10.2–10.4) [11–16]. The association of ACC with BWS/IHH is also well confirmed (Table 10.3) [17]. Less clear is the association of ACC with FAP, MEN1, and NF1, which will be discussed in this overview as well as in the following chapters (Table 10.3). BWS/IHH patients present with ACC in early childhood, LFS patients usually present in childhood or adolescence and occasionally in young adults, and NF1 can present with ACC in adult life (Table 10.3) [15, 18–22]. MEN1 and FAP patients almost invariably present later in life, and at least in some cases an adrenal abnormality had already been confirmed before progression to a lesion with obvious malignant characteristics [4–7, 23–27]. In LFS and BWS/IHH, ACC can be the presenting malignancy, while in all others the syndrome diagnosis is usually already established and other symptoms or tumors are already present. Aside from the mentioned syndromes, descriptions of ACC as part of an inherited syndrome are very rare. It is worthwhile mentioning that there are reports of at least two cases of ACC in patients with Lynch syndrome and one with Werner syndrome [28–30]. ACC can also occur in patients with congenital adrenal hyperplasia [31].

The evidence presented in the following sections has been derived from a careful review of standard literature and textbooks as well as literature searches in Pubmed and Google scholar. In some cases personal communications and resources were used and are marked accordingly.

Table 10.3 Adrenal characteristics of syndromes reported to occur with ACC. Summary of adrenocortical phenotype and clinical data of ACC in cases of genetic syndromes in which ACC has been observed. Data are based on available case reports and patient series

Syndrome	Adrenocortical phenotype	Number reported	Association with ACC	Median size (cm)	Median age (years)	Age distribution (years)
Beckwith-Wiedemann syndrome (BWS) [17, 35, 74]	Adrenocortical cytomegaly, adrenal hyperplasia, adrenal cysts, ACC	Multiple	Established	N/A	<10	<10
Isolated hemihyperplasia (IHH) [17, 18, 20, 76]	Adenoma, ACC, possibly adrenocortical cytomegaly	Multiple	Established	N/A	<10	<10
Li-Fraumeni syndrome (LFS) [15, 16, 19]	ACC	Multiple	Part of diagnostic criteria	N/A	Female: 11.5 Male: 3	Female: 0.5–38 Male: 2–3.5
Familial adenomatous polyposis (FAP) [16, 23–25, 27, 50, 51, 54]	Adenoma (7.4–13%), unilateral and bilateral, functional lesions reported (14.3), ACC(?)	5	Not established	8.3 (5–10)	31	14–63
Neurofibromatosis type 1 (NF1) [21, 22, 80]	ACC(?)	4	Not established	1 ACC: 23	N/A	2–46 1 patient 46
Multiple endocrine neoplasia type 1 (MEN1) [4–7, 59]	36–55% with hyperplasia, adenoma (unilateral and bilateral), functional lesions reported, ACC(?)	6	Not established (max 2.6–6% of patients with adrenocortical lesions)	9.4 (7–15)	33	16–50

10.1 Syndromes Associated with Adrenocortical Cancer

10.1.1 The Overgrowth Syndromes: BWS and IHH

BWS and IHH are two of a myriad of slightly differing overgrowth syndromes, such as Simpson-Golabi-Behmel syndrome, Perlman syndrome, Proteus syndrome, Sotos syndrome. [17] Of these syndromes, only BWS and IHH have been shown to be associated with ACC and more specifically with childhood ACC [17]. It is still a matter of debate whether these two syndromes truly represent two different syndromes or two entities on the scale of one syndrome spectrum. Both diseases commonly show alterations of the *IGF2/H19* locus (see Chapters 14 and 15).

In his first report on this condition, Beckwith, for whom the syndrome is named in part, highlighted the characteristic cytomegaly of a hyperplastic adrenal cortex [32, 33]. The first description of adrenocortical cytomegaly in patients with the syndrome, which later became known as BWS and IHH, predates Beckwith's original description by 8 years [34]. Beatty and Hawes analyzed autopsies for adrenocortical cytomegaly and reported an association with isolated hemihypertrophy, omphalocele, and macroglossia [34]. The reason for this peculiar adrenocortical morphological alteration is unknown. Benign adrenal lesions can also occur in BWS patients [17]. Adenomas and hyperplasia have been described, but their number is exceeded by reports of large adrenal cysts, which are otherwise rather rare in the general population [17].

Soon after Beckwith and Wiedemann described the syndrome, it became evident that a minority of these patients are prone to develop certain childhood cancers with a higher frequency than observed in the general population [17]. These tumors commonly include Wilms tumor, hepatoblastoma, and ACC, but adrenomedullary tumors, specifically neuroblastomas and occasionally pheochromocytomas, have also been reported [17]. While an early analysis suggested that ACCs represented 15.6% of malignancies, a recent analysis states that ACCs comprise 7% of all reported malignancies in BWS [17, 35]. The association of BWS and ACC has mainly been confirmed by retrospective studies. The only large prospective study did not show any ACCs [36]. The cancer risk is mainly confined to childhood and adolescence, and only a minority (~8.8%) of BWS patients develop cancers [17]. The overall frequency of ACC in BWS is ~0.7%, which is rather low but still strikingly increased when compared to the estimated childhood ACC frequency of 0.3 per million in the general population [20, 37] (see Chapter 28).

The association between IHH and ACC has also been well established. The tumor spectrum of IHH and BWS has a significant overlap; the overall tumor frequency in one large study of 168 affected children was 5.9% and therefore slightly lower than in BWS [18]. ACC comprises 16% of all IHH-related tumors [17].

Genetic alterations, such as mutations or altered methylation, of the *IGF2/H19* locus lead to an increased IGF2 production in BWS/IHH [38]. Further support that this mechanism may play a significant role in carcinogenesis of sporadic ACCs comes from recent gene expression array studies, all of which find upregulation of IGF2 as one of the most prominent alterations in ACCs compared to benign lesions and normal adrenocortical tissue [39, 40].

Table 10.4 Diagnostic criteria for the main syndromes discussed in this chapter. Current diagnostic criteria for Beckwith-Wiedemann syndrome, idiopathic hemihyperplasia, Li-Fraumeni syndrome, familial adenomatous polyposis, neurofibromatosis type 1, multiple endocrine neoplasia type 1 are summarized. [a]Chompret criteria are not diagnostic criteria, but identify individuals for whom genetic testing would be recommended

Beckwith-Wiedemann syndrome (BWS)	Isolated hemihyperplasia (IHH)	Li-Fraumeni syndrome (LFS)	Familial adenomatous polyposis (FAP)	Neurofibromatosis type 1 (NF1)	Multiple endocrine neoplasia type 1 (MEN1)
DeBaun et al. (1998) [36]: Diagnosed by a physician AND at least two of the five common features associated with BWS • macroglossia • macrosomia • midline abdominal wall defects • ear creases/ear pits • neonatal hypoglycemia	*Clericuzio & Martin (2009)* [76]: • IHH should be apparent "from the end of the bed." • The asymmetry can be due to differences in the growth of bone and/or soft tissue • Diagnosis made by a clinical geneticist experienced in the differentiation of IHH from other causes of body asymmetry (including regional body undergrowth, seen for example with mild fibular hemimelia and hemiatrophy)	*Classic LFS* [16]: Patient with sarcoma before 45 years *AND* first-degree relative with cancer before 45 years *AND* first- or second-degree relative with any cancer before 45 years or with sarcoma at any age *Chompret* [12, 13][a]: Patient with sarcoma, brain tumor, breast cancer, or ACC before 36 years *AND* • at least one first- or second-degree relative with cancer (other than breast cancer if the patient has breast cancer) before 46 years	*Classic FAP* [49, 79]: One hundred or more colorectal adenomatous polyps, usually before age 40 years *OR* fewer than 100 adenomatous polyps and a relative with FAP *Gardner syndrome*: Colonic adenomatous polyposis, osteomas, and soft tissue tumors (epidermoid cysts, fibromas, desmoid tumors) *Turcot syndrome*: Colonic adenomatous polyposis and CNS tumors, usually medulloblastoma.	*NIH criteria* [75]: Two or more of the following features: • Six or more café au lait macules (>5 mm in prepubertal and >15 mm in postpubertal individuals • Two or more neurofibromas of any type or one plexiform neurofibroma • Freckling in the axillary or inguinal regions (Crowe's sign)	*MEN1* [73]: two of the three major manifestations: • parathyroid, • pancreatic neuroendocrine • pituitary tumors OR one major proband manifestation in a family member

Table 10.4 (continued)

Beckwith-Wiedemann syndrome (BWS)	Isolated hemihyperplasia (IHH)	Li-Fraumeni syndrome (LFS)	Familial adenomatous polyposis (FAP)	Neurofibromatosis type 1 (NF1)	Multiple endocrine neoplasia type 1 (MEN1)
Elliot et al. (1994) [74]: Three major features • anterior abdominal wall defect • macroglossia • pre- and/or post-natal overgrowth (>90th centile) OR two major plus three minor findings • ear pits • nevus flammeus • neonatal hypoglycemia • nephromegaly • hemihyperplasia deBaun Elliot et al. 1994	• The following diagnoses should be ruled out: • Other overgrowth syndromes (including BWS, proteus syndrome, NF1, mosaic trisomy 8) • Other disorders associated with vascular malformations (including Klippel-Trenaunay syndrome, megalencephaly-cutis marmorata telangiectatica congenita)	• *OR* a relative with multiple primaries at any age • *OR* a patient with multiple primary tumors, two of which are sarcoma, brain tumor, breast cancer, and/or ACC, with an initial cancer before the age of 36 years, regardless of the family history • *OR* patient with ACC at any age, regardless of the family history For families that do not conform to classic LFS:	*Attenuated FAP (AFAP* [78]): No family member with more than 100 polyps before age 30 years AND • At least two individuals with 10 to 99 adenomas diagnosed after age 30 years	• Optic glioma • Two or more Lisch nodules (iris harmartomas) • A distinctive osseous lesion such as sphenoid dysplasia or thinning of long bone cortex with or without pseudoarthrosis • A first-degree relative (parent, sibling, or offspring) with NF1 by the above criteria	

Table 10.4 (continued)

Beckwith-Wiedemann syndrome (BWS)	Isolated hemihyperplasia (IHH)	Li-Fraumeni syndrome (LFS)	Familial adenomatous polyposis (FAP)	Neurofibromatosis type 1 (NF1)	Multiple endocrine neoplasia type 1 (MEN1)
		Birch [11]: Patient with any childhood cancer or sarcoma, brain tumor, or ACC before 45 years *AND* a first- or second-degree relative with a typical LFS-related cancer (sarcoma, breast cancer, brain tumor, leukemia, or ACC) at any age *AND* a first- or second-degree relative in the same genetic lineage with any cancer before 60 years *Eeles* [14]: Two different tumors that are part of extended LFS in first- or second-degree relative at any age (sarcoma, breast cancer, brain tumor, leukemia, ACC, melanoma, prostate cancer, and pancreatic cancer)	• OR one individual with 10–99 adenomas diagnosed after age 30 years and a first-degree relative with colorectal cancer with a few adenomas Gardner syndrome and Turcot syndrome are subvariants of classical FAP.		

10.1.2 Li–Fraumeni Syndrome

LFS is a rare syndrome. Recent estimations suggest a prevalence of 1:20,000 (Tables 10.3 and 10.4) [15]. The inheritance of LFS was first described in 1967, and in 1990 *TP53* was identified as the gene mutated in LFS [10, 41]. Subsequently, somatic mutations in the *TP53* gene were found in roughly 50% of all cancers, and multiple other mutations were identified negatively impacting the p53 pathway by either interfering with its upstream or downstream signaling events or by over-expression of negative modulators of p53 activity [42]. There are several different criteria used to diagnose LFS [11–16, 42]. Almost all of them include ACC as a disease-specific neoplasia (Table 10.4). Recently, LFS patients with mutations in genes other than *TP53* (e.g., *CHK2*) have been described [43]. To our knowledge to date, ACC has not been described in LFS families with mutations other than *TP53*.

Childhood ACCs commonly occur as part of the LFS with classical *TP53* mutations, but several low-penetrance alleles have been identified causing only ACC, but no other classical LFS-associated neoplasias (see Chapters 11, 12, 28) [37, 42]. Roughly, 1 out of 10 carriers of these low-penetrance alleles develop ACC [37, 42]. Interestingly, only a few adult cases of ACC have been described in LFS [15]. In sporadic adult ACC, *TP53* mutations can be found in about 20–70% of cases [44–46]. Furthermore, nuclear or cellular p53 accumulation can be found in the striking majority of adult ACC cases, but not adrenocortical adenomas, underscoring the importance of the disturbance of this pathway in adrenocortical carcinogenesis [45].

ACC is the third to fifth most common tumor in LFS. with a frequency of 6.5–9.9% [13, 15]. ACC is of special importance because it specifically can be the first tumor to be diagnosed in LFS patients. The median age of onset has been reported between 3 and 11.5 years of age [15, 19]. As ACC is usually a rare tumor in childhood, the diagnosis should immediately raise the suspicion for LFS, and childhood ACC patients often serve as index cases. Some of the proposed LFS diagnostic criteria may have slightly overemphasized the role of ACC in making the diagnosis of LFS. For example, Chompret et al. and more recently Gonzalez et al. suggest that ACCs at any age warrant an evaluation a diagnostic work-up for LFS [12, 15]. Due to the fact that childhood ACC is a classical index neoplasia of LFS, most studies are skewed towards analysis of ACC patients at a young age. To date evidence for adult ACC as part of LFS is sparse, but further studies need to be conducted to prove or disprove the relationship between adult ACC and LFS.

10.1.3 Familial Adenomatous Polyposis

There are two syndromes closely related to FAP, which should be defined here. While FAP refers to the presence of multiple, usually >100 colonic polyps, Gardner syndrome is defined as FAP with certain extracolonic manifestations, such as osteomas, epidermoid cysts, and desmoid tumors. Turcot syndrome is FAP together with CNS tumors, such as medulloblastomas. FAP, Gardner syndrome and Turcot syndrome are caused by inactivating mutations in the *APC* gene (Tables 10.2–10.4) [47–49].

The *APC* gene codes for a protein that sequesters the transcriptional activator β-catenin in the cytoplasm, rendering it inactive. Nuclear translocation and activation of β-catenin represent the endpoint of the WNT-signaling pathway and lead to the transcription of β-catenin/WNT-signaling activated genes. Loss of function mutations of *APC* consequently lead to autonomous target gene activation by β-catenin.

There are several large studies that document adrenocortical pathologies in FAP patients. The overall risk to develop an adrenocortical adenomas (ACA) ranges from 7.4% to 13% in different studies, roughly double that in the normal population [50, 51]. The risk to develop functional lesions is not clear. There is a significant number of case reports of adenomas producing cortisol or aldosterone in FAP patients [52, 53]. In the two largest studies only 2/162 and 0/107 FAP patients showed evidence of adrenocortical hyperfunction [50, 51]. Whether there is an increased risk for the development of ACC is still unclear. Interestingly, there are at least seven reports of FAP patients carrying malignant adrenocortical lesions in the literature, of which three describe the same patient from the Cleveland Clinic [23–27, 50, 54]. Therefore the total number of reported patients is five. One of the tumors had an unusual sex cord-like differentiation, another one is described as a cortisol-, and possibly androgen-secreting tumor and two tumors were nonfunctional. For one lesion there is no comment on functionality. Two of the ACCs had undergone classic loss of heterozygosity (LOH) at the APC locus [25, 27]. LOH has also been observed in adrenocortical adenomas associated with FAP [55, 56]. Taking into account the current estimation of a prevalence of FAP as 1:7,500, the subpopulation within FAP patients that actually develop ACC seems to be negligible [57]. Nevertheless, there is substantial evidence for frequent somatic mutations of β-catenin within benign and malignant tumors of the adrenal cortex [39, 58]. None of the published patients had developed ACC as an index manifestation of FAP. All had been diagnosed with FAP earlier and most of them had undergone prophylactic bowel surgery. Potentially, all colonic polyps represent premalignant lesions, but only one or a few will progress to an overt colon cancer. Like the colonic polyps, the common adrenocortical adenomas may represent premalignant lesions, but because of their much lower number and possibly less exposure to additional carcinogens chances to develop an ACC are significantly lower. Therefore, a certain bias may exist that FAP patients in the past did not reach the age to develop ACC, but diagnosis of ACC may become more frequent in the future with increasing awareness of the disease, increasing patient survival and surveillance, and prophylactic treatment.

10.1.4 Multiple Endocrine Neoplasia Type 1

Mutations in the *MENIN* gene cause MEN1, a syndrome which primarily comprised parathyroid, pancreatic, and pituitary tumors (Tables 10.2–10.4) [59]. The syndrome was first described by Paul Wermer in 1954 [8]; the *MENIN* gene was cloned in 1997, includes 10 exons and is located on chromosome 11q13 [60]. The knock out mouse model manifests some of the features observed in human patients [61]. With regards to the adrenal gland, *Menin* knock out mice develop tumors, which are referred to as adrenocortical cancers, but most likely represent tumors of unknown malignant potential, as the authors do not mention any metastasis, invasion, or mitotic counts [61].

There is slightly more evidence for an association of ACC with MEN1 than with FAP. As with FAP, there is a clear association with benign lesions with a frequency that ranges between 36 and 55% [5, 7, 62]. Hyperplasias (uni- or bilateral) represent most of the adrenocortical pathologies, followed by adenomas and rare ACCs. Most of these tumors are nonfunctional, but hypercortisolism, feminization, and even aldosterone production have been reported [59, 63, 64]. Two studies have focused on the frequency of functional lesions. The first study reports one cortisol-secreting adenoma, one virilizing ACC and one pheochromocytoma in 21 of 38 MEN1 patients with adrenal lesions [5]. The second study, analyzing patients with Zollinger Ellison syndrome (ZES) and MEN1, details two cortisol-secreting adenomas and one pheochromocytoma in 48 of 107 MEN1 patients with adrenal lesions [62]. A total of six ACC cases in association with MEN1 have been reported, four of which are reported in one larger study [4–7], suggesting that as many as 22% of adrenal lesions may be malignant and that the overall lifetime risk of ACC in MEN1 patients may be as high as 6% [5]. Other studies suggest a lifetime risk in a range of 2.6% [7]. The association is also mentioned in the most recent version of the "*Concise Handbook of Familial Cancer Susceptibility Syndromes*" [65]. However, taking the overall prevalence of MEN1 into account, which is estimated about 1:5,000 to 1:30,000, the total number of six reported cases is rather small (see discussion in Introduction) [2, 3]. Therefore, the actual risk for MEN1 patients to develop an ACC may be lower than estimated by these single studies. The majority of reported ACCs have been functional lesions leading to hypercortisolism, virilization, or feminization. In all cases ACCs developed after diagnosis of the syndrome, and in at least two cases an adrenal lesion was already known, but over the time of follow-up progressed significantly in size which warranted surgery [5, 6]. Interestingly, it has been suggested that adrenocortical tumors predominantly arise in patients with pancreatic endocrine tumors [7, 62]. This observation may link the IGF-system to ACCs in MEN1. This may also explain the observation that none of the studies analyzing sporadic ACC found a bona fide LOH as a mechanism underlying carcinogenesis [66]. Classical LOH of the 11q13 locus, which includes the *MENIN* gene, occurs frequently in sporadic adrenocortical tumors, but almost invariably the remaining *MENIN* allele is intact and *MENIN* mRNA levels are normal [67]. No classical LOH was found in any MEN1-associated adrenocortical tumors, except for one aldosterone-producing adenoma [6, 63, 68]. This may further support the hypothesis that, at least with respect to adrenocortical lesions, *MENIN* may not serve as a classical tumor suppressor gene. Perhaps other changes, such as endocrine factors secreted by, for example, pancreatic tumors may fuel adrenocortical growth and consequently emergence of adrenocortical hyperplasia, adenomas, and possibly ACC. In one case an ACA was identified in a patient, who subsequently developed a carcinoid of the lung. Therefore a benign adrenal lesion, but not an ACC, is more likely to be the presenting lesion in MEN1 [69].

10.1.5 Neurofibromatosis Type 1

Hereditary neurofibromatosis type 1 is caused by mutations in the neurofibromin gene, which consists of 57 exons encoding a protein that has GTPase activity and thereby regulates RAS activity, inhibiting cellular growth and proliferation. *NF1*, together with *VHL*, *SDHx*, and *RET* germline mutations, have been well recognized to predispose individuals to the development of pheochromocytoma [70]. The frequency of developing these tumors within the NF1 patient population is estimated to be 0.1–5.7% [70]. In a study analyzing 27 sporadic pheochromocytomas, one patient could be identified having a germline NF1 mutation without having been previously diagnosed with this syndrome [71]. It was determined retrospectively that this patient displayed classical symptoms and signs of NF1. The overall risk to develop a malignant adrenocortical lesion is not well established. The literature mentions four different cases of ACC in the setting of NF1, one of which is a case report of a metastasized ACC leading to virilization and Cushing's syndrome in a 3-year-old female [22]. Another case report describes an ACC in a 2-year old female with virilization [80]. The two other ACCs were observed in a large study by Sorensen et al. during long-term follow-up of 212 patients [21]. Interestingly, this study identifies another three patients with pheochromocytoma. Therefore, according to this large study ACC may be almost as common as pheochromocytoma in these patients. On the contrary, the total report of four cases in a disease with a prevalence of ~1:3000 is not convincing [72]. In conclusion, while ACC is included in the differential diagnosis of an adrenocortical lesion of any NF1 patient, future analysis will need to assess the real ACC frequency within NF1 patients.

10.2 Screening for Germline Mutations in Adrenocortical Cancer Patients

An important question that arises in the clinical setting is when to recommend genetic counseling and testing for a germline mutation. As always in clinical practice, a thorough history and physical examination are important to identify possible genetic syndromes. In general, genetic testing of adult ACC patients for NF1, MEN1, and FAP should not be recommended, as evidence for an association of these syndromes with ACC is currently unconvincing. Furthermore, to date in all patients reported with both conditions, the syndromes had been diagnosed before the time of ACC diagnosis. There are no studies that prove ACC to be the single or first manifestation of these syndromes. However, in the presence of a typical family history or other clinical and pathological findings, genetic testing may be warranted (e.g., for FAP in a patient with coexisting multiple colon polyps or for MEN1 in a patient with coexisting hyperparathyroidism). NF1 almost always is a clinical diagnosis and can be readily identified by a medical geneticist. Physical examination and medical history will also identify most patients with an overgrowth syndrome, and the diagnosis can usually be made on a clinical basis. Furthermore, because the sensitivity of genetic testing for these conditions is limited by the diversity of possible genetic mutations, clinical findings and family history remain paramount in establishing these diagnoses.

Diagnosis of LFS may be more difficult as the family history and/or patient history are the only clues to diagnosis. Furthermore, because certain *TP53* alleles have different penetrance, a child with ACC may be the only affected family member. Other tumors of the LFS spectrum are somewhat more common in the general population than ACC and do not immediately raise the clinical suspicion for LFS. Therefore, ACC frequently serves as an index neoplasia. As pointed out earlier, there are several clinical criteria for the diagnosis of LFS. According to Chompret et al. and another recent analysis, ACC at any age qualifies for a clinical suspicion for LFS [12, 15]. While this conclusion is valid for all published studies, it is clearly biased by the analysis of primarily childhood and adolescence ACC. Interestingly, the more recent studies report an older age of median onset and an age distribution up to 38 years of age [15]. Therefore, any family with a child or adolescent with ACC should be recommended to undergo genetic counseling and genetic testing for *TP53* mutations or other LFS-like associated mutations. However, in contrast with LFS, so far no ACC has been described in LFS-like cases. Strictly reading the current LFS criteria and taking into account recent reports of older patients (up to 38 years) harboring *TP53* mutations, the same recommendation for genetic counseling and testing may be made for adults with ACC. The evidence for testing adult ACC patients is much lower. However, to overcome the current lack of evidence, genetic analysis, particularly as part of research studies, should be encouraged.

In summary, if a syndrome for which an association with ACC has been suggested is clinically suspected, clinicians should proceed with confirmatory tests and genetic counseling. Without any symptoms or signs that may suggest a hereditary syndrome and in the absence of a significant family history, there is only evidence for genetic testing in ACC patients for LFS, especially in cases diagnosed during childhood and adolescence.

10.3 Screening and Surveillance of Patients with Hereditary Syndromes Predisposing to Adrenocortical Cancer

For all syndromes discussed above, with the exception of LFS, guidelines for clinical surveillance are in place [20, 36, 49, 73–75]. However, there are no specific recommendations for any of these syndromes that specifically focus on the surveillance or detection of adrenocortical lesions. Given the potential association of these syndromes with increased risk for ACC, it is imperative that clinicians are aware of the possibility of adrenocortical lesions. Thus, they should look for any hormone-production abnormality that can be identified in clinical exam, history, and basic laboratory evaluations. In addition, because not all lesions will be hormone-producing, clinicians should consider imaging to identify adrenocortical lesions, specifically in the case of LFS families. When employing imaging for screening, clinicians should whenever possible rely on techniques that do not employ ionizing radiation. Most other patients with ACC-associated syndromes undergo imaging surveillances for abdominal tumors, which most likely will cover the adrenal glands too. For MEN1 patients annual CT or MRI imaging of the pancreas is recommended, and for BWS/IHH patients ultrasound screening for Wilms tumor and hepatoblastoma is recommended [20, 73, 76]. Both approaches can sufficiently visualize the area of the adrenal glands as well. With MEN1 a special focus should be on patients with a concurrent pancreatic lesion, because of the suggestion that these patients may be more likely to develop an adrenocortical lesion [7]. Neither the guidelines for NF1 or FAP include any abdominal imaging procedure [49, 75]. Regarding NF1 no abdominal imaging is recommended, but regular assessment for pubertal development is recommended, which would possibly detect virilizing tumors as well [75]. Due to the increased risk of renal artery stenosis (2%) and pheochromocytoma regular blood pressure measurements are recommended, which could possibly detect cortisol- or aldosteorone-related hypertension as well [75]. The current FAP surveillance guidelines do mention adrenocortical adenomas as a manifestation of the disease, but do not make recommendations for detection or surveillance of adrenocortical lesions [49]. One publication specifically discusses the surveillance of adrenocortical tumors, which basically follow the suggested NIH-guidelines for incidentally discovered adrenal masses (see Chapter 5) [77].

If an adrenal lesion is found in these syndromes diagnostic work-up should follow the guidelines used for the evaluation of incidentally discovered adrenal masses, although per definition these lesions would technically not be defined as incidentally discovered adrenal masses. The only difference is that work-up should be done under the premise of a higher pre-test probability for ACC, a functional adenoma (e.g., FAP) and/or pheochromocytoma (e.g., NF1).

References

1. Bilimoria KY (2008) Adrenocortical carcinoma in the United States: treatment utilization and prognostic factors. Cancer 113(11):3130–3136
2. Agarwal SK (2004) Molecular pathology of the MEN1 gene. Ann N Y Acad Sci 1014: 189–198
3. Gardner D (2007) Multiple endocrine neoplasia. In: Gardner D (ed) Greenspan's basic and clinical endocrinology, D.a.S. McGraw-Hill: New York
4. Langer P (2002) Adrenal involvement in multiple endocrine neoplasia type 1. World J Surg 26(8):891–896
5. Waldmann J (2007) Adrenal involvement in multiple endocrine neoplasia type 1: results of 7 years prospective screening. Langenbecks Arch Surg 392(4):437–443
6. Skogseid B (1992) Clinical and genetic features of adrenocortical lesions in multiple endocrine neoplasia type 1. J Clin Endocrinol Metab 75(1):76–81

7. Skogseid B (1995) Adrenal lesion in multiple endocrine neoplasia type 1. Surgery 118(6):1077–1082
8. Wermer P (1954) Genetic aspects of adenomatosis of endocrine glands. Am J Med 16(3): 363–371
9. Fraumeni JF Jr, Miller RW (1967) Adrenocortical neoplasms with hemihypertrophy, brain tumors, and other disorders. J Pediatr 70(1):129–138
10. Li FP , Fraumeni JF Jr (1969) Soft-tissue sarcomas, breast cancer, and other neoplasms. A familial syndrome? Ann Intern Med 71(4):747–752
11. Birch JM (1994) Prevalence and diversity of constitutional mutations in the p53 gene among 21 Li-Fraumeni families. Cancer Res 54(5):1298–1304
12. Chompret A (2001) Sensitivity and predictive value of criteria for p53 germline mutation screening. J Med Genet 38(1):43–47
13. Chompret A (2000) P53 germline mutations in childhood cancers and cancer risk for carrier individuals. Br J Cancer 82(12):1932–1937
14. Eeles RA (1995) Germline mutations in the TP53 gene. Cancer Surv 25:101–124
15. Gonzalez KD (2009) Beyond Li Fraumeni Syndrome: clinical characteristics of families with p53 germline mutations. J Clin Oncol 27(8):1250–1256
16. Li FP (1988) A cancer family syndrome in twenty-four kindreds. Cancer Res 48(18): 5358–5362
17. Lapunzina P (2005) Risk of tumorigenesis in overgrowth syndromes: a comprehensive review. Am J Med Genet C Semin Med Genet 137C(1):53–71
18. Hoyme HE (1998) Isolated hemihyperplasia (hemihypertrophy): report of a prospective multicenter study of the incidence of neoplasia and review. Am J Med Genet 79(4): 274–278
19. Olivier M (2003) Li-Fraumeni and related syndromes: correlation between tumor type, family structure, and TP53 genotype. Cancer Res 63(20):6643–6650
20. Tan TY, Amor DJ (2006) Tumour surveillance in Beckwith-Wiedemann syndrome and hemihyperplasia: a critical review of the evidence and suggested guidelines for local practice. J Paediatr Child Health, 2006. 42(9):486–490
21. Sorensen SA et al (1986) Long-term follow-up of von Recklinghausen neurofibromatosis. Survival and malignant neoplasms. N Engl J Med 314(16):1010–1015
22. Wagner AS et al (2005) Pediatric adrenal cortical carcinoma: brain metastases and relationship to NF-1, case reports and review of the literature. J Neurooncol 75(2):127–133
23. Marshall WH et al (1967) Gardner's syndrome with adrenal carcinoma. Australas Ann Med 16(3):242–244
24. Painter TA, Jagelman DG (1985), Adrenal adenomas and adrenal carcinomas in association with hereditary adenomatosis of the colon and rectum. Cancer 55(9): 2001–2004
25. Seki M (1992) Loss of normal allele of the APC gene in an adrenocortical carcinoma from a patient with familial adenomatous polyposis. Hum Genet 89(3):298–300
26. Traill Z et al (1995) Adrenal carcinoma in a patient with Gardner's syndrome: imaging findings. AJR Am J Roentgenol 165(6):1460–1461
27. Wakatsuki S (1998) Adrenocortical tumor in a patient with familial adenomatous polyposis: a case associated with a complete inactivating mutation of the APC gene and unusual histological features. Hum Pathol 29(3):302–306
28. Broaddus RR (2004) Unusual tumors associated with the hereditary nonpolyposis colorectal cancer syndrome. Mod Pathol 17(8):981–989
29. Berends MJ (2000) Adrenocortical adenocarcinoma in an MSH2 carrier: coincidence or causal relation? Hum Pathol 31(12):1522–1527
30. Takazawa R (2004) Unusual double primary neoplasia: adrenocortical and ureteral carcinomas in Werner syndrome. Urol Int 72(2):168–170
31. Varan A (2000) Adrenocortical carcinoma associated with adrenogenital syndrome in a child. Med Pediatr Oncol 35(1):88–90

32. Beckwith J (1963) Extreme cytomegaly of the adrenal fetal cortex, omphalocele, hyperplasia of kidneys and pancreas, and Leydig-cell hyperplasia: Another syndrome? Western Society for Pediatric Research, Los Angeles, CA
33. Beckwith JB (1955) Vignettes from the history of overgrowth and related syndromes. Am J Med Genet 79(4):238–248
34. Beatty EC Jr, Hawes CR (1955) Cytomegaly of the adrenal gland. AMA Am J Dis Child 89(4):463–467
35. Wiedemann H (1983) Tumours and Hemihypertrophy associated with Wiedemann-Beckwith syndrome. Eur J Pediatr 141:129
36. DeBaun MR (2002) Epigenetic alterations of H19 and LIT1 distinguish patients with Beckwith-Wiedemann syndrome with cancer and birth defects. Am J Hum Genet 70(3): 604–611
37. Figueiredo BC (2006) Penetrance of adrenocortical tumours associated with the germline TP53 R337H mutation. J Med Genet 43(1):91–96
38. Weksberg R et al (2005) Beckwith-Wiedemann syndrome. Am J Med Genet C Semin Med Genet 137C(1):12–23
39. Giordano TJ (2009) Molecular classification and prognostication of adrenocortical tumors by transcriptome profiling. Clin Cancer Res 15(2):668–676
40. Giordano TJ (2003) Distinct transcriptional profiles of adrenocortical tumors uncovered by DNA microarray analysis. Am J Pathol 162(2):521–531
41. Malkin D (1990) Germ line p53 mutations in a familial syndrome of breast cancer, sarcomas, and other neoplasms. Science 250(4985):1233–1238
42. Zambetti GP (2007) The p53 mutation "gradient effect" and its clinical implications. J Cell Physiol 213(2):370–373
43. Bell DW (1999) Heterozygous germ line hCHK2 mutations in Li-Fraumeni syndrome. Science 286(5449):2528–2531
44. Barzon L (2001) Molecular analysis of CDKN1C and TP53 in sporadic adrenal tumors. Eur J Endocrinol 145(2):207–212
45. Reincke M (1994) p53 mutations in human adrenocortical neoplasms: immunohistochemical and molecular studies. J Clin Endocrinol Metab 78(3):790–794
46. Reincke M (1996) p53 mutations in adrenal tumors: Caucasian patients do not show the exon 4 "hot spot" found in Taiwan. J Clin Endocrinol Metab 81(10):3636–3638
47. Gardner EJ (1951) A genetic and clinical study of intestinal polyposis, a predisposing factor for carcinoma of the colon and rectum. Am J Hum Genet 3(2):167–176
48. Turcot J et al (1959) Malignant tumors of the central nervous system associated with familial polyposis of the colon: report of two cases. Dis Colon Rectum 2:465–468
49. Vasen HF (2008) Guidelines for the clinical management of familial adenomatous polyposis (FAP). Gut 57(5):704–713
50. Marchesa P (1997) Adrenal masses in patients with familial adenomatous polyposis. Dis Colon Rectum 40(9):1023–1028
51. Smith TG (2000) Adrenal masses are associated with familial adenomatous polyposis. Dis Colon Rectum 43(12):1739–1742
52. Alexander GL et al (2000) Primary aldosteronism in a patient with familial adenomatous polyposis. Mayo Clin Proc 75(6):636–637
53. Beuschlein F (2000) Cortisol producing adrenal adenoma--a new manifestation of Gardner's syndrome. Endocr Res 26(4):783–790
54. Arvanitis ML (1990) Mortality in patients with familial adenomatous polyposis. Dis Colon Rectum 33(8):639–642
55. Blaker H (2004) Analysis of somatic APC mutations in rare extracolonic tumors of patients with familial adenomatous polyposis coli. Genes Chromosomes Cancer 41(2):93–98
56. Hosogi H (2009) Biallelic APC inactivation was responsible for functional adrenocortical adenoma in familial adenomatous polyposis with novel germline mutation of the apc gene: report of a case. Jpn J Clin Oncol 39(12):837–846

57. Offit K (1998) Clinical cancer genetics. 1st ed. 1998, New York: Wiley-Liss. 125–148
58. Tissier F (2005) Mutations of beta-catenin in adrenocortical tumors: activation of the Wnt signaling pathway is a frequent event in both benign and malignant adrenocortical tumors. Cancer Res 65(17):7622–7627
59. Schussheim DH (2001) Multiple endocrine neoplasia type 1: new clinical and basic findings. Trends Endocrinol Metab 12(4):173–178
60. Chandrasekharappa SC (1997) Positional cloning of the gene for multiple endocrine neoplasia-type 1. Science 276(5311):404–407
61. Crabtree JS (2001) A mouse model of multiple endocrine neoplasia, type 1, develops multiple endocrine tumors. Proc Natl Acad Sci U S A 98(3):1118–1123
62. Gibril F (2004) Multiple endocrine neoplasia type 1 and Zollinger-Ellison syndrome: a prospective study of 107 cases and comparison with 1009 cases from the literature. Medicine (Baltimore) 83(1):43–83
63. Beckers A (1992) Aldosterone-secreting adrenal adenoma as part of multiple endocrine neoplasia type 1 (MEN1): loss of heterozygosity for polymorphic chromosome 11 deoxyribonucleic acid markers, including the MEN1 locus. J Clin Endocrinol Metab 75(2):564–570
64. Trump D (1996) Clinical studies of multiple endocrine neoplasia type 1 (MEN1). Qjm 89(9):653–669
65. Lindor NM (2008) Concise handbook of familial cancer susceptibility syndromes – second edition. J Natl Cancer Inst Monogr, 2008(38):1–93
66. Schulte KM (2000) Complete sequencing and messenger ribonucleic acid expression analysis of the MEN I gene in adrenal cancer. J Clin Endocrinol Metab 85(1):441–448
67. Schulte KM (1999) MEN I gene mutations in sporadic adrenal adenomas. Hum Genet 105(6):603–610
68. Vortmeyer AO (1999) Multiple endocrine neoplasia type 1: atypical presentation, clinical course, and genetic analysis of multiple tumors. Mod Pathol 12(9):919–924
69. Gortz B (1999) MEN1 gene mutation analysis of sporadic adrenocortical lesions. Int J Cancer 80(3):373–379
70. Karagiannis A (2007) Pheochromocytoma: an update on genetics and management. Endocr Relat Cancer 14(4):935–956
71. Bausch B (2006) Comprehensive mutation scanning of NF1 in apparently sporadic cases of pheochromocytoma. J Clin Endocrinol Metab 91(9):3478–3481
72. Rasmussen SA, Friedman JM (2000) NF1 gene and neurofibromatosis 1. Am J Epidemiol 151(1):33–40
73. Brandi ML (2001) Guidelines for diagnosis and therapy of MEN type 1 and type 2. J Clin Endocrinol Metab 86(12):5658–5671
74. Elliott M (1994) Clinical features and natural history of Beckwith-Wiedemann syndrome: presentation of 74 new cases. Clin Genet 46(2):168–174
75. Ferner RE (2007) Guidelines for the diagnosis and management of individuals with neurofibromatosis 1. J Med Genet 44(2):81–88
76. Clericuzio CL, Martin RA (2009) Diagnostic criteria and tumor screening for individuals with isolated hemihyperplasia. Genet Med 11(3):220–222
77. Ferrandez A (2006) An evidence-based, multidisciplinary approach to the clinical considerations, management, and surveillance of adrenal lesions in familial adenomatous polyposis: report of three cases. Dis Colon Rectum 49(11):1781–1790
78. Nielsen M (2007) Germline mutations in APC and MUTYH are responsible for the majority of families with attenuated familial adenomatous polyposis. Clin Genet 71(5):427–433
79. Gardner EJ, Richards RC (1953) Multiple cutaneous and subcutaneous lesions occurring simultaneously with hereditary polyposis and osteomatosis. Am J Hum Genet 5(2):139–147
80. Fienman NL, Yakovac WC (1970) Neurofibromatosis in childhood. J Pediatr 76(3):339–346.

Chapter 11
Li–Fraumeni Syndrome

David Malkin

11.1 Clinical Definition of LFS

In 1969, a remarkable cancer predisposition syndrome was reported by Li and Fraumeni. Using a classical epidemiologic approach, they retrospectively evaluated 280 medical charts and 418 death certificates of children diagnosed with rhabdomyosarcoma in the United States from 1960 to 1964 [1, 2]. Five families were identified in whom a second child had developed a soft tissue sarcoma. In addition, a high frequency of diverse cancer types were observed among the first- and second degree adult relatives along one ancestral line of each proband with cancer rates considerably in excess of those expected by chance alone. In addition to soft tissue sarcomas and pre-menopausal breast cancers, carcinomas of the lung, skin, pancreas or adrenal cortex, leukemia, and various brain tumors were also observed. Multiple metachronous primary neoplasms were also observed in several family members. Li and Fraumeni suggested that the occurrence of diverse neoplasms in these families might represent a counterpart of the tendency for a single individual to develop multiple primary tumors, and that these families represented a previously undescribed familial cancer syndrome, with transmission suggestive of an autosomal dominant gene.

Based on prospective analysis of 24 families, the "classic" Li-Fraumeni syndrome (LFS) (OMIM #151623) pedigree was defined as a proband with sarcoma diagnosed under age 45 years, who has a first-degree relative with any cancer under 45 years, plus another first- or second-degree relative with either any cancer under 45 years or a sarcoma at any age [3]. An example of a "classic" LFS family is shown in Fig. 11.1. To date, more than 400 LFS families have been reported. As more families have been ascertained, the list of possible or probable component tumors has been expanded to include choroid plexus carcinoma, gastric cancer, lymphoma, melanoma, germ cell tumor, Wilms tumor, and colorectal cancer [4]. Families

D. Malkin (✉)
Division of Hematology/Oncology, Department of Pediatrics, The Hospital for Sick Children, University of Toronto, 555 University Avenue, Toronto, ON M5G 1X8, Canada
e-mail: david.malkin@sickkids.ca

G.D. Hammer, T. Else (eds.), *Adrenocortical Carcinoma*,
DOI 10.1007/978-0-387-77236-3_11,

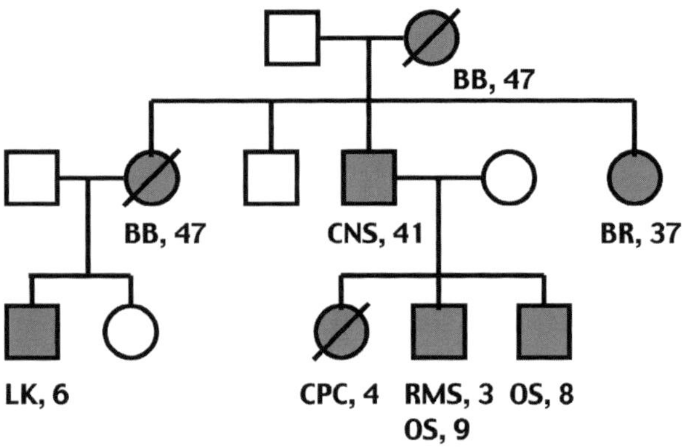

Fig. 11.1 Pedigree of a family with LFS. *Filled circles/squares* represent affected members; *slashes* represent deceased family members. *Numbers* represent age at diagnosis. BB, bilateral breast cancer; CNS, brain tumor; BR, unilateral breast cancer; LK, leukemia; CPC, choroid plexus carcinoma; RMS, rhabdomyosarcoma; OS, osteosarcoma

that do not conform to the criteria of classic LFS have been termed "LFS-Like (LFS-L)" [5]. These families were initially defined on the basis of a proband with any childhood cancer or sarcoma, brain tumor or adrenocortical carcinoma (ACC) diagnosed under 45 years of age with one first- or second-degree relative with a typical LFS cancer diagnosed at any age, plus a first- or second-degree relative in the same parental lineage with any cancer diagnosed under the age of 60 years. Chompret et al. [6] refined this definition further as: (1) a proband with a characteristic LFS tumor (sarcoma, brain tumor, breast cancer, adrenocortical carcinoma) before 36 years who has at least one first- or second-degree relative with a characteristic LFS tumor (other than breast cancer, if the proband has a breast cancer) before 46 years or; (2) a proband with multiple tumors, two of which represent characteristic LFS tumors and the first of which occurred before 36 years, or; (3) a proband with ACC whatever the age of onset or family history. Recently, this definition has again been modified, reflecting more comprehensive genotyping studies (see below) of kindred. The "Revised Chompret" criteria [7] increase the age of tumor onset, and focus on unique subsets of pediatric cancers for which genetic testing in the absence of a family history should be considered. Among these is adrenocortical carcinoma. In addition to the wide spectrum of tumor types observed in LFS, Hisada and colleagues showed that gene carriers are at significant risk of developing multiple synchronous or metachronous non-therapy-induced neoplasms [8]. Furthermore, affected individuals in these families who survived their first tumor are prone to develop second cancers, particularly if exposed to radiation therapy. In a retrospective study of 200 cancer-affected carriers of *TP53* germline mutations, 15% developed a second cancer, 4% a third cancer, and 2% a fourth cancer, with survivors of childhood malignancies being those with the highest risk of developing additional malignancies [8]. The overall relative risk of occurrence of a second cancer was 5.3 (95% CI = 2.8–7.8), with a cumulative probability of second cancer occurrence of 57%.

11.2 Cancer Risk Patterns in LFS Families

Even prior to identification of the gene associated with the majority of LFS cases, epidemiologic studies defined remarkable cancer-risk patterns within families. In a hospital-based analysis, the lifetime cancer risk of gene mutation carriers was estimated to be 73% in males and nearly 100% in females, with the high risk of breast cancer accounting for the difference. The specific risk for males is 19, 27, and 54% before the age of 15, 16–45 years, and >45years, respectively. The risk for females is 12, 82 and 100% before the age of 15, 16–45 years, and >45years, respectively [9]. A study by Hwang et al. [10] described the cancer risk in kindreds ascertained on the basis of childhood soft tissue sarcomas. Cancer risk was determined for gene mutation carriers and non-carriers who had been followed for greater than 20 years. Among the carriers, 12, 35, 52, and 80% developed cancer by ages 20, 30, 40, and 50 years, respectively. The most common cancers were breast cancer and soft tissue sarcomas. The 3201 non-carriers had a cumulative risk of 0.7, 1.0, 2.2, and 5.1% for the same ages, which is almost identical to that of the general population. While the number of carriers was similar in males and females, the cancer risks were not. The observed cancer risk was significantly higher in female carriers than males and, in contrast to the previous study presented, was not due to the incidence of breast cancer. At every age analyzed, females had a significantly higher incidence of cancer ($p < 0.001$). The specific cumulative risks for female carriers was found to be 18, 49, 77, and 93% by ages 20, 30, 40, and 50 years, compared with cumulative risks of 10, 21, 33, and 68% in male carriers at the same ages. Even after excluding sex-specific cancers (breast, ovarian, and prostate cancer), a higher female cancer risk was observed, including a higher risk for brain and lung cancer. Notwithstanding the intense interest in this unusual and highly penetrant syndrome, it was 20 years from its first description before the etiology of LFS was discovered.

11.3 The TP53 Tumor Suppressor

The *TP53* gene encodes a nuclear phosphoprotein, first identified in 1979 when it was observed that Simian polyomavirus (*SV40*) infection or transformation of mouse cells stimulated the synthesis or enhanced the stability of a 53 kDa protein of unknown function. This protein bound the large T antigen of SV40 and accumulated in the nuclei of chemically induced sarcomas and other transformed cells [11–13]. The human *TP53* gene is approximately 20 kb, contains 11 exons, and expresses a 2.8 kb mRNA transcript, which encodes a protein of 393 amino acids. The gene is located on the short arm of human chromosome 17 band 13.1 [14]. Extensive characterization of the TP53 gene and protein has been described and is depicted in Fig. 11.2. The gene has five phylogenetically conserved functional domains. The first domain is within the first and untranslated exon of the gene. The other four

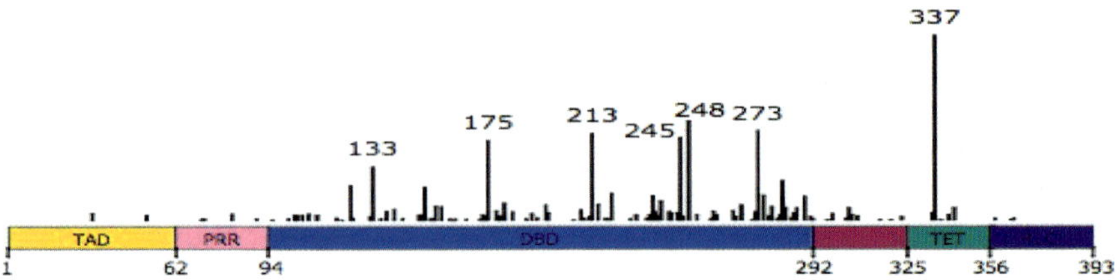

Fig. 11.2 Relative frequency of germline mutations in *p53* by codon adjacent to the primary structure of the p53 protein. TAD: Transactivation domain; PRR: proline-rich region; DBD: DNA-binding domain; TET: tetramerization domain; REG: regulatory domain. (Adapted from IARC database, Revision 14, November 2009)

domains are spanned by codons 129–146, 171–179, 234–269, and 270–287, which are within exons 4, 5, 7, and 8, respectively [15, 16]. Other biologically important regions include two SV40 large T antigen-binding sites, a nuclear localization signal, a transactivation signaling domain, an oligomerization domain, and several phosphorylation sites [17–21].

The TP53 protein is a tumor suppressor that plays key roles in cellular response pathways for cell cycle control, apoptosis, genomic stability, senescence, differentiation, and angiogenesis. Wild-type TP53 is expressed at low steady-state levels within cells. The regulation of TP53 occurs by various post-translational mechanisms including protein stability and degradation mediated by molecules such as calpain and Mdm2 [22, 23]. TP53 can become activated by multiple intracellular and extracellular mediators, which include both DNA-damaging and non-DNA-damaging agents. Signals of DNA damage can include DNA strand breaks, "bulky" DNA lesions, and nucleotide pool depletion. Signals of non-DNA damage can include markers of cellular stress such as hypoxia, changes in pH, antioxidants, as well as cold and heat shock. The actions of TP53 are carried out not only by the protein itself but also through its ability to interact and change the expression of specific target genes. Once activated, the protein begins to accumulate in the nucleus and undergoes modifications including conformational changes, phosphorylation of sites in both the C and N terminal domains, and acetylation of lysines, all of which can alter the function of the protein [24]. As well, a number of proteins have been identified that regulate TP53 function, including ABL which can bind to and stabilize the protein in response to DNA damage by preventing ubiquitination by Mdm2 and nuclear export [25].

As a transcription factor, TP53 can both upregulate and downregulate the expression of other genes. TP53 upregulates the expression of genes involved in cell cycle arrest and apoptosis pathways, such as cyclin-dependent kinase inhibitor *p21* (*CDKN1A*) and *BAX1*, respectively. With respect to cell cycle arrest, the TP53 protein and related family members inhibit cell cycle progression by initiating arrest at the G1, S, and G2 checkpoints in response to a variety of stress signals. These checkpoints are vital for the prevention of transmission of genetically unstable material to daughter cells and are regulated by the activation of cyclin-dependent kinase (CDK) complexes. TP53 also downregulates other genes that contribute to cell cycle progression at the G1 checkpoint. TP53 can also initiate G2/M arrest by upregulating genes such as *p21* (*CDKN1A*), *GADD45*, and *14-3-3σ* (*SFN*), all of which are involved in disrupting and inhibiting the cyclinB/cdc2 complex needed for progression to the mitosis phase of the cell cycle [26, 27]. By preventing cell cycle progression in response to DNA damage signals, TP53 functions to maintain genomic integrity [28].

In addition to its role in cell cycle control, TP53 also plays an important role in apoptotic pathways. TP53 induces apoptosis, in times of cellular stress, through mitochondrial depolarization and sensitization of cells to apoptotic inducers. As mitochondria are responsible for the release of many pro-apoptotic factors, the integrity of the mitochondrial membrane plays a central role in regulating apoptosis. TP53 can thus regulate apoptotic pathways by modulating the expression of genes involved in modifying mitochondrial permeability [29], or by sensitizing cells to apoptosis through increasing the expression of cellular death receptors, such as *FAS* and *KILLER/DR5* (*TNFRSF10B*) [30, 31]. As a regulator of apoptosis, TP53 is a cellular gatekeeper, constantly surveying cellular stress.

11.4 *TP53* Gene Inactivation

Alteration of TP53 function most frequently occurs through inactivating mutations of amino acid residues that alter the protein's structural or functional integrity leading to genomic instability. Inactivation of TP53 function occurs via several mechanisms including alterations in the DNA sequence, changes in protein conformation, and binding of cellular proteins to the TP53 protein. DNA sequence alterations include missense mutations, deletions, and nonsense mutations that prevent the protein from forming tetrameric complexes required to bind specific DNA sequences [32]. Studies of representative mutants from *TP53* mutation "hotspot" regions show that the majority of mutants lose TP53's ability to bind TP53 target-binding sites and thus can no longer activate the expression of target genes [18–33]. In fact, 80% of point mutations occur in the DNA-binding region. Interestingly, missense mutations, the most common genetic change in *TP53*, markedly prolong the half-life of the TP53 protein. Thus, "positive" expression of the gene/protein (as commonly visualized by immunostaining techniques) occurs with missense mutations even when the protein's function is diminished [34]. Mutations in the DNA sequence can also lead to changes in protein conformation that expose epitopes altering the protein's functions. It is also possible that these mutations can affect areas other than the mutated site in functionally important domains downstream [32]. Mutations that cause changes in protein conformation affect normal TP53 function, as these functions also rely on proper conformation and oligomerization of the protein [35]. A "dominant negative" complex forms, as the mutant TP53 tetramers no longer properly bind to target DNA sequences or transcriptionally activate target genes.

TP53 function can also be compromised through the binding of other cellular proteins to the TP53 protein itself. For example, viral oncogenes such as the *SV40* T-antigen, the *E1B* adenovirus gene, and the *E6* human papilloma virus gene, all encode proteins that bind to TP53 and prevent the expression of various TP53 target genes [35]. As well, binding of the *Mdm2* gene product inhibits the transactivation of genes by the TP53 molecule. In fact, *Mdm2* overexpression has been found in human sarcomas, and consequent TP53 dysfunction has been suggested as a culprit in this malignant process [36].

Inactivating mutations of *TP53* and disruptions of the TP53 protein are observed in some fraction of virtually every sporadically occurring malignancy. In fact, as of November 2009, the IARC *TP53* Mutation Database identified the existence of 26,597 somatic mutations reported in 1769 original publications, 535 germline mutations reported in 2197 publications, as well as functional information on 2314 mutant proteins (http://www-p53.iarc.fr/index.html).

11.5 TP53 and the LFS

In 1990, a candidate gene approach was taken to determine the underlying genetic lesion in LFS [37]. Based on earlier observations that somatic mutations of *TP53* were observed in greater than 50% of sporadic human cancers [38], and that *TP53* transgenic mice carrying mutant *TP53* alleles developed a wide spectrum of malignancies [39], *TP53* was examined in the constitutional DNA of LFS kindreds. While heterozygous point mutations were initially detected in 5 of 5 families, numerous subsequent studies have since shown that only 60–80% of "classic" LFS families harbor detectable germline *TP53* mutations [4, 40, 41], while the majority of LFS-like families do not harbor detectable *TP53* mutations in the coding regions of the gene [42, 43]. Studies in the United States and in Europe have suggested that germline *p53* mutations occur at the rate of about 1:5,000 individuals [44]. The lack of 100% concordance between *TP53* mutations and the classic phenotype may be explained in several ways, including post-translational TP53 alterations, complete *TP53* deletion, the effects of modifier genes, or alterations of other genes influencing the phenotype generated by the presence of specific germline alterations. Recently, lesions within introns or the regulatory regions of the gene have been identified, although their functional significance is unclear. The spectrum of mutations detected in the germline reflects those found in sporadic tumors; the majority occurs within the DNA-binding domain of the gene, primarily confined to highly conserved regions (Fig.11.2). However, it is important to note that of the germline mutations found to date, few are located outside the coding regions of exons 5–8 [45]. The most common mutations found in both sporadic tumors and in the germline are in codons 175, 245, 248, 273, and 282, although their order of frequency varies between the two groups [43; http://www-p53.iarc.fr/index.html].

Functional analysis of the germline *TP53* mutations has been carried out to establish the significance of these mutations and structural features of the corresponding TP53 proteins. In vitro analysis of TP53 alterations reveals that not all are associated with the inhibition of growth arrest, apoptosis, transcriptional activation, or an increased cancer risk. In fact, it is believed that in humans, the limited organ or target cell specificity of *TP53* mutations may be due to varying genetic backgrounds, acquisition of subsequent gene alterations in target tissues, or the influence of epigenetic or environmental factors. Importantly, these studies determined that certain *TP53* mutations might change the amino acid sequence in a conserved domain, yet are not associated with an increased risk of cancer [46]. As well, these studies were able to explain the functional significance of heterozygous germline mutations, such as those at codon 245, by showing the transdominant effect of some mutant *TP53* alleles on wild-type *TP53* DNA binding and T-antigen binding [47].

11.6 The Role of Other Genes in LFS

The absence of detectable germline *TP53* mutations in some LFS families has suggested the involvement of other genes, but this hypothesis remains controversial. Numerous genes involved in TP53 pathway, apoptosis, or cell cycle control, such as *TP63* [48], *BCL10* [49], *BAX* [50], *p14ARF* (*CDKN2A*) [51, 52], *PTEN* [51, 53], and *CHEK1* [54, 55], have been considered as candidate genes for LFS, but all these studies have provided negative results. Germline mutations of *CHEK2*, encoding a kinase able to phosphorylate Cdc25c and TP53, were initially reported in one LFS family and two families suggestive of LFS [54], but one alleged mutation, 1422delT, was subsequently shown to be on a duplicated exon [56]. The two other reported mutations, Ile157Thr and 1100delC, found in a total of four families suggestive of LFS [54, 55], were subsequently shown to be polymorphisms, whose allele frequency has been respectively estimated to 0.12–1.4% and 2.4% in European populations, and which confer an increased risk for breast, prostate, and thyroid cancer [55, 57, 58]. These data argue against any major involvement of *CHEK2* mutations in LFS. A linkage to chromosome 1q23 was reported in a LFS family [59], but the implication of a second locus in LFS remains to be confirmed.

11.7 Modifier Genes in LFS

The variability in age of onset and type of cancer among LFS families suggests the effects of modifier genes on the underlying mutant *TP53* genotype. Analysis of mutant genotype-phenotype correlations reveals intriguing observations. Nonsense, frameshift, and splice mutations yield truncated or nonfunctional proteins that are commonly associated with early-onset cancers, particularly brain tumors [42]. Missense mutations in the *TP53* DNA-binding domain are frequently observed in the setting of breast and brain tumors, while ACCs are the only group that are associated with mutations in the non-DNA-binding loops. Age of onset modifiers have also now been established. Recently, the *MDM2*-SNP309 polymorphism has been shown to be a plausible candidate as a genetic modifier in *TP53*-mutated cancers and in LFS [35, 60]. *MDM2* is a key negative regulator of TP53, targeting

TP53 towards proteasomal degradation. The SNP309 T>G variant, located in the first intron of *MDM2*, increases Sp1 transcription factor binding and, consequently, *MDM2* expression levels. The mean age of tumor onset in *MDM2* SNP309 carriers is significantly less than that observed in patients homozygous for the T allele [61]. The common *TP53* codon 72Arg polymorphism has been shown to have a higher affinity towards MDM2 compared with the 72Pro isoform leading to a higher degree of TP53 degradation. The mean age of tumor onset in *TP53* codon 72Arg allele carriers is significantly less than that of Pro:Pro variant carriers [61]. Furthermore, a cumulative effect is observed when both the *MDM2* SNP309 and the *TP53* 72Arg isoform coexist [60, 61], suggesting that the early onset conferred by the *MDM2* SNP309 polymorphism is amplified by presence of the *TP53* codon 72Arg polymorphism. However, this confluence of genetic modifiers does not fully explain the observed differences in cancer phenotypes of individuals with the same *TP53* genotype, especially within the same family. The observation of genetic anticipation in LFS [62] suggests a role of additional "hits" or higher mutator phenotypes with successive generations within these families. The earlier age of onset of cancers with subsequent generations in mutant *TP53* LFS families suggests genetic anticipation. This observation can be explained by accelerated telomere attrition from generation to generation, which may be a useful predictive marker of tumor age of onset [63, 64]. Thus, while germline *TP53* mutations establish the baseline risk of tumor development in LFS, a complex interplay of modifying genetic cofactors likely defines the specific phenotypes of individual patients.

Three *TP53* polymorphisms are in linkage disequilibrium within a 312 bp stretch of genomic DNA, including a SNP in intron 2 (PIN2), a 16 bp duplication in intron 3 (PIN3), and the SNP at codon 72 (PEX4). In a population of LFS patients harboring a unique mutation at codon 337, PIN3 has a significant effect on age of onset, with carriers of one minor allele (16 bp duplication) developing their first cancer, on average, 17.1 years later than carriers of two major (non-duplicated) alleles [65]. Haplotype analysis combining the three polymorphisms demonstrated that PEX4 (codon 72) has no independent effect. Further studies are needed to determine whether the effect of PIN3 is particularly important in R337H carriers, or if it is a general effect in all germline *TP53* mutation carriers. Recently, using high-resolution SNP/CNV array technologies, it has been demonstrated that *TP53* mutation carriers harbor a higher frequency of DNA copy number variable regions in their genome, and that these regions frequently encompass cancer genes [66, 67]. The increased copy number variable regions may be a reflection of the underlying genomic instability conferred by the *TP53* mutations in these individuals.

11.8 The Unique Brazilian LFS-*TP53* Codon 337 Mutation Phenotype

In Brazil, a specific germline mutation at codon R337H (c.1010 G>A, genomic nucleotide number 17588) in exon 10, encoding the oligomerization domain of *TP53*, was first identified in children with ACC in families with no reported history of cancer [68, 69]. Based on the analysis of four hypervariable loci on the short arm of chromosome 17, it had been concluded that the mutation might have arisen independently in different patients, perhaps due to an environmental mutagen. However, using two *TP53* intragenic hypervariable loci in a larger group of cases and controls, Pinto et al. [11] suggested that a founder effect was statistically probable. The allele frequency of R337H in the population of Southeast and Southern Brazil is about 15 times higher than any other single *TP53* mutation associated with LFS [70]. At pH in the low to normal physiological range (up to 7.5), the mutant protein forms normal oligomers and retains its suppressor function. However, at high physiologic pH, the histidine replacing arginine at codon 337 becomes deprotonated and is unable to donate a hydrogen bond critical for protein dimerization. This prevents TP53 from assembling into a functional transcription factor. This unique biochemical feature might contribute to the particular features of R337H families, which often show incomplete penetrance and heterogeneous tumor patterns [71].

Analysis of tumor patterns in R337H carriers and their families revealed all the common features of LFS/LFL, clearly establishing that this mutant predisposes to a wide spectrum of multiple cancers. In R337H carriers, the penetrance at age 30 is less than 20% (compared to about 50% in "classical" LFS). However, the penetrance over lifetime is about 90%, similar to "classical" LFS. Interestingly, the mutation appears to be particularly prevalent in Southeast and Southern Brazilian populations where the allele frequency is suggested to be about 0.0015 [72].

The high prevalence of a rare mutation raised the question of a possible founder effect among Brazilian family's carriers of the same alteration. Using a dense panel of SNPs encompassing the whole *TP53* gene revealed the presence of a rare haplotype, with a probability that the mutation arose by independently on this haplotype of less than 10^{-8}[73], establishing the existence of a founder effect. Given the high population density in these areas, mutations might be present in several hundred thousand subjects, and could explain the high frequency of many cancers including colorectal cancer and the greater than 15-fold increase in childhood adrenocortical cancer in the Brazilian population.

11.9 Functional Models of Germline *TP53* Mutations

Since the initial identification of germline *TP53* mutations in LFS, in vitro transfection of tumor cell lines with plasmids carrying human germline *TP53* mutations indicated that mutations compromise the ability of TP53 to inhibit the growth of malignant cells in vitro and to transactivate reporter plasmids containing TP53-binding sites [74, 75]. To systematically evaluate the effects of *TP53* mutations on the transcriptional activity of the protein, which underlies its ability to control cell cycle, apoptosis, and DNA repair, functional assays in yeast were developed [76, 77]. The FASAY (Functional Analysis of Separated Allele in Yeast) is now widely used to detect germline or somatic *TP53* mutations. The assay is based on the co-transformation of a reporter yeast strain with PCR-amplified *TP53* cDNA (between codons 53 and 364), derived from patients lymphocytes, a gapped expression vector linearized between codons 67 and 346, and the cloning of the cDNAs by homologous recombination. The activation by wild-type TP53 of the reporter system, containing the ADE2 open reading frame cloned downstream of TP53-binding sites, changes the color of the yeast colonies (red to white). Heterozygote inactivating mutations yield about 50% red colonies. FASAY analysis of lymphocytes from LFS patients harboring germline *TP53* mutations has demonstrated that all the missense mutations result in a loss of function. Missense mutations confer oncogenic properties in vitro, and this gain of function could be explained either by the ability of mutant *TP53* to transactivate inappropriate target genes involved in cell cycle [78] or by a transdominant negative effect whereby missense mutants interfere with the DNA binding of the wild-type protein [79]. Therefore, although the common biological effect of germline *TP53* mutations is a loss of function, it is likely that some missense mutations may have a dual effect.

Furthermore, analysis of LFS fibroblasts or lymphocytes harboring heterozygous *TP53* mutation has revealed striking differences with normal cells, in term of chromosomal stability, apoptotic response to ionizing radiations, G2 arrest after DNA damage, and gene expression profiles [80–83]. This strongly suggests that heterozygous *TP53* mutations have a biological effect contributing to genetic instability and therefore facilitating the appearance of a second hit.

11.10 Mouse Models of LFS

In 1992, homozygous knockout mice with a germline *p53* deletion were shown to be developmentally normal, but highly susceptible to early tumors [84]. Subsequent *p53* null mice with different deletions of the *p53* allele showed similar tumorigenic phenotypes [41, 85, 86]. The majority of *p53* null mice developed T and B cell lymphomas within 6 months of age [84, 87]. Genetically, the *p53* null heterozygous mice are a model for a significant fraction of LFS germline mutations that are functionally null for TP53 [43]. A closer genetic model for LFS, however, was the *p53* mutant heterozygous mice, since affected LFS individuals are invariably heterozygous rather than homozygous for mutant *TP53*.

Given the genetic similarity between the *p53* heterozygous null mice and the subset of LFS lineages with null mutations, it is of interest to explore phenotypic similarities. Approximately 50% of heterozygous null *p53* mice succumb to tumors by 18 months of age [87, 88]. On a lifespan basis of 36 months for C57BL/6 mice, this is not too dissimilar from the 50% incidence that has been observed for affected members of LFS families, with a 50% incidence of cancers by age 30. With respect to tumor spectrum, like the LFS families, the *p53* null heterozygous mice not only exhibit high numbers of osteosarcomas and soft tissue sarcomas but also display high numbers of B cell lymphoma/leukemia, a tumor type only weakly associated with LFS. In contrast to the high frequency of breast cancers in LFS, there were few mammary carcinomas in the *p53* null heterozygous mice, though this may be largely due to the predominantly C57BL/6 background of the study population [87], as C57BL/6 mice are highly resistant to mammary carcinomas [89]. When the *p53* null allele was backcrossed into a mammary tumor susceptible Balb/c background, 55% of the female heterozygotes developed mammary adenocarcinomas [89]. Thus, strain-associated modifier genes may greatly influence the types of tumors arising in the *p53*-deficient mice. It also suggests that appropriate manipulation of the strain background in the *p53* heterozygous mice could be exploited to generate a mouse with similar tumor spectra as LFS patients.

In general, tumor suppressor genes such as *TP53* are considered to be recessive. In those familial syndromes resulting from inheritance of a single defective tumor suppressor allele, loss or mutation of the second allele is often observed in the tumors that arise in these syndromes. *TP53* appears to be an exception to this rule. While mutation and loss of both *TP53* alleles occur quite frequently in sporadically arising cancers, the tumors arising in LFS patients often retain a structurally intact wild-type *TP53* allele [90]. Interestingly, two third of the tumors in those patients inheriting missense mutations in the central DNA-binding domain of TP53 show retention of a wild-type *TP53* allele [90]. The tumors from those families with functionally null *TP53* germline mutations invariably exhibit loss of the remaining wild-type *TP53* allele. There is evidence that many *TP53* missense mutants can behave in a dominant negative manner and functionally inactivate wild-type TP53 forms [91]. Thus, selective pressure for loss of the wild-type allele in the tumor is reduced. In those LFS patients with a null *TP53* allele, it is expected that there would be higher selective pressure for loss of the remaining wild-type allele. Such results in humans would imply that all of the tumors from the *p53* null heterozygous mice should exhibit loss of the wild-type *p53* allele. In fact, only about half of the *p53* null heterozygous mouse tumors do exhibit loss of the wild-type *p53* allele [92]. These tumors tend to arise sooner and are more aggressive than those heterozygote tumors that retain wild-type *p53* [92]. However, tumors from heterozygous mice with germline missense *p53* mutations invariably retain their wild-type *p53* allele, more consistent with the LFS observations. The retention of wild-type *p53* in the *p53* null heterozygous tumors indicates that in mice, unlike in humans, reduction of *p53* dosage is sufficient to promote tumorigenesis, though loss of both alleles certainly accelerates tumor formation. In humans, functional (via dominant negative mutant TP53 effects) or structural loss of wild-type TP53 seems to be a prerequisite for tumor formation. Such species differences are consistent with generally higher constraints on oncogenic transformation of human cells compared to mouse cells [93]. They are also consistent with the fact that *p53* mutations are relatively rare in spontaneous and carcinogen-induced tumors in mice, in considerable contrast to spontaneous tumors in humans. Thus, humans and mice may harbor some fundamental differences in their requirement for disabling TP53 function in the path to tumorigenesis.

The development of mice with a *p53* null allele, as described above, has been instrumental in our understanding of TP53 function in tumorigenesis. However, the majority of individuals with LFS that inherit *TP53* mutations inherit missense mutations (>80%). The increased incidence of *TP53* missense mutations in LFS patients and in somatic tumors suggests additional oncogenic properties of mutant TP53.

Four mouse models have now been generated, using "knock in" technology, that contain specific missense mutations in *p53*. The first mouse contained the $p53^{R172H}$ mutation, which corresponds to the $p53^{R175H}$ hotspot mutation in human cancers, but expressed low levels of mutant *p53* due to an additional splicing abnormality [94]. Nevertheless, heterozygous mice with this mutation developed tumors that were highly metastatic as compared to the rare occurrence of metastasis in $p53^{+/-}$ mice, and suggested for the first time that *p53* missense mutations could confer a gain of function even when expressed at low levels. The same $p53^{R172H}$ mutation expressed at appropriate levels recapitulated these data and yielded additional insights into the role of *p53* missense mutations [95, 96].

Mice inheriting the $p53^{R172H}$ mutation were studied in two different backgrounds [95, 96]. In both backgrounds, a metastatic phenotype in heterozygous mutant mice was obvious although the presence of metastasis did not alter survival. Additionally, in the $129S_4$/Sv background, mice heterozygous for the $p53^{R172H}$ mutation showed a twofold increase in the number of osteosarcomas and a slight increase in the number of carcinomas as compared to the $p53^{+/-}$ mice [96]. These data have important implications for human disease in that they indicate that mutant p53 has additional activities not represented by loss of *p53* even though both result in loss of p53 transcriptional activity.

Additional insights into the function of missense mutations came from the generation of another *p53* mutation, the $p53^{R270H}$ mutation, which corresponds to the human $p53^{R273H}$ hotspot mutation. An important difference between mutations is that the $p53^{R172H}$ mutation represents a conformational mutant while the $p53^{R270H}$ mutation represents a contact mutant. In the $129S_4$/Sv background, $p53^{R270H}$ heterozygous mice showed increased tumor burden, increased incidence of carcinomas and hemangiomas, and a metastatic phenotype as compared to $p53^{+/-}$ mice. Thus, different *p53* alleles show different tumor spectra. Whether different *p53* mutations give rise to different spectra in humans will be difficult to decipher due to the inherent differences in humans.

The availability of mice with one mutant and one wild-type *p53* allele allowed an evaluation of the dominant-negative nature of mutant p53. The lack of differences in survival of *p53* heterozygous and mutant heterozygous mice indicates that the presence of mutant p53 has no effect on wild-type p53 activity in terms of longevity [95]. Additionally, heterozygous $p53^{R172H}$ mutant mice could not rescue the p53-dependent phenotype of *Mdm2* null mice, again suggesting that wild-type *p53* was not inactivated by the presence of mutant p53. In contrast, p53-dependent apoptosis in the developing nervous system of $p53^{R172H/+}$ mice resembled that of *p53* null mice, suggesting that in this case wild-type p53 was inactivated by mutant p53. Thus, only in some cases does mutant p53 function as a dominant negative. This may be due to the observation that mutant p53 in normal mouse tissues is unstable and therefore unable to function as a dominant negative isoform. The stability of mutant TP53 in normal LFS samples is yet to be determined.

Lastly, a rare human *TP53* mutation corresponding to an Arg-to-Pro substitution at amino acid 172 has also been made available by knock in of a point mutation [97]. This mutation occurs in human cancers, but has not yet been identified in LFS patients. However, this mutation separates the apoptotic from cell cycle arrest functions of p53 and has yielded exciting results. Cells from mice homozygous for the $p53^{R172P}$ mutation are unable to initiate p53-dependent apoptosis and thus resemble *p53* null cells. Importantly, $p53^{R172P}$ homozygous mutant cells retain the ability to induce cell cycle arrest and maintain a stable genome. Homozygous mutant mice show a dramatic delay of tumorigenesis as compared to $p53^{-/-}$ mice, suggesting that the ability to suppress the cell cycle is also an important tumor-suppressing activity. Thus, the cell cycle arrest function of p53 is also important in the inhibition of tumorigenesis.

The generation of mice with specific missense mutations in *p53* suggests that the inheritance of *p53* mutations as opposed to those mutations that lead to loss of p53 will lead to a worse prognosis. Moreover, different missense mutations may have different effects. Other underlying genetic modifying factors that contribute to the age of onset and the kinds of tumors that develop in LFS patients may also be modeled in mice and offer insight into the human condition.

11.11 Medical and Ethical Considerations

Presymptomatic molecular testing for *TP53* germline mutations in members of LFS kindreds has been met with significant controversy. Because of the variable expressivity, the diverse tumor spectrum, and lack of clear clinical surveillance, preventative, or treatment recommendations, it is unclear how to manage the detection of a *TP53* mutation carrier. It has been suggested that women who carry *TP53* mutations should begin screening for breast cancer in their mid-20s, given that the average age of onset is 31 years [10]. Recently, use of PET-CT as a clinical surveillance modality has been reported, identifying presymptomatic lesions in adults [98], and anecdotal reports of presymptomatic detection of childhood cancers, in particular ACC, have also been noted [99, 100]. The concept of predictive genetic testing of a child for a disease that may (or may not) occur in young adulthood challenges our perception of the ethics of disclosure of genetic test results, where the potential beneficiary of these results may wish to uphold the right to "not know." Notwithstanding these considerations, presymptomatic and even prenatal genetic testing for *TP53* is being performed in carefully selected and counseled situations, taking into account the particular balance of beneficence and harm [101–104].

Although predisposition testing may identify asymptomatic carriers, and allow institution of preventive or surveillance programs where available, such testing is associated with the following caveats that must be considered: (a) the genetic heterogeneity of cancer predisposition; (b) the technical difficulty inherent to gene testing and to test interpretation; and (c) the psychosocial impact of testing. Both variable degrees of penetrance and expressivity for many conditions, including LFS, suggest that other genetic events play an important role in defining the particular cancer phenotype of individual members of families. This variability makes predictions of clinical disease and specific susceptible target organs difficult and complicates the design of adequate screening programs.

The technical aspects involved in predisposition gene testing and interpretation are complex. Some tests are only available through research settings where results are made less immediately available, and confirmation of results is less well controlled than in clinically certified laboratories. Databases are now available to facilitate identification of clinical and research laboratories performing specific genetic tests (e.g., www.genetests.org). Furthermore, such testing, particularly of novel genes, tends to be expensive, and the physician may need to make extra effort to obtain insurance coverage of testing. Given the complexity, genetic testing should only be undertaken by a physician or genetic counselor fully capable of interpreting these results.

Genetic testing for LFS may have profound psychological and emotional impact on patients, and may be further complicated by relationships with parents and other family members [105]. Issues of the "vulnerable child syndrome" in affected carriers and "survivor guilt" in unaffected, non-carrier siblings raise complex psychosocial concerns that may be beyond the general purview of the pediatric or medical oncologist. Furthermore, lessons from studies in adults have demonstrated that although patients learning of their increased risk of disease usually do well, they may experience feelings of shock, depression, grief, altered self-esteem, or even guilt. Limited studies in children, parents, and families have yet to clarify the impact of predictive testing for cancer in children.

In an attempt to address these issues, guidelines for testing have been established by both the American Society of Human Genetics [106, 107] and the American Society of Clinical Oncology [108]. These guidelines form a useful foundation on which to build practical testing parameters as better defined genotype to phenotype correlations are generated. A recent comprehensive study from France explores the perceptions of two groups of genetic services providers for the usage of prenatal diagnosis (PND) and pre-implantation genetic diagnosis (PIGD). As parents now routinely discuss these options in planning future pregnancies, the need to engage a multidisciplinary team in these discussions is key to providing parents and families the necessary tools with which to make these ethically challenging decisions [94, 102, 109]. While some studies suggest the benefits to predictive genetic testing for children are still not substantial, further evaluations from different perspectives will continue to evolve this field [101].

Based on many of the preceding arguments, several recommendations established in 1992 for LFS [110] are still applicable to genetic testing in family cancer syndromes that include children. The quality of information provision on cancer genetics is directly related to the knowledge of professionals and their ability to communicate this to a patient and family, regardless of their specialty [111]. The multidisciplinary approach taken by several groups [109, 112], involving pediatric and medical oncologists, clinical geneticists, genetic counselors, psychologists, and ethicists in establishing cancer genetics clinics and programs whose primary focus is to serve children with cancer and their families, provides an intriguing and novel mechanism to optimize care of these families and advance our understanding of the role of genetics in the etiology of childhood cancer in general and LFS in particular.

References

1. Li FP, Fraumeni Jr JF (1969) Soft-tissue sarcomas, breast cancer, and other neoplasms. A familial syndrome? Ann Intern Med 71(4):747–752
2. Li FP, Fraumeni JF Jr (1969) Rhabdomyosarcoma in children: epidemiologic study and identification of a familial cancer syndrome. J Natl Cancer Inst 43:1365–1373
3. Li FP et al (1988) A cancer family syndrome in twenty-four kindreds. Cancer Res 48: 5358–5362
4. Nichols KE et al (2001) Germ-line p53 mutations predispose to a wide spectrum of early-onset cancers. Cancer Epidemol Biomark Preven 10(2):83–87
5. Birch JM et al (1994) Prevalence and diversity of constitutional mutations in the *p53* gene among 21 Li-Fraumeni families. Cancer Res 54:1298–1304
6. Chompret A et al (2001) Sensitivity and predictive value of criteria for p53 germline mutation screening. J Med Genet 38:43–47
7. Tinat J et al (2009) version of the Chompret criteria for Li-Fraumeni syndrome. J Clin Oncol 27(26):e108–109
8. Hisada M et al (1998) Multiple primary cancers in families with Li-Fraumeni syndrome. J Natl Cancer Inst 90:606–611
9. Wu CC et al (2006) Joint effects of germ-line p53 mutation and sex on cancer risk in Li-Fraumeni syndrome. Cancer Res 66:8287–8292
10. Hwang SJ et al (2003) Germline p53 mutations in a cohort with childhood sarcoma: sex differences in cancer risk. Am J Hum Genet 72:975–983
11. DeLeo AB et al (1979) Detection of a transformation-related antigen in chemically induced sarcomas and other transformed cells of the mouse. Proc Natl Acad Sci USA 76:2420–2424
12. Lane DP, Crawford LV (1979) T antigen bound to a host protein in SV40-transformed cells. Nature 278:261–263
13. Linzer DI, Levine AJ (1979) Characterization of a 54 K Dalton cellular SV40 tumor antigen present in SV40-transformed cells and uninfected embryonal carcinoma cells. Cell 417: 43–52
14. McBride OW et al (1986) The gene for human p53 cellular tumor antigen is located on chromosome 17 short arm (17p13). Proc Natl Acad Sci USA 83:130–134
15. Soussi T (2007) Oncogene. p53 alterations in human cancer: more questions than answers. 26:2145–2156
16. Soussi T et al (1990) Structural aspects of the p53 protein in relation to gene evolution. Oncogene 5:945–952
17. Addison C et al (1990) The p53 nuclear localization signal is structurally linked to a p34cdc2 kinase motif. Oncogene 5:423–426
18. Farmer G et al (1992) Wild-type p53 activates transcription in vitro. Nature 358:83–86
19. Jenkins JR et al (1988) Two distinct regions of the murine p53 primary amino acid sequence are implicated in stable complex formation with simian virus 40 T antigen. J Virol 62: 3903–3906
20. Meek DW, Eckhart W (1988) Phosphorylation of p53 in normal and simian virus 40-transformed NIH3T3 cells. Mol Cell Biol 8:461–465
21. Milner J. Medcalf EA (1991) Cotranslation of activated mutant p53 with wild-type drives the wild-type p53 protein into the mutant conformation. Cell 65:765–774
22. Kubbutat MH, Vousden KH (1997) Proteolytic cleavage of human p53 by calpain: a potential regulator of protein stability. Mol Cell Biol 17:460–468
23. Kubbutat MH et al (1997) Regulation of p53 stability by Mdm2. Nature 387:299–303

24. Jayaraman L, Prives C (1999) Covalent and noncovalent modifiers of the p53 protein. Cell Mol Life Sci 55:76–87
25. Sionov RV et al (2001) c-Abl regulates p53 levels under normal and stress conditions by preventing its nuclear export and ubiquitination. Mol Cell Biol 21:5869–5878
26. Hermeking LC et al (1997) 14-3-3 sigma is a p53-regulated inhibitor of G2/M progression. Mol Cell 1:3–11
27. Zhan Q et al (1999) Association with Cdc2 and inhibition of Cdc2/Cyclin B1 kinase activity by the p53-regulated protein Gadd45. Oncogene 18:2892–2900
28. Lane DP (1992) p53, guardian of the genome. Nature 358:15–16
29. Rosse T et al (1998) Bcl-2 prolongs cell survival after Bax-induced release of cytochrome c. Nature 391:496–499
30. Muller M et al (1998) p53 activates the CD95 (APO-1/Fas) gene in response to DNA damage by anticancer drugs. J Exp Med 188:2033–2045
31. Wu GS et al (1997) KILLER/DR5 is a DNA damage-inducible p53-regulated death receptor gene. Nature Genet 17:141–143
32. Vogelstein B. Kinzler KW. (1994) Tumor-suppressor genes. X-rays strike p53 again. Nature 370:174–175
33. Kern SE et al (1992) Oncogenic forms of p53 inhibit p53-regulated gene expression. Science 256:827–830
34. Kern SE et al (1991) Identification of p53 as a sequence-specific DNA-binding protein. Science 252:827–830
35. Ruijs MWG et al (2006) The single nucleotide polymorphism 309 in the MDM2 gene contributes to the Li-Fraumeni syndrome and related phenotypes. Eur J Human Genet [adv online pub]
36. Oliner JD et al (1992) Amplification of a gene encoding a p53-associated protein in human sarcomas. Nature 358:80–83
37. Malkin D et al (1990) Germ line p53 mutations in a familial syndrome of breast cancer, sarcomas, and other neoplasms. Science 250:1233–1238
38. Baker SJ et al (1989) Chromosome 17 deletions and p53 gene mutations in colorectal carcinomas. Science 244:217–221
39. Lavigueur A et al (1989) High incidence of lung, bone, and lymphoid tumors in transgenic mice overexpressing mutant alleles of the p53 oncogene. Mol Cell Biol 9:3982–3991
40. Kleihues P et al (1997) Tumors associated with p53 germline mutations: a synopsis of 91 families. Am J Pathol 150:1–13
41. Tsukada T et al (1993) Enhanced proliferative potential in culture of cells from p53-deficient mice. Oncogene 8:3313–3322
42. Olivier M et al (2003) Li-Fraumeni and related syndromes: correlation between tumor type family structure, and TP53 genotype. Cancer Res 63:6643–6650
43. Varley JM, Germline (2003) TP53 mutations and Li-Fraumeni syndrome. Human Mutation 21:313–320
44. Lalloo F et al (2003) Prediction of pathogenic mutations in patients with early-onset breast cancer by family history. Lancet 361:1101–1102
45. Quesnel S et al (1999) p53 compound heterozygosity in a severely affected child with Li-Fraumeni syndrome. Oncogene 18:3970–3978
46. Gannon JV et al (1990) Activating mutations in p53 produce a common conformational effect. A monoclonal antibody specific for the mutant form. EMBO J 9:1595–1602
47. Srivastava S et al (1993) Several mutant p53 proteins detected in cancer-prone families with Li-Fraumeni syndrome exhibit transdominant effects on the biochemical properties of the wild-type p53. Oncogene 8:2449–2456
48. Bougeard G et al (2001) Detection of 11 germline inactivating TP53 mutations and abse nce of TP63 and HCHK2 mutations in 17 French families with Li-Fraumeni or Li-Fraumeni-like syndrome. J Med Genet 38(4):253–257
49. Stone JG et al (1999) Analysis of Li-Fraumeni syndrome and Li-Fraumeni-like families for germline mutations in Bcl10. Cancer Lett 147:185–189

50. Barlow JW et al (2004) Germline BAX alterations are infrequent in Li-Fraumeni Syndrome. Cancer Epid Biomark Prev 13:1403–1406
51. Burt EC et al (1999) Exclusion of the genes CDKN2 and PTEN as causative gene defects in Li-Fraumeni syndrome. Br J Cancer 80:9
52. Portwine C et al (2000) Absence of p16^{INK4a} alterations in p53 wild-type Li-Fraumeni syndrome families. J Med Genet 37:e13
53. Brown LTR et al (2000) Identification of a novel *PTEN* intronic deletion in Li-Fraumeni syndrome and its effect on RNA processing. Cancer Genet Cytogenet 123:65
54. Bell DW et al (1999) Heterozygous germ line hCHK2 mutations in Li-Fraumeni syndrome. Science 286:2528–2531
55. Vahteristo P et al (2001) p53, CHK2, and CHK1 genes in Finnish families with Li-Fraumeni syndrome: further evidence of CHK2 in inherited cancer predisposition. Cancer Res 61(15):5718–5722
56. Sodha N et al (2000) Screening hCHK2 for mutations. Science 289:359
57. Cybulski C et al (2008) Constitutional CHEK2 mutations are associated with a decreased risk of lung and laryngeal cancers. Carcinogenesis 29:762–765
58. Meijers-Heijboer H et al (2002) Low-penetrance susceptibility to breast cancer due to CHEK2(*)1100delC in noncarriers of BRCA1 or BRCA2 mutations. Nature Genet 31:55–59
59. Bachinski LL et al (2005) Genetic mapping of a third Li-Fraumeni syndrome predisposition locus to human chromosome 1q23. Cancer Res 65:427–431
60. Bond GL et al (2006) MDM2 SNP309 accelerates tumor formation in a gender-specific and hormone-dependent manner. Cancer Res 66:5104
61. Bougeard G et al (2006) Impact of the MDM SNP309 and p53 Arg72Pro polymorphism on age of onset in Li-Fraumeni syndrome. J Med Genet 43:531–533
62. Trkova M et al (2002) Is there anticipation in the age at onset of cancer in families with Li-Fraumeni syndrome? J Hum Genet 47(8):381–386
63. Tabori U et al (2007) Younger age of cancer initiation is associated with shorter telomere length in Li-Fraumeni syndrome. Cancer Res 67(4):1415–1418
64. Trkova M et al (2007) Telomere length in peripheral blood cells of germline TP53 mutation carriers is shorter than that of normal individuals of corresponding age. Cancer. 110(3): 694–702
65. Marcel V et al (2009) TP53 PIN3 and MDM2 SNP309 polymorphisms as genetic modifiers in the Li-Fraumeni syndrome: impact on age at first diagnosis. J Med Genet 46: 766–772
66. Shlien A et al (2008) Excessive genomic DNA copy number variation in the Li-Fraumeni cancer predisposition syndrome. Proc Natl Acad Sci USA 105(32):11264–11269
67. Shlien A, Malkin D (2009) Copy number variations and cancer. Genome Med 1(6):62–67
68. Figueiredo BC et al (2006) Penetrance of adrenocortical tumours associated with the germline TP53 R337H mutation. J Med Genet 43(1):91–96
69. Ribeiro RC et al (2001) An inherited p53 mutation that contributes in a tissue-specific manner to pediatric adrenal cortical carcinoma. Proc Natl Acad Sci USA 98:9330–9335
70. Achatz MI et al (2007) The TP53 mutation, R337H, is associated with Li-Fraumeni and Li-Fraumeni-like syndromes in Brazilian families. Cancer Lett 245(1–2):96–102
71. DiGiammarino EL et al (2002) A novel mechanism of tumorigenesis involving pH-dependent destabilization of a mutant p53 tetramer. Nat Struct Biol 9(1):12–16
72. Palmero EI et al (2007) Detection of R337H, a germline TP53 mutation predisposing to multiple cancers, in asymptomatic women participating in a breast cancer screening program in Southern Brazil. Cancer Lett 261: 21–25
73. Garritano S et al (2010) Detailed haplotype analysis at the TP53 locus in p.R337H mutation carriers in the population of Southern Brazil: evidence for a founder effect. Human Mut 31(2):143–150
74. Frebourg T et al (1992) Germ-line mutations of the p53 tumor suppressor gene in patients with high risk for cancer inactivate the p53 protein. Proc Natl Acad Sci 89:6413–6417

75. Frebourg T et al (1992) A functional screen for germ line p53 mutations based on transcriptional activation. Cancer Res 52:6967–6968
76. Flaman JM et al (1995) A simple p53 functional assay for screening cell lines, blood, and tumors. Proc Natl Acad Sci 92:3963–3967
77. Ishioka C et al (1993) Screening patients for heterozygous p53 mutations using a functional assay in yeast. Nature Genet 5:124–129
78. Weisz L et al (2004) Transactivation of the EGR1 gene contributes to mutant p53 gain of function. Cancer Res 64:8318–8327
79. Willis A et al (2004) Mutant p53 exerts a dominant negative effect by preventing wild-type p53 from binding to the promoter of its target genes. Oncogene 23:2330–2338
80. Boyle JM et al (1998) Chromosome instability is a predominant trait of fibroblasts from Li-Fraumeni families. Br J Cancer 77:2181–2192
81. Camplejohn RS et al (1995) A possible screening test for inherited p53-related defects based on the apoptotic response of peripheral blood lymphocytes to DNA damage. Br J Cancer 72:654–662
82. Goi K et al (1998) DNA damage-associated dysregulation of the cell cycle and apoptosis control in cells with germ-line p53 mutation. Cancer Res 57:1895–1902
83. Yoon DS et al (2002) Variable levels of chromosomal instability and mitotic spindle checkpoint defects in breast cancer. Am J Pathol 161:391–397
84. Donehower LA et al (1992) Mice deficient for p53 are developmentally normal but susceptible to spontaneous tumours. Nature 356:215–221
85. Jacks T et al (1994) Tumor spectrum analysis in p53-mutant mice. Curr Biol 4:1–7
86. Purdie CA et al (1994) Tumour incidence, spectrum and ploidy in mice with a large deletion in the p53 gene. Oncogene 9:603–609
87. Donehower LA (1996) The p53-deficient mouse: a model for basic and applied cancer studies. Semin Cancer Biol 7:269–278
88. Harvey M et al (1993) Spontaneous and carcinogen-induced tumorigenesis in p53-deficient mice. Nat Genet 5:225–229
89. Kuperwasser C et al (2000) Development of spontaneous mammary tumors in BALB/c p53 heterozygous mice. A model for Li-Fraumeni syndrome. Am J Pathol 157: 2151–2159
90. Varley JM et al (2001) Characterization of germline TP53 splicing mutations and their genetic and functional analysis. Oncogene 20:2647–2654
91. Chene P (1998) In vitro analysis of the dominant negative effect of p53 mutants. J Mol Biol 281:205–209
92. Venkatachalam S et al (1998) Retention of wild-type p53 in tumors from p53 heterozygous mice: reduction of p53 dosage can promote cancer formation. Embo J 17:4657–4667
93. Rangarajan A, Weinberg RA (2003) Opinion: Comparative biology of mouse versus human cells: modelling human cancer in mice. Nat Rev Cancer 3:952–959
94. Liu G et al (2000) High metastatic potential in mice inheriting a targeted p53 missense mutation. Proc Natl Acad Sci USA 97:474–4179
95. Lang GA et al (2004) Gain of function of a p53 hot spot mutation in a mouse model of Li-Fraumeni syndrome. Cell 119:861–872
96. Olive KP et al (2004) Mutant p53 gain-of-function in two mouse models of Li-Fraumeni syndrome. Cell, 119:847–860
97. Liu G et al (2004) Chromosome stability, in the absence of apoptosis, is critical for suppression of tumorigenesis in Trp53 mutant mice. Nat Genet 36:63–68
98. Masciari S et al (2008) F18-fluorodeoxyglucose positron emission tomography/computed tomography screening in Li-Fraumeni syndrome. J Amer Med Assoc 299(11):1315–1319
99. Hwang SM et al (2008) Genetic counseling can influence the course of a suspected familial cancer syndrome patient: from a case of Li-Fraumeni like syndrome with a germline mutation in the TP53 gene. Korean J Lab Med 28(6):493–497

100. Lin MT et al (2009) Early detection of adrenocortical carcinoma in a child with Li-Fraumeni syndrome. Pediatr Blood Cancer 52(4):541–544
101. Evans DG et al (2010) Childhood predictive genetic testing for Li-Fraumeni syndrome. Fam Cancer 9(1):65–69
102. Lammens C et al (2009) Attitudes towards pre-implantation genetic diagnosis for hereditary cancer. Fam Cancer 8(4):457–464
103. Peterson SK et al (2008) Psychological functioning in persons considering genetic counseling and testing for Li-Fraumeni syndrome. Psychooncology 17(8):782–789
104. Schwarzbraun T et al (2009) Predictive diagnosis of the cancer-prone Li-Fraumeni syndrome by accident: new challenges through whole genome array testing. J Med Genet 46(5): 341–344
105. Croyle RT et al (1997) Psychologic aspects of cancer genetic testing—A research update for clinicians. Cancer 80:569–575
106. Statement of the American Society of Clinical Oncology (1996) Genetic testing for cancer susceptibility. J Clin Oncol 14:1730–1736
107. Statement of the American Society of Human Genetics (1994) Genetic testing for breast and ovarian cancer predisposition. Am J Hum Genet 55:i–iv
108. American Society of Clinical Oncology (2003) Policy statement update: genetic testing for cancer susceptibility. J Clin Oncol 21:2397–2406
109. Julian-Reynier C et al (2009) Professionals assess the acceptablity of preimplantation genetic diagnosis and prenatal diagnosis for managing inherited predisposition to cancer. J Clin Oncol 27(27):4475–4480
110. Li FP et al (1992) Recommendations on predictive testing for germ line p53 mutations among cancer-prone individuals. J Natl Cancer Inst 84:1156–1160
111. Chorley W, MacDermot K (1997) Who should talk to patients with cancer about genetics? BMJ 314:441
112. Malkin D et al (1999) Establishment of a dedicated cancer genetics program in a tertiary pediatric centre. Am J Hum Genet 65(4):A386

Chapter 12
TP53 Molecular Genetics

Gerard P. Zambetti and Raul C. Ribeiro

The TP53 tumor suppressor normally functions as a transcription factor within a stress response signaling pathway to activate genes that block cell proliferation, repair DNA, inhibit angiogenesis, and induce apoptotic cell death. Collectively, TP53 limits the growth and survival of abnormal cells. It is therefore not surprising that *TP53* is the most frequently mutated gene detected in human cancer. Pediatric adrenocortical tumors (ACC) are rare, usually aggressive malignancies that are often associated with inherited or de novo mutations in the *TP53* tumor suppressor gene. Recent molecular and biochemical analyses of childhood ACC have revealed new insight into *TP53* genotype–phenotype relationships and the factors that cooperate with the loss of TP53 functions to promote tumorigenesis. This chapter will review the TP53 signaling pathway and its clinical implications to pediatric and adult ACC and cancer in general.

12.1 The Pre-eminent Tumor Suppressor

TP53 was discovered by the Lane and Levine groups in 1979 by virtue of its ability to bind the SV40 DNA tumor virus large T antigen [1, 2]. For nearly a decade, the field generated compelling data that *TP53* functions as an oncogene; however, there was one minor complication – these studies inadvertently relied on a mutant allele, ironically isolated from a normal liver library. We now know that wild-type TP53 is an essential tumor suppressor that is commonly inactivated in human cancer (for review see [3]). Indeed, approximately 50% of all tumors are associated with *TP53* mutations, and those tumors retaining normal *TP53* alleles have often undergone other genetic and biochemical changes that interfere with *TP53* expression or function. It is therefore reasonable to propose that TP53 is inactivated by direct or indirect mechanisms in most, if not all, human cancers. In support of such

G.P. Zambetti (✉)
Department of Biochemistry, St. Jude Children's Research Hospital, 262 Danny Thomas Place, Memphis, TN 38105, USA
e-mail: gerard.zambetti@stjude.org

G.D. Hammer, T. Else (eds.), *Adrenocortical Carcinoma*,
DOI 10.1007/978-0-387-77236-3_12,

a critical requirement for TP53 as a tumor suppressor, mice that lack TP53 develop lymphoma, sarcoma, and other tumor types with full penetrance by 6 months of age [4, 5]. Consistent with the *p53*-knockout mice, people who are born with a *TP53* mutation are at a remarkably high risk for a variety of cancers such as sarcomas, breast carcinomas, brain tumors, and ACC at a very young age [6]. Carriers are also predisposed to developing multiple tumors. For example, Nutting et al. [7] reported a patient with a germline *TP53* mutation (R273C) who developed 17 primary independent tumors. This condition where *TP53* mutations are inherited and associated with increased risk for malignancy is referred to as Li-Fraumeni Syndrome. The role for TP53 in preventing cancer is unequivocal.

12.2 Transcription Is Key

Human *TP53* encodes a 393 amino acid protein that exhibits strong sequence-specific DNA-binding activity mediated by its central core domain (aa102–300) (Fig. 12.1). The N-terminus is acidic and contains two transactivation domains that interact with transcription-associated factors (aa1–80). The function of the C-terminus is multipurpose and contains a series of nuclear localization signals, a dimerization and oligomerization domain, and a negative regulatory domain. TP53 forms dimers of dimers and the tetramer is the active complex that binds DNA to regulate transcription (see [8]).

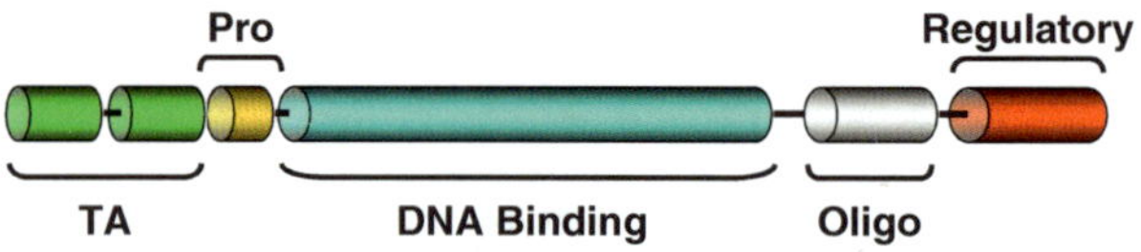

Fig. 12.1 Schematic diagram of the TP53 tumor suppressor protein. Human TP53 is 393 amino acids and the N-terminus consists of two transcription activation domains (TA; aa1–42 and 43–62). The proline-rich domain (Pro; aa65–97) influences TP53 apoptotic activity and tumor suppressor function [9, 10]. The central core domain (aa102–292) binds DNA in a sequence-specific manner. Most inherited and spontaneously arising mutations occur within the DNA-binding domain [11]. The oligomerization domain (Oligo; aa323–356) allows TP53 to form dimers and tetramers, which are the transcriptionally active form of the tumor suppressor. Within the C-terminus are three conserved nuclear localization signals (predominant active motif at aa313–322) to ensure proper targeting of the protein to the nucleus where it functions to regulate transcription [12]. The C-terminal tail of TP53 also acts as a negative regulator of TP53 activity and is controlled by posttranslational modifications during cell stress

It is estimated that more than 100 TP53-responsive target genes have been identified to date. Several of these genes have been demonstrated to play an in vivo physiological role in mediating TP53 activities. TP53 functions as a sensor of stress (e.g., DNA damage, hypoxia, or hyperproliferation due to oncogene activation) to block the growth of the cell or to induce apoptosis. A key TP53 target that blocks cell cycle progression is $p21^{CIP1}(CDKN1A)$, which is a universal cyclin kinase inhibitor [13, 14]. It is considered that TP53 induction of $p21^{CIP1}$ provides the time to repair the damage or to wait-out the inhospitable condition. Alternatively, TP53 eliminates abnormal cells by triggering apoptosis largely through the induction of *PUMA* (p53 upregulated modulator of apoptosis), a BH3-only proapoptotic Bcl2 family member [15–17]. Indeed, *PUMA*$^{-/-}$ mice are essentially as resistant as *p53*-knockout mice to DNA damage and other forms of stress [18, 19]. There is strong data supporting the hypothesis that TP53-mediated apoptosis is its primary function for blocking tumorigenesis. Surprisingly, however, the *PUMA*-deficient mice are not inherently cancer-prone, suggesting that P53 control of cell cycle arrest as well as its other activities (e.g., cellular senescence, inhibition of angiogenesis and DNA repair) are also significant in maintaining normal cell growth and blocking tumor development.

Analysis of more than 25,000 human tumors demonstrated that most *TP53* mutations occur within the DNA-binding domain, with several codons (e.g., 175, 245, 248, 273, 282) being more frequently altered than others [11]. These sites are referred to as hotspot mutations and they do not arise by chance. They are selected during tumorigenesis for their ability to abrogate TP53 DNA binding and transcriptional regulation [20]. For example, the common R248W mutation disrupts a DNA contact point, whereas the R175H substitution causes a catastrophic unfolding of the protein. In either case, the TP53 mutant protein fails to bind DNA and activate target gene expression and, therefore, is unable to regulate cell proliferation and survival.

12.3 The TP53 Signaling Pathway: Loops Within Loops

TP53 operates within an intricate signaling pathway that responds to abnormal conditions (Fig. 12.2). But to understand and appreciate how this pathway is controlled and suppresses tumorigenesis, one first needs to recognize how TP53 activities are normally downregulated at the end of a pathophysiological response. *HDM2* (*Mdm2* in mouse) was initially identified as an oncogene [21] and subsequently as a TP53-binding protein that blocks TP53 function [22]. It is now established that *HDM2*, which encodes an E3-ubiquitin ligase [23], is a critical downstream target gene of TP53 that serves to limit TP53 function through a negative feedback loop [24–26] (Fig. 12.2). As TP53 levels increase in response to cell stress, *HDM2* expression concomitantly becomes elevated, resulting in enhanced TP53 turnover and diminished activity. The importance of the balance between TP53 and HDM2 is clearly based on genetically engineered mouse models. Whereas *p53*-knockout mice are born at near Mendelian frequency and are highly tumor prone, deletion of *Mdm2* results in early embryonic lethality [27, 28]. The failure of *Mdm2*-knockout embryos to survive past E4.5–6.5 of gestation is due to uncontrolled p53 activity, which was genetically proven by completely rescuing *Mdm2*-deficient mice on a *p53*-knockout background. The double knockout animals exhibit a similar tumor susceptibility phenotype as the *p53*-null mice. The clinical relevance of this regulatory loop to human disease is illustrated by the findings that *HDM2* is amplified and

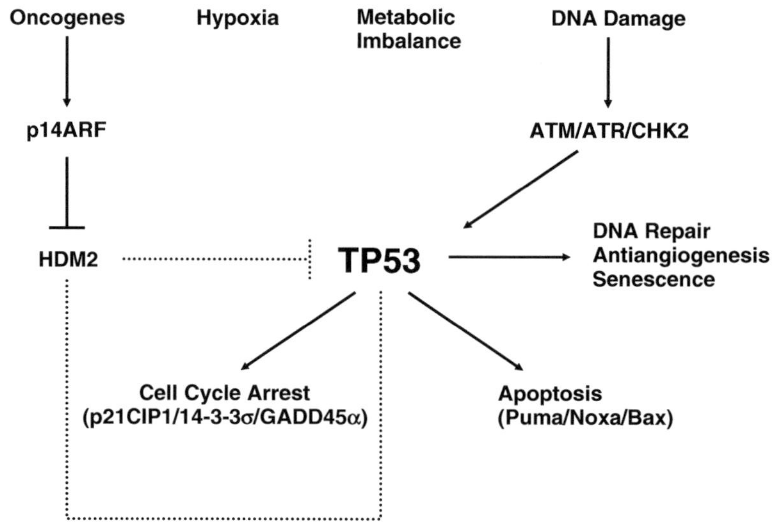

Fig. 12.2 The TP53 tumor suppressor signaling pathway. TP53 is maintained at low levels in normal cells. Upon cellular stress, TP53 becomes activated by phosphorylation mediated by kinases (ATM/ATR/CHK2) or through the induction of $p14^{ARF}$*(CDKN2A)*. In both cases, HDM2 binding to TP53 is suppressed and TP53 is free to regulate downstream target genes that elicit cell cycle arrest, senescence, DNA repair, apoptosis, or the suppression of angiogenesis. The pathway is downregulated through an elegant negative feedback mechanism controlled by the induction of *HDM2*, which in turn targets TP53 for protein degradation

overexpressed in tumors (e.g., approximately 30% of sarcomas), which retain wild-type p53 alleles [29–31].

Different stresses induce TP53 activity in slightly different ways. For example, DNA damage caused by UV, reactive oxygen species, or chemotherapeutic agents activates PI3-related kinases, such as ATM or ATR, and in turn CHK2 kinase, which phosphorylate key serines within the N-terminus of TP53 [32] (Fig. 12.2). These phosphorylations inhibit HDM2 binding and consequently lead to a cascade of additional post-translational modifications that activate TP53 DNA binding, specific target gene expression, and cell cycle arrest and/or apoptosis [33–35]. By contrast, deregulation of protooncogenes such as c-*MYC* leads to inappropriate cellular proliferation, which triggers the induction of $p14^{ARF}$*(CDKN2A)* ($p19^{Arf}$ in mouse), a product of the *INK4a* locus [36–38] (Fig. 12.2). ARF binds HDM2 and antagonizes its E3 ubiquitin ligase activity, resulting in the stabilization and activation of TP53 [39, 40, 41]. In turn, TP53 downregulates *ARF* expression through an ill-defined negative feedback mechanism [36, 37, 42]. Consistent with ARF playing an important role as an upstream activator of TP53, $p19^{Arf}$-knockout mice are highly prone to sarcomas and other tumors that maintain wild-type p53 status [43]. Similarly, spontaneous human tumors that retain wild-type p53 alleles have frequently lost $p14^{ARF}$ expression through gene mutation, deletion, or silencing [44, 45].

12.4 Acquired and Inherited *TP53* Mutations

Mutation of *TP53* compromises essential cell cycle and apoptotic checkpoints, and consequently promotes tumorigenesis. But what causes *TP53* mutations? Individuals can acquire mutations within *TP53* and throughout our genome over time, which helps to explain why cancer usually affects the elderly. Epidemiology studies have identified some important risk factors such as benzo[a]pyrene, a tobacco carcinogen, which can selectively form adducts at specific codons within *TP53* that are commonly mutated in human lung cancers [46]. Similarly, aflatoxin B1, a dietary mutagen produced by certain strains of *Aspergillus*, induces a G:C to T:A transversion at codon 249, resulting in an arginine to serine substitution [47, 48]. Ser249 was detected in hepatocellular carcinomas arising in geographic areas associated with high levels of aflatoxin B1 and an increased incidence of hepatitis B virus infection. DNA damage caused by ultraviolet light B has also been correlated with specific *TP53* mutations at dipyrimidine sites that are found in skin carcinomas [49–51]. These are just a few examples of the recognized carcinogens that can generate signature mutations which are associated with human cancers. We are a product of our environment and our tumor risk can be influenced by what we eat, drink, and breathe.

A hallmark feature of tumor suppressor genes is that one allele undergoes mutation and the other is selected against by deletion, gene conversion, or other means. This process is referred to as loss of heterozygosity (LOH) and is what usually occurs when *TP53* is targeted in cancer. The fact that the TP53 protein forms a tetramer, inactive DNA-binding missense mutants can attenuate wild-type TP53 function and alleviate the requirement for the tumor to undergo LOH, which is occasionally observed [52–54].

As discussed above, *TP53* mutations can also be inherited and these genetic alterations have been linked to Li-Fraumeni Syndrome (LFS). Carriers of a mutant *TP53* allele develop diverse and multiple malignancies at a young age. One such tumor type found within LFS families is childhood ACC [55]. Given the rarity of pediatric ACC (1 in 3 million) and its strong association with LFS, it has been proposed that childhood ACC could be a bellwether indicator for an underlying constitutional *TP53* mutation. Usually, in these cases it is evident from querying the family medical history, whereby the maternal or paternal side has a remarkably high incidence of cancer at early ages.

12.5 *TP53* Mutations in Childhood and Adult Adrenocortical Tumors

A large primary pediatric ACC cohort has been studied through an IRB-approved International Tumor Registry and Tissue Bank (www.stjude.org). Blood and tumor genomic DNA from these patients and their families is subjected to comprehensive sequence analysis covering the entire coding region of *TP53*, including all splicing sites and a significant proportion of the intronic regions. Many earlier studies characterized *TP53* status in ACC where only the DNA-binding region (exons 5–8) was surveyed. As illustrated by the finding of the 337His mutation (see below) [56], which now represents the most commonly inherited *TP53* alteration reported in the IARC database (www-p53.iarc.fr), screening only the DNA-binding domain would have missed this important mutation.

By sequencing the entire coding region, *TP53* mutations in 27 of 31 primary childhood adrenocortical carcinomas (87%) and 7 of 12 adenomas (58%) were uncovered. Similar results were previously published by Varley and coworkers [57] and more recently by Gonzalez and colleagues [58], who reported that approximately 80% of patients with adrenocortical carcinoma under the age of 18 had a *TP53* germline mutation. Some of these genetic alterations were observed in families that were not associated with an increased risk of cancer, suggesting the existence of low-penetrant *TP53* mutant alleles. Therefore, a constitutional *TP53* mutation should be considered in cases where a child presents with an ACC, even when arising outside the context of LFS.

The incidence of *TP53* mutations in adult ACC is far less clear. For example, 3 of 15 primary adrenocortical carcinomas were found to harbor a *TP53* mutation, but this study only tested exons 5–8 by single-strand-conformation-polymorphism analysis followed by direct sequence confirmation [59]. A subsequent study that also restricted its analysis to the DNA-binding domain identified *TP53* mutations in 0/5 adenomas and 3/11 carcinomas [60]. By contrast, screening the entire coding region by SSCP and/or by direct sequencing revealed somatic *TP53* mutations in 6/7 functioning adrenocortical carcinomas, 1/3 non-functioning adrenocortical carcinomas, and 1/4 suspect nonfunctioning adrenocortical carcinomas [61]. Bertherat and colleagues [62] also sequenced the entire coding region of *TP53* in 36 ACC that underwent 17p13 LOH and detected mutations in only 33% of the cases. Notably, those tumors with a mutation in *TP53* were larger (640 g vs. 185 g) and were associated with a worse prognosis in terms of shorter disease-free survival. Collectively, these findings implicate *TP53* inactivation in the genesis of the majority of childhood and a significant proportion of adult adrenocortical tumors. Consistent with this hypothesis, deletion of *p53* in the adrenocortical dysplasia (acd) mouse accelerates tumor onset with a shift towards the development of carcinomas [63]. It is expected that the generation and characterization of genetically engineered mouse models will continue to be invaluable for challenging the molecular defects observed in human ACC.

12.6 Low-Penetrance Mutant *TP53* Alleles

The prevalence of pediatric ACC in the southern states of Brazil, in particular Parana and Sao Paulo, is 10–15 times higher than worldwide estimates. Although, the vast majority of these affected children are not from tumor-prone families, nearly all have the same germline *TP53* missense mutation (codon 337, Arg to His substitution)

[56]. In each case, the 337His mutation was identified in at least one parent, with one exception [64], and a substantial number of relatives. The oldest carrier was 88 years of age and cancer-free. Interestingly, several families were enrolled on study with two siblings who developed ACC, which is truly remarkable in light of its normal incidence of 1 in 3 million. It is now recognized that approximately 1 in every 375 individuals in the general population in southern Brazil are carriers of the 337His mutation ([65], Figueredo, personal communication). The 337His mutation significantly increases the risk of childhood ACC in a rather tissue-restricted manner without being associated with LFS [56, 66, 67].

Interestingly, the mutation is within the oligomerization domain, specifically at an important salt bridge that stabilizes complex formation. Extensive biological analyses (e.g., DNA binding, promoter-reporter, cell cycle arrest, apoptosis, and colony reduction assays) to determine the consequence of the Arg337His mutation on TP53 function failed to demonstrate any significant loss in activity [56]. In retrospect, these negative results are entirely consistent with the low frequency of tumor development in the majority of the Brazilian families. Analysis of the primary tumors, however, provides strong evidence that the 337His mutant is defective, at least within the microenvironment of the adrenal tumor itself. Each ACC sample ($n = 15$) exhibited LOH where the wild-type allele was selected against and the missense protein was expressed at high levels in the nucleus. Intuitively, if the 337His protein was active, the proliferation and survival of the ACC would be seriously compromised. Furthermore, biophysical analyses demonstrated that the 337His mutant is structurally unstable in a pH-dependent manner, indicating that the missense mutation is not simply a polymorphism [68, 69]. It is speculated that the unique pH-dependent nature of the 337His structure, and presumably function, lies at the heart of its specificity for predisposing carriers to pediatric ACC. It may well be that the marked tissue remodeling of the adrenal gland during human embryogenesis and shortly after birth may also sensitize this tissue to small perturbations in TP53 activity. Additional studies will be required to challenge these hypotheses.

In pediatric ACC patients several other novel germline *TP53* mutations that display varying degrees of activity have also been identified. Perhaps one of the most intriguing is the 175Leu mutant, which represents a hotspot variant [70]. Codon 175 is the third most commonly mutated site in *TP53* and almost invariably exists as an arginine to histidine substitution. The abnormal histidine residue inappropriately participates in binding zinc and consequently causes catastrophic misfolding of the protein [20]. The 175His mutant is completely inactive for tumor suppression, and individuals who have inherited this mutation are associated with LFS and are at extremely high risk of cancer. By contrast, the TP53-175Leu mutant exhibits a wild-type conformation [71] and a substantial level of tumor suppressor function [70]. Consistent with at least partial TP53 activity, family members who are carriers of the 175Leu mutation have remained tumor-free. These findings provide a strong argument that not all mutations are equal, either biochemically, functionally, or clinically. Remarkably, this concept of haploinsufficient mutants also applies when the same codon is differentially targeted, resulting in two different amino acid substitutions, such as 175His and 175Leu. Genetically engineered mouse models harboring germline *p53* mutations clearly confirm this concept. For example, mice that express the 172His mutant (equivalent to human 175His), which is functionally inactive, develop tumors at a rate that is indistinguishable to *p53*-knockout mice [72]. Tumor latency in mice expressing the 172Pro mutant, which exhibits a normal conformation and is partially active in transcription and cell cycle arrest properties, is markedly delayed [73]. Therefore, there exists a clinically relevant genotype–phenotype relationship with respect to *TP53* mutations and tumor risk. This spectrum of activities and tumor susceptibility is referred to as the "TP53 gradient effect" [74]. In general, the higher percentage of tumor suppressor activity, which can be influenced by genetic background (see below), is associated with a lower risk of cancer in terms of penetrance, age of onset, and tumor spectrum.

12.7 Genetic Modifiers

A subset of the Brazilian families (7 of 30 cohorts) with the germline 337His mutation had an elevated number of breast, brain, and other tumor types in addition to ACC. An independent study also found an increased prevalence and diversity of tumors in families associated with the 337His mutation [65]. What sets these families apart from the majority of the others who are essentially only at risk for childhood adrenocortical tumors? To begin addressing this issue, a group of southern Brazilian women who developed breast cancer at a young age were screened for the 337His mutation [75]. Three of 123 affected women were found to be carriers, which represents a statistically significant tenfold increase in frequency. As expected, the analysis of more than 200 normal control age-matched women from the same region failed to identify a carrier. Interestingly, characterization of the three breast tumor tissues from the carriers demonstrated that each underwent LOH by deleting the 337His mutant allele, not the wild-type allele. Furthermore, one of the women also developed a malignant brain tumor. In this case, the tumor underwent LOH by convention where the wild allele was eliminated; however, the remaining 337His allele suffered a second site mutation in the DNA-binding domain. Collectively, these results demonstrate that 337His can elevate tumor risk beyond just ACC, but retains sufficient activity to still be selected against during tumorigenesis.

Detailed molecular analyses of the three 337His-positive women who developed breast cancer revealed that they also carried several polymorphisms within *TP53* and *HDM2* that are recognized to lower TP53 expression and activity [75]. For example, PIN3 is a 16 base pair duplication within intron 3 of *TP53* that reduces expression by approximately 50% [76]. PIN3 is associated with increased risk of breast and ovarian cancer, presumably due to diminished TP53 tumor suppressor activity [77–80]. Haplotype studies by our group and others indicate that the PIN3 polymorphism is likely associated with the wild-type allele. It is therefore understandable why the 337His allele, which retains full expression and significant activity, would be selected against during tumorigenesis rather than the compromised "wild-type" *TP53/PIN3* allele. The SNP309 polymorphism in *HDM2* creates an SP1 transcription factor-binding site, which enhances *HDM2* expression [81]. In turn, increased levels of HDM2 protein further repress TP53 activity. Consistent with these findings, SNP309 was shown to accelerate tumor onset in LFS families [81, 82]. It has been proposed that 337His predisposes carriers to childhood ACC, and in combination with other genetic alterations that further impact *TP53* expression and/or function, such as PIN3 and SNP309, contributes to the development of breast, brain, and other tumor types. Scientists are only now beginning to understand and appreciate how polymorphisms within the TP53 signaling pathway affect TP53 tumor suppressor activity and cancer risk. Defining these TP53 genotype–phenotype relationships will be important for genetic counseling purposes and for making informed clinical decisions.

12.8 Concluding Thoughts

Inactivation of *TP53* lies at the heart of most human cancers. In the vast majority of cases this occurs directly by mutating *TP53*. However, alternative mechanisms such as amplification of *HDM2* or its related family member *HDMX*, loss of *ARF*, or mutation of the *ATM/ATR/CHK2* signaling pathway must also be considered. In general, tumors that have suffered a *TP53* mutation are more aggressive and less responsive to treatment (see [83]). Restoration of TP53 function in these tumors may improve treatment, and some studies at least provide a proof-of-principle that this may be possible [84]. More promising approaches include small molecule inhibitors that interfere with HDM2 binding to wild-type TP53 [85]. Obviously, this mentality fits with tailored treatments and will depend on the genetics that drive the growth and survival of the particular tumor. Inheritance of *TP53* mutations clearly has long-term consequences on the health of the carriers and knowing the risk of a particular mutation could influence clinical management. For example, a woman who has a constitutional 175His mutation may be counseled to undergo a prophylactic double mastectomy due to the incredibly high risk of developing breast cancer [86, 87]. Would the physician in consultation with the patient consider this possibility if the mutation was the 175Leu substitution [70]?

Recognizing that a patient carries a *TP53* mutation could provide an opportunity to closely monitor the individual for the first signs of cancer. Indeed, this is already occurring in the cases of the Brazilian children with the 337His mutation. Identification of carriers has led to earlier detection and surgical intervention with improved prognosis. It has also been reported that germline carriers of *TP53* mutations may be susceptible to treatment-induced malignancies, such as sarcomas and other solid tumors arising within the field of radiation [88]. Therefore, how the patient is treated should be an important clinical consideration. Carriers of germline *TP53* mutations should also avoid known cancer risk factors such as tobacco, alcohol, and UV/sunburn.

This year (2009) marks the 30th anniversary of the discovery of TP53. Our understanding of how TP53 functions as a tumor suppressor has advanced significantly since its inception. Indeed, there are presently more than 50,000 published studies on TP53 and despite this incredible wealth of knowledge, we are still hampered by our inability to correct *TP53* genetic defects. Given the remarkable technical advances in cancer research and gene therapy, answers to these problems may lie just around the corner.

References

1. Linzer DI, Levine AJ (1979) Characterization of a 54 K dalton cellular SV40 tumor antigen present in SV40-transformed cells and uninfected embryonal carcinoma cells. Cell17:43–52
2. Lane DP, Crawford LV (1979) T antigen is bound to a host protein in SV40-transformed cells. Nature 278:261–263
3. Vousden KH, Prives C (2009) Blinded by the Light: the growing complexity of p53. Cell 137:413–431
4. Donehower LA et al (1992) Mice deficient for p53 are developmentally normal but susceptible to spontaneous tumours. Nature 356:215–221
5. Jacks T et al (1994) Tumor spectrum analysis in p53-mutant mice. Curr Biol. 4:1–7
6. Malkin D et al (1990) Germ line p53 mutations in a familial syndrome of breast cancer, sarcomas, and other neoplasms. Science 250:1233–1238
7. Nutting C et al (2000) A patient with 17 primary tumours and a germ line mutation in TP53: tumour induction by adjuvant therapy? Clin Oncol 12:300–304
8. Zambetti GP (2005) P53 tumor suppressor pathway and cancer. Springer, New York
9. Murphy ME (2006) Polymorphic variants in the p53 pathway. Cell Death Differ 13:916–920
10. Walker KK, Levine AJ (1996) Identification of a novel p53 functional domain that is necessary for efficient growth suppression. Proc Natl Acad Sci USA 93:15335–15340
11. Petitjean A et al (2007) Impact of mutant p53 functional properties on TP53 mutation patterns and tumor phenotype: lessons from recent developments in the IARC TP53 database. Hum Mutat 28:622–629
12. Shaulsky G et al (1990) Nuclear accumulation of p53 protein is mediated by several nuclear localization signals and plays a role in tumorigenesis. Mol Cell Biol 10:6565–6577
13. Deng C et al (1995) Mice lacking p21CIP1/WAF1 undergo normal development, but are defective in G1 checkpoint control. Cell 82:675–684
14. el-Deiry WS et al (1993) WAF1, a potential mediator of p53 tumor suppression. Cell 75: 817–825
15. Han J et al (2001) Expression of bbc3, a pro-apoptotic BH3-only gene, is regulated by diverse cell death and survival signals. Proc Natl Acad Sci USA 98:11318–11323
16. Nakano K, Vousden KH (2001) PUMA, a novel proapoptotic gene, is induced by p53. Mol Cell 7:683–694
17. Yu J et al (2001) PUMA induces the rapid apoptosis of colorectal cancer cells. Mol Cell 7:673–682
18. Jeffers JR et al (2003) Puma is an essential mediator of p53-dependent and -independent apoptotic pathways. Cancer Cell 4:321–328
19. Villunger A et al (2003) p53- and drug-induced apoptotic responses mediated by BH3-only proteins puma and noxa. Science 302:1036–1038
20. Cho Y et al (1994) Crystal structure of a p53 tumor suppressor-DNA complex: understanding tumorigenic mutations. Science 265:346–355
21. Fakharzadeh SS et al (1991) Tumorigenic potential associated with enhanced expression of a gene that is amplified in a mouse tumor cell line. EMBO J 10:1565–1569

22. Momand J et al (1992) The mdm-2 oncogene product forms a complex with the p53 protein and inhibits p53-mediated transactivation. Cell 69:1237–1245
23. Honda R et al (1997) Oncoprotein MDM2 is a ubiquitin ligase E3 for tumor suppressor p53. FEBS Lett 420:25–27
24. Barak Y et al (1993) mdm2 expression is induced by wild type p53 activity. EMBO J 12: 461–468
25. Barak Y et al (1993) Regulation of mdm2 expression by p53: alternative promoters produce transcripts with nonidentical translation potential. Genes Dev 8:1739–1749
26. Wu X et al (1993) The p53-mdm-2 autoregulatory feedback loop. Genes Dev 7:1126–1132
27. Jones SN et al (1995) Rescue of embryonic lethality in Mdm2-deficient mice by absence of p53. Nature 378:206–208
28. Montes de Oca Luna R et al (1995) Rescue of early embryonic lethality in mdm2-deficient mice by deletion of p53. Nature 378:203–206
29. Momand J, Zambetti GP (1997) Mdm-2: "big brother" of p53. J Cell Biochem 64:343–352
30. Momand J et al (1998) The MDM2 gene amplification database. Nucleic Acids Res 26: 3453–3459
31. Oliner JD et al (1992) Amplification of a gene encoding a p53-associated protein in human sarcomas. Nature 358:80–83
32. Appella E, Anderson CW (2001) Post-translational modifications and activation of p53 by genotoxic stresses. Eur J Biochem 268:2764–2772
33. Kussie PH et al (1996) Structure of the MDM2 oncoprotein bound to the p53 tumor suppressor transactivation domain. Science 274:948–953
34. Sakaguchi K et al (1998) DNA damage activates p53 through a phosphorylation-acetylation cascade. Genes Dev 12:2831–2841
35. Shieh SY et al (1997) DNA damage-induced phosphorylation of p53 alleviates inhibition by MDM2. Cell 91:325–334
36. de Stanchina E et al (1998) E1A signaling to p53 involves the p19(ARF) tumor suppressor. Genes Dev 12:2434–2442
37. Quelle DE et al (1995) Alternative reading frames of the INK4a tumor suppressor gene encode two unrelated proteins capable of inducing cell cycle arrest. Cell 83:993–1000
38. Zindy F et al (1998) Myc signaling via the ARF tumor suppressor regulates p53-dependent apoptosis and immortalization. Genes Dev 12:2424–2433
39. Honda R, Yasuda H (1999) Association of p19ARF with Mdm2 inhibits ubiquitin ligase activity of MDM2 for tumor suppressor p53. EMBO J 18:22–27
40. Kamijo T et al (1998) Functional and physical interactions of the ARF tumor suppressor with p53 and Mdm2. Proc Natl Acad Sci USA 95:8292–8297
41. Zhang Y et al (1998) ARF promotes MDM2 degradation and stabilizes p53: ARF-INK4a locus deletion impairs both the Rb and p53 tumor suppression pathways. Cell 92:725–734
42. Bates S et al (1998) E2F-1 regulation of p14ARF links pRB and p53. Nature 395:124–125
43. Kamijo T et al (1997) Tumor suppression at the mouse INK4a locus mediated by the alternative reading frame product p19ARF. Cell 91:649–659
44. Sherr CJ (2001) The INK4a/ARF network in tumour suppression. Nat Rev Mol Cell Biol 2:731–737
45. Williams RT, Sherr CJ (2008) The INK4-ARF (CDKN2A/B) locus in hematopoiesis and BCR-ABL-induced leukemias. Cold Spring Harb Symp Quant Biol 73:461–467
46. Denissenko MF et al (1996) Preferential formation of benzo[a]pyrene adducts at lung cancer mutational hotspots in P53. Science 274:430–432
47. Bressac B et al (1991) Selective G to T mutations of p53 gene in hepatocellular carcinoma from southern Africa. Nature 350:429–431
48. Hsu IC et al (1991) Mutational hotspot in the p53 gene in human hepatocellular carcinomas. Nature 350:427–428
49. Brash DE et al (1991) A role for sunlight in skin cancer: UV-induced p53 mutations in squamous cell carcinoma. Proc Natl Acad Sci USA 88:1012–1048

50. Kress S et al (1992) Carcinogen-specific mutational pattern in the p53 gene in ultraviolet B radiation-induced squamous cell carcinomas of mouse skin. Cancer Res 52:6400–6403
51. Ziegler A et al (1993) Mutation hotspots due to sunlight in the p53 gene of nonmelanoma skin cancers. Proc Natl Acad Sci USA 90:4216–4220
52. Chen PL et al (1990) Genetic mechanisms of tumor suppression by the human p53 gene. Science 250:1576–80
53. Friedman PN et al (1993) The p53 protein is an unusually shaped tetramer that binds directly to DNA. Proc Natl Acad Sci USA 90:3319–3323
54. Hinds PW et al (1990) Mutant p53 DNA clones from human colon carcinomas cooperate with ras in transforming primary rat cells:a comparison of the “hot spot” mutant phenotypes. Cell Growth Differ 1:571–580
55. Kleihues P et al (1997) Tumors associated with p53 germline mutations: a synopsis of 91 families. Am J Pathol 150:1–13
56. Ribeiro RC et al (2001) An inherited p53 mutation that contributes in a tissue-specific manner to pediatric adrenal cortical carcinoma. Proc Natl Acad Sci USA 98:9330–9335
57. Varley JM et al (1999) Are there low-penetrance TP53 Alleles? Evidence from childhood adrenocortical tumors. Am J Hum Genet 65:995–1006
58. Gonzalez KD et al (2009) Beyond Li Fraumeni Syndrome: clinical characteristics of families with p53 germline mutations. J Clin Oncol 27:1250–1256
59. Ohgaki H et al (1993) p53 mutations in sporadic adrenocortical tumors. Int J Cancer 54: 408–410
60. Reincke M et al (1994) p53 mutations in human adrenocortical neoplasms: immunohistochemical and molecular studies. J Clin Endocrinol Metab 78:790–794
61. Barzon L et al (2001) Molecular analysis of CDKN1C and TP53 in sporadic adrenal tumors. Eur J Endocrinol 145:207–212
62. Libè R et al (2007) Somatic TP53 mutations are relatively rare among adrenocortical cancers with the frequent 17p13 loss of heterozygosity. Clin Cancer Res 13:844–850
63. Else T et al (2009) Genetic p53 deficiency partially rescues the adrenocortical dysplasia phenotype at the expense of increased tumorigenesis. Cancer Cell 15:465–476
64. Latronico AC et al (2001) An inherited mutation outside the highly conserved DNA-binding domain of the p53 tumor suppressor protein in children and adults with sporadic adrenocortical tumors. J Clin Endocrinol Metab 86:4970–4973
65. Achatz MI et al (2007) The TP53 mutation, R337H, is associated with Li-Fraumeni and Li-Fraumeni-like syndromes in Brazilian families. Cancer Lett 245:96–102
66. Figueiredo BC et al (2006) Penetrance of adrenocortical tumours associated with the germline TP53 R337H mutation. J Med Genet 43:91–96
67. Ribeiro RC et al (2007) Germline TP53 R337H mutation is not sufficient to establish Li-Fraumeni or Li-Fraumeni-like syndrome. Cancer Lett 247:353–355
68. DiGiammarino EL et al (2002) A novel mechanism of tumorigenesis involving pH-dependent destabilization of a mutant p53 tetramer. Nat Struct Biol 9:12–16
69. Galea C et al (2005) Disruption of an intermonomer salt bridge in the p53 tetramerization domain results in an increased propensity to form amyloid fibrils. Protein Sci 14:2993–3003
70. West AN et al (2006) Identification of a novel germ line variant hotspot mutant p53-R175L in pediatric adrenal cortical carcinoma. Cancer Res 66:5056–5062
71. Ory K et al (1994) Analysis of the most representative tumour-derived p53 mutants reveals that changes in protein conformation are not correlated with loss of transactivation or inhibition of cell proliferation. EMBO J 13:3496–3504
72. Liu G et al (2000) High metastatic potential in mice inheriting a targeted p53 missense mutation. Proc Natl Acad Sci USA 97:4174–4179
73. Liu G et al (2004) Chromosome stability, in the absence of apoptosis, is critical for suppression of tumorigenesis in Trp53 mutant mice. Nat Genet 36:63–68
74. Zambetti GP (2007) The p53 mutation “gradient effect” and its clinical implications. J Cell Physiol 213:370–373

75. Assumpção JG et al (2008) Association of the germline TP53 R337H mutation with breast cancer in southern Brazil. BMC Cancer 8:357
76. Gemignani F et al (2004) A TP53 polymorphism is associated with increased risk of colorectal cancer and with reduced levels of TP53 mRNA. Oncogene 23:1954–1956
77. Costa S et al (2008) Importance of TP53 codon 72 and intron 3 duplication 16 bp polymorphisms in prediction of susceptibility on breast cancer. BMC Cancer 8:32
78. Wang-Gohrke S et al (1998) p53 germline polymorphisms are associated with an increased risk for breast cancer in German women. Anticancer Res 18:2095–2099
79. Wang-Gohrke S et al (1999) Intron variants of the p53 gene are associated with increased risk for ovarian cancer but not in carriers of BRCA1 or BRCA2 germline mutations. Br J Cancer 81:179–183
80. Wang-Gohrke S et al (2002) Intron 3 16 bp duplication polymorphism of p53 is associated with an increased risk for breast cancer by the age of 50 years. Pharmacogenetics 12:269–272
81. Bond GL et al (2004) A single nucleotide polymorphism in the MDM2 promoter attenuates the p53 Tumor Suppressor pathway and accelerates tumor formation in humans. Cell 119:591–602
82. Bougeard G et al (2006) Impact of the MDM2 SNP309 and p53 Arg72Pro polymorphism on age of tumour onset in Li-Fraumeni syndrome. J Med Genet 43:531–533
83. Brosh R, Rotter V (2009) When mutants gain new powers: news from the mutant p53 field. Nat Rev Cancer 9:701–713
84. Boeckler FM et al (2008) Targeted rescue of a destabilized mutant of p53 by an in silico screened drug. Proc Natl Acad Sci USA 105:10360–10365
85. Vassilev LT et al (2004) In vivo activation of the p53 pathway by small-molecule antagonists of MDM2. Science 303:844–848
86. Evans DG, Lalloo F (2002) Risk assessment and management of high risk familial breast cancer. J Med Genet 39:865–871
87. Moule RN et al (2006) Genotype phenotype correlation in Li-Fraumeni syndrome kindreds and its implications for management. Familial Cancer 5:129–133
88. Hisada M et al (1998) Multiple primary cancers in families with Li-Fraumeni syndrome. J Natl Cancer Inst 90:606–611

Chapter 13
Telomeres and Telomerase in Adrenocortical Carcinoma

Tobias Else and Peter J. Hornsby

Telomeres are the outer ends of chromosomes and consist of noncoding hexameric repeats of DNA (TTAGGG). There are two main challenges inherently connected to these structures. First, they need to be protected by special mechanisms to prevent their recognition as DNA breaks by DNA surveillance mechanisms and potential processing by the DNA repair machinery. Second, due to the semiconservative mechanism of DNA replication using RNA primers, small stretches of telomeric sequences are lost with each cell division. This is referred to as the "end-replication problem". The first challenge is met by a specialized structure of the telomere and its association with protein factors that prevent its recognition as damaged DNA and regulate the access of the DNA repair machinery. In the absence of mechanisms to overcome the end-replication problem, the ongoing loss of telomere sequences in somatic cells ultimately leads to critically short and dysfunctional telomeres that will lead to signaling events, resulting in the removal of these cells from the pool of proliferating cells by mechanisms such as senescence, crisis, or potentially apoptosis. These mechanisms prevent the accumulation of telomere dysfunction-induced genomic aberrations. Telomere shortening can be overcome, e.g., in stem cell compartments and malignant cells, by telomere maintenance mechanisms (TMMs). TMMs either involve the action of telomerase, a ribonucleoprotein that adds telomeric repeats to the telomere or involve alternative TMMs (ALT), the molecular bases of which need yet to be determined. There is experimental and observational evidence that telomeres and telomerase play a role in carcinogenesis in general and in the adrenal cortex in particular. When there is inactivation of checkpoint mechanisms, which normally would induce apoptosis or senescence, critically short or dysfunctional telomeres can set off processes of genome shuffling, such as breakage-fusion-bridge cycles (BFBs), leading to the loss or amplification of genomic material. BFBs and their morphological correlate, anaphase bridges, are important hallmarks of the stage of crisis. Crisis, like senescence, is a terminal state

T. Else (✉)
Department of Internal Medicine – Division of Metabolism, Endocrinology & Diabetes, University of Michigan Health System, University of Michigan, Domino's Farms, Lobby C, Suite 1300, 24 Frank Lloyd Wright Drive, PO Box 451, Ann Arbor, MI 48106, USA
e-mail: telse@med.umich.edu

G.D. Hammer, T. Else (eds.), *Adrenocortical Carcinoma*,
DOI 10.1007/978-0-387-77236-3_13, © Springer Science+Business Media, LLC 2011

in which cells will persist and eventually die by presumably unspecific mechanisms. Only very rarely, clones may emerge and bypass crisis and acquire TMMs. TMMs can have a dual role with regards to tumorigenesis. Depending on the timing of activation of these mechanisms, before or after the acquisition of genomic alterations (meaning before or after crisis), they can either act as an antitumorigenic mechanism by preventing the occurrence of critically short telomeres or help maintaining a malignant phenotype by stabilizing the genome at later stages of tumorigenesis, thereby providing the basis of immortality.

This chapter will focus on the basic principles of telomere and telomerase in cellular physiology and will then detail the knowledge of this field pertinent to adrenocortical carcinoma (ACC). Telomere pathophysiology involves the action of p53, a main gatekeeper of the DNA surveillance and repair machinery, as well as other factors in this pathway. Therefore, telomere biology is closely connected to the pathophysiology of inherited cancer syndromes like Li-Fraumeni syndrome (LFS).

13.1 The End-Replication Problem and Telomerase

Telomeres are composed of hexameric telomeric repeats. With every round of DNA replication, telomeres shorten by roughly 40–100 bp [1]. The reason for this is depicted in Fig. 13.1. While leading strand synthesis by DNA polymerases is carried out to completion, lagging strand synthesis depends on small randomly priming RNA fragments. This on average leads to a loss of telomeric sequences of the emerging chromosome copy. Over consecutive rounds of chromosome replication, this leads to telomere shortening [2]. Cells that experience critical telomere shortening progress to an irreversible cell cycle arrest termed senescence or initiate programmed cell death, termed apoptosis [3–5]. Both mechanisms are commonly induced by p53-sensitive signaling pathways [6, 7]. In human fibroblast cultures, this state is mirrored by a gradual slowing of cell proliferation until the entire population enters senescence. It occurs after a number of population doublings characteristic for the cell type, often in the range of 50 as for human skin fibroblasts. It is also known as the Hayflick limit [8, 9]. The process of telomere shortening is often referred to as a main mechanism of cellular aging. However, this is mainly a theoretical consideration with only little direct evidence that telomere shortening can result in senescence in vivo [10].

In stem cell compartments, such as the hematopoietic system, the basal layer of the skin and germ cell epithelia, as well as in embryonic stem cells, the activity of the specialized ribonucleoprotein telomerase overcomes the issue of excessive telomere shortening [11–13]. Telomerase consists of an RNA component, which harbors a telomeric repeat template, and a protein subunit with reverse transcriptase activity [14, 15]. This enzyme acts by adding telomeric repeats to the chromosome ends in a 5' to 3' direction. The lagging strand is then synthesized in the usual way by the DNA polymerase using RNA primers. This mechanism prevents shortening

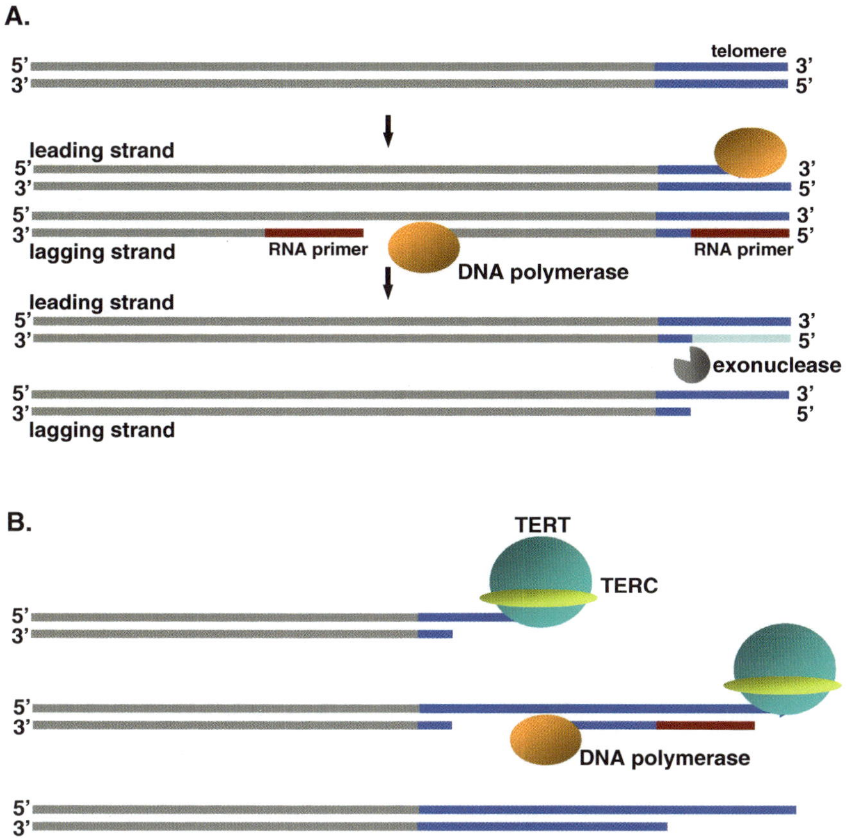

Fig. 13.1 Model of telomere shortening and telomerase activity. (**a**) Telomere shortening. A 3'-overhang is created by the lagging strand synthesis after excision of the RNA primer resulting in a shortened telomere. 3'-synthesis of the leading strand can be carried to completion by the DNA polymerase. A 3'-overhang is created by a yet unidentified mechanism, most likely a 5'-exonuclease. After a certain number of cell divisions, telomeres become critically short and induce cellular senescence or apoptosis. (**b**) Telomere maintenance. Telomerase, consisting of the protein (TERT) and RNA (TERC) subunit, extends telomeres by adding telomeric repeats (TTAGGG) in the 3'-direction. The DNA polymerase can then synthesize the lagging strand. This process can maintain telomere length or lead to telomere lengthening (Figure modified from Else [45])

of telomeres and the progression to a length based dysfunctional state and ensures a life time replenishment of tissues. Telomerase activity distinguishes somatic cell types from stem cells such as embryonic stem cells [16]. On the basis of sequence similarities, evolutionary evidence, and an overlap in functional characteristics, it is hypothesized that the telomerase reverse transcriptase shares a common ancestry with the reverse transcriptase of retrotransposons [17].

It is estimated that >90% of malignant human tumors have TMMs. The vast majority of malignant tumors (90%) exploit telomerase as a mechanism of telomere length maintenance, rendering them resistant to telomere-based crisis induced by excessive telomere shortening [18]. The remaining tumors use ALT, which maintains telomere length and integrity in a telomerase-independent manner [19]. The underlying molecular mechanisms of this process are less well understood. These seem to depend on the action of DNA helicases (e.g., WRN and BLM) and most likely employ an exchange of telomere sequences between chromosomes and possibly extrachromosomal telomeric DNA [20, 21].

As pointed out earlier, telomerase activity can theoretically also serve as an anti-cancer mechanism. While this seems to be a paradox, it can be explained by the different timing of acquisition of telomerase activity. When telomerase is expressed at early stages of carcinogenesis, i.e., premalignant stages, it may prevent the occurrence of dysfunctional telomeres induced by telomere shortening, ensuring genomic and telomere integrity and protecting the cell from acquisition of oncogenic mutations through BFBs.

13.2 Telomeres

Telomeres play a key role in the maintenance of genome stability and therefore need to meet one main challenge. They need to avoid being recognized as a DNA break by the DNA surveillance and repair machinery. This task is ensured by two mechanisms. Telomere DNA forms a specialized structure, the so-called T-loop, where the 3' single-stranded overhang loops back and intercalates ("hides") into an opening of the double-stranded telomeric DNA, called the D-loop [22]. The 3' single-stranded overhang results from lagging strand synthesis as described above (Fig. 13.2, Table 13.1). The 3' single-stranded overhang of the leading strand

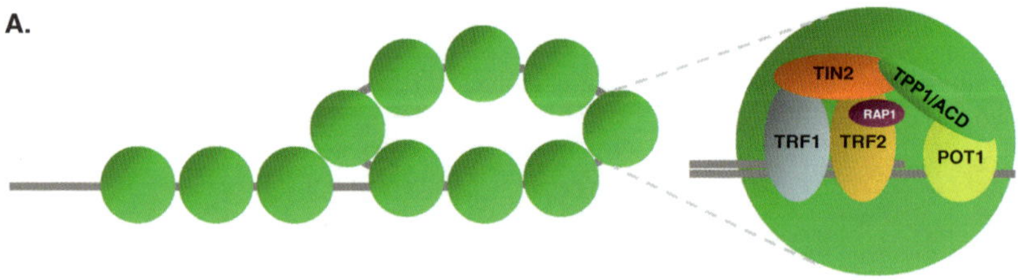

Fig. 13.2 The telomere cap complex (shelterin complex). Multiple shelterin complexes can be found at the telomere DNA T-loop and exist in different compositions to serve the multiple functions of the telomere, protect it from recognition, and processing by the DNA surveillance machinery. On the right a "magnified" model of the telomere cap complex (shelterin complex) bound to the end of the telomere is shown. (POT1, protection of telomeres 1; ACD, adrenocortical dysplasia homolog (TPP1/ACD); TERT, telomerase reverse transcriptase; TERF2IP, TERF2-interacting protein (RAP1); TERF2, telomeric repeat-binding factor 2 (TRF2); TERF1, telomeric repeat-binding factor 1 (TRF1); TINF2, TRF1-interacting nuclear factor 2 (TIN2)) (Figure modified from Else [45])

Table 13.1 Telomere-associated proteins (chromosomal location, function, associated hereditary diseases)

Gene	Chromosomal location	Function	Associated diseases
POT1	*7q31.33*	Shelterin component	None reported
ACD/TPP1	*16q22.1*	Shelterin component	None reported
TRF1	*8q13*	Shelterin component	None reported
TRF2	*16q22.1*	Shelterin component	None reported
RAP1	*16q23.1*	Shelterin component	None reported
TIN2	*14q12*	Shelterin component	Sporadic DC, autosomal dominant DC, Hoyeraal Hreidarsson
TERC	*3q26.2*	Telomerase RNA component	Sporadic and hereditary IPF, sporadic and hereditary aplastic anemia, hereditary liver cirrhosis, autosomal dominant DC
TERT	*5p15.33*	Telomerase protein subunit, catalytic subunit	Sporadic and hereditary IPF, sporadic and hereditary aplastic anemia, hereditary liver cirrhosis, autosomal dominant DC
DKC1	*Xq28*		X-linked DC, Hoyeraal Hreidarsson
NOP10	*15q14-15q15*		Autosomal recessive DC
NHP2	*5q35.3*		Autosomal recessive DC

is produced by a putative exonuclease, which to date has not been definitively identified. Furthermore, telomeres are bound by a complex of six main proteins [23]. This complex, also termed shelterin, forms the telomere cap, which further prevents the recognition of telomeric DNA as a DNA double-strand break and regulates telomerase access. The shelterin complex consists of six different core proteins, which either bind to telomeric DNA or serve as interconnectors between DNA-bound shelterin complex proteins (Table 13.1). TRF1 and TRF2 bind directly to double-stranded telomeric repeats [24, 25]. POT1 binds to the single-stranded 3'-overhang [26]. The remaining three components of this complex bind to DNA-bound factors and form several different configurations, which are proposed to serve different functions [27]. RAP1 binds to TRF2, TIN2 binds to TRF1 and TRF2, and TPP1/ACD serves as an interconnector between TIN2 and POT1 [28–33]. The importance of these factors is underscored by the fact that deficiency of most of the shelterin components renders telomeres dysfunctional and induces signaling events leading to the induction of senescence or apoptosis [6, 34–36]. Dysfunctional telomeres can therefore either arise from critical decrease in number of telomeric repeats or from shelterin component deficiency [3, 4, 6]. Whether apoptosis or senescence is induced by telomere dysfunction seems to be dependent on cell type and degree of telomere dysfunction [37, 38]. In human cells in the presence of functional checkpoints, telomere dysfunction leads to signaling events inducing senescence as the main non-replicative state [5]. Experimental data, at least in the murine organism and in cell culture experiments with overwhelming sudden telomere dysfunction (e.g., induced by transduction with a dominant negative isoform of TRF2) also suggests the possibility of apoptosis induction [6, 37, 39, 40]. However, it remains unclear, whether telomere dysfunction-induced apoptosis plays a significant role in in vivo tumor prevention. The lack of detection may also be due to the usual transient character of apoptosis in tissues. Cells in final static states such as crisis and senescence accumulate, and can rather easily be detected, while apoptotic cells may escape analysis as cell remains are readily eliminated, e.g. by macrophages. In the adrenal cortex senescence seems to be the major mechanism. Dysfunctional telomeres can be detected as TIFs in tissue sections, where telomere hybridization signals co-localize with factors of the DNA surveillance machinery, such as γH2AX or 53BP1 [36]. Dysfunctional telomeres activate ATM and ATR phosphorylation followed by a subsequent signaling cascade that activates p53 to stall the cell cycle and induce apoptosis or senescence [6, 7]. A hallmark of senescence induction is the activation of p21, which lies downstream of p53 signaling, but is also characterized by the activation of p16, which plays, at least in human cells, an adjunct role in response to dysfunctional telomeres [41, 42]. The non-replicative state of senescence is also referred to as M1 (mortality stage 1) [43].

In the absence of sufficient checkpoints that would act to detect dysfunctional telomeres, cells bypass the stage of senescence and enter a state called crisis [43]. Crisis is characterized by chromosomal end-to-end fusions, leading to aneuploidy, and by mitotic catastrophe, leading to an arrest in mitosis [44]. Therefore, crisis represents a second terminal state, which is also referred to as M2 (mortality stage 2) [43]. Only extremely rarely clones will manage to escape this stage and give rise to a fully malignant tumor. These clones must acquire: (1) alterations leading to malignant transformation (e.g., via transient BFBs, see below) and (2) TMMs for genomic stabilization to acquire immortality (e.g., telomerase activity).

In summary, telomeres may play two different roles in carcinogenesis depending on the presence or absence of sufficient checkpoints of telomere and DNA integrity. In the presence of these checkpoints, telomere dysfunction induces removal of cells from the pool of proliferating cells and serves as an anti-cancer mechanism. On the other hand, in the absence of these checkpoints dysfunctional fusogenic telomeres may serve as a starting point for BFBs and lead to the acquisition of a pro-cancer genome. However, it is important to mention that BFBs leading to genomic rearrangements, which provide the cell with TMMs, are very likely rare events and therefore crisis still acts as a tumor suppressor mechanism.

13.3 Telomere-Based Model of Carcinogenesis

There are two main steps in order to acquire a full malignant phenotype in the telomere-based model of carcinogenesis. The first event leads to the acquisition of a pro-cancer genome while the second event stabilizes telomeres and prevents crisis-based growth arrest [45–47].

As described above, dysfunctional telomeres usually signal to induce preferentially senescence and possibly apoptosis. This is of course only true in cells with proficient DNA surveillance machinery and intact checkpoint mechanisms. Therefore, most of our knowledge of dysfunctional telomere-induced carcinogenesis stems from animal models and human syndromes deficient in main DNA surveillance signaling factors, such as p53 or ATM, as well as proteins necessary for telomere maintenance and integrity. The two main mouse models are homozygous *Terc* $^{-/-}$ mice, which acquire telomere dysfunction in late generations due to excessive telomere shortening, and adrenocortical dysplasia (*acd*) mice, which are deficient in the shelterin component Tpp1/Acd [48–52]. *Terc*$^{-/-}$ mice tend to develop cancers at late generations and old age [53]. Additional p53 deficiency of *Terc*$^{-/-}$ mice leads to an acceleration of tumor incidence compared to *Terc*$^{+/+}$/*p53*$^{-/-}$ mice [49, 51]. On the contrary, *acd* mice exhibit signs of telomere dysfunction already within the first generation and do not develop tumors unless they are challenged with a second event such as p53 deficiency [48, 54, 55]. *p53*$^{-/-}$/*acd* mice develop cancer at a significantly earlier age than *p53*$^{-/-}$ mice, which carry the *wt Tpp1/Acd* allele, and which have intact telomeres. In both animal models it has been shown that tissues display a higher degree of telomere dysfunction as evidenced by the occurrence of telomere dysfunction-induced foci (TIFs). Tissues and tumors from these mice show an increase in anaphase bridges. These are morphological correlates of telomere fusions, which can serve as a starting point for BFBs. BFBs are thought to be the main mechanism leading to genomic alterations in the setting of telomere dysfunction (Fig. 13.3). In case of checkpoint deficiency, e.g., absence of p53, cells with dysfunctional telomeres, either as a result of critical shortening (e.g., *Terc*$^{-/-}$) or due to deficiency of a shelterin component (*acd* mice), fail to undergo apoptosis or senescence [3, 4, 37]. The uncapped telomeres are recognized by the DNA repair machinery and are fused by cellular ligases (e.g., as part of non-homologous end-joining processes (NHEJ)) resulting in dicentric chromosomes. These chromosomal alterations can be observed in metaphase spreads of mouse embryonic fibroblasts from several shelterin-deficient animals [35, 54, 56–58]. During mitosis those dicentric chromosomes may be pulled to the opposite poles of the emerging daughter cells, and in anaphase these chromatin strings can be observed as anaphase bridges. Eventually, these dicentric chromosomes break at a location that is not necessarily the former fusion point. As a result, the genome of one of the daughter cells will have genomic gains and the other one losses. The new DNA breaks can serve again as starting points for BFBs, leading to further amplification or losses of genetic loci [59, 60]. The genomic alterations can be either visualized by spectral karyotyping or analyzed by comparative genomic hybridization [48, 49, 61]. Both available mouse models of telomere dysfunction have been subjected to these analyses and show

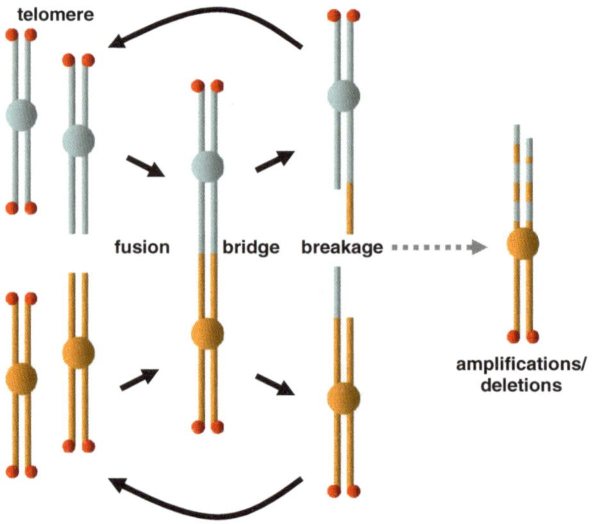

Fig. 13.3 Model of genomic shuffling by breakage fusion bridge (BFB) cycles. Dysfunctional telomeres (absent red circles) fuse and form dicentric chromosomes. During cell division, the fused chromosomes are pulled to the two different poles of the emerging daughter cells. During anaphase these can be observed as anaphase bridges, chromosomal material spanning from one daughter cell to the other. Eventually, a break occurs and creates another open (unprotected) end, which can serve as a new starting point for a subsequent BFB. Ultimately, this process leads to genomic amplifications and deletions (Figure modified from Else [45])

typical translocations and genomic copy number changes, which are in accordance with presumed BFBs.

There is growing evidence from the analysis of human pathologies that telomere dysfunction and the subsequent development of genomic aberrations take place in early malignant or premalignant lesions [62]. Recent studies have focused on breast cancer and colon cancer [63–66]. Both tumors have well-defined histological stages of carcinoma progression from premalignant stages. During the development of breast cancer genomic instability occurs at a very early stage, during the progression from usual ductal hyperplasia to ductal carcinoma in situ [63]. In human colon cancer as well as in the *Apc^min^* mouse model, telomere-based genomic instability has been detected at the stage of high-grade dysplasia and carcinoma in situ but not in adenomas [64, 67].

In the second step of the telomerase-based model of tumorigenesis, malignant cells acquire telomerase activity or an alternative TMM [47, 63, 68]. Genomic alterations resulting from end-to-end fusions in most incidences will lead to crisis and mitotic arrest [43]. Only very rarely clones will escape and bypass the stage of crisis and acquire telomerase activity or ALT [69]. These TMMs lead to a stabilization of telomeres and provide the emerging clone with an indefinite potential to proliferate without undergoing telomere dysfunction-based crisis. Indeed, roughly 90% of human cancers are positive for telomerase activity [18]. In breast cancer, telomerase activity can first be detected during the progression from usual ductal hyperplasia to ductal carcinoma in situ, presumably shortly after the acquisition of genomic alterations necessary for progression to a malignant phenotype [63].

In summary, in order to give rise to an immortal malignant cell clone, this clone will need to bypass senescence through some kind of checkpoint deficiency and acquire a malignant phenotype, possibly through further genomic alterations generated by BFBs. This genomic instability due to dysfunctional telomeres seems to parallel early stages of progression from pre-malignant to malignant lesions. Of note, sufficient telomerase activity as a preventive mechanism is absent during this phase, underscoring the potential importance of telomerase activity as an anti-cancer mechanism. While these genomic aberrations lead to a malignant phenotype, immortality is acquired by later activation of telomerase activity (or ALT).

13.4 Telomerase in Experimental Adrenocortical Carcinoma

TERT-expressing vectors have been employed in several tissue-engineering experiments involving xenografts in immunodeficient mice. Human or bovine adrenocortical cells transduced with a *TERT* expression vector, when transplanted under the renal capsule, produce sufficient hormones to prevent death of adrenalectomized mice [70] (Fig. 13.5). It is noteworthy that these cells do not form tumors. Therefore, the simple introduction of telomerase activity into a normal telomerase-negative cell does not induce a malignant phenotype. When this xenotransplant model was applied to test different oncogene requirements for malignant transformation, an important observation was made. In the past, experiments with human fibroblasts and other human cell types had shown that the minimal requirement for a full malignant tumor-forming phenotype was the inactivation of the retinoblastoma (pRB) and p53 tumor-suppressor pathways (for example, by the action of viral proteins such as SV40 LT), acquisition of a constitutive mitogenic signal provided by oncogenic Ras, and perturbation of protein phosphatase 2A by SV40 ST as well as introduction of telomerase activity [71–73]. In all these experiments cells were transplanted or injected into the subcutaneous tissue of immunodeficient nude mice. However, when adrenocortical cells (or fibroblasts) of human or bovine origin were transplanted under the kidney capsule, transduction with *SV40 LT* and oncogenic *Ras* were sufficient to induce a fully malignant phenotype – there was no necessity for telomerase activity [74, 75]. A thorough analysis of these tumor cells did not show acquisition of any telomere maintenance mechanism, neither telomerase activity nor alternative telomere lengthening. These experiments challenged the paradigm that telomerase activity or other telomere maintenance mechanisms are needed for a malignant transformation, and clearly showed that telomere maintenance mechanisms are not necessary for a malignant phenotype of adrenocortical cells. Two other roles of telomerase were identified in subsequent experiments. First, telomerase is sufficient to induce immortality, and second, it was hypothesized that telomerase may play a role in malignant transformation different from its role in telomere maintenance. Transduction with *SV40 LT* and oncogenic *Ras* were sufficient to induce a malignant phenotype, but these cell clones lacked immortality [75]. When tumors of these cells were harvested, diluted, and serially transplanted, tumor growth ceased and transplanted cells entered a stage of crisis after a definite number of serial transplantations. An immortal phenotype with an "indefinite" number of serial transplantation could be induced when telomerase activity was conferred by transducing *TERT* additionally into these cells, consistent with the concept that TMMs are necessary for immortality (Fig. 13.4). However, this does not explain why *TERT* is needed for a malignant phenotype of fibroblasts when transplanted subcutaneously. A possible explanation is that *TERT* serves different functions aside from its role at the telomere. There is accumulating evidence that there is an alternative *TERT* function in stem cell physiology, independent of telomeres. It has been shown in several experiments that ectopic *TERT* alters overall gene expression patterns of different cell types, which cannot simply be explained by its role at the telomere [76–79].

In summary, telomerase activity or TMMs are not necessary to induce a malignant phenotype in the setting of xenotransplantation under the kidney capsule, but

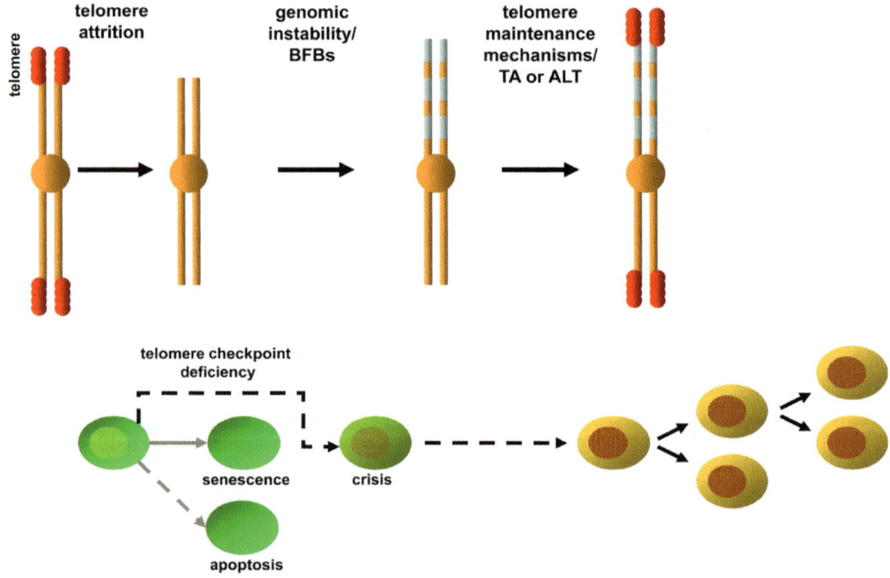

Fig. 13.4 Telomere-focused model of tumorigenesis. Dysfunctional telomeres, either as a consequence of telomere decapping or resulting from telomere shortening, will be recognized by the DNA surveillance machinery and induce senescence (M1) or apoptosis (telomeres are shown as red circles). In the setting of checkpoint deficiency, such as p53 deficiency, chromosomes may fuse and start BFBs, leading to a shuffling of the genome and genomic amplifications and deletions. These cells usually enter the state of crisis (M2), a terminal non-proliferative state. Only very rarely a clone will gain a mechanism of telomere maintenance (TMM, either telomerase-dependent or independent). TMMs stabilize the genome and the emerging cancer cells acquire independence of telomere shortening-induced senescence or apoptosis (Figure modified from Else [45])

they are necessary to induce immortality and "indefinite" tumor growth/cell proliferation. They are therefore important for the maintenance of a malignant tumor phenotype. Moreover, telomerase may present an interesting therapeutic target. Though inhibition of telomerase or TMMs is unlikely to lead to tumor shrinkage, it still may stall tumor growth, stop tumor progression, and may induce a crisis state of tumor cells. Additional non-telomere functions of telomerase need to be further investigated.

13.5 Human Syndromes with Defects in Telomere Physiology

To date, only dyskeratosis congenita (DC) and various variations of this syndrome can clearly be attributed to defects in telomere physiology; however, there are several other syndromes that impact telomere physiology as well as other cellular DNA surveillance, repair and replication mechanisms [80, 81]. None of these syndromes, with the exception of LFS, have been reported to be associated with ACC. This may be due to the fact that these patients usually succumb to other kinds of malignancies, and ACC may be as rare in these patients as in the general population.

The main syndromes are DC and related disorders (e.g., aplastic anemia, idiopathic pulmonary fibrosis), which are caused by mutations in the telomerase subunits *TERC* or *TERT* (autosomal dominant), a telomerase-associated protein, *DKC* (X-linked recessive), the shelterin complex component *TIN2* (autosomal dominant), or other genes encoding parts of the telomerase holoenzyme (e.g., *NOP10*) [80, 82–86]. All of these gene products serve functions at the telomere. DC is mainly inherited in an autosomal-dominant, an autosomal-recessive, or an X-chromosomal recessive fashion. Depending on the gene mutated and on the gene mutation, there is a great variation of severity and of organs affected, ranging from isolated aplastic anemia or idiopathic pulmonary fibrosis to the severe Hoyeraal-Hreidarsson syndrome [87]. *TERT* and *TERC* mutations vary in their penetrance and human pedigrees. These mutations seem to be subjected to genetic anticipation, which means that the severity of the phenotype increases and the age of onset decreases over generations [87]. The main clinical features of DC are refractory anemia and bone marrow failure, presumably due to exhaustion of stem cell compartments, and early onset of tumors [88]. The spectrum of malignancies is mainly dominated by squamous cell cancer of the head and neck and skin, but other neoplasias such as gastrointestinal neoplasms and lymphoma have also been described [89].

ACC is one of the disease-defining neoplasms in LFS [90, 91]. Most interestingly, it has recently been shown that the age of first tumor manifestation is correlated with telomere length, meaning the shorter the telomere, the earlier a patient within the same LFS pedigree will manifest disease [92]. Though this study did not focus on LFS patients with ACC in particular, it nevertheless links LFS to telomere pathophysiology and telomere shortening, which can be interpreted as a pro-oncogenic mechanism in these patients.

13.6 Telomerase and Adrenocortical Carcinoma

Shortly after the discovery of telomerase activity, it became clear that this mechanism is heavily exploited by malignant tumors. Roughly 90% of all human tumor samples are telomerase positive [18]. Later, several tumor entities were described that did not display telomerase activity, yet maintained telomere integrity and length [19]. Most of these samples had very long telomeres, by far exceeding the usual length of human telomeres of ~5 kb, and also showed a distribution over a wide range of lengths. This mechanism was termed ALT. Classical examples of tumor entities that use ALT are liposarcoma, glioblastoma, and osteosarcoma [93–95]. While the mechanisms underlying telomere length maintenance by telomerase activity are mostly understood, the mechanisms underlying ALT are still enigmatic [20, 21]. Interestingly, one of the first reports describing surrogate parameters of ALT, i.e., long telomeres and the immunohistochemical co-localization of a bright telomere signal with PML bodies, included several adrenal tumors [19]. Unfortunately, these adrenal tumors were not further specified with regard to their histology and clinical behavior. Several studies have surveyed TMMs in benign and malignant adrenocortical tumors [96–102]. All but one study focused on telomerase activity alone [97]. Most studies find telomerase activity in the majority of malignant lesions and not in benign neoplasms or normal adrenal tissue. The study by Mannelli et al. also finds telomerase activity in 9 of 11 benign lesions, but states that telomerase activity was significantly lower when compared to ACC [100]. Bamberger et al. also found low levels of telomerase activity in all samples, including normal adrenal control tissue [96]. This study employed an ELISA-based method; with this method it is difficult to determine a threshold cut-off for telomerase activity. This is usually very easy using the traditional radioactive telomere repeat amplification protocol (TRAP) assay, which gives a clearly negative or positive result. On average, they detected higher levels of telomerase activity in ACC vs. normal tissue, and telomerase activity was higher in 6 of 7 ACCs when compared to benign adenomas. Though results from these different studies are difficult to compare for several reasons, such as differences in material preparation, differences in clinical descriptions and differences in methods measuring telomerase activity, it seems to be clear that most malignant lesions are positive for telomerase activity while most benign lesions are not (Table 13.2). ALT seems to play a minor role in ACCs, but is present in a subset of ACCs either together with telomerase activity or as the only TMM [97]. This further supports a role for TMMs in maintaining immortality in ACC. This assumption also makes TMMs an interesting potential therapeutic target. Several telomerase inhibitors have shown anti-tumor activity in in vitro and in vivo experiments and the first compounds are progressing to phase I clinical trials [103, 104].

13.7 Telomeres and Adrenocortical Carcinoma

There is growing evidence that telomere dysfunction may play a role in adrenocortical tumorigenesis as well [45, 48]. Unfortunately, the small sample sizes available

Table 13.2 Studies of telomere maintenance mechanisms in ACC

Author	Year	Sample size[a]	ACC	ACA	NL	
Kinoshita et al. [111]	1997	27	NA	1/13	0/7	Positive sample had some malignant features
Hirano et al. [98]	1998	75	2/2	2/32	0/27	
Teng et al. [102]	1998	33	1/1	1/12	0/10	Weak activity in the positive ACA
Bamberger et al. [96]	1999	45	7/7	15/15	5/5	Higher level in ACC vs. ACA and NL, quantitative PCR-based assay[b]
Mannelli et al. [100]	2000	21	7/7	9/11	0/3	Higher levels in ACCs vs. ACA
Else et al. [97]	2008	38	21/24	0/11	0/3	1 ACC positive for ALT, 2 ACC indeterminate
Total			40/41	28/94	5/55	

[a]Total sample size includes other tumors tested in these studies (e.g., pheochromocytoma, lymphoma)

[b]The employed method does not distinguish positive vs. negative activity as well as the traditional radioactive TRAP method

for adrenocortical tumors have so far precluded a thorough analysis as has been done for other tumors, such as breast cancer. Another problem is that the molecular events leading to malignant lesions in other tissues have been very well described; the adenoma to carcinoma progression of colon cancer is a classical example. Interestingly, despite the high incidence of benign adrenocortical tumors, there is no convincing evidence that these tumors may present precursor lesions for ACC. The frequency of progression of adrenocortical adenomas to ACC is basically unknown, if it exists at all. Despite these limitations and differences from other tumor entities, there are currently several lines of evidence arguing for a possible role of telomere dysfunction in adrenocortical tumorigenesis. In general, ACCs show a high degree of aneuploidy and genomic diversity, which can be explained by some event furthering genomic instability; telomere-induced genomic instability is one possible explanation (see Chapter 9). Observational studies using gene expression arrays show significant differences in expression of genes encoding shelterin complex components between benign lesions and ACC [45, 105]. While this may reflect general alterations in telomere physiology, it may also suggest a direct role of disproportional expression of these factors in inducing telomere dysfunction and subsequently genomic instability. Several studies of other malignancies, such as T-cell leukemia, B-CLL, gastric cancer, non-small cell lung cancer, and breast cancer have shown alterations in expression levels of shelterin component-coding genes [106–110]. Probably, the most direct evidence comes from the *acd* mouse, which develops

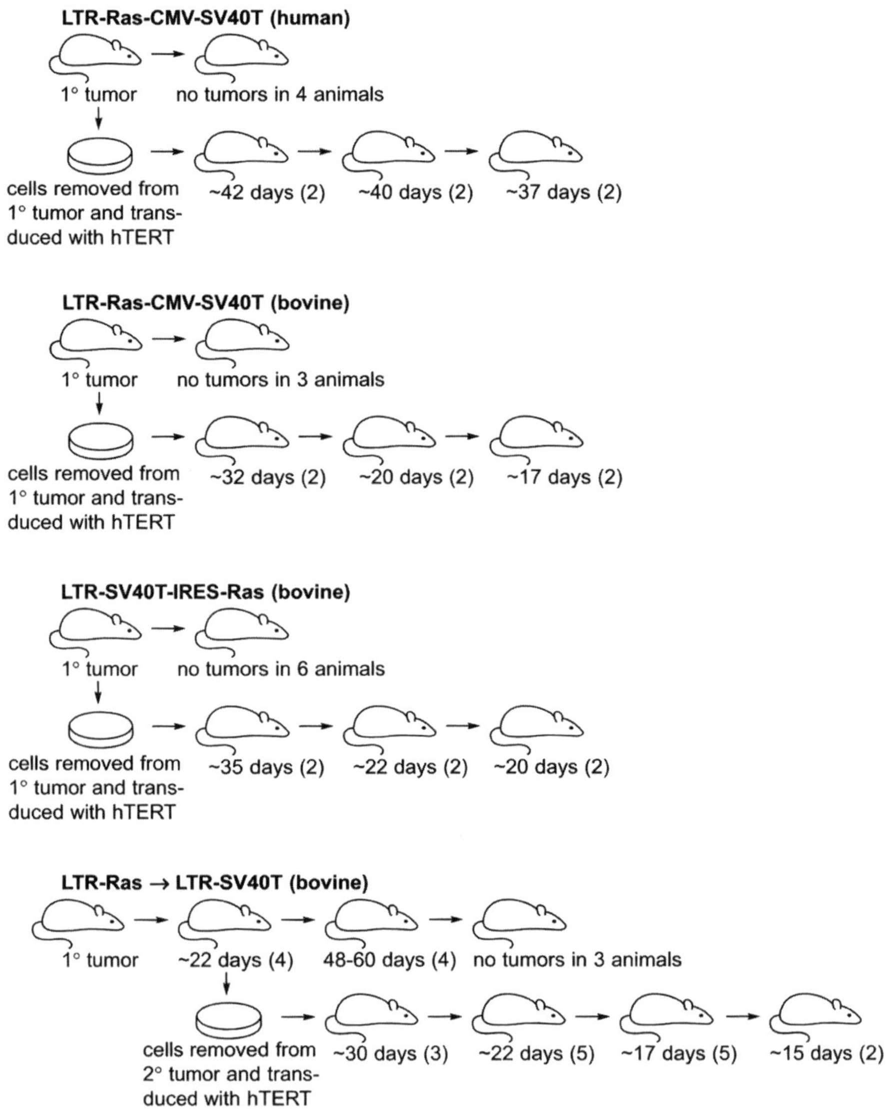

Fig. 13.5 Experimental restoration of tumorigenicity by hTERT. Representative experiments are shown in which cells isolated from telomerase-negative tumors, formed from $Ras^{G12V}/SV40TAg$-transduced human and bovine adrenocortical cells, were transduced with *TERT* and retransplanted into immunodeficient mice. After establishment of the 1° tumor, 2° and subsequent tumors were formed by subcutaneous implantation of tumor fragments. The retroviruses used are indicated. The times shown are the number of days after transplantation before the tumor reached a diameter of 0.5 cm (Figure from Sun et al. [75])

telomere dysfunction-induced genomic alterations. In p53-proficient *acd* mice, dysfunctional telomeres lead to the induction of senescence in adrenococortical cells. About 5% of *p53* heterozygous *acd* mice develop bona fide ACC as evidenced by *Sf1* expression [48]. Though ACCs occur only in a small proportion of these animals, it is still noteworthy in light of the lack of the extreme rarity of this cancer in any other mouse model. Furthermore, it provides evidence that dysfunctional telomeres are sufficient to induce ACCs. However, it does not answer the question of whether telomere dysfunction is involved in human adrenocortical tumorigenesis.

References

1. Harley CB et al (1990) Telomeres shorten during ageing of human fibroblasts. Nature 345(6274):458–460
2. Levy MZ et al (1992) Telomere end-replication problem and cell aging. J Mol Biol 225(4):951–960
3. Bodnar AG et al (1998) Extension of life-span by introduction of telomerase into normal human cells. Science 279(5349):349–352
4. Lee HW et al (1998) Essential role of mouse telomerase in highly proliferative organs. Nature 392(6676):5569–574
5. Deng Y et al (2008) Telomere dysfunction and tumour suppression: the senescence connection. Nat Rev Cancer 8(6):450–458
6. Karlseder J et al (1999) p53- and ATM-dependent apoptosis induced by telomeres lacking TRF2. Science 283(5406):1321–1325
7. Artandi SE, Attardi LD (2005) Pathways connecting telomeres and p53 in senescence, apoptosis, cancer. Biochem Biophys Res Commun 331(3):881–890
8. Hayflick L (1965) The limited in vitro lifetime of human diploid cell strains. Exp Cell Res 37:614–636
9. Hayflick L, Moorhead PS (1961) The serial cultivation of human diploid cell strains. Exp Cell Res 25:585–621
10. Hornsby PJ (2001) Cell proliferation in mammalian aging. In: Masoro EJA, Austad SN (eds) Handbook of the biology of aging. Academic, San Diego, CA, pp 207–266
11. Taylor RS et al (1996) Detection of telomerase activity in malignant and nonmalignant skin conditions. J Invest Dermatol 106(4):759–765
12. Weng NP et al (1996) Regulated expression of telomerase activity in human T lymphocyte development and activation. J Exp Med 183(6):2471–2479
13. Wright WE et al (1996) Telomerase activity in human germline and embryonic tissues and cells. Dev Genet 18(2):173–179
14. Greider CW, Blackburn EH (1987) The telomere terminal transferase of Tetrahymena is a ribonucleoprotein enzyme with two kinds of primer specificity. Cell 51(6):887–898
15. Morin GB (1989) The human telomere terminal transferase enzyme is a ribonucleoprotein that synthesizes TTAGGG repeats. Cell 59(3): 521–529
16. Thomson JA et al (1998) Embryonic stem cell lines derived from human blastocysts. Science 282(5391):1145–1147
17. Curcio MJ, Belfort M (2007) The beginning of the end: links between ancient retroelements and modern telomerases. Proc Natl Acad Sci USA 104(22):9107–9108
18. Kim NW et al (1994) Specific association of human telomerase activity with immortal cells and cancer. Science 266(5193):2011–2015
19. Bryan TM et al (1997) Evidence for an alternative mechanism for maintaining telomere length in human tumors and tumor-derived cell lines. Nat Med 3(11):1271–1274
20. Muntoni A, Reddel RR (2005) The first molecular details of ALT in human tumor cells. Hum Mol Genet 14(Spec No. 2):R191–196
21. Bhattacharyya S et al (2010) Unwinding protein complexes in ALTernative telomere maintenance. J Cell Biochem 109(1):7–15
22. Griffith JD et al (1999) Mammalian telomeres end in a large duplex loop. Cell 97(4):503–514

23. de Lange T (2005) Shelterin: the protein complex that shapes and safeguards human telomeres. Genes Dev 19(18):2100–2110
24. Chong L et al (1995) A human telomeric protein. Science 270(5242):1663–1667
25. Broccoli D et al (1997) Human telomeres contain two distinct Myb-related proteins, TRF1 and TRF2. Nat Genet 17(2):231–235
26. Baumann P, Cech TR (2001) Pot1, the putative telomere end-binding protein in fission yeast and humans. Science 292(5519):1171–1175
27. Liu D et al (2004) Telosome, a mammalian telomere-associated complex formed by multiple telomeric proteins. J Biol Chem 279 (49):51338–51342
28. Houghtaling BR et al (2004) A dynamic molecular link between the telomere length regulator TRF1 and the chromosome end protector TRF2. Curr Biol 14(18):1621–1631
29. Kim SH et al (1999) TIN2, a new regulator of telomere length in human cells. Nat Genet 23(4):405–412
30. Li B et al (2000) Identification of human Rap1: implications for telomere evolution. Cell 101(5):471–483
31. Liu D et al (2004) PTOP interacts with POT1 and regulates its localization to telomeres. Nat Cell Biol 6(7):673–680
32. Ye JZ et al (2004) TIN2 binds TRF1 and TRF2 simultaneously and stabilizes the TRF2 complex on telomeres. J Biol Chem 279(45):47264–47271
33. Ye JZ et al (2004) POT1-interacting protein PIP1: a telomere length regulator that recruits POT1 to the TIN2/TRF1 complex. Genes Dev 18(14):1649–1654
34. Guo X et al (2007) Dysfunctional telomeres activate an ATM-ATR-dependent DNA damage response to suppress tumorigenesis. Embo J 26(22):4709–4719
35. Hockemeyer D et al (2006) Recent expansion of the telomeric complex in rodents: Two distinct POT1 proteins protect mouse telomeres. Cell 126(1):63–77
36. Takai H et al (2003) DNA damage foci at dysfunctional telomeres. Curr Biol 13(17): 1549–1556
37. Karlseder J (2003) Telomere repeat binding factors: keeping the ends in check. Cancer Lett 194(2):189–197
38. Lechel A et al (2005) The cellular level of telomere dysfunction determines induction of senescence or apoptosis in vivo. EMBO Rep 6(3):275–281
39. Goytisolo FA et al (2001) The absence of the dna-dependent protein kinase catalytic subunit in mice results in anaphase bridges and in increased telomeric fusions with normal telomere length and G-strand overhang. Mol Cell Biol 21(11):3642–3651
40. van Steensel B et al (1998) TRF2 protects human telomeres from end-to-end fusions. Cell 92(3):401–413
41. Brown JP et al (1997) Bypass of senescence after disruption of p21CIP1/WAF1 gene in normal diploid human fibroblasts. Science 277(5327):831–834
42. Jacobs JJ, de Lange T (2005) p16INK4a as a second effector of the telomere damage pathway. Cell Cycle 4(10): 1364–1368
43. Shay JW, Wright WE (2005) Senescence and immortalization: role of telomeres and telomerase. Carcinogenesis 26(5):867–874
44. Acilan C et al (2007) DNA repair pathways involved in anaphase bridge formation. Genes Chromosomes Cancer 46(6):522–531
45. Else T (2009) Telomeres and telomerase in adrenocortical tissue maintenance, carcinogenesis, and aging. J Mol Endocrinol 43(4):131–141
46. Hornsby PJ (2007) Senescence as an anticancer mechanism. J Clin Oncol 25(14):1852–1857
47. Ju Z, Rudolph KL (2006) Telomeres and telomerase in cancer stem cells. Eur J Cancer 42(9):1197–1203
48. Else T et al (2009) Genetic p53 deficiency partially rescues the adrenocortical dysplasia phenotype at the expense of increased tumorigenesis. Cancer Cell 15(6):465–476
49. Artandi SE et al (2000) Telomere dysfunction promotes non-reciprocal translocations and epithelial cancers in mice. Nature 406(6796):641–645
50. Blasco MA et al (1997) Telomere shortening and tumor formation by mouse cells lacking telomerase RNA. Cell 91(1):25–34

51. Chin L et al (1999) p53 deficiency rescues the adverse effects of telomere loss and cooperates with telomere dysfunction to accelerate carcinogenesis. Cell 97(4):527–538
52. Keegan CE et al (2005) Urogenital and caudal dysgenesis in adrenocortical dysplasia (acd) mice is caused by a splicing mutation in a novel telomeric regulator. Hum Mol Genet 14(1):113–123
53. Rudolph KL et al (1999) Longevity, stress response, and cancer in aging telomerase-deficient mice. Cell 96(5):701–712
54. Else T et al (2007) Tpp1/Acd maintains genomic stability through a complex role in telomere protection. Chromosome Res 15(8):1001–1013
55. Hockemeyer D et al (2007) Telomere protection by mammalian Pot1 requires interaction with Tpp1. Nat Struct Mol Biol 14(8):754–761
56. Hande MP et al (1999) Telomere length dynamics and chromosomal instability in cells derived from telomerase null mice. J Cell Biol 144(4):589–601
57. He H et al (2006) POT1b protects telomeres from end-to-end chromosomal fusions and aberrant homologous recombination. Embo J 25(21):5180–5190
58. Wu L et al (2006) Pot1 deficiency initiates DNA damage checkpoint activation and aberrant homologous recombination at telomeres. Cell 126(1):49–62
59. Murnane JP (2006) Telomeres and chromosome instability. DNA Repair (Amst) 5 (9-10):1082–1092
60. Murnane JP, Sabatier L (2004) Chromosome rearrangements resulting from telomere dysfunction and their role in cancer. Bioessays 26(11):1164–1174
61. O'Hagan RC et al (2002) Telomere dysfunction provokes regional amplification and deletion in cancer genomes. Cancer Cell 2(2):149–155
62. Gordon KE et al (2003) High levels of telomere dysfunction bestow a selective disadvantage during the progression of human oral squamous cell carcinoma. Cancer Res 63(2): 458–467
63. Chin K et al (2004) In situ analyses of genome instability in breast cancer. Nat Genet 36(9):984–988
64. Rudolph KL et al (2001) Telomere dysfunction and evolution of intestinal carcinoma in mice and humans. Nat Genet 28(2):155–159
65. Meeker AK, Argani P (2004) Telomere shortening occurs early during breast tumorigenesis: a cause of chromosome destabilization underlying malignant transformation? J Mammary Gland Biol Neoplasia 9(3):285–296
66. Meeker AK et al (2004) Telomere shortening occurs in subsets of normal breast epithelium as well as in situ and invasive carcinoma. Am J Pathol 164(3):925–935
67. Plentz RR et al (2003) Telomere shortening of epithelial cells characterises the adenoma-carcinoma transition of human colorectal cancer. Gut 52(9):1304–1307
68. Herbert BS et al (2001) Telomerase and breast cancer. Breast Cancer Res 3(3):146–149
69. Maser RS, DePinho RA (2002) Connecting chromosomes, crisis, and cancer. Science 297(5581):565–569
70. Thomas M, Hornsby PJ (1999) Transplantation of primary bovine adrenocortical cells into scid mice. Mol Cell Endocrinol 153(1-2):125–136
71. Hahn WC et al (1999) Creation of human tumour cells with defined genetic elements. Nature 400(6743):464–468
72. Zhao JJ, Roberts TM (2004) W.C. Hahn, Functional genetics and experimental models of human cancer. Trends Mol Med 10(7):344–350
73. Hahn WC, Weinberg RA (2002) Modelling the molecular circuitry of cancer. Nat Rev Cancer 2(5):331–341
74. Sun B et al (2006) The minimal set of genetic alterations required for conversion of primary human fibroblasts to cancer cells in the subrenal capsule assay. Neoplasia 7(6):585–593
75. Sun B et al (2004) Progressive loss of malignant behavior in telomerase-negative tumorigenic adrenocortical cells and restoration of tumorigenicity by human telomerase reverse transcriptase. Cancer Res 64(17): 6144–6151
76. Choi J et al (2008) TERT promotes epithelial proliferation through transcriptional control of a Myc- and Wnt-related developmental program. PLoS Genet 4(1):e10

77. Sarin KY et al (2005) Conditional telomerase induction causes proliferation of hair follicle stem cells. Nature 436(7053):1048–1052
78. Venteicher AS et al (2008) Identification of ATPases pontin and reptin as telomerase components essential for holoenzyme assembly. Cell 132(6):945–957
79. Park JI et al (2009) Telomerase modulates Wnt signalling by association with target gene chromatin. Nature 460(7251):66–72
80. Walne AJ, Dokal I (2009) Advances in the understanding of dyskeratosis congenita. Br J Haematol 145(2):164–172
81. Savage SA, Alter BP (2009) Dyskeratosis congenita. Hematol Oncol Clin North Am 23(2):215–231
82. Armanios M et al (2005) Haploinsufficiency of telomerase reverse transcriptase leads to anticipation in autosomal dominant dyskeratosis congenita. Proc Natl Acad Sci U S A 102(44):15960–15964
83. Heiss NS et al (1998) X-linked dyskeratosis congenita is caused by mutations in a highly conserved gene with putative nucleolar functions. Nat Genet 19(1):32–38
84. Savage SA et al (2008) TINF2, a component of the shelterin telomere protection complex, is mutated in dyskeratosis congenita. Am J Hum Genet 82(2):501–509
85. Vulliamy T et al (2001) The RNA component of telomerase is mutated in autosomal dominant dyskeratosis congenita. Nature 413(6854):432–435
86. Armanios MY et al (2007) Telomerase mutations in families with idiopathic pulmonary fibrosis. N Engl J Med 356(13):1317–1326
87. Armanios M (2009) Syndromes of telomere shortening. Annu Rev Genomics Hum Genet 10:45–61
88. Kirwan M, Dokal I (2009) Dyskeratosis congenita, stem cells and telomeres. Biochim Biophys Acta 1792(4):371–379
89. Alter BP et al (2009) Cancer in dyskeratosis congenita. Blood 113(26):6549–6557
90. Li FP et al (1988) A cancer family syndrome in twenty-four kindreds. Cancer Res 48(18):5358–5362
91. Gonzalez KD et al (2009) Beyond Li Fraumeni Syndrome: clinical characteristics of families with p53 germline mutations. J Clin Oncol 27(8):1250–1256
92. Tabori U et al (2007) Younger age of cancer initiation is associated with shorter telomere length in Li-Fraumeni syndrome. Cancer Res 67(4):1415–1418
93. Costa A et al (2006) Telomere maintenance mechanisms in liposarcomas: association with histologic subtypes and disease progression. Cancer Res 66(17):8918–8924
94. Hakin-Smith V et al (2003) Alternative lengthening of telomeres and survival in patients with glioblastoma multiforme. Lancet 361(9360):836–838
95. Johnson JE et al (2005) Multiple mechanisms of telomere maintenance exist in liposarcomas. Clin Cancer Res 11(15):5347–5355
96. Bamberger CM et al (1999) Telomerase activity in benign and malignant adrenal tumors. Exp Clin Endocrinol Diabetes 107(4):272–275
97. Else T et al (2008) Evaluation of telomere length maintenance mechanisms in adrenocortical carcinoma. J Clin Endocrinol Metab 93(4):1442–1449
98. Hirano Y et al (1998) Telomerase activity as an indicator of potentially malignant adrenal tumors. Cancer 83(4):772–776
99. Kinoshita H et al (1998) Telomerase activity in adrenal cortical tumors and pheochromocytomas with reference to clinicopathologic features. Urol Res 26(1):29–32
100. Mannelli M et al (2000) Telomerase activity is significantly enhanced in malignant adrenocortical tumors in comparison to benign adrenocortical adenomas. J Clin Endocrinol Metab 85(1):468–470
101. Orlando C, Gelmini S (2001) Telomerase in endocrine and endocrine-dependent tumors. J Steroid Biochem Mol Biol 78(3):201–214
102. Teng L et al (1998) Telomerase activity in the differentiation of benign and malignant adrenal tumors. Surgery 124(6):1123–1127

103. Chen H et al (2009) Strategies targeting telomerase inhibition. Mol Biotechnol 41(2): 194–199
104. Zimmermann S, Martens UM (2007) Telomeres and telomerase as targets for cancer therapy. Cell Mol Life Sci 64(7–8):906–921
105. Giordano TJ et al (2009) Molecular classification and prognostication of adrenocortical tumors by transcriptome profiling. Clin Cancer Res 15(2):668–676
106. Bellon M et al (2006) Increased expression of telomere length regulating factors TRF1, TRF2 and TIN2 in patients with adult T-cell leukemia. Int J Cancer 119(9):2090–2097
107. Kondo T et al (2004) Expression of POT1 is associated with tumor stage and telomere length in gastric carcinoma. Cancer Res 64(2):523–529
108. Lin X et al (2006) Expression of telomere-associated genes as prognostic markers for overall survival in patients with non-small cell lung cancer. Clin Cancer Res 12(19):5720–5725
109. Poncet D et al (2008) Changes in the expression of telomere maintenance genes suggest global telomere dysfunction in B-chronic lymphocytic leukemia. Blood 111(4):2388–2391
110. Salhab M et al (2008) The expression of gene transcripts of telomere-associated genes in human breast cancer: correlation with clinico-pathological parameters and clinical outcome. Breast Cancer Res Treat 109(1):35–46
111. Kinoshita H et al (1998) Telomerase activity in adrenal cortical tumors and pheochromocytomas with reference to clinicopathologic features. Urol Res 26(1):29–32

Chapter 14
Beckwith–Wiedemann Syndrome

Michael DeBaun and Jennifer Horst

Beckwith-Wiedemann syndrome (BWS) (OMIM 130650) is a disease of prenatal overgrowth, congenital malformations, and predisposition to cancer. The syndrome was independently described by J.B. Beckwith, an American pathologist, at the annual meeting of the Western Society for Pediatric Research in 1963 [1] and H.R. Wiedemann, a German pediatrician, in 1964 [2]. This disease was initially referred to as the EMG syndrome for its most prominent clinical features that distinguished the syndrome from other congenital malformations: exomphalos, macroglossia, and gigantism. Beckwith also emphasized the pathological finding of cytomegaly of the adrenal cortex [3]. Children with BWS are 600 times more likely than other children to develop certain childhood cancers, particularly Wilms tumor, hepatoblastoma, neuroblastoma, and adrenocortical carcinoma. Evidence reveals an increased risk for cancer during childhood (especially before age four); however, less data are available to document the risk of cancer in adults.

BWS is one of the most commonly recognized overgrowth syndromes. However, the exact incidence of BWS is unknown because of the marked variability in the syndrome's presentation and the lack of widely accepted diagnosis criteria. The number of reported infants born with BWS most likely underestimates the real prevalence, because clinical features may be subtle and often missed. BWS has been documented in a variety of ethnic groups and occurs equally in males and females. It has been estimated to occur in approximately 1 in 13,700 live births [4] or 300 children in the United States each year.

14.1 Diagnosis

Infants with BWS may have multiple congenital anomalies, including macroglossia, macrosomia, midline abdominal wall defects (omphalocele, diastasis recti, and umbilical hernia), ear pits or creases, and neonatal hypoglycemia. A consensual

M. DeBaun (✉)
Division of Pediatric Hematology-Oncology, Department of Pediatrics, Washington University School of Medicine, 660 South Euclid Avenue, Box 8067, St. Louis, MO 63110-1093, USA
e-mail: debaun_m@kids.wustl.edu

G.D. Hammer, T. Else (eds.), *Adrenocortical Carcinoma*,
DOI 10.1007/978-0-387-77236-3_14, © Springer Science+Business Media, LLC 2011

clinical definition for BWS has been challenged by the lack of standard diagnostic criteria that have been independently verified in patients who have either genetic or epigenetic mutations. In an attempt to standardize the classification of BWS, DeBaun et al. defined a patient as having BWS when a clinical diagnosis of BWS is made by a physician in a child with at least two of the five common features associated with BWS (macroglossia, macrosomia, midline abdominal wall defects, ear creases/ear pits, neonatal hypoglycemia) [5]. When these diagnostic criteria were used for The BWS Registry at the National Cancer Institute (NCI) and correlated with molecular analyses, approximately 7 of 10 clinically defined cases of BWS had evidence of genetic or epigenetic mutations [5]. These findings suggest that other genetic or epigenetic mutations not yet identified are responsible for the disease in approximately one third of children with BWS. An alternative definition of BWS was introduced by Elliot et al. who classified BWS by the presence of either three major features (anterior abdominal wall defect, macroglossia, or pre- and or post-natal overgrowth (>90th centile)) or two major plus three minor findings (ear pits, nevus flammeus, neonatal hypoglycemia, nephromegaly, or hemihyperplasia) [6]. To date there has not been a clinical study correlating the clinical definition of BWS as defined by Elliot with a known genetic or epigenetic mutations associated with BWS. Given the variation among individuals with BWS and the lack of a simple diagnostic test, identifying BWS can be difficult.

14.2 Clinical Features

The BWS Registry was established in 1994 at the Genetic Epidemiology Branch of the National Cancer Institute (NCI). In the BWS Registry, only 13% of the children had all five of the most common features associated with BWS. Based on the data from the BWS Registry, the most common clinical or laboratory features associated with BWS are shown in Table 14.1 [5].

Other features of BWS include craniofacial abnormalities with prominent occiput, maxillary hypoplasia with a broad nasal bridge, and nevus flammeus of the head. Premature infants with BWS may initially have normal facial features, but later develop macroglossia and other facial features associated with BWS [7]. Asymmetry of the extremities or face with or without cleft lip or palate has also been reported in children with BWS. In a study by Gerber et al., asymmetry of length or girth was defined as greater than 10% discrepancy between the right and left sides [8]. Asymmetric overgrowth of the limbs, trunk, face, cranium, or entire body is known as hemihyperplasia, which can occur as an isolated finding or in association with several malformation syndromes. Children with BWS can have asymmetry of the limbs or face, as well as joint laxity, scoliosis, and thoracic cage abnormalities [8]; these features were best characterized in a study of 388 children with BWS where the rate of hemihypertrophy was 12.5% [9].

Table 14.1 Clinical features associated with BWS

Clinical finding	Observed incidence (%)
Macroglossia	94
Abdominal wall defects	74
Ear pits or ear grooves	68
Hemangiomas, nevus flammeus	63
Neonatal hypoglycemia	52
Born premature	50
Undescended testes	44
Polyhydramnios during pregnancy	43
Hearing loss	12
Cliteromegaly	9
Hypospadias	8
Significant hypoglycemia beyond the neonatal period	4

Another striking feature of BWS as reported by Beckwith in his first case series description, is adrenocortical cytomegaly, which is almost invariably present in BWS patient autopsies [10, 11]. The cause of adrenal cytomegaly is unknown, but the feature is shared with other syndromes, such as adrenal hypoplasia congenita (AHC) with cytomegaly with hypogonadotropic hypogonadism caused by *DAX1* mutations. AHC with cytomegaly is also a main clinical characteristic of the IMAGe syndrome and can be found associated with other congenital abnormalities (e.g., monochromosome 7 syndrome) or as an incidental finding in pediatric autopsies, where it can globally or focally affect the adrenal cortex. Mainly because of the occurrence in pediatric cases and because of the resemblance of the adrenal cytomegaly to fetal adrenocortical cells, some authors have favored the theory that adrenocortical cytomegaly may represent complete or focal persistence of fetal adrenocortical cells. Currently there is no proof for this theory and certainly other explanations can be entertained. While it is unknown whether adrenal cytomegaly results in changes of adrenocortical function in BWS patients, in view of the lack of reported adrenal insufficiency or overt hyperfunction of the adrenal cortex (in the absence of adrenocortical carcinoma (ACC)), such an association appears unlikely.

Studies have found that isolated hemihyperplasia (IH) is an independent risk factor for the development of cancer during childhood [12]. Given the clinical overlap of IH with BWS and the high rate of cancer in patients with IH, children with IH are currently counseled to receive the same cancer screening recommendation as patients with BWS. Despite similarities between BWS and IH, it remains unclear whether these two syndromes represent differing phenotypes of the same genotype or are these two separate syndromes with different genotypes. While some data suggest that IH may simply reflect the tail end of a spectrum of methylation defects in the BWS clinical continuum [13], Neimitz et al. demonstrated that children with IH and BWS with Wilms tumor had different epigenotype changes [14]. Specifically, children with IH and Wilms tumor have a much lower frequency of *H19* mutations, 20% (3/15) compared to 79% (11/14) in children with

BWS and Wilms tumor, this is consistent with a hypothesis that IH is the result of a different genetic or epigenetic mutation than BWS but acts in a common causal molecular pathway. However, data published by Martin et al. suggested that children with IH may reflect cases at the tail end of the spectrum of methylation defects in the BWS clinical continuum [13]. Together these data suggest that there are two groups of children with IH: the first group represents part of the BWS spectrum while the second group is genetically distinct from BWS.

Children with BWS can present both malignant and nonmalignant manifestations of renal disease. Wilms tumor and nephroblastomatosis are the malignant and premalignant manifestations of renal disease in children with BWS. Nonmalignant renal disease, such as multiple caliceal cysts or diverticulae, hydronephrosis, and medullary cysts, can be confused with Wilms tumor and/or nephroblastomatosis. In 152 patients with BWS, 45 nonmalignant renal abnormalities were identified: medullary cysts (13%), caliceal diverticulae (1%), hydronephrosis (12%), and nephrolithiasis (6.4%) [15]. The incidence and rate of progression of these nonmalignant renal conditions is unknown; although, several patients in the BWS Registry developed ESRD.

14.3 Genetics

The genetic causes of BWS are extremely complex and include various cytogenetic, molecular, and epigenetic alterations in chromosomal band 11p15 [16]. Although chromosomal rearrangement and genetic mutations on 11p15 are associated with BWS, the majority of alterations (>70%) observed in patients with BWS involve errors in gene imprinting and methylation in one of the two 11p15 domains [5]. Epigenetic modifications in the following six genes located on 11p15 have been observed in patients with BWS: insulin-like growth factor 2 (*IGF2*) and *H19* in one domain and *LIT1*, *CDKN1C* (also called *p57KIP2*), and *KvLQT1* in the other domain (Fig. 14.1). Over five distinct errors involving 11p15 have been identified among patients with BWS. These include (1) abnormal methylation of *LIT1*, (2) abnormal methylation of *H19* with reciprocal biallele expression of *IGF2*, (3) paternal uniparental disomy (UPD) of 11p15, (4) abnormal methylation of both LIT1 and H19 with no UPD and (5) *CDKN1C* gene mutation.

While transmission to future offspring is a concern expressed by most family members and patients, (due to the range of mutations that are responsible for BWS, as well as the significant proportion of patients with no definable mutation) inheritance of BWS is not easily evaluated. Wangler et al. did not find evidence to support an autosomal dominant inheritance pattern [17], although some families had a pattern of inheritance suggestive of autosomal dominance. Because all known cases of UPD involve somatic mosaicism, only when a child with BWS has UPD can the family of a patient with BWS be told that the recurrence risk is similar to the general population (1/13,700).

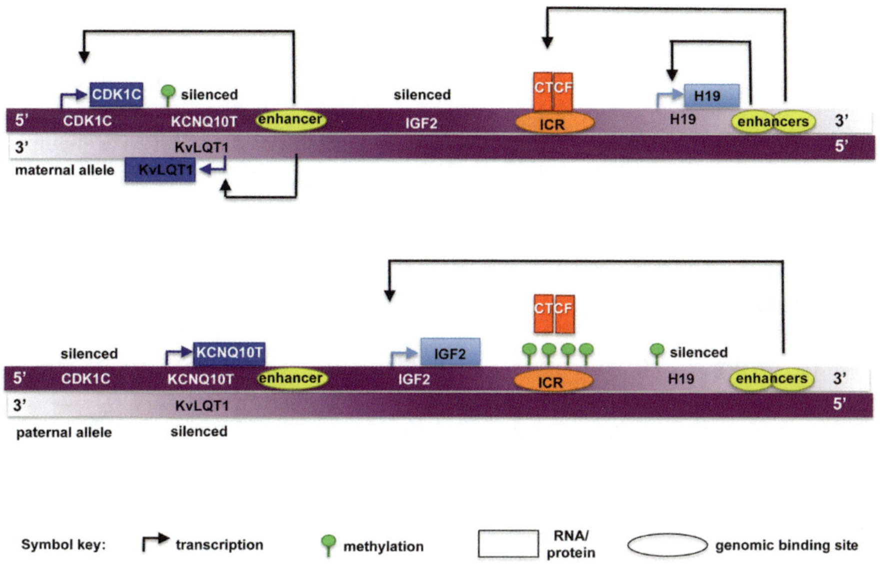

Fig. 14.1 Schematic of the *IGF2* imprinted locus. *IGF2* and *H19* are coordinately regulated by a shared set of enhancers. *CDKN1C* and *KvLQT1* are also coordinately regulated by a separate shared set of enhancers. Methylation of the H19 DMR silences *H19* and activates *IGF2*. Methylation of KvDMR1 silences *KCNQ1OT* and activates *CDKN1C*

14.4 Cancer

While historic studies reported a 7% prevalence of cancer in patients with BWS [9], more recent analyses suggest that approximately 12% of children with BWS develop cancer before 10 years of age [18]. Specifically, among children with BWS, the risk of developing cancer is age-related, with the highest risk occurring in children younger than 4 years of age. Cancer risk decreases dramatically after 4 years of age and by 10 years of age the risk approaches that of the general population [18]. The BWS Registry (http://bws.wustl.edu) retrospectively followed 183 children with BWS who had no history of cancer for 482 person-years during the first 4 years of life [18]. During this time period (age 0–4), 13 children developed cancer (6 Wilms tumor, 5 hepatoblastoma, 2 neuroblastoma), corresponding to 0.027 cancers per patient-year and a 10.8% risk of cancer during the first 4 years of life. This confers a risk 676 times greater than the baseline population risk. A group of children were also followed up to 10 years of age for a total of 204 patient-years. During this time period, one patient developed cancer, corresponding to 0.0049 cancers per patient-year and a 2.9% risk of cancer between 4 and 10 years of life. The two most common cancers in this group include Wilms tumor and hepatoblastoma [18]. Other cancers that occur with an increased frequency in this population include rhabdomyosarcoma, neuroblastoma, and adrenocortical carcinoma [9, 18, 19].

The usefulness of cancer screening in children with BWS has been demonstrated in retrospective and anecdotal studies. With approximately 1 of 8 children with BWS developing cancer, the risk is high enough to warrant cancer screening in order to improve survival and/or decrease morbidity associated with cancer treatment. Both Wilms tumor and hepatoblastoma, the two most common cancers in BWS, meet the criteria for cancer screening. In the case of Wilms tumor, cure rates are over 90% for localized disease and more than 70% for advanced disease; however, the radiation and chemotherapy necessary to treat advanced stage WT can have significant, long-term consequences that impact the child's health. Choyke et al. demonstrated that abdominal ultrasonography at intervals of 4 months or less is effective at reducing the occurrence of late-stage WT; thus this cancer screening protocol is implemented to reduce treatment-related morbidity [20]. Ultrasonography is the optimal screening tool because it is noninvasive, widely available, relatively inexpensive, and does not involve radiation. There is no evidence that screening CT scans of the abdomen are superior to renal ultrasonography. In a cost-effectiveness analysis, McNeil and colleagues demonstrated that abdominal sonography in children with BWS is a reasonable cancer screening program [21].

Similar to Wilms tumor, hepatoblastoma can be identified by abdominal ultrasound; however, an abdominal ultrasound does not image the entire liver. Clericuzio et al. [22] published a case series of five patients with BWS who were identified with early-stage hepatoblastoma (stage 1). In all five cases, alpha-fetoprotein (AFP) levels were elevated in serial evaluations at 8 week intervals. The expected proportion was found in a series of 182 children with hepatoblastoma, where two thirds of the tumors were stage III or IV at presentation [23]. Early detection of hepatoblastoma is critical as stages I and II (91% 5-year event-free survival) have a much better prognosis compared with stages III and IV (64 and 25% 5-year event-free survival) [22]. Taken together, these studies provide a compelling rationale to use renal sonography to screen for Wilms tumor in an interval of 4 months or less and (AFP) to screen for hepatoblastoma at intervals of 6–12 weeks.

Children with BWS are also at increased risk of developing adrenocortical carcinoma; however, screening for adrenocortical carcinoma does not meet the minimum requirements of cancer screening discussed by DeBaun et al. [24]. These authors describe five principles for cancer screening in children: (1) Early treatment or detection should result in a decreased mortality and morbidity, (2) Age-specific incidence should be high enough to warrant screening, (3) The population at risk should be easily identified, (4) The natural history of the cancer should be known, and (5) the screening test must be easy to administer, acceptable, and accessible to the target population [24]. The exact prevalence of ACC in BWS is poorly documented. In a survey of 388 children with BWS, Wiedemann reported five adrenocortical carcinomas [9]. Sotelo-Avila et al. reported four cases of ACC amongst a total number of 17 tumors (10 WT, 4 ACC, 1 hepatoblastoma, 1 glioblastoma, and 1 rhabdomyosarcoma) [19]. However, both of these studies enrolled patients on the basis of cancer referral; therefore, a referral bias exists. In contrast, the BWS Registry, where there is no referral bias, did not report any cases of ACC [18]. However, taken the close relationship between IH and BWS and the possibility that IH may represent a specific phenotype of the BWS spectrum, it is worthwhile mentioning that a prospective study of IH patients found two ACCs in 162 study subjects. Though the incidence of adrenocortical cancer may be low, the association can still be regarded highly specific, taken the rarity of this cancer in the overall population. Nevertheless, given the observation that the kidneys are screened for WT every 3 months until at least 4 years of age, visualization of the adrenals is prudent and therefore recommended. In the event that a mass is visualized, then appropriate referral to a tertiary care medical center with expertise in the management of cancer is warranted.

References

1. Beckwith JB (1963) Extreme cytomegaly of the adrenal fetal cortex, omphalocele, hyperplasia of kidneys and pancreas, and Leydig cell hyperplasia – another syndrome? Paper presented at annual meeting of the Western society for pediatric research, Los Angeles, Nov 11
2. Wiedemann HR (September 1964) Familial malformation complex with umbilical hernia and macroglossia – a "new syndrome?" (in French). J de génétique humaine 13:223–232
3. Beckwith JB (1998) Vignettes from the history of overgrowth and related syndromes. Am J Med Gen 79:238–248
4. Thorburn MJ et al (1970) Exomphalos-Macroglossia-Gigantism syndrome in Jamaican infants. Amer J Dis Child 119:316–321
5. DeBaun MR et al (2002) Epigenetic alterations of H19 and LIT1 distinguish patients with Beckwith-Wiedemann syndrome with cancer and birth defects. American J Hum Genet 70(3):604–611
6. Elliott M et al (1994) Clinical features and natural history of Beckwith-Wiedemann syndrome: presentation of 74 new cases. Clin genet 46(2):168–174
7. Motokura T et al (1991) A novel cyclin encoded by a bcl1-linked candidate oncogene. Nature 350:512–515
8. Gerber LH et al (2000) Joint laxity, scoliosis and thoracic cage abnormalities in children with Beckwith-Wiedemann syndrome. European J Pediatr 160(2):143–144
9. Wiedemann HR (1983) Tumors and hemihypertrophy associated Wiedemann-Beckwith syndrome. Eur J Pediatr 141:129
10. Irving IM (1967) Exomphalos with macroglossia: a study of eleven cases. J Pediatr Surg 2(6):499–507
11. Weksberg R et al (2010) Beckwith-Wiedemann Syndrome. Eur J Hum Genet 18:8–14
12. Hoyme HE et al (1998) Isolated hemihyperplasia (hemihypertrophy): report of a prospective multicenter study of the incidence of neoplasia and review. Am J Med Genet 9:274–278
13. Martin RA et al (2005) Lit1 and H19 Methylation Defects in Isolated Hemihyperplasia. Am J of Med Genet 134A:129–131
14. Niemitz E et al (2005) Children with idiopathic hemihypertrophy and Beckwith-Wiedemann syndrome have different constitutional epigenotypes associated with Wilms tumor. Am J Hum Genet 77:887–891
15. Choyke PL et al (1998) Nonmalignant renal disease in pediatric patients with Beckwith-Wiedemann syndrome. AJR 1711:733–737
16. Weksberg R et al (2005) Beckwith-Wiedemann syndrome. Am J Med Genet C Semin Med Genet 137C(1):12–23
17. Wangler M et al (2005) Inheritance pattern of Beckwith–Wiedemann syndrome is heterogeneous in 291 families with an affected proband. Am J Med Genet 137A:16–21
18. DeBaun M, Tucker MA (1998) Cancer during the first four years of life in children from the Beckwith Wiedemann Syndrome Registry. J Pediatr (132):398–400

19. Sotelo-Avila F et al (1980) Complete and incomplete forms of Beckwith-Wiedemann syndrome: their oncogenic potential. J Pediatr 96:47–50
20. Choyke PL et al (1999) Screening for Wilms tumor in children with Beckwith-Wiedemann syndrome or idiopathic hemihypertrophy. Med Pediatr Oncol 32:196–200
21. McNeil DE et al (2001) Screening for Wilms tumor and hepatoblastoma in children with Beckwith-Wiedemann syndromes: a cost-effective model. Med Ped Oncol 37:349–356
22. Clericuzio C et al (2003) Serum alpha-fetoprotein screening for hepatoblastoma in children with Beckwith-Wiedemann Syndrome or Isolated hemihyperplasia. J Pediatr 143:270–272
23. Ortega JA et al (2000) Randomized comparison of cisplatin/vincristine/fluorouracil and cisplatin/continuous infusion doxorubicin for treatment of pediatric hepatoblastoma: a report from the Children's Cancer Group and the Pediatric Oncology Group. J Clin Oncol 18: 2665–2675
24. DeBaun M et al (1996) Screening for Wilms' tumor in children with high-risk congenital syndromes: considerations for, an intervention trial. Med Pedia Oncol 27:15421

Chapter 15
The Insulin-Like Growth Factor System in Adrenocortical Growth Control and Carcinogenesis

Christian Fottner, Ina M. Niederle, and Matthias M. Weber

In recent years there has been growing evidence for a central role of the insulin-like growth factor (IGF) system in tumorigenesis and tumor growth. IGFs inhibit apoptosis, induce transformation, and promote tumor growth in many types of malignancies. Previously published data indicate that the IGF system is a major regulator of normal adrenocortical growth and development. Additionally, increased levels of Insulin–like growth factor II (IGF2), IGF-binding protein 2 (IGFBP2), and IGF1-receptor (IGF1R) are frequent findings in ACC that correlate with a malignant tumor phenotype. Altogether, there is substantial evidence for a major role of the IGF system in controlling adrenocortical growth and carcinogenesis.

15.1 The IGF System

The IGFs are polypeptides that play key roles in cellular metabolism, differentiation, proliferation, transformation, and apoptosis during normal development and malignant growth. Both IGF1 and IGF2 are structurally related to proinsulin and secreted in an endocrine and paracrine/autocrine manner. Both proteins mainly mediate their mitogenic effects by binding to the IGF1R, a transmembrane tyrosine kinase receptor with a high sequence homology to the insulin receptor [1]. IGF1R exhibits high affinity for both IGFs. The structurally distinct IGF2/mannose-6-phosphate receptor (IGF2R), which preferentially binds IGF2 and which has no tyrosine kinase activity, is believed to exert a growth suppressive function by internalization and degradation of extracellular IGF2 [2]. To date, the function of the IGF2 receptor still remains unclear in many aspects. The IGFs also exhibit a high binding affinity to at least six specific IGF-binding proteins (IGFBP1 – 6), a family of structurally different peptides that are synthesized locally by most tissues and secreted in tissue-specific patterns. This secretion is in part regulated by other hormones. Based on their high

M.M. Weber (✉)
Schwerpunkt Endokrinologie und Stoffwechselerkrankungen, I. Medizinische Klinik und Poliklinik, Universitätsmedizin, Johannes Gutenberg Universität Mainz, Langenbeckstrasse 1, 55131 Mainz, Germany
e-mail: mmweber@uni-mainz.de

G.D. Hammer, T. Else (eds.), *Adrenocortical Carcinoma*,
DOI 10.1007/978-0-387-77236-3_15,

affinity for IGFs, these peptides serve as autocrine and/or paracrine modulators of IGF action. Moreover, in addition to exerting both inhibitory and stimulatory effects on IGF action, IGFBPs have been shown to have ligand-independent effects as well [2, 3].

There is a growing body of evidence that the IGF system controls growth and proliferation of several types of cancer [4]. Epidemiological observations indicate that circulating IGF1 levels are positively associated with an increased risk for the development of several common tumors like breast, colorectal, lung, prostate, and ovarian cancer, to mention only a few. Additionally, high expression of *IGF2* and *IGFBP2* as well as an increased proteolysis of IGFBP3 are found in various types of cancer [5, 6]. IGFs bind with high affinity to the IGF1R, a tyrosine kinase receptor that transduces signals to the nucleus and mitochondria primarily via the mitogen-activated protein kinase (MAPK) and PI3K/Akt pathways. IGF1R signaling has been shown to contribute to each stage of cancer progression: malignant transformation, tumor growth, local invasion, distant metastases, and resistance to treatment [7]. Finally, circulating IGF1 may facilitate cancer development though it likely does not participate in cancer induction. In addition to direct contributions to tumor growth and carcinogenesis, IGF1 may promote cancer indirectly through interactions with oncogenes, tumor suppressors, and other hormones, especially the sex steroids in breast and prostate cancers, and through interaction with IGFBPs [8]. In addition to their roles in IGF transport, the six IGFBPs regulate cell activity in various ways. By sequestering IGFs away from the type IGF1R, they inhibit mitogenesis, differentiation, survival, and other IGF-stimulated events. IGFBP proteolysis can reverse this inhibition or generate IGFBP fragments with novel bioactivity. Alternatively, IGFBP interaction with cell or matrix components may concentrate IGFs near their receptor, enhancing IGF activity.

15.2 The Role of the IGF System in the Normal Adult Adrenal Gland

15.2.1 Insulin-Like Growth Factors

IGF1 and IGF2 play important roles in the control of growth and function of the adrenal gland. The genes for both IGF ligands and their receptors, as well as specific IGF-binding protein genes, are expressed in the adrenal gland of various species [9–11].

In the human fetal adrenal gland very high levels of *IGF2* mRNA and protein (but almost no IGF1) are found, while in the adult adrenal gland both *IGF*s are expressed at similar levels [12]. In situ hybridization of human fetal adrenal glands shows that *IGF2* is expressed in high abundance in all cortical cells while *IGF1* is only detectable in the adrenal capsule. In cultured fetal human adrenocortical cells *IGF2* mRNA is upregulated by ACTH. IGF2 is a potent mitogen in fetal adrenocortical cells and acts cooperatively with other growth factors like EGF and FGF [9, 13]. Thus, IGF2 is assumed to mediate ACTH-induced adrenal growth during prenatal life [9]. Furthermore, IGF2 seems to play a role in steroidogenesis of the fetal adrenal gland. It is expressed in a coordinated manner with steroidogenic enzymes [14, 15]. In cultured human fetal adrenal cells both IGFs equipotently enhance basal as well as ACTH-induced steroidogenesis, but do not affect ACTH receptor (*MC2R*) expression [16]. IGF1 and IGF2 preferentially stimulate fetal adrenal androgen synthesis as indicated by the selective induction of the androgenic enzyme P450c17 [9, 17, 18]. Taken together, these findings have lead to the hypothesis that IGF2 is responsible for adrenal growth and differentiation during prenatal life, while IGF1 acts mainly in the postnatal period [12]. This is in accordance to the dominant role of IGF1 in mediating whole body growth after birth while IGF2 serum and tissue levels show a strong decline postnatally. Furthermore, IGF2 is a poor promoter of whole body growth as shown after continuous infusion in the hypophysectomized rat or in transgenic mice with transgenic expression of *IGF2* [19–23].

In adult bovine and human adrenal cortex, IGF1 and IGF2 both stimulate basal as well as ACTH-induced steroid biosynthesis by upregulating steroidogenic key enzymes and, in contrast to fetal adrenocortical cells, *MC2R* expression [14, 15]. This stimulation is time- and dose-dependent and androgen biosynthesis is preferentially stimulated [24]. Interestingly, in adult bovine and human adrenocortical cells IGF2 has a significant stronger stimulatory effect on basal and ACTH-induced steroidogenesis. The steroidogenic effect of both IGF1 and IGF2 is mediated through interaction with the IGF1R. This is somewhat surprising since the IGF1R exhibits a higher affinity for IGF1 as compared to IGF2. However, incubation studies with mutated IGF ligands with altered affinities for IGFBPs demonstrate that the stronger steroidogenic effect of IGF2 can be explained by interaction with locally produced IGFBPs [24, 25]. The stronger androgenic potency of IGF2 in the adult human adrenal gland is especially prominent at low physiological concentrations of IGF2 and IGF1 [24].

Compared to other species, the human adrenal gland is unique in its ability to secrete androgens such as dehydroepiandrosterone (DHEA), its sulfate (DHEA-S), and androstenedione. The IGF system has been implicated as a possible trigger for adrenarche, which is characterized by the prepubertal rise in adrenal androgen secretion that is not accompanied by an increase in cortisol secretion and independent of the gonads or gonadotropins [26]. From ontogenetic studies of *IGF1*, *IGF2*, and *IGF1R* expression and immunolocalization in human adrenal tissues from early infancy to late puberty, it was proposed that IGF1 and IGF2 could be involved in the postnatal mechanism of adrenal progenitor cell proliferation and migration, which play an important role in adrenal zonation and adrenarche [27]. Furthermore, a positive correlation between DHEA-S and IGF1 serum levels has been reported [28], and various states of hyperandrogenemia such as polycystic ovary syndrome have been associated with an activation of the IGF1R by IGFs or high levels of circulating insulin [29].

In this context, it is interesting to notice that an intra-fetal infusion of IGF1 in sheep can induce growth of both the adrenocortical and the adrenomedullary cells, resulting on one hand in a significant increase in cell size in the zona glomerulosa and in the zona fasciculata, as well as in the catecholamine-producing medullary cells. On the other hand, IGF1 infusion could neither stimulate the expression of the steroidogenic or catecholamine-synthetic enzymes nor stimulate fetal plasma cortisol concentrations, resulting in a dissociation of adrenal growth and function [30].

15.2.2 IGF Receptors

The presence of both types of IGF receptors has been identified in adult and fetal human adrenal glands by PCR, in situ hybridization, autoradiography, and immunohistochemistry [31–35]. Binding studies with normal adult human adrenocortical tissue revealed the presence of intact IGF1Rs with a single class of high-affinity IGF1-binding sites with a dissociation constant (Kd) of 0.16 nmol/l, and a receptor concentration (RC) of 19.2 nmol/kg protein. As expected, IGF1 bound with an eightfold lower affinity and insulin with more than 100-fold lower affinity to the IGF1R. Furthermore, the presence of intact IGF2R receptors with single class of high-affinity binding sites for IGF2 (Kd 2,2 nmol/l, RC 1137 nmol/kg protein) and no affinity for IGF1 or insulin was demonstrated [36]. In the adult adrenal cortex, both IGFRs and the insulin receptor are expressed in all zones at a similar level [12, 33] During fetal and early postnatal periods, the *IGF1R* in the human adrenal cortex is predominantly expressed in the subcapsular zona glomerulosa [37].

Currently, all mitogenic and differentiating effects of IGF1 and IGF2 in the fetal and adult adrenal gland have been shown to be mediated through interaction of the ligands with the IGF1R [15, 36, 38]. The presence of the IGF2R receptor has been demonstrated in bovine and human adrenal glands and its expression does not seem to be differentially regulated during fetal and postnatal development of the adrenal gland [11, 36, 39]. The physiological role of the IGF2R receptor, which only binds IGF2 and does not transduce a signal, remains unclear. It is assumed, however, that by mediating the clearance and inactivation of IGF2, it may play a role as a tumor suppressor in the adrenal gland [40].

15.2.3 IGF-Binding Proteins

The biological effects of IGF1 and IGF2 are modulated in vivo by at least six high-affinity IGFBPs (IGFBP1-6) that, depending on the cellular context, are able to stimulate or inhibit IGF signaling through a variety of mechanisms and have been shown to exert also IGF-independent actions [41]. In adult and fetal human adrenocortical cells and tissue, the expression of all six high-affinity *IGFBPs* has been shown [24, 41–43]. Furthermore, conventional and two-dimensional Western ligand blotting and immunoblotting revealed the secretion of IGFBP1-5 by human adrenocortical cells in primary culture [43, 44], while no significant secretion of IGFBP6 could be detected. In adult adrenocortical cells, the expression and secretion of *IGFBPs* are differentially regulated by ACTH, steroids, and IGFs [24, 42, 44]. While ACTH specifically stimulates *IGFBP1* and *IGFBP4*, IGF1 and IGF2 preferentially induce the expression and secretion of adrenocortical *IGFBP3* and IGFBP5. In contrast to the forementioned IGFBPs, no regulatory factors of adrenal IGFBP2 and IGFBP4 secretion or expression have been described in normal adrenocortical cells [24, 42, 43]. Analogous to human adrenocortical cells, an induction of *IGFBP1* by ACTH and of *IGFBP3* by IGFs has been demonstrated in bovine adrenocortical cells [42]. The stimulation of *IGFBP1* by ACTH seems to be specific for the adult adrenal gland, since no regulation of *IGFBP*s by ACTH in fetal human adrenocortical cells has been described [32].

The physiological significance of adrenal IGFBP secretion is unknown. However, since IGFs are potent stimulators of adrenocortical cell function and IGFBPs are modulators of the cellular responsiveness to IGFs, changes in of *IGFBP* expression may represent an important feedback mechanism of IGF-dependent adrenocortical cell growth and differentiated function.

In adult human adrenocortical cells, locally produced IGFBPs have a greater inhibitory effect on IGF1- vs. IGF2-mediated steroidogenesis [24, 43]. The fact that in this primary cell culture system a truncated IGF1 analog with reduced affinity for IGFBPs had increased steroidogenic potency supports the hypothesis that the stronger steroidogenic effect of IGF2 as compared to IGF1 is due to a modulatory effect of locally produced IGFBPs [42, 45]. Although a preferential interaction of IGF1 with an inhibitory IGFBP could explain the divergent steroidogenic potency of IGF1 and IGF2, this was not the case for locally produced IGFBP1 since this binding protein has been recently shown to inhibit the steroidogenic action of IGF2 and to potentiate the effect of IGF1 at least in primary cultures of bovine adrenocortical cells [25]. This unexpected divergent effect of IGFBP1 on IGF2-induced steroidogenesis is not due to its phosphorylation status, which in other cell systems is known to significantly influence the binding affinity of IGFBP1 to its ligands IGF1 and IGF2. The mechanism of the divergent effect of IGFBP1 in adrenocortical cells remains unknown. An attractive hypothesis involves the regulated degradation of IGFBPs by specific proteases. Specifically, adrenocortical proteolytic activity may play a role in regulating IGF1 action by cleavage of IGFBPs into fragments with lower affinity for IGFs. These lower-affinity IGFBP fragments have been demonstrated to allow increased levels of free IGFs to activate the IGFR and induce specific biological effects. IGFBP-proteases for all of the six IGFBPs have been described [46], with recent data demonstrating a specific IGFBP1 protease in human amniotic fluid [47]. In adrenocortical cells, the divergent effect of IGFBP1 on IGF-induced steroidogenesis could be explained by a different induction of IGFBP1 proteases by IGF1 and IGF2. A similar mechanism, with preferential induction of an IGFBP-protease by IGF2 but not by IGF1, has been reported in cultured human fibroblasts [48], where an IGF2-induced IGFBP protease leads to an increased level of bioavailable IGF2 and subsequent enhanced steroidogenic effect of IGF2 compared to IGF1.

In contrast to its role on IGF-induced differentiated function, the endocrine effects of IGFBPs on IGF1-induced growth and proliferation of adrenocortical cells are predominantly inhibitory. In *IGF2*- and *GH/IGF1*-transgenic mice, IGF overexpression induces adrenal enlargement and elevated corticosterone serum levels, presumably by a direct mitogenic effect of IGFs on adrenocortical fasciculata cells [49]. This observed IGF-induced growth-promoting effect is abolished by simultaneous overexpression of *IGFBP2*, providing evidence for an inhibitory effect of this IGFBP in vivo. Additionally, in the double *GH/IGFBP2*- transgenic mice, GH-induced hypertrophy (but not GH-induced hyperplasia) of zona fasciculata cells is completely abolished by *IGFBP2* overexpression, indicating differential regulation of adrenocortical hypertrophy and hyperplasia by the GH/IGF1 axis [50, 51]. Moreover, the growth-inhibiting effect of IGFBPs in the adrenal gland is further supported by data, showing a significantly stronger growth-promoting effect of long R^3 IGF1 (LR^3IGF1), an IGF1-analog that has much reduced affinities for IGF-binding proteins [52]. Importantly, the inhibitory effect of IGFBP2 on adrenocortical cell growth is not observed in *IGFBP2*-transgenic mice without concomitant IGF hypersecretion, indicating that this observed effect is not an IGF1-independent effect exerted by IGFBP2 itself but rather an inhibitory effect of IGFBP2 on IGF-dependent actions.

15.3 Specific Role of the IGF System in Adrenocortical Tumorigenesis

15.3.1 IGF1

In vitro, IGF1 is mitogenic in fetal and adult adrenocortical cells from different species [53], and in vivo infusion of IGF1 into guinea pigs causes an increase in the fractional weight of the adrenal glands [52]. In growth hormone (*GH*)-overexpressing transgenic mice characterized by elevated IGF1 serum levels, an enlargement of the adrenal glands with an increase in zona fasciculata cell number and size and an elevated corticosterone secretion has been reported [49], supporting an important role of the GH/IGF axis for adrenal growth and function. While *IGF1* is expressed in ACCs as shown by microarray analysis and immunohistochemistry, most studies do not show very high *IGF1* expression in adrenal tumors [45, 54–57]. Increased levels of IGF2 and IGFBP2 are associated with malignancy in sporadic adrenocortical tumors. On the contrary, there is no increase in IGF1 protein in ACC specimens when compared to both normal and adenomatous adrenal tissue [57, 58] (for overview see Table 15.1). While one immunohistochemical study

Table 15.1 Alterations of the IGF system in adrenal tumors

Gene/protein	Alteration	Prevalence (tumors)	Reference
IGF1	High mRNA levels	0/18 adenomas 0/23 carcinomas	De Fraipont et al. [55]
	High mRNA levels	0/15 adenomas 0/4 carcinomas	Ilvesmäki et al. [32]
	>50% cells positive immunohistochemical staining	1/23 adenomas 21/64 carcinomas	Kamio et al. [33]
IGF2	High mRNA levels	0/15 adenomas 5/6 carcinomas	Ilvesmäki et al. [32]
	High mRNA levels	2/17 adenomas 5/6 carcinomas	Gicquel et al. [59]
	High mRNA levels	0/35 adenomas 25/29 carcinomas	Giquel et al. [60, 61]
	High protein levels	1/9 adenomas 9/9 carcinomas	Boulle et al. [58]
	High mRNA levels	10/11 carcinomas	Giordano et al. [62]
	Strong IGF2-IHC staining	4/64 adenomas 33/67 carcinomas	Erickson et al. [63]
	High mRNA levels	4/4 pediatric carcinomas	Wilkin et al. [64]
	Gene upregulation in microarray analysis	51-fold in 6 pediatric carcinomas 31-fold in 17 pediatric adenomas 270-fold in 14 adult carcinomas	Almeida et al. [65]
		75% of 24 carcinomas 10% of 33 adenomas	De Fraipont et al. [66]
		20-fold in 5 pediatric adenomas and 18 carcinomas Increased immature big IGF2 protein	West et al. [67]
		Three- to sevenfold in 10 carcinomas vs. 10 adenomas	Slater et al. [68]
		20-fold upregulation in 34 malignant vs. 58 benign adrenal tumors	De Reyniès et al. [69]
		Upregulation vs. adenoma and normal in 28/33 carcinomas	Giordano et al. [70]
		135- to 430-fold upregulation in 7 carcinomas vs. 13 adenomas	Velázquez-Fernández et al. [71]

Table 15.1 (continued)

Gene/protein	Alteration	Prevalence (tumors)	Reference
IGFIR	Increased receptor concentration	0/8 adenomas 3/4 carcinomas	Weber et al. [36]
	Increased IHC staining	9/23 adenomas 40/64 carcinomas	Kamio et al. [33]
	Increased IHC staining	Medium-high in 18/24 carcinomas Negative-low in 12/22 adenomas and in 3/4 normal glands	Barlaskar et al. [72]
	Microarray analysis	Fourfold downregulation in 10 carcinomas vs. normal	Slater et al. [68]
	Microarray analysis	1.6-fold downregulation in 34 malignant vs. 58 benign adrenal tumors	De Reyniès et al. [69]
IGF2R	LOH	2/25 adenomas 11/29 carcinomas	Leboulloux et al. [73]
	Microarray analysis	80-fold upregulation in 7 carcinomas vs. 13 adenomas	Velázquez-Fernández et al. [71]
IGFBP2	Increased protein concentration in tumor tissue	0/9 adenomas 8/9 carcinomas	Boulle et al. [58]
	Increased serum concentration	0/36 healthy controls 2/13 complete remission 23/28 metastatic disease	Boulle et al. [74]
IGFBP6	Microarray analysis	Fourfold downregulation in 10 carcinomas vs. normal	Slater et al. [68]
		Upregulation in 7 carcinomas vs. 13 adenomas	Velázquez-Fernández et al. [71]
	Northern blot analysis	Lower mRNA Levels in 9 ACC vs. normal and 9 adenoma	Boulle et al. [58]
IGFBP3	Microarray analysis	Threefold upregulation in 10 carcinomas vs. normal (not confirmed by PCR)	Slater et al. [68]
		Upregulation in 7 carcinomas vs. 13 adenomas	Velázquez-Fernández et al. [71]
IGFBP5	Microarray analysis	Two- to sixfold downregulation in 34 malignant vs. 58 benign adrenal tumors	De Reyniès et al. [69]

demonstrates an increased percentage of cells expressing *IGF1* in ACC (greater than 50% of the cells stain positive for IGF1 in 83% of ACCs vs. only 10 ± 50% IGF1-positive cells in the majority of normal adrenocortical tissue samples (75%) and adrenal adenoma samples (64%), the preponderance of data suggest that while

IGF1 is an important physiological mediator of the adult adrenal gland, it is not a major regulator of adrencortical tumorigenesis. [75].

15.3.2 IGF2

A strong expression of *IGF2* is a dominant finding in ACC, occurring in approximately 80–90% of all adult ACCs (see Table 15.1). Messenger RNA levels of *IGF2* usually are elevated more than 100-fold as compared to normal or adenomatous adrenocortical tissue [32, 55, 57, 63, 76]. In gene expression profiling of sporadic ACCs *IGF2* has been shown to be the single most upregulated transcript [62, 70–72] (see Chapter 29).

While one genome-wide profiling study of 85 sporadic adult adrenal tumors found no differential *IGF2* gene expression in ACC compared to ACA and normal adrenal tissue, such findings taken together with the overwhelming data on *IGF2* expression in adult ACC probably reflect the methodological problems of these microarray techniques including different microarray platforms, sample size, clinical follow-up data, and composition of the cohort [77]. Indeed, higher IGF2 levels in adrenal tumors are usually associated with a more malignant phenotype with high expression of *IGF2* being associated with both a fivefold increased risk for the recurrence of sporadic ACCs [61] and a shorter disease-free survival [69]. It is intriguing that in contrast to adult ACCs only a 20-fold upregulation of *IGF2* overexpression is observed in childhood adrenal tumors [64, 67], the upregulation does not discriminate between adenomas and carcinomas and accordingly did not predict clinical outcome [67, 78]. Whether this reflects a unique biology of pediatric vs. adult ACC remains unclear. It is intriguing to speculate that the relative high *IGF2* expression in adult tumors vs. pediatric tumors reflects the low baseline expression of *IGF2* in normal adult adrenocortical tissue compared to the high *IGF2* in fetal adrenal tissue. Specifically , the *IGF2* expression pattern of adult ACCs resembles fetal adrenocortical tissue and shows a high degree of similarity to childhood tumors, supporting a hypothesis that adult adrenocortical tumors might arise from adrenal stem cells (common progenitor cells of the adrenocortical fetal zone) or undergo dedifferentiation (fetal reprogramming) as they develop (see Chapters 17 and 28).

Using the cDNA microarray technique in a series of clinically well-characterized adult adrenocortical tumors, two independent and specifically regulated clusters of genes (the *IGF2* cluster and the steroidogenesis cluster) have been identified as good predictors of malignancy [66]. Upregulation of the so-called *IGF2* cluster is found in 75% of ACCs and includes: in addition to *IGF2*, the two mitogenic FGF receptor genes (*FGFR1* and *FGFR4*); two members of the TGFß gene family (*TGFβ2*, and *TGFβR*), which are strong inhibitors of steroidogenesis; *MSTR1* encoding a receptor for macrophage-stimulating 1 receptor, which mediates mitogenic effects in adrenomedullary PC12 cells; the *KCNQ1OT1* gene, which is involved in the regulation of parental imprinting of the 11p15 region; and *GAPD*, which is upregulated through hypoxia and apoptosis. In contrast, the steroidogenesis cluster activity is suppressed in 81% of carcinomas. *IGF2* expression alone has not been shown to be predictive of metastases in adult ACCs [65] and does not correlate with overall survival in one cohort study of 124 patients with metastatic disease [79]. However, when high *IGF2* cluster expression and low steroidogenesis gene cluster expression are combined, a significant lower recurrence-free survival rate is found, which is equivalent to the recurrence-free survival rate in tumors with Weiss scores ≥ 4 [66]. Similarly, in a recent gene expression study of 153 unilateral adrenocortical tumors, the prediction of malignancy and survival based on *IGF2* expression was less accurate than the combined expression of the two cell-cycle-associated genes *DLG7* and *PINK1* [80]. Clearly, other mutations are cooperating with IGF1R activation in the pathogenesis and maintenance of ACC.

IGF2 mRNA is apparently translated efficiently into IGF2 protein in ACC samples, since significantly stronger immunostaining for IGF2 and 14-fold higher concentrations of IGF2 protein have been found in ACC [32, 58, 64]. Northern blotting analysis showed the same *IGF2* mRNA species (4.8 and 6/2.2 kb, transcribed from promotor 4 and 3, respectively) in normal and tumorous adrenal tissue, with a preferential use of promotor P3 in tumoral tissue [59]. However, the majority of adult and pediatric adrenocortical tumors grossly express immature forms of "big" IGF2 [58, 67], which are also the major forms of *IGF2* found in the normal fetal adrenal cortex [81]. In contrast to the marked increase in serum IGFBP2, no elevated serum levels of IGF2 were observed in patients with malignant or metastatic adrenocortical tumors despite the marked increase in tumoral *IGF2* [58, 59].

This data argue for a paracrine or autocrine effect of IGF2 on ACC cells. NCI-H295R cells that most closely resemble adult ACCs secrete large amounts of IGF2 and IGFBP2. IGF2 has been shown to be mitogenic through interaction with the endogenously expressed *IGF1R* [40]. Moreover, both IGF1 and IGF2 have been shown to be mitogenic through interaction with the IGF1R in various adrenocortical cell lines including the mouse tumor cell line Y1, the adult human ACC cell line NCI-H295R, and in a pediatric adrenocortical adenoma cell line [53, 65, 72]. In human fetal adrenal glands IGF2 and fibroblast growth factor-2 (FGF2) have a cooperative mitogenic effect [82]. FGF2 seems to be an important modulator of posttranslational processing of IGF2 in NCI-H295R cells, leading to an increase in secreted pro-IGF2 (of about 18 kDa) and a strong decrease in the mature 7.5 kDa IGF2 [58].

When IGF2 is overexpressed in the liver, isolated endocrine effects of IGF2 alone have been evaluated. In vivo, the effects of elevated levels of IGF2 on adrenal growth and function have been evaluated in *PEPCK-IGF2* mice that express *IGF2* postnatally under a transgenic construct. These *IGF2*-transgenic mice exhibit four- to sixfold higher IGF2 serum levels, elevated serum IGFBP2 levels, and a local overexpression of *IGF2* in the adrenal gland. Morphologically, they show a normal body weight and appearance and only subtle changes in organ growth [83]. The adrenal glands, however, were significantly enlarged, which was mainly due to a 50% increase in the number of zona fasciculata cells, while cell volume and zonation of transgenic adrenal glands remained unchanged. The hyperplasia of the zona fasciculata was paralleled by an enhanced steroidogenesis with twice the basal and ACTH-induced corticosterone levels of controls. When normalized for adrenal weight, the corticosterone secretion was similar in both groups, suggesting that the increased serum levels of corticosterone are mainly caused by a direct mitogenic effect of IGF2 on adrenocortical cells. Although it can not be completely ruled out that an endocrine effect of elevated IGF2 serum levels is responsible for the enlarged adrenal gland in this transgenic mouse model, it seems likely that the trophic effects are exerted by locally expressed IGF2. This is supported by the fact that systemic IGF2 is a poor mediator of postnatal growth in other *IGF2* transgenic mouse models. In these mice total body weight and adrenal weight are normal or reduced despite grossly elevated serum IGF2 levels, but tissue-specific trophic effects were associated with local *IGF2* expression [20, 84–86]. Furthermore, no growth effect was observed after infusion of IGF2 in hypophysectomized rats [19] or in adult rodents with IGF2-producing tumors [22].

Similar to the findings in *PEPCK-IGF2* mice, enlarged adrenal glands and elevated corticosterone serum levels have been reported in mice with transgenic expression of bovine or human *GH* [87]. Interestingly, the enlargement of the adrenal glands in *PEPCK-GH* mice, which was presumably induced through elevated IGF1 levels, was due to a combination of hyperplasia and hypertrophy of zona fasciculata cells [49]. It is of importance, however, that *PEPCK-IGF2* mice did not show any increased frequency of adrenal tumors, thus indicating that IGF2 by itself is not sufficient for malignant transformation of adrenocortical cells, and that additional factors are required for adrenal tumorigenesis [88], supporting similar conclusions of both the genetic profiling and the cell line studies detailed above.

The importance of IGF2 as a potential tumor-promoting factor – not only for ACC – is supported by the fact that several mechanisms exist which limit the bioactivity of IGF2 during adult life. On the epigenetic level, the *IGF2* gene is maternally imprinted, resulting in inactivation of the maternal *IGF2* gene and exclusive expression of the paternal allele. Furthermore, the expression of *IGF2* is under the control of several tumor-suppressor genes like Wilms tumor-suppressor gene *WT1*. On the protein level IGF2 is inactivated through binding to the IGF2R receptor, resulting in internalization and degradation of IGF2. An additional level of regulation is the interaction with IGFBPs which – depending on the cellular context – can have either inhibitory or stimulating effects on IGF2 bioactivity and which themselves are additionally regulated in their bioactivity by specific IGFBP-proteases. Many of these factors are altered in genetic syndromes associated with adrenal tumors and in sporadic ACC and thus may contribute to the IGF2 deregulation. Possible mechanisms are *IGF2* dosage effects (LOH, UPD), loss of tumor-suppressor genes on the maternal chromosome 11, germline or somatic *TP53* mutations, and changes in IGF2 gene methylation [60, 61].

Of particular relevance are abnormalities in the imprinted 11p15 region (involving the maternally imprinted *IGF2* gene and the paternally imprinted *p57KIP2* and *H19* genes) that are frequently found in ACCs and are highly specific for malignancy [89]. Alterations at the 11p15 gene locus, which result in a strong expression of *IGF2*, are loss of heterozygosity with loss of the maternal and duplication of the paternal allele and less frequently loss of imprinting (LOI) with a paternal-like expression of the maternal allele. In adult patients with nonmetastatic sporadic ACC, 11p15 LOH is a strong predictor for a shorter disease-free survival (relative risk ratio: 9) [61]. Similar genetic and epigenetic alterations of the 11p15 locus with a strong overexpression of *IGF2* have been implicated in the pathogenesis of the Beckwith-Wiedemann syndrome, an overgrowth disorder with increased risk of childhood tumors including ACCs (see Chapter 14) The fact that the predictive value of 11p15 LOH is stronger than that of *IGF2* overexpression indicates that in this region additional molecular changes like a loss of maternally expressed tumor-suppressor genes contribute to adrenal tumorigenesis [61]. Two candidate tumor-suppressor genes are *p57KIP2* and *H19*, which also map to the 11p15.5 region but which are – in contrast to *IGF2* – paternally imprinted. Thus, genetic alterations with loss of the maternal and duplication of the paternal 11p15 allele can result not only in the overexpression of the paternally expressed *IGF2*-gene but also in the functional loss of the maternally expressed *p57KIP2* and *H19* genes [59, 60, 64, 90, 91]. The gene *H19* encodes an mRNA that is not translated into a protein and has been postulated to act as a tumor-suppressor gene. *p57KIP2* is a known suppressor of the cell cycle progression and is thought to play an important role in the Beckwith-Wiedemann syndrome [92]. A decreased expression of *H19* and *p57KIP2* is a frequent and specific finding in ACCs [60, 90, 93]. It seems likely that loss of function of these putative tumor-suppressor genes contributes to the highly malignant phenotype of these tumors. Furthermore, these genes might be involved in the regulation of *IGF2* gene expression or mRNA stability, since a strong negative correlation between *p57KIP2* and *IGF2* mRNA has been found [90] and *H19* mRNA has been shown to decrease steady-state *IGF2* mRNA levels [64] (see Fig. 15.1).

Other factors which might be involved in the mechanism of *IGF2* overexpression in ACCs are novH, *IGF2* gene methylation, and the 5′ VNTR of the insulin gene. The minisatellite DNA polymorphism of a variable number of tandem repeats (VNTR) in the 5′-flanking region of the human insulin gene also is located in the 11p15 region [94, 95]. In 3 of 4 pediatric ACCs, only the short class I Insulin 5′ VNTR alleles, which are associated with an increased *IGF2* expression, were found [64]. In addition, demethylation of the *IGF2* gene has been demonstrated in pediatric ACCs [64], suggesting that alterations of the methylation status might be involved in *IGF2* overexpression and dysregulation of the imprinted 11p15 region, as it has been shown in other tumors [57, 96]. NovH (nephroblastoma overexpressed) belongs to the CCN (CNTF/CYR61/NOV) family of proteins which is part of the IGFBP superfamily, and seems to play a role as a negative regulator of cell growth and adhesion. In ACCs, the *novH* gene is significantly decreased, and there is an inverse correlation with the *IGF2* mRNA concentration [97, 98].

15.4 IGF Receptors

15.4.1 The IGF1R

The presence of the intact IGF1R has been demonstrated in adrenal tumors of the cortex and medulla both on the mRNA and the protein level [32]. Similar to other tissues, the mitogenic effects of both IGF1 and IGF2 seem to be mediated through interaction with the IGF1R. Elevated IGF1R levels have been described in adult ACCs compared to hyperplasias, adenomas, and normal adrenals [33, 36]. In competition binding studies and Scatchard plot analysis, a single class of high-affinity binding sites with a dissociation constant (Kd) of 0.16 nmol/l was reported. In contrast, three out of four hormonally active ACCs showed a significantly increase in specific IGF1 binding with a three- to fourfold increase in IGF1R concentration compared to normal adrenocortical tissue. In accordance with the above study, a strong expression of the *IGF1R* has been found by immunohistochemistry in 8/21 ACCs, but none of the adenomas investigated [36]. The fact that the binding affinity and electrophoretic mobility of the IGF1R was unaltered in ACCs suggests expression of functionally intact *IGF1Rs* in these tumors [36]. This is supported by the demonstration of an increased IGF1R signaling in ACCs by immunoblot analysis and human tissue microarray staining of activated phospho-IGF1R and phospho-Akt^{Ser473} [72]. In this study a significant shift to a high-intensity staining for activated IGF1Rs and downstream signaling proteins has been observed in 24 ACCs as compared to 22 adenomas and 4 normal adrenocortical samples.

In contrast to the strong expression of functionally active *IGF1R*s on the protein level, an expression of *IGF1R* could be demonstrated only in pediatric ACCs by quantitative real-time PCR [65], while in adult ACCs a similar or even lower *IGF1R* mRNA level was reported [32, 65, 68, 80]. Therefore, the expression of *IGF1Rs* and increase in signaling through the receptor in adult ACCs might be due to alterations in posttranslational processing, internalization, and/or degradation of the IGF1R. In the pediatric cohort, high expression of *IGF1R* was a predictor of metastases [65].

The mechanism responsible for enhanced *IGF1R* expression in ACC remains unclear. Expression of the *IGF1R* is regulated by a variety of factors including growth factors, oncogenes, and tumor-suppressor genes such as *TP53* [99–102]. In normal cells, expression of wild-type *TP53* was shown to inhibit *IGF1R* gene expression, whereas loss of function p53 upregulates *IGF1R* expression in several different tumors [103, 104]. In ACC, loss-of-function mutations within the conserved regions of p53 have been found in approximately 30% of malignant ACCs, whereas mutations are rarely found in benign adrenocortical adenomas, suggesting a role for p53 later in adrenocortical carcinogenesis [105] (see Chapters 9, 10, 11 and 12). Thus, *TP53* mutations may represent one possible mechanism for the high expression of *IGF1R* in a late stage of adrenocortical tumorigenesis. However, no correlation has been found between *p53* mutations and expression level of *IGF1R* in pediatric ACC [65]. Furthermore, the elevated IGF2 concentration in adrenal malignancies might contribute to the expression of *IGF1R* in these tumors. It has been shown in CaCo2 human colon carcinoma cells that stable high expression of *IGF2* results in an increased *IGF1R* expression with increased proliferation and anchorage-independent growth [106], and a positive correlation between the expression of *IGF2* and *IGF1R* has been reported in colorectal carcinomas [107].

High expression of the *IGF1R* has been demonstrated in a variety of malignant tumors like colon, breast, and lung cancer [41, 108], and strong evidence indicates that the IGF1R plays a pivotal role in tumorigenesis. Interestingly, alterations in the IGF system also seem to play an important role in tumors originating from the adrenal medulla or sympathetic ganglia, like pheochromocytomas or neuroblastomas. High levels of the IGF1R in neuroblastoma cells result in resistance to apoptosis, leading to unregulated growth [109]. *IGF2* [110] and *IGFBP2* [111] are widely expressed in human neuroblastomas, possibly enhancing and/or modulating IGF1R activation, and expression of *IGF2* mRNA and peptide has been described in human pheochromocytomas [112, 113]. Furthermore, a significant two- to threefold overexpression of the *IGF1R* mRNA and protein level has been recently reported in the majority of 16 human pheochromocytomas using RT-PCR and binding studies [114]. The mitogenic effect of IGF2 is dependent on the presence of the intact IGF1R [41, 108]. Interaction with the IGF1R has been shown to mediate the steroidogenic and mitogenic effect of IGF1 and IGF2 in the adult human adrenal gland [24, 43]. Therefore, high local levels of IGF2 in combination with elevated IGF1R concentrations would be predicted to represent an autocrine stimulatory loop, thus contributing to adrenocortical tumorigenesis. Increased expression of the human *IGF1R* promotes ligand-dependent neoplastic transformation in a variety of different cell systems [41, 44]. In contrast, absence or decreased levels of the IGF1R prevents malignant growth and transformation in vitro and in vivo, and has been demonstrated to confer resistance to oxidative stress and even extends lifespan [107, 115, 116].

In rat pheochromocytoma PC12 cells, IGF1R has been shown to be important for the stimulation of cell replication [117] and the IGFs are potent mitogens stimulating cell proliferation three times over basal. IGF1 was ten times more potent in stimulating DNA synthesis than IGF2, suggesting that these effects are mediated by the IGF1R [118, 119]. Moreover, binding affinities to the IGF1R correlate directly with the ability of IGF1 and IGF2 to completely prevent apoptosis in PC12 cells [120]. In these cells, promotion of cell growth and proliferation by IGF1 is exerted by the ERK pathway [121], whereas for prevention of apoptosis the phosphatidylinositol-3 kinase pathway is involved [122].

In the mouse adrenocortical tumor cells Y1 overexpression of the human *IGF1R* results in an increased IGF-dependent cell proliferation and antagonizes the antiproliferative effect of ACTH in vitro [53]. On the other hand, the inhibition of the IGF1R signaling results in significant antiproliferative effects in mouse and human adrenocortical cell lines [65, 72]. Treatment of adult human adrenocortical tumor cells NCI-H295 and a pediatric adrenal adenoma cell line with the selective IGF1R kinase inhibitor NVP-AEW541 induced a time- and dose-dependent inhibition of IGF2-induced cell proliferation and survival and an induction of apoptosis in these cells. Interestingly, the NCI-H295 cells exhibited a very high sensitivity to the antimitotic effects of IGF1R kinase inhibition, which was comparable with that of the most sensitive cell lines such as Ewing's sarcoma and neuroblastoma cell lines [65]. The NCI-H295 cell line most closely reflects human ACC due to its constitutional expression of high *IGF2* levels, the presence of *IGF1R*, and an active IGF-induced mitogenic signaling. The antiproliferative effects of the small molecule inhibitor NVP-AEW541 and the fully human monoclonal IGF1R antibody IMC-A12 in NCI-H295 cells were dependent on the presence of IGFIRs, since no significant antimitotic effect of these agents was observed in the human adrenocortical cell line RL251, which expresses only minimal amounts of IGF1R [72]. In vivo, treatment of NCI-H295 xenografted athymic nude mice with NVP-AEW541 or IMC-A12 for 21 days was well tolerated and resulted in a significant reduction in tumor size, intratumoral suppression of IGF1R signaling, as measured by reduced levels of phosphorylated Akt^{Ser473}, and in a clear decrease in tumor vascularity which was paralleled by an 1.6-fold decrease in *VEGF* expression in the tumor. Furthermore, the combined treatment of NCI-H295 cells with IGF1R antagonists and mitotane resulted in a synergistic antiproliferative effect in vitro and in vivo in tumor xenografts [72].

15.4.2 The IGF2/Mannose-6-Phosphate (IGF2R)*-Receptor*

Little information is available on the role of the IGF2R in the pathogenesis of adrenocortical tumors. The IGF2R is a single chain transmembrane multiligand-binding glycoprotein that binds and degrades IGF2 and mediates the activation of the growth inhibitor TGFß (transforming growth factor ß). Therefore, it has been assumed to play an important role as a tumor suppressor. In vitro, an antiproliferative effect of the IGF2R receptor has been demonstrated in choriocarcinoma and in colorectal cells, which depend in their growth on IGF2 [123, 124]. Mice lacking functional IGF2R have high levels of circulating IGF2, are approximately 30% larger than their wild-type littermates, and show perinatal lethality. This fetal overgrowth is mediated through interaction of IGF2 with the IGF1R since it is not seen in mice that in addition lack functional IGF2 or the IGF1R [125–127]. Abnormalities of the *IGF2R* like LOH, missense mutations which often lead to reduced IGF2 binding, and microsatellite instability have been demonstrated in various cancers [80, 128–131].

Recently, it has been shown that the IGF2R also might play an important role in the pathogenesis of ACCs. Abnormal fetal imprinting of the *IGF2R* with marked repression of the paternal allele has been described in 50% of Wilms tumors, a carcinoma which shares many common mechanisms with ACCs, including high *IGF2* expression [132]. Furthermore, in adrenocortical tumors, loss of heterozygosity at the *IGF2R* locus was detected in 15 of 57 (26%) informative tumors and was more frequent in malignant (58%) than in benign tumors (9%). Although inactivation of the remaining allele by mutations or abnormal fetal imprinting was not evaluated, this data support the hypothesis that IGF2R may function as a tumor suppressor in the adrenal gland [73]. In contrast, microarray analysis has demonstrated an 80-fold upregulation of *IGF2R* mRNA in 7 ACCs as compared to 13 adrenal adenomas [71]. Therefore, the exact role of the IGF2R in adrenocortical tumorigenesis remains unknown.

15.5 IGFBPs

In normal adrenocortical cells the predominant IGFBPs are IGFBP1, -3 and -5, which are regulated by IGFs and ACTH. In contrast, adrenocortical tumors show a characteristic change in IGFBP expression pattern, with significantly higher IGFBP2 levels in malignant as compared to benign tumors. In ACC, almost all detectable IGF-binding protein consists of IGFBP2, whereas in normal adrenocortical cells only 12% of all IGFBPs are IGFBP2, which does not show specific regulation [24, 25, 43, 44, 133]. Apart from IGFBP2, no differences in the secretion of other IGFBPs were found in human adrenocortical tumors [58, 74]. At the mRNA-level however, microarray analysis of ACC did show conflicting results. While one study reports upregulation of *IGFBP6* in ACCs vs. adenomas [71], two other studies demonstrate lower *IGFBP6* mRNA levels in ACC [58, 68]. Similar results with mRNA downregulation have been reported for *IGFBP5* with two- to sixfold lower levels in 34 malignant vs. 58 benign adrenocortical tumors [80]. In contrast, microarray analysis of *IGFBP3* did show a slight upregulation in two studies [68, 71]. The pathophysiological significance of these microarray results is unclear. There are no data demonstrating a significant alteration of these IGFBPs at the protein level either in the serum of patients with ACC or in tumor tissues. Thus, a relevance of these alterations remains questionable.

However, elevated levels of IGFBP2 are consistently demonstrated in patients with ACC. In more than 80% of patients with metastasized ACC significantly higher plasma levels of IGFBP2 are found as compared to a normal control group. In these patients, plasma IGFBP2 levels correlate positively with tumor burden and are inversely correlated with survival and predict a more aggressive clinical phenotype. In contrast, there was no significant difference in plasma IGFBP2 concentration between patients with complete remission, localized disease, and healthy controls [58, 74]. Accordingly increased IGFBP2 levels have been demonstrated in NCI-H295R cells both in vitro and in vivo in a tumor xenograft immunoincompetent nude mouse model [40, 134]. Despite elevated levels of IGFBP2 protein in malignant tumor tissue, no increase in *IGFBP2* mRNA levels has been detected, suggesting a posttranscriptional mechanism in the regulation of IGFBP2 abundance in ACC [58].

Increased serum IGFBP2 levels are not only found in patients with ACC but can also be found frequently in patients suffering from various kinds of malignancies, including lung, colorectal, ovarian, prostate and CNS cancer, as well as in patients with lymphoid tumors and in children suffering from Wilms tumor [4]. In several of these malignant tumors, (colorectal, breast, prostate, or ovarian cancer), serum IGFBP2 levels correlate positively with tumor markers and tumor stage and are inversely correlated with survival. In glioblastoma and breast cancer patients, elevated IGFBP2 levels correlate with decreased sensitivity to chemotherapy and increased tolerance to radiation therapy. Additionally, they are highly prognostic for metastasis and recurrent disease and are generally thought to reflect tumor burden. However, serum IGFBP2 levels are most probably not indicative of an increased cancer risk, because in these tumors serum IGFBP2 levels are normal before the diagnosis of cancer, as it is the case in patients with ACC [135, 136].

Clinical data are paralleled by many in vitro studies that show *IGFBP2* overexpression in different cancer cell lines like Y1 and NCI-H295R, MCF-7, CACO-2, LNCaP, and C6 cell lines among others [137]. In these tumor models, IGFBP2 has been found to modulate gene expression and subsequent proliferation, cell adhesion, cell migration, and apoptosis through both IGF-dependent and IGF-independent mechanisms [138]. However, the functional significance of elevated IGFBP2 levels in ACC and the exact mechanisms leading to increased *IGFBP2* expression remain unclear. Until recently, IGFBP2 has been postulated to be a negative regulator of normal somatic growth, most probably by sequestering IGFs from their receptors [139]. In transgenic mice, overexpression of *IGFBP2* leads to a strong inhibition of GH/IGF1-induced adrenocortical hypertrophy, but has no effect on adrenal hyperplasia. This selective inhibition of cell size increase is an interesting new facet in the spectrum of mechanisms by which IGFBP2 may affect cell growth and differentiation [49, 139]. However, the inhibitory effect of IGFBP2 on adrenocortical cell growth is not observed in *IGFBP2* transgenic mice without concomitant IGF-hypersecretion, indicating that this observed effect is not an IGF-independent effect exerted by IGFBP2 itself but rather an inhibitory effect of IGF-dependent action by binding excess free IGFs. However, in vitro, murine IGFBP2 in Y1 cells is associated with significant morphological alterations, enhanced cell proliferation, and increased colony formation as compared to control transfected cells. The enhanced proliferation of IGFBP2-secreting clones was independent of exogenous IGFs or the presence of a blocking IGF1R antibody aIR-3 [139, 140]. Additionally, recent data show that inhibition of IGFBP2 with specific antibodies significantly reduced cell proliferation in the human ACC cell line NCI-H295R [141]. These data suggest that elevated levels of IGFBP2 in the tumor can contribute to the highly malignant phenotype of ACC by both IGF-dependent and IGF-independent mechanisms, most probably involving auto/paracrine mechanisms.

While the exact mechanism of the observed high expression of *IGFBP2* in ACC is still unknown, the physiologic regulation of *IGFBP2* expression is highly complex and influenced by multiple hormones and growth factors [142]. Known hormonal regulators of *IGFBP2* expression include GH, IGF1, TGF-beta, interleukin-1, estradiol, glucocorticoids, insulin, follicle-stimulating hormone, and, of particular interest with regard to ACC, IGF2. Postnatal transgenic expression of *IGF2* results in elevated circulating IGFBP2 serum levels, thus activation of the *IGFBP2* promoter by IGF2 could be one explanation for the observed IGFBP2 levels in patients with ACC. However, increased *IGFBP2* expression is not a phenomenon confined to ACC, therefore additional regulatory mechanisms applying for many different types of cancer may be involved. Induction of antioxidative mechanisms could be a possible mechanism, since elevated *IGFBP2* expression has been found after exposing various cancer cell lines to oxidative stress [143, 144]. IGFs also induce expression of hypoxia-inducible factor-1α (*HIF1α*), which could be involved in the control of *IGFBP2* expression. *HIF1α*-deficient embryonic stem cells show reduced *IGFBP2* expression. Furthermore, astrocytomas and glioblastomas show increased *HIF1α* expression paralleled by increased IGFBP2 levels. In these cells IGFBP2 induced DNA damage repair and therapeutic resistance to radiation therapy [145]. Notably, the redox-regulated transcription factor NFκB can bind the *IGFBP2* promoter region at four distinct positions [146] and NFκB has been found to activate *IGFBP2* expression in lung cancer cells under oxidative stress. Additionally, recent data indicate that high *IGFBP2* expression results in elevated catalase activities in ACC cells [147]. Since catalase controls intracellular hydrogen peroxide levels, which represents an important intracellular signaling molecule, a new link between IGFBP2 and intracellular signaling processes might be established. It is tempting to speculate that IGFBP2 activates defense mechanisms against oxidative stress and thereby contributes to the highly malignant phenotype of many cancers characterized by high expression of *IGFBP2*. Additionally, a protein-kinase A (PKA)-dependent regulation of *IGFBP2* is observed in primary pigmented nodular adrenocortical disease and the ACC cell line NCI-H295R [141]. In these cell systems, increased *IGFBP2* expression is the result of loss-of-function mutations in *PRKAR1A*, which encodes the 1α regulatory subunit of PKA, thus causing PKA inhibition. It is known that PKA and/or cAMP act as a coordinator of growth and proliferation in the adrenal cortex. Moreover, it has been shown that components of the cAMP signaling pathway can be altered to various degrees in adrenocortical tumors and that the ACTH-cAMP-protein kinase A and Wnt pathways are also implicated in adrenocortical tumorigenesis. Therefore, the frequently observed alterations in the PKA signaling pathway could be another explanation for the observed increase in *IGFBP2* expression in adrenocortical tumors [148, 149]. Further results show not only increased *IGFBP2* expression in various tumor cells but also increased proteolysis of IGFBP2, thus facilitating IGF2 bioavailability in the cancer microenvironment. In several different tumor cell lines like prostate, ovarian, or colon cancer cells increased concentrations of matrix-metallo-proteinases (MMP) have been described, which are able to cleave IGFBP2, resulting in the release of bioactive IGF and the promotion of cell growth and motility [150, 151], Whether the frequently observed overexpression of *IGFBP2* in malignant tumors indicates a role of IGFBP2 in the initiation or progression of cancer remains unknown. In human breast cancer cells, Perks et al. have shown that IGFBP2 and IGF2 are able to regulate the phosphatase and tensin homolog deleted on chromosome 10 (PTEN). PTEN is a dual function protein and lipid phosphatase and one of the most frequently mutated tumor-suppressor genes [152, 153]. It dephosphorylates the phospholipids generated by the oncogenic phosphatidylinositol-3 kinase (P13-kinase) and its protein phosphatase activity can suppress mitogen-activated protein kinase (MAPK) signaling. PTEN can therefore antagonize the mitogenic action of many growth factors. IGF2 is one of the few known regulators of PTEN [152] with a tightly controlled feedback loop in which IGF2 can enhance *PTEN* expression and, conversely, PTEN can suppress *IGF2* expression [154, 155]. Moreover, in MCF-7 breast cancer cells, the IGF2 blocking effects of PTEN seem to be dependent on the presence of locally produced IGFBP2 [153].

These data show that an increase in IGFBP2 could block the feedback response of PTEN that protects from overstimulation by IGF2, which could then contribute to tumor progression and the development of resistance to therapeutic interventions. Serum IGFBP2 levels are potential biomarkers of PTEN status and consecutive PI3K/Akt pathway activation in brain and prostate cancer patients [156, 157]. In addition, activation of PI3K can induce *IGFBP2*, whereas inhibition of mTOR with rapamycin reduces *IGFBP2* expression, thus indicating that IGFBP2 levels reflect PI3K/Akt/mTOR signaling pathway activity [158]. Furthermore, IGFBP2 induces cell proliferation by sequentially activating the extracellular signal-regulated kinases Raf, MEK, ERK1/2 and the stress-activated protein kinase/*c*-Jun N-terminal kinase (SAPK/JNK) pathway in human epithelial ovarian cancer cells [159]. Recent data show that IGFBP2 is not only able to contribute significantly to tumor progression but is also involved directly in cancer development. In a glial-specific transgenic mouse model, the combined expression of *IGFBP2* or *Akt* with *K-Ras* or *PDGF-β* could induce malignant brain tumors, indicating that combined activation of these two pathways are relevant mechanisms in brain cancer development. Additionally, in ex vivo experiments, blockade of Akt by an inhibitor led to decreased viability of cells coexpressing *IGFBP2*, providing evidence that IGFBP2 plays a key role in activation of the Akt pathway and collaborates with K-Ras or PDGF-β in the progression and development of cancer [156].

15.6 Summary and Conclusion

Clinically silent adrenocortical adenomas are the most frequent abnormalities of the adrenal gland. In contrast, ACC is a rare tumor with an extremely poor prognosis. The factors that are responsible for the frequent occurrence of benign adrenocortical tumors and the rare malignant transformation are not known. However, recent progress has been achieved in the understanding of adrenal tumorigenesis by mapping and identification of the genes responsible for several hereditary tumor syndromes associated with the formation of benign and malignant adrenocortical tumors like the Li-Fraumeni – and the Beckwith-Wiedemann-syndrome, and by microarray analysis of the genetic alterations in sporadic ACCs.

Alterations of the gene locus 11p15.5 and high expression of *IGF2* is a dominant finding in ACC, occurring in approximately 90% of malignant tumors but in almost none of the benign adenomas. Higher IGF2 levels are associated with a more malignant phenotype of these tumors, and overexpression of *IGF2* is associated with an increased risk of recurrence and metastasis. Similarly, high expression of the *IGF1R* has been described in ACC but not in adrenocortical hyperplasias or adenomas. The IGF1R has also been shown to be a biomarker for pediatric ACC, functioning as a predictor of metastasis in these patients. The functional significance and the exact mechanisms and cofactors of the strong and specific overexpression of *IGF2* and the *IGF1R* in the majority of ACCs are only partly understood until today. However, the mitogenic effect of IGF2 is dependent on the presence of an intact IGF1R, and interaction with the IGF1R has been shown to mediate the steroidogenic and mitogenic effects of IGF1 and IGF2 in the adult human adrenal gland. IGFs are potent mitogens regulating growth and apoptosis through interaction with the IGF1R, and overexpression of the human IGF1R promotes ligand-dependent neoplastic transformation in a variety of different cell systems. It is evident, therefore, that high local levels of IGF2 in combination with elevated IGF1R concentrations could represent an autocrine stimulatory loop, contributing to adrenocortical tumorigenesis and the highly malignant phenotype of this rare type of cancer. In addition to the overexpression of *IGF2* and the *IGF1R*, increased levels of IGFBP2 protein have been found in advanced human ACC. Patients with ACC show significantly elevated IGFBP2 serum–concentrations, and IGFBP2 levels correlate positively with tumor burden and are inversely correlated with survival. Although high concentrations of IGFBP2 are a frequent finding in a variety of malignant tumors, the functional significance of elevated IGFBP2 levels in malignant disease has been unclear. Until recently, IGFBP2 has been believed to be mainly a negative regulator of normal somatic growth, most probably by sequestering IGFs from their receptors. However, this effect seems to be confined to its endocrine effects on IGF-dependent function. It is now increasingly recognized that IGFBP2 can act locally via auto and/or paracrine mechanisms in an IGF-independent way, by directly regulating mitogenic post-receptor signaling pathways of tumor cells. Recently published data suggest that IGFBP2 plays an important role in PI3K signaling, and the suppression of IGFBP2 may also have selective anticancer activity or can serve as a tool to monitor response to other PI3K pathway inhibitors. Furthermore, IGFBP2 seems to be not only a modulator of IGF/IGF1R-signaling but also a pleiotropic factor that has important effects on cellular proliferation, motility, and interaction with extracellular matrix and transcription (Fig. 15.1).

It is interesting to note that a similar profile of the IGF system has been observed in the fetal adrenal gland, comparable to those observed in ACC, raising speculations that adrenocortical tumorigenesis reflects a lack of physiologic fetal gland regression, where IG2 is believed to regulate fetal adrenal growth. However, the fact that mice transgenic for *IGF2* or *IGFBP2* in the adrenal gland do not show an increased frequency of adrenal tumors suggests that IGF2 or *IGFBP2* may function in cancer progression, but not as initiation factors in adrenocortical tumorigenesis. This is supported by the clinical observation that changes in the IGF system seem to be a rather late event in the transition of the frequent benign adrenal adenomas to the rare but highly malignant ACC and that these changes are associated with an advanced stage of the disease, a poor clinical prognosis, and a high risk of recurrence. Therefore, it is most likely that circulating IGF via interaction with the IGF1R may facilitate cancer development but does not cause cancer to form. In addition to direct contributions to tumor growth and carcinogenesis,

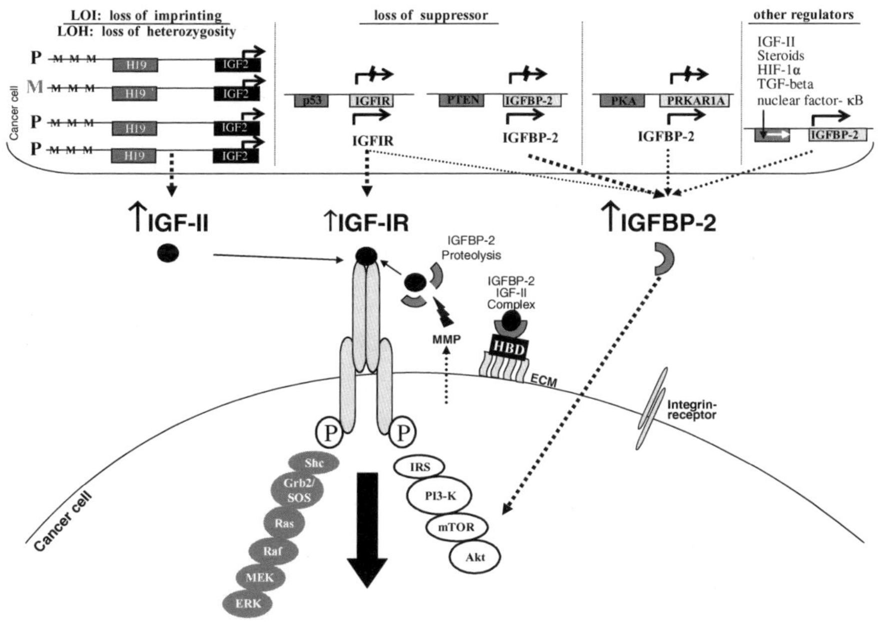

Fig. 15.1 Schematic overview of the postulated effects of the IGF system on adrenocortical tumor growth and carcinogenesis. *HIF-1α* hypoxia-inducible factor 1α; *MMP* matrix metallo proteinase; *ECM* extracellular matrix; *HBD* heparin-binding domain

IGFs may promote cancer indirectly through interactions with oncogenes and tumor suppressors as it has been shown in ACC and various other malignancies.

In conclusion, there now is ample evidence for an important role of the IGF system in adrenocortical tumorigenesis with an overexpression of *IGF2*, an increased IGF1R signaling and increased *IGFBP2* expression in the majority of ACCs. Taking into account that the pharmacological interruption of the IGF1R signaling in human adrenocortical tumor cells has a strong anti-proliferative effect in vitro and in vivo and that this effect is at least additive to the antitumor effect of the standard treatment with mitotane, it is tempting to speculate that IGF1R or inhibitors of post-receptor signaling pathways of the IGF1R-like mTOR-inhibitors will represent an effective therapy for these highly malignant tumors in the future. This hypothesis is currently tested in a randomized, multi-institutional clinical phase II and phase III trials in the US and Europe in patients with ACC.

References

1. Schutt BS et al (2004) Integrin-mediated action of insulin-like growth factor binding protein-2 in tumor cells. J Mol Endocrinol 32:859–68
2. Baserga R (1995) The IGFIR: a key to tumor growth? Cancer Res 555:249–252

3. Macaulay VM (1992) Insulin-like growth factors and cancer. Br J Cancer 65:311–320
4. Samani AA et al (2007) The role of the IGF system in cancer growth and metastasis: overview and recent insights. Endocr Rev 28:20–47
5. Doerr ME, Jones JI (1996) The roles of integrins and extracellular matrix proteins in the insulin-like growth factor I-stimulated chemotaxis of human breast cancer cells. J Biol Chem 271:2443–7
6. Khandwala HM et al (2000) The effects of insulin-like growth factors on tumourigenesis and neoplastic growth. Endocrine Reviews 21:215–244
7. Chitnis MM et al (2008) The type 1 insulin-like growth factor receptor pathway. Clin Cancer Res 14:6364–70
8. Pollak MN (2008) Insulin and insulin-like growth factor signalling in neoplasia. Nat Rev Cancer 8:915–28
9. Mesiano S, Jaffe RB (1997) Development and functional biology of the primate fetal adrenal cortex. Endocr Rev 18:378–403
10. Penhoat A et al (1988) Characterization of insulin-like growth factor I and insulin receptors on cultured bovine adrenal fasciculata cells. Role of these peptides on adrenal cell function. Endocrinology 122:2518–1526
11. Weber MM et al (1994) Identification and characterization of insulin-like growth factor I (IGF1) and IGF2/mannose-6-phosphate (*IGF2R*) receptors in bovine adrenocortical cells. Eur J Endocrinol 130:165–170
12. Penhoat A et al (1994) Regulation of adrenal cell-differentiated functions by growth factors. Horm Res 42:39–43
13. Mesiano S et al (1992) Mitogenic action, regulation and localization of insulin-like growth factors in the human fetal adrenal gland. J Clin Endocrinol Metab 76:968–976
14. Han VK et al (1992) Insulin-like growth factor-II (IGF2) messenger ribonucleic acid is expressed in steroidogenic cells of the developing ovine adrenal gland: evidence of an autocrine/paracrine role for IGF2. Endocrinology 131:1300–1309
15. Voutilainen R, Miller WL (1987) Coordinate tropic hormone regulation of mRNAs for insulin-like growth factor II and the cholesterol side-chain-cleavage enzyme, P450scc [corrected], in human steroidogenic tissues. Proc Natl Acad Sci USA 84: 1590–1594
16. Mesiano S et al (1997) Insulin-like growth factors augment steroid production and expression of steroidogenic enzymes in human fetal adrenal cortical cells: Implications for adrenal androgen regulation. J Clin Endocrinol Metab 82:1390–1396
17. L'Allemand D et al (1996) Insulin-like growth factors enhance steroidogenic enzyme and corticotropin receptor messenger ribonucleic acid levels and corticotropin responsiveness in cultured human adrenocortical cells. J Clin Endocrinol Metab 81:3892–3897
18. Pham-Huu-Trung MT et al (1991) Effects of insulin-like growth factor-I (IGF1) on enzymatic activity in human adrenocortical cells. Interactions with ACTH. J Steroid Biochem Molec Biol 39:903–909
19. Glasscock GF et al (1992) Effects of continuous infusion of insulin-like growth factor I and II, alone and in combination with thyroxine or growth hormone, on the neonatal hypophysectomized rat. Endocrinology 130:203–210
20. Rogler CE et al (1994) Altered body composition and increased frequency of diverse malignancies in insulin-like growth factor-II transgenic mice. J Biol Chem 260:13779–13784
21. Rainey WE et al (2002) The adrenal genetic puzzle: how do the fetal and adult pieces differ? Endocr Res 28:611–622
22. Wilson DM et al (1987) Transplantation of IGF2 secreting tumours in to nude rodents. Endocrinology 120:1896–1901
23. Ward A et al (1994) Disproportionate growth in mice with IGF2 transgenes. Proc Natl Acad Sci USA 91:10365–10369
24. Fottner C et al (1998) Regulation of steroidogenesis by insulin-like growth factors (IGFs) in adult human adrenocortical cells: IGF1 and more potently IGF2 preferentially enhance

androgen biosynthesis through interaction with the IGFIR and IGF-binding proteins. J Endocrinol 158:409–417
25. Fottner C et al (2007) The divergent effect of insulin-like growth factor binding protein (IGFBP-) 1 on the steroidogenic effect of IGF1 and IGF2 in bovine adrenocortical cells is not due to its phosphorylation status. Growth Hormone and IGF-Research 13:219
26. Miller WL (1999) The molecular basis of premature adrenarche: a hypothesis. Acta Pediatr Suppl 88:60–66
27. Baquedano MS et al (2005) Expression of the IGF System in Human Adrenal Tissues from Early Infancy to Late Puberty: Implications for the Development of Adrenarche. Pediatr Res 58:451–458
28. Kasayama S et al (2007) Independent association between insulin-like growth factor-I and dehydroepiandrosterone sulphate in women in middle adulthood. Clin Endocrinol 66: 797–802
29. Barbieri RL et al (1986) Insulin stimulates androgen accumulation in incubations of ovarian stroma obtained from women with hyperandrogenism. J Clin Endocrinol Metab 62:904–910
30. Ross JT et al (2007) Intrafetal insulin-like growth factor-I infusion stimulates adrenal growth but not steroidogenesis in the sheep fetus during late gestation. Endocrinology 148: 5424–5432
31. Han VK et al (1987) Cellular localization of somatomedin (insulin-like growth factor) messenger RNA in the human fetus. Science 236:193–197
32. Ilvesmäki V et al (1993) Insulin-like growth factors (IGFs) and their receptors in adrenal tumors: high IGF2 expression in functional ACCs. J Clin Endocrinol Metab 77:852–8
33. Kamio T et al (1991) Immunoreactivity and receptor expression of insulin-like growth factor I and insulin in human adrenal tumors. Am J Pathol 138:83–91
34. Shigematsu K et al (1989) Receptor autoradiographic localization of insulin-like growth factor-I (IGF1) binding sites in human fetal and adult adrenal glands. Life Sci 45:383–389
35. Pillion DJ et al (1988) Distribution of receptors for insulin and insulin-like growth factor I (somatomedin C) in the adrenal gland. Biochem Biophys Res Commun 154:138–145
36. Weber MM et al (1997) Insulin-like growth factor receptors in normal and tumorous adult human adrenocortical glands. Eur J Endocrinol 136:296–303
37. Belgorosky A et al (2009) Expression of the IGF and the aromatase/estrogen receptor systems in human adrenal tissues from early infancy to late puberty: Implications for the development of adrenarche. Rev Endocr Metab Disord 10:51–61
38. Weber MM et al (1998) Adrenocortical and adrenomedullary cells, In: Bidey ES (ed) Endocrine cell culture, Cambridge University Press, Cambridge
39. Coulter CL (2005) Fetal adrenal development: insight gained from adrenal tumors, Trends in Endocrinology and Metabolism 16:235–242
40. Logie A et al (1999) Autocrine role of IGF2 in proliferation of human ACC NCL H295R cell line. J Mol Endocrinol 23:23–32
41. LeRoith D, Roberts Jr CT (2003) The Insulin-like growth factor system and cancer. Cancer letters 195:127–137
42. Fottner C et al (1999) Characterization of Insulin-like growth factor binding proteins (IGFBPs) secreted by bovine adrenocortical cells in primary culture: Regulation by Insulin-like growth factors (IGFs) and adrenocorticotropin (ACTH). Hormone and Metabolism Res 31:203–208
43. Fottner C et al (2001) Identification and characterization of Insulin-like growth factor binding protein-expression and – secretion by adult human adrenocortical cells: Differential regulation by IGFs and adrenocorticotropin. J Endocrinol 168:465–474
44. Grimberg A, Cohen P (2000) Role of insulin-like growth factors and their binding proteins in growth control and carcinogenesis. J Cell Physiol 183:1–9
45. Weber MM et al (1995) Insulin-like growth factor II (IGF2) is more potent than IGF1 in stimulating cortisol secretion from cultured bovine adrenocortical cells: Interactions with the IGFIR and IGF-binding proteins. Endocrinology 136:3714–3720

46. Maile LA, Holly JM (1999) Insulin-like growth factor binding protein (IGFBP) proteolysis: occurrence, identification, role and regulation. Growth Horm IGF Res 9:85–95
47. Miell JP et al (1997) Insulin-like growth factor binding protein concentration and post-translational modification in embryological fluid. Mol Hum Reprod 3: 343–349
48. Conover CA, De Leon DD (1994) Acid-activated insulin-like growth factor-binding protein-3 proteolysis in normal and transformed cells. Role of cathepsin D. J Biol Chem 269: 7076–7080
49. Hoeflich A et al (2002) Insulin-like growth factor binding protein-2 (IGFBP-2) separates hypertrophic and hyperplastic effects of Growth Hormone (GH)/IGF1 excess on adrenocortical cells in vivo. FASEB-J 16:1721–1731
50. Hoeflich A et al (1999) Overexpression of insulin-like growth factor-binding protein-2 in transgenic mice reduces postnatal body weight gain. Endocrinology 140:5488–5496
51. Weber MM et al (1999) Postnatal overexpression of insulin-like growth factor II in transgenic mice is associated with adrenocortical hyperplasia and enhanced steroidogenesis. Endocrinology 140:1537–1543
52. Conlon MA et al (1995) Long R3 Insulin-like growth factor I (IGF1) infusion stimulates organ growth but reduces plasma IGF1, IGF2 and IGF binding protein concentrations in the guinea pig. J Endocrinol 146:247–253
53. Weber MM et al (2000) The role of the insulin-like growth factor (IGF) system in adrenocortical tumourigenesis. Eur J Clin Invest 30:69–75
54. Boulle N et al (2000) Fibroblast growth factor-2 inhibits the maturation of pro-insulin-like growth factor-II (Pro-IGF2) and the expression of insulin-like growth factor binding protein-2 (IGFBP-2) in the human adrenocortical tumor cell line NCI-H295R. Endocrinology 141:3127–3136
55. De Fraipont F et al (2002) Transcription profiling of benign and malignant adrenal tumors by cDNA macro-array analysis. Endocr Res 28: 785–786
56. Edgren M et al (1997) Biological characteristics of ACC: a study of p53, IGF, EGF-r, Ki-67 and PCNA in 17 ACCs. Anticancer Res 17: 1303–1310
57. Schneid H et al (1992) Abnormalities of insulin-like growth factor (IGF1 and IGF2) genes in human tumor tissue. Growth Regulation 2:45–54
58. Boulle N et al (1998) Increased levels of insulin-like growth factor II (IGF2) and IGF-Binding Protein-2 are associated with malignancy in sporadic adrenocortical tumors. J Clin Endocrinol Metab 83: 1713–1720
59. Gicquel C et al (1994) Rearrangements at the 11p15 locus and overexpression of insulin-like growth factor-II gene in sporadic adrenocortical tumors. J Clin Endocrinol Metab 78: 1444–1453
60. Gicquel C et al (1997) Structural and functional abnormalities at 11p15 are associated with the malignant phenotype in sporadic adrenocortical tumors: Study on a series of 82 tumors. J Clin Endocrinol Metab 82:2559–2565
61. Gicquel C et al (2001) Molecular markers and long-term recurrences in a large cohort of patients with sporadic adrenocortical tumors. Cancer Res 61:6762–6767
62. Giordano TJ et al (2003) Distinct transcriptional profiles of adrenocortical tumors uncovered by DNA microarray analysis. Am J Pathol 162:521–531
63. Erickson LA et al (2001) Pathological features and expression of insulin-like growth factor-2 in adrenocortical neoplasms. Endocr Pathol 12:429–435
64. Wilkin F et al (2000) Pediatric adrenocortical tumors: molecular events leading to Insulin-like growth factor II gene overexpression. J Clin Endocrinol Metab 85:2048–2056
65. Almeida MQ et al (2008) Expression of insulin-like growth factor-II and its receptor in pediatric and adult adrenocortical tumors. J Clin Endocrinol Metab 93: 3524–3531
66. De Fraipont F et al (2005) Gene expression profiling of human adrenocortical tumors using complementary deoxyribonucleic Acid microarrays identifies several candidate genes as markers of malignancy. J Clin Endocrinol Metab 90:1819–1829

67. West AN et al (2007) Gene expression profiling of childhood adrenocortical tumors. Cancer Res 67: 600–608
68. Slater EP et al (2006) Analysis by cDNA microarrays of gene expression patterns of human adrenocortical tumors. Eur J Endocrinol 154:587–598
69. De Reyniès A et al (2009) Gene expression profiling reveals a new classification of adrenocortical tumors and identifies molecular predictors of malignancy and survival. J Clin Oncol 27:1108–1115
70. Giordano TJ et al (2009) Molecular classification and prognostication of adrenocortical tumors by transcriptome profiling. Clin Cancer Res 15:668–676
71. Velázquez-Fernández D et al (2005) Expression profiling of adrenocortical neoplasms suggests a molecular signature of malignancy. Surgery 138:1087–1094
72. Barlaskar FM et al (2009) Preclinical targeting of the type I insulin-like growth factor receptor in ACC. J Clin Endocrinol Metab 94:204–212
73. Leboulleux S et al (2001) Loss of heterozygosity at the mannose-6-phosphate/insulin-like growth factor II receptor locus: a frequent but late event in adrenocortical tumorigenesis. Eur J Endocrinol 144:163–168
74. Boulle N et al (2001) Evaluation of plasma insulin-like growth factor binding protein-2 as a marker for adrenocortical tumors. Eur J Endocrinol 144:29–36
75. Faical S et al (1998) Immunodetection of Insulin-like growth factor I (IGF1) in normal and pathological adrenocortical tissue. Endocr Pathol 9:63–70
76. Gicquel C et al (1995) Recent advances in the pathogenesis of adrenocortical tumours. Eur J Endocrinol 133:133–144
77. Fernandez-Ranvier GG et al (2008) Identification of biomarkers of ACC using genomewide gene expression profiling. Arch Surg 143:841–846
78. Rosati R et al (2008) High frequency of loss of heterozygosity at 11p15 and IGF2 overexpression are not related to clinical outcome in childhood adrenocortical tumors positive for the R337H TP53 mutation. Cancer Genet Cytogenet 186:19–24
79. Assié G et al (2007) Prognostic Parameters of Metastatic ACC. J Clin Endocrinol Metab 92:148–154
80. De Souza AT et al (1995) M6P/IGF2R gene is mutated in human hepatocellular carcinomas with loss of heterozygosity. Nature Genet. 11:447–449
81. Hill D. Relative abundance and molecular size of immunoreactive insulin-like growth factors I and II in human fetal tissues (1990) Early Hum Dev 21:49–58
82. Mesiano S et al (1993) Mitogenic action, regulation, and localization of insulin-like growth factors in the human fetal adrenal gland. J Clin Endocrinol Metab 76:968–976
83. Wolf E et al (1994) Consequences of postnatally elevated insulin-like growth factor-II in transgenic mice: endocrine changes and effects on body and organ growth. Endocrinology 135:1877–1886
84. Blackburn A et al (1997) Actions and interactions of growth hormone and insulin-like growth factor-II: body and organ growth of transgenic mice. Transgenic Res 6: 213–222
85. van Buul-Offers SC et al (1995) Overexpression of human insulin-like growth factor-II in transgenic mice causes increased weight of the thymus. J Endocrinol 144:91–502
86. Zaina S et al (2003) Shortened life span, bradycardia, and hypotension in mice with targeted expression of an Igf2 transgene in smooth muscle cells. Endocrinology 144:2695–2703
87. Cecim M et al (1991) Elevated corticosterone levels in transgenic mice expressing human or bovine growth hormone genes. Neuroendocrinology 53:313–316
88. Wolf E et al (1998) What is the function of IGF2 in postnatal life? Answers from transgenic mouse models. Growth Horm IGF Res 8:185–193
89. Libé R, Bertherat J (2005) Molecular genetics of adrenocortical tumours, from familial to sporadic disease. Eur J Endocrinol 153:477–487
90. Liu J et al (1995) H19 and insulin-like growth factor-II gene expression in adrenal tumors and cultured adrenal cells. J Clin Endocrinol Metab 80:492–496

91. Toretsky JA, Helman LJ (1996) Involvement of IGF2 in human cancer. J Endocrinol 149:367–372
92. Kirschner LS (2002) Signaling pathways in ACC. Ann N Y Acad Sci 58:222–239
93. Bourcigaux N et al (2000) High expression of cyclin E and G1 CDK and loss of function of p57KIP2 are involved in proliferation of malignant sporadic adrenocortical tumors. J Clin Endocrinol Metab 85:322–330
94. Paquette J et al (1998) The INS 5′ variable number of tandem repeats is associated with IGF2 expression in humans. J Biol Chem 273:14158–14164
95. Yano T et al (1989) Genetic changes in human ACCs. J Natl Cancer Inst 81:518–523
96. Schneid H et al (1993) Parental allele specific methylation of the human insulin-like growth factor-II gene and Beckwith Wiedemann syndrome. J Med Genet 30:353–362
97. Martinerie C et al (2001) Altered expression of novH is associated with human adrenocortical tumorigenesis. J Clin Endocrinol Metab 86:3929–3940
98. Thibout H et al (2003) Characterization of human NOV in biological fluids: an enzyme immunoassay for the quantification of human NOV in sera from patients with diseases of the adrenal gland and of the nervous system. J Clin Endocrinol Metab 88:327–336
99. Makos Wales B et al (1995) p53 activates expression of HIC-1, a new candidate tumor suppressor gene on 17p13.3. Nat Med 1:570–582
100. Neuberg M et al (1997) The p53/IGF-1 receptor axis in the regulation of programmed cell death. Endocrine 7:107–9
101. Werner H, Le Roith D (2000) New concepts in regulation and function of the insulin-like growth factors: implications for understanding normal growth and neoplasia. Cell Mol Life Sci. 57:932–42
102. Werner H et al (2000) Regulation of the insulin-like growth factor-I receptor gene by oncogenes and antioncogenes: implications in human cancer. Mol Genet Metab 71:315–20
103. Girnita L et al (2000) Increased expression of insulin-like growth factor I receptor in malignant cells expressing aberrant p53:functional impact. Cancer Res 60:5278–5283
104. Werner H et al (1996) Wild type and mutant p53 differentially regulate transcription of the insulin-like growth factor I receptor gene. Proc Natl Acad Sci USA 93:8318–8323
105. Reincke M et al (1994) p53 mutations in human adrenocortical neoplasms: immunohistochemical and molecular studies. J Clin Endocrinol Metab 78:790–796
106. Hoeflich A et al (1996) Coordinate expression of insulin-like growth factor II (IGF2) and IGF2/mannose-6-phosphate receptor mRNA during differentiation of human colon carcinoma cells (caco-2). Eur J Endocrinol 135:49–59
107. Weber MM et al (2002) Overexpression of the insulin-like growth factor I receptor in human colon carcinomas. Cancer 95:2086–2095
108. Rubin R, Baserga R (1995) Insulin-like growth factor I receptor. Its role in cell proliferation, apoptosis, and tumourigenicity. Lab Invest 73:311–331
109. Singleton JR et al (1996) Insulin-like growth factor I receptor prevents apoptosis and enhances neuroblastoma tumorigenesis. Cancer Res 56:4522–4529
110. Sullivan KA et al (1995) Insulin-like growth factor II in the pathogenesis of human neuroblastoma. Am J Pathol 147:1790–1798
111. Menouny M et al (1997) Role of insulin-like growth factor binding protein-2 and its limited proteolysis in neuroblastoma cell proliferation: modulation by transforming growth factor-beta and retinoic acid. Endocrinology 138:683–690
112. Gelato MC, Vassalotti J (1990) Insulin-like growth factor II: possible local growth factor in pheochromocytoma. J Clin Endocrinol and Metabol 7:1168–1174
113. Haselbacher GK et al (1987) Insulin-like growth factor II in human adrenal pheochromocytomas and Wilms tumors: expression at the mRNA and protein level. PNAS 84:1104–1106
114. Fottner C et al (2006) Overexpression of the insulin-like growth factor I receptor on human pheochromocytomas. J Mol Endocrinol 36:279–287
115. Holzenberger M et al (2003) IGFIR regulates lifespan and resistance to oxidative stress in mice. Nature 421:182–187

116. Lithgow G, Gill MS (2003) Cost-free longevity in mice? Nature 421:125–127
117. Dahmer MK et al (1989) Characterization of insulin-like growth factor-I receptors in PC12 pheochromocytoma cells and bovine adrenal medulla. J Neurochem 53:1036–1042
118. Dahmer MK, Perlman RL (1988) Insulin and insulin-like growth factors stimulate deoxyribonucleic acid synthesis in PC12 pheochromocytoma cells. Endocrinology 22:2109–2113
119. Nielsen FC, Gammeltoft S (1988) Insulin-like growth factors are mitogens for rat pheochromocytoma PC 12 cells. Biochem Biophys Res Commun 154:1018–1023
120. Forbes BE et al (2002) Characteristics of binding of insulin-like growth factor (IGF)-I and IGF2 analogues to the type 1 IGF receptor determined by BIAcore analysis. Eur J Biochem 269:961–968
121. Foncea R et al (1997) Insulin-like growth factor-I rapidly activates multiple signal transduction pathways in cultured rat cardiac myocytes. J Biol Chem 272:19115–9124
122. Kulik G et al (1997) Antiapoptotic signalling by the insulin-like growth factor I receptor, phosphatidylinositol 3-kinase, and Akt. Mol Cell Biol 17:1595–1606
123. O'Gorman DB et al (1999) Decreased insulin-like growth factor-II/mannose-6-phosphate receptor expression enhances tumorigenicity in JEG-3 cells. Cancer Res 59:5692–5694
124. Souza RF et al (1999) Expression of the wild-type insulin-like growth factor II receptor gene suppresses growth and causes death in colorectal carcinoma cells. Oncogene 18: 4063–4068
125. Lau MM et al (1994) Loss of the imprinted IGF2/cation-independent mannose 6-phosphate receptor results in fetal overgrowth and perinatal lethality. Genes and Development 8: 2953–2963
126. Ludwig T et al (1996) Mouse mutants lacking the type 2 IGF receptor (IGF2R) are rescued from perinatal lethality in Igf2 and Igf1r null backgrounds. Developmental Biology 177:517–535
127. Wang Z et al (1994) Regulation of embryonic growth and lysosomal targeting by the imprinted IGF 2/Mpr gene. Nature 372:464–467
128. Hankins GR et al (1996) M6P/IGF2 receptor: a candidate breast tumor suppressor gene. Oncogene 12:2003–2009
129. Oates AJ et al (1998) The mannose 6-phosphate/insulin-like growth factor 2 receptor (M6P/IGF2R), a putative breast tumor suppressor gene. Breast Cancer Res Treat 47: 269–281
130. Ozturk M (1999) Genetic aspects of hepatocellular carcinogenesis. Seminars in Liver Disease 19:235–242
131. Scott CD, Firth SM (2004) The role of the M6P/IGF2 receptor in cancer: tumor suppression or garbage disposal? Horm Metab Res 36, 261–71
132. Xu Y et al (1997) Aberrant imprinting of the insulin-like growth factor II receptor gene in Wilms' tumor. Oncogene 14:1041–1046
133. Ilvesmäki V et al (1992) Insulin-like growth factor binding proteins in the human adrenal gland. Mol Cell Endocrinol 97:71–79
134. Logie A et al (2000) Establishment and characterization of a human ACC xenograft model. Endocrinology 141:3165–3171
135. Baxter RC, Martin JL (1989) Binding proteins for the insulin-like growth factors: structure, regulation and function. Prog Growth Factor Research 1:49–68
136. Holly J, Perks C (2006) The role of Insulin-like growth factor binding proteins. Neuroendocrinology 83:154–160
137. Pollak MN (2004) Insulin-like growth factors and neoplasia. Nat Rev Cancer 4:505–18
138. Pollak MN et al (2004) Insulin-like growth factors and cancer. Nat Rev Cancer 14:277–286
139. Hoeflich A et al (2001) Insulin-like growth factor binding protein 2 in tumorigenesis: protector or promoter? Cancer Res 61:8601–8610
140. Hoeflich A et al (2000) Overexpression of insulin-like growth factor-binding protein 2 results in increased tumorigenic potential in Y-1 adrenocortical tumor cells. Cancer Res 60: 834–838

141. Shi Z et al (2007) Primary pigmented nodular adrenocortical disease reveals insulin-like growth factor binding protein-2 regulation by protein kinase A. Growth Horm IGF Res 17:113–121
142. Engstrom W et al (1987) Expression of growth regulatory genes in primary human testicular neoplasms. Int J Androl 10:79–84
143. Cazals V et al (1994) Insulin-like growth factors, their binding proteins, and transforming growth factor-1 in oxidant-arrested lung alveolar epithelial cells. J Biol Chem 269: 14111–14117
144. Wang D et al (1994) Insulin-like growth factor-binding protein-2: the effect of human chorionic gonadotropin on its gene regulation and protein secretion and its biological effects in rat Leydig cells. Mol Endocrinol 8:69–76
145. Becher OJ et al (2008) IGFBP2 is overexpressed by pediatric malignant astrocytomas and induces the repair enzyme DNA-PK. J Child Neurol 23:1205–1213
146. Besnard V et al (2001) Distinct patterns of insulin-like growth factor binding protein (IGFBP)-2 and IGFBP-3 expression in oxidant exposed lung epithelial cells. Biochem Biophys Acta 1538:47–58
147. Hoeflich A et al (2003) Increased activity of catalase in tumor cells overexpressing IGFBP-2. Horm Metab Res 35:816–821
148. Iliopoulos D et al (2009) MicroRNA signature of primary pigmented nodular adrenocortical disease: clinical correlations and regulation of Wnt signaling. Cancer Res 69:3278–3282
149. Stratakis CA (2009) New genes and/or molecular pathways associated with adrenal hyperplasias and related adrenocortical tumors. Mol Cell Endocrinol 300:152–157
150. Miyamoto S et al (2007) Matrix metalloproteinase-7 triggers the matricrine action of insulin-like growth factor-II via proteinase activity on insulin-like growth factor binding protein 2 in the extracellular matrix. Cancer Sci 98:685–91
151. Rorive S et al (2008) Matrix metalloproteinase-9 interplays with the IGFBP2-IGFII complex to promote cell growth and motility in astrocytomas. Glia 56:1679–1690
152. Cazals V et al (1999) Role for NF-KB in mediating the effects of hyperoxia on IGF-binding protein 2 promoter activity in lung alveolar epithelial cells. Biochim Biophys Acta 1448:349–362
153. Perks CM et al (2007) IGF2 and IGFBP-2 differentially regulate PTEN in human breast cancer cells. Oncogene 26:5966–5972
154. Hwang PH et al (2005) PTEN/MMAC1 enhances the growth inhibition by anticancer drugs with downregulation of IGF2 expression in gastric cancer cells. Exp Mol Med 37:391–398
155. Moorehead RA et al (2003) Insulin-like growth factor-II regulates PTEN expression in the mammary gland. J Biol Chem 278:50422–50427
156. Dunlap SM et al (2007) Insulin-like growth factor binding protein 2 promotes glioma development and progression. PNAS 104:11736–11741
157. Kang-Park S, Lee YI (2003) PTEN modulates insulin-like growth factor II (IGF2)-mediated signaling; the protein phosphatase activity of PTEN downregulates IGF2 expression in hepatoma cells. FEBS Lett 545:203–208
158. Martin JL, Baxter RC (2007) Expression of insulin-like growth factor binding protein-2 by MCF-7 breast cancer cells is regulated through the phosphatidylinositol 3-kinase/AKT/mammalian target of rapamycin pathway. Endocrinology 148:2532–41
159. Chakrabarty S, Kondratick L (2006) Insulin-like growth factor binding protein-2 stimulates proliferation and activates multiple cascades of the mitogen-activated protein kinase pathways in NIH-OVCAR3 human epithelial ovarian cancer cells. Cancer Biol Ther 5:189–197

Chapter 16
WNT/β-Catenin Signaling in Adrenocortical Carcinoma

Sébastien Gaujoux, Frédérique Tissier, and Jérôme Bertherat

The WNT/β-catenin signaling pathway plays a major role in the development of various tissues, including the adrenal cortex. β-Catenin fulfills a dual role as a structural component in cell–cell adhesion and as the key transcription cofactor of T-cell factor/lymphoid enhancer factor (TCF/LEF). Activation of the WNT/β-catenin signaling pathway leads to β-catenin activation and subsequent translocation to the nucleus. Genetic alterations of a component of the WNT/β-catenin signaling pathway were initially identified in familial adenomatous polyposis coli (FAP). Over the past decades, these findings have been extended to a variety of other cancers. FAP patients usually have a germline mutation of the *APC* (adenomatous polyposis coli) gene that leads to the activation of the WNT/β-catenin signaling pathway. In addition to a significant increase in colon cancer risk, they develop adrenocortical adenomas (ACAs) and possibly adrenocortical cancers (ACCs). Molecular studies of these patients have shown that in affected tissues, somatic mutations of *APC* occur in addition to the omnipresent germline *APC* mutation, following the classical principle of loss of heterozygosity (LOH). Somatic activating mutations of the β-catenin (*CTNNB1*) gene causing an activation of the WNT/β-catenin signaling pathway have been identified in various cancers, especially colon and liver tumors. More recently, various studies have suggested an activation of the WNT/β-catenin signaling pathway in adrenocortical tumors (ACTs), ACAs, and ACCs. The physiology of the WNT/β-catenin signaling pathway will be summarized in order to explain its alterations in adrenal tumors and its potential importance in adrenal tumorigenesis. Increased understanding of the WNT/β-catenin signaling pathway could ultimately lead to new therapeutic approaches.

J. Bertherat (✉)
Endocrinology, Metabolism and Cancer Department, Institut Cochin, Descartes University, INSERM U567, CNRS UMR8104, Paris, France; Reference center for rare adrenal disorders, Assistance Publique Hôpitaux de Paris, Hôpital Cochin, Paris Descartes University, 27 Rue du Faubourg Saint-Jacques, 75014 Paris, France
e-mail: jerome.bertherat@cch.aphp.fr

G.D. Hammer, T. Else (eds.), *Adrenocortical Carcinoma*,
DOI 10.1007/978-0-387-77236-3_16, © Springer Science+Business Media, LLC 2011

16.1 The WNT/β-Catenin Signaling Pathway

16.1.1 Molecular Mechanisms of the Canonical WNT/β-Catenin Signaling Pathway

β-Catenin plays a crucial role in two major cellular processes. It is present at the cell membrane where it is a part of cell–cell adhesion complexes [1–3] and in the cytoplasm and nucleus where it is a key component of the cellular WNT/β-catenin signaling pathway [4–7]. The membrane-bound β-catenin interacts with the cytoplasmic domain of E-cadherin. This allows an additional direct interaction of β-catenin with actin via α-catenin (Fig. 16.1). This membrane pool is stable. On the other hand, the cytoplasmic pool of β-catenin is unstable. In the absence of WNT ligands, β-catenin is tethered to a complex of the tumor suppressor APC, axis inhibitor 1 (AXIN), Wilms tumor gene on the X chromosome (*WTX*) [8], and two serine/threonine kinase, glycogen synthase kinase 3β (GSK3β) and casein kinase 1

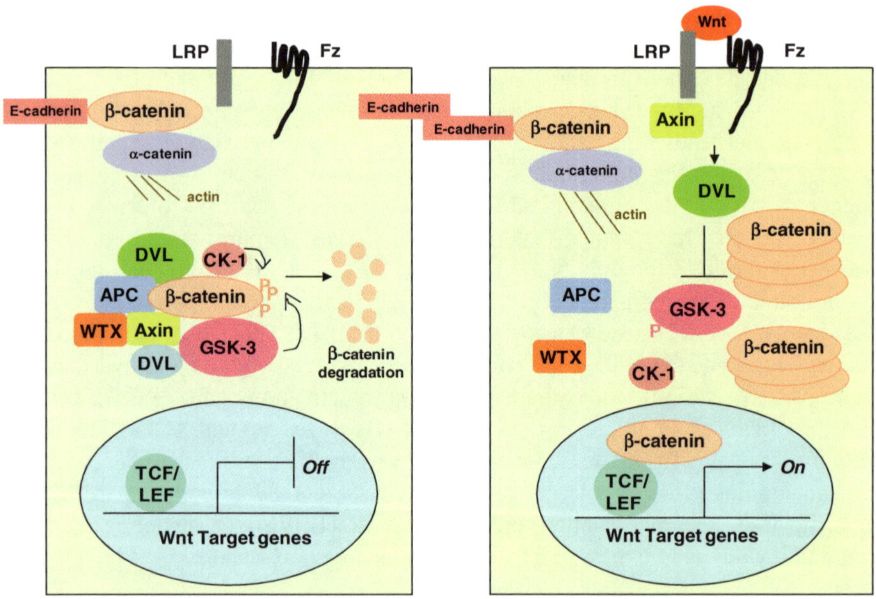

Fig. 16.1 The canonical Wnt/β-catenin signaling pathway. In the absence of Wnt signaling (*left*), β-catenin is in a complex with axin, APC, and GSK3β and gets phosphorylated and targeted for degradation. β-Catenin also exists in a cadherin-bound form and regulates cell–cell adhesion. In the presence of Wnt signaling (*right*), β-catenin is uncoupled from the degradation complex and translocates to the nucleus, where it binds TCF/LEF transcription factors, thus activating target genes. In steroidogenic tissues, β-catenin interacts with steroidogenic factor-1 (SF1) and influences transcription of SF1-dependent genes ; Abbreviations are as follows: GSK3β: glycogen synthase kinase 3-β kinase; *APC*: adenomatous polyposis coli; FZ: family of seven transmembrane receptor (Frizzled); Dsh: Dishevelled; TCF/LEF: T-cell factor/lymphoid enhancer factor; *WTX*: Wilms Tumor gene on the X chromosome, SF1: steroidogenic factor-1

(CK1) [1] (Fig. 16.1). β-Catenin is phosphorylated by CK1α, isoform of CK1, at serine 45 [9] and subsequently by GSK3β at threonine 41, serine 37, and serine 33 [9]. Phosphorylated β-catenin allows the recruitment of β-transducin repeat-containing protein (βTrCP), which is an initiating protein of the process of ubiquitination and degradation by the proteasome [10, 11]. On the other hand, in the presence of a WNT ligand, the WNT/β-catenin signaling pathway will be activated by ligand binding to a complex of a Frizzled (FZ) family receptor and one of their coreceptors, low-density lipoprotein receptor-related protein 5 (LRP5) or LRP6. Thereafter, a cascade of events will lead to the dissociation of the complex, allowing a cytoplasmic accumulation of β-catenin [4]. In the next step, β-catenin will be targeted to the nucleus by PYGO and Legless/BCL9 [12]. Within the nucleus, β-catenin serves as a key cofactor for the TCF/LEF family of transcription factors [13], leading to the final activation of WNT/β-catenin signaling pathway target genes [4].

16.1.2 Components of the WNT/β-Catenin Signaling Pathway

WNT/β-catenin signaling results in accumulation of β-catenin through various interlinked mechanisms [14]. The ongoing discovery of new signaling components over the past decades has resulted in an increasingly complex signaling network [8], which can be roughly divided into several processes segregated in unique cellular compartments.

16.1.2.1 Initiation of the WNT/β-Catenin Signaling Pathway at the Cell Membrane

The presence of a WNT ligand will lead to its binding to a receptor complex, which is comprised of FZ family receptor and one of the coreceptors LRP5 or LRP6. Activation of the WNT/β-catenin signaling pathway by WNT ligands can only occur when FZ and LRP are complexed to WNT [4]. Several mechanisms can antagonize WNT/β-catenin signaling at this level. The binding of WNT ligands to FZ receptors can be inhibited by soluble factors, such as WNT inhibitory factor 1 (WIF1), Cerberus, and secreted FZ-related protein (sFRP). These factors serve as antagonists of WNT/β-catenin signaling by direct sequestration of WNT ligands. Members of the Dickkopf family (DKK1, DKK2) inhibit WNT/β-catenin signaling together with the KRM1 and KRM2 gene products via a different mechanism. They block WNT ligands after interaction with the LRP coreceptors, leading to endocytosis of LRPs [4, 15].

The binding of a WNT ligand to FZ–LRP5/6 leads to the activation of dishevelled (DVL or DSH), which in turn phosphorylates and activates GSK3β, thereby inhibiting β-catenin phosphorylation. The cytoplasmic part of LRPs binds to AXIN and facilitates the dissociation of the sequestration complex, resulting in a release of β-catenin [16]. As a result of this signaling cascade, the cytosolic pool of β-catenin increases.

16.1.2.2 WNT/β-Catenin Signaling Events in the Cytoplasm

DVL and β-catenin are associated with the degradation complex, which consists of the following main components: APC, GSK3β, CK1, and WTX as well as some additional factors that modulate the WNT/β-catenin signaling [4, 5].

Dishevelled

DVL serves as an interface of the WNT/β-catenin signaling between the cell membrane and the APC/GSK3β/AXIN complex, which in the absence of active WNT/β-catenin signaling promotes the destruction of β-catenin [7]. DVL disrupts this complex by binding to AXIN [17], leading to inhibition of GSK3β [18]. As a result of GSK3β inhibition, β-catenin phosphorylation by GSK3β is inhibited [19] and GSK3β itself is routed to degradation by the proteasome [19].

β-Catenin

β-Catenin was initially discovered in association with its role in cell–cell adhesion [2]. It contains a total of 781 amino acids (AA). Its primary structure is defined by an amino-terminal domain of approximately 100 AA, a central region of 500 AA, which is comprised of several repeat sequence, the so-called armadillo repeats (Arm repeats), and a carboxy-terminal domain of about 150 AA (Fig. 16.2). The amino-terminal domain contains the binding site for α-catenin [20, 21] and the phosphorylation consensus sites for GSK3β [22]. It is important for rate control of intracellular accumulation and activation of β-catenin [23]. The central region containing the Arm repeats contains the binding sites for cadherins [21], APC [21, 24], and the TCF/LEF family of transcription factors [25]. In addition, it serves as a part of the α-catenin binding site [26]. The carboxy-terminal region harbors the transactivation domain required for the gene transactivation by the β-catenin/TCF complex. Therefore, this domain is indispensable for the transcriptional control of target genes

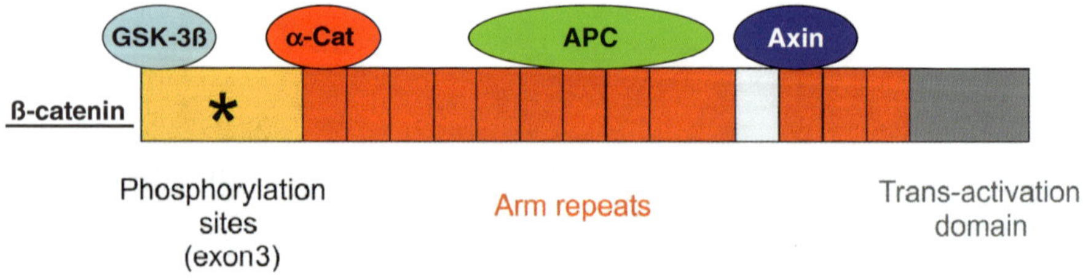

Fig. 16.2 β-Catenin protein structure. The figure shows the amino acids of the β-catenin protein. The amino-terminal domain of about 100 AA, a central region of about 500 AA containing repeated sequence named "Armadillo repeats" (Arm repeats) and a carboxy-terminal domain of about 150 AA. Most somatic β-catenin mutations occur in phosphorylation site encoded by exon 3 of the gene indicated by the star (∗). Major partner proteins interecalating with β-catenin are shown—GSK3β: glycogen synthase kinase 3-β kinase; α-Cat: α-catenin, APC: adenomatous polyposis coli, and axin

[27–29]. The β-catenin gene symbol is *CTNNB1*. It is located at 3p22-3p21 [30, 31]. It is comprised of 16 exons and 15 introns [32].

Axin

AXIN was initially identified as an inhibitor of the WNT/β-catenin signaling during embryogenesis [33]. Two different proteins have been identified: AXIN1 (AXIN) and AXIN2 (alternatively named conductin or axil) [34]. These proteins contain an amino-terminal regulator of G-protein signaling (RGS) domain, a central domain, and a carboxy-terminal dishevelled and axin binding domain (DIX) [35]. The amino-terminal RGS domain binds to APC. The central domain facilitates the binding to β-catenin and GSK3β. The carboxy-terminal DIX domain mediates dimerization with protein phosphatase 2A (PP2A) [36] and CK1 [37]. The two *AXIN* genes, *AXIN1* and *AXIN2*, are considered tumor suppressor genes [34, 38]. Their loci are respectively located at 16p13.3 [33] and 17p24 [39]. *AXIN1* and *AXIN2* each have 10 exons [39]. AXIN directly binds to APC, β-catenin, GSK3β, and DVL [7]. It serves as a scaffold for assembling GSK3β, CK1, APC, and β-catenin. AXIN in concert with APC stimulates phosphorylation of β-catenin using GSK3β. In the absence of active WNT/β-catenin signaling, this mechanism inhibits the cytoplasmic accumulation of β-catenin [4]. AXIN1 is essential for β-catenin degradation. It is constitutively expressed and regulates the maintenance of basal WNT/β-catenin signaling [34]. AXIN2 is expressed in response to active β-catenin activation and its main role is to limit the duration and intensity of the WNT/β-catenin signaling [40–42].

Adenomatous Polyposis Coli

APC is a large protein of 2843 AA [43, 44]. It contains an amino-terminal domain with an oligomerization domain and an Arm repeats domain, a central region containing repeats of 15 and 20 AA, and a carboxy-terminal domain [35]. The Arm repeats bind PP2A [36]. The 20 AA repeats facilitate binding of β-catenin [24], leading to β-catenin sequestration and degradation [35]. *APC* is frequently mutated in colorectal carcinomas associated with FAP [44, 45]. It is located at 5q21 and consists of 21 exons [35, 44]. Its tumor suppressor activity is due to its role as a tonic suppressor of β-catenin activation in the absence of WNT/β-catenin signaling.

Casein Kinase 1 and Glycogen Synthase 3β

In the absence of WNT/β-catenin signaling, the serine/threonine kinase CK1 initiates β-catenin phosphorylation at serine 45 [15]. The serine/threonine kinase GSK3β phosphorylates different components of the Wnt/β-catenin signaling pathway, including β-catenin at threonine 41, serine 37, and serine 33, as well as APC and AXIN [4, 9, 46, 47]. β-Catenin phosphorylation is enhanced in the presence of AXIN [15]. There is some evidence that PP2A may serve as an antagonist of GSK3β activity [36].

Wilms Tumor Gene on the X Chromosome

The importance of *WTX* has only been recently explored. It is located on chromosome X at the locus Xq11.1 and considered a tumor suppressor gene, initially shown to be dysregulated in Wilms tumor [48]. It was subsequently found to operate through WNT/β-catenin signaling, downregulating its activity by forming a complex with β-catenin, AXIN, APC, and βTrCP [49]. *WTX*, alternatively named *FAM132B* or *AMER1*, encodes a protein of 1135 amino acids. *WTX* is deleted or mutated not only in 7–29% of Wilms tumors [48, 50, 51] but also in sclerosing skeletal dysplasia [52]. Due to its localization on chromosome X, *WTX* is inactivated in an unusual manner: *WTX* mutations in the single X chromosome in male tissues as well as mutations in the active X chromosome in female tissues cause gene inactivation and loss of tumor suppressor characteristics [48, 50, 54]. The interaction of β-catenin with WTX in a complex with AXIN1, βTrCP2, and APC [49, 53] promotes its proteasomal degradation [49]. In addition to this repressive action on WNT/β-catenin signaling pathway, WTX also regulates the distribution of APC between the microtubular cytoskeleton and the plasma membrane [53], suggesting an additional tumor suppressor function of WTX independent of direct effects on β-catenin.

Other Components of the Cytoplasmic WNT/β-Catenin Signaling Pathway

There are additional activating factors such as FRODO that interacts with DVL and additional inhibiting factors such as diversin that bind to AXIN at the same sites as GSK3β [15].

16.1.2.3 Nuclear Components of the WNT/β-Catenin Signaling Pathway

The TCF/LEF family transcription factors are the central nuclear partners of β-catenin, serving as the terminal effectors of WNT-mediated transcription. The TCF/β-catenin complex proteins are associated with a variety of additional transcriptional inhibitors or activators in the nucleus [15] and hence integrate the WNT pathway with multiple other signaling pathways.

The T-Cell Factor/Lymphoid Enhancer Factor Family Transcription Factors

The members of the TCF/LEF family of transcription factors (TCF1, LEF1, TCF3, and TCF4) contain different functional domains, including a high mobility group (HMG) domain that binds to DNA and a β-catenin binding domain [4, 29]. In the absence of WNT/β-catenin signaling, TCF/LEF partners as transcription suppressor through interaction with Groucho [54, 55], which maintains chromatin condensation [56]. In the presence of WNT/β-catenin signaling, TCF/LEF dissociates from Groucho, binds β-catenin, and recruits the coactivator, the cyclic AMP response element-binding protein (CBP) [5, 57], to ultimately stimulate TCF/LEF-dependent target gene transcription [5, 58, 59]. Several factors interfere with WNT/β-catenin signaling at the nuclear level by different mechanisms. As mentioned above, Groucho binds to TCF/LEF and inhibits transcription. The inhibitor of β-catenin and

T-cell factor (ICAT) binds to the Arm repeats of β-catenin and inhibits interactions with TCF/LEF and CBP.

Other Nuclear Factors of the WNT/β-Catenin Signaling Pathway

There are additional transcriptional activators that interact with the WNT/β-catenin signaling pathway, such as the chromatin remodeling complex of SWI/SNF and Legless/BCL9. Legless/BCL9 recruits PYGO to facilitate the targeting of β-catenin to the nucleus.

16.1.3 The WNT/β-Catenin Signaling Pathway Target Genes

Numerous target genes of the WNT/β-catenin signaling pathway have been identified and can be viewed at the Internet site of Roel Nusse (http://www.stanford.edu/~rnusse/pathways/targets.html). The majority of these genes contain binding sites for TCF/LEF. These genes are involved in several different biological processes [5], including organismal and cellular development [60, 61], cell proliferation and cell cycle control (c-myc or cyclin D1) [62–64], angiogenesis (VEGF) [65], invasion, and cellular migration (metalloproteinase matrilysin (MMP-7)) [66–68].

Some partners of the WNT/β-catenin signaling, such as AXIN2, are themselves target genes of the WNT/β-catenin signaling pathway [5].

16.2 The WNT/β-Catenin Signaling Pathway in Familial Adenomatous Polyposis Coli

In 1991, the tumor suppressor adenomatous polyposis coli (*APC*) encoded by the FAP locus was identified by molecular cloning [44, 45]. Further analyses revealed involvement of this tumor suppressor gene not only in tumors from FAP patients but also in sporadic colon cancer. Later, its binding to β-catenin and its major role in the canonical Wnt/β-catenin pathway were identified. WNT/β-catenin pathway activation has since been observed in various cancers [4, 5, 69], most notably cancers of the digestive tract (Table 16.1) [70–72]. Additionally, it was found that there is an increased incidence of adrenal tumors in FAP patients [73–76]. This observation together with additional recent evidence suggests that the WNT/β-catenin signaling pathway might be involved in adrenal cortex tumorigenesis.

16.3 The WNT/β-Catenin Signaling Pathway in the Adrenal Cortex and in Adrenocortical Tumors

16.3.1 Adrenal Cortex Development

The WNT/β-catenin signaling pathway participates in various developmental processes during embryogenesis. A crucial role of β-catenin, presumably as part of

Table 16.1 Frequency of somatic *CTNNB1*, *APC*, *AXIN1*, and *AXIN2* mutations in various digestive cancers

Type of tumors	Frequency of *CTNNB1* mutations	Frequency of *APC* mutations	Frequency of *Axin1* and *2* mutations
Esophageal squamous cell carcinoma	0–4%	NA	NA
Esophageal adenocarcinoma	0%	2%	NA
Gastric adenoma	NA	76%	NA
Gastric adenocarcinoma	0–26%	4%	
Colorectal adenocarcinoma	16%	34–72%	*Axin1*: 11–21% *Axin2*: 10–25%
With MSI	0–25%	20%	
Without MSI	0–1%		
Hepatoblastoma	13–89%	69%	*Axin1*: 5–7%
Liver adenoma	0–30%	NA	NA
Hepatocarcinoma	12–41%	0%	*Axin1*: 5–10% *Axin2*: 3%
Desmoid tumor	25–54%	21–50%	NA
Nephroblastoma (Wilms tumor)	14–39%	NA	NA
Solid-pseudopapillary tumor of the pancreas (Frantz tumor)	90%	NA	NA
Acinus cell pancreatic carcinoma	NA	18%	NA

the canonical WNT signaling, has recently been demonstrated by Kim et al. in both embryonic development of the adrenal cortex and maintenance of the adult gland [77]. In mice harboring a complete genetic inactivation of β-catenin in the embryonic adrenal gland, most of the adrenal gland disappears by E18.5, with a significant decrease in the expression of the transcription factor, steroidogenic factor-1 (*Sf1*), and the steroidogenic enzymes *Cyp11a1* and *3βHsd*. In mice with partial inactivation of β-catenin, while no adrenal defects were observed during embryonic life, at 45 weeks postpartum, a thinning and disorganization of the adrenal cortex, increased apoptosis, and decreased expression of *Sf1* and steroidogenic markers were observed. This is in keeping with the important convergent actions of *Sf1* and WNT signaling in the regulation of gene expression [78]. The impairment of proliferation in the embryonic adrenal cortex of β-catenin-deficient mice is consistent with clinical observations, suggesting that constitutive activation of β-catenin due to somatic mutation in adult adrenal glands could be involved in the pathogenesis of benign and malignant adrenal cortical tumors [79, 80].

16.3.2 Adrenocortical Diseases

Studies of tumor clonality and chromosomal rearrangements have shown a major role of genetic alterations in adrenocortical tumors [81–85]. Studies of rare hereditary syndromes predisposing to adrenocortical tumors, such as Carney complex [86], Li–Fraumeni [84], or Beckwith–Wiedemann syndromes [87], have been very important to identify key genetic alterations involved in familial as well as sporadic adrenocortical tumors [88]. More recently, studies suggest that the WNT/β-catenin signaling pathway plays an important role in sporadic adrenocortical tumorigenesis. β-Catenin gene (*CTNNB1*) mutations are found in a significant number of ACAs and ACCs (Table 16.2) [89–92]. This is emphasized by the frequent observation of nuclear and/or cytoplasmic β-catenin localization by immunohistochemistry in ACAs, ACCs, and primary pigmented nodular adrenocortical disease (PPNAD). The extramembranous localization of β-catenin suggests activation of the WNT/β-catenin pathway in adrenal tumors and is in accordance with the presence of β-catenin-activating mutation in a subset of these tumors. At present, β-catenin-activating mutations are the most frequent genetic defect observed both in sporadic ACA and ACC [90, 92]. While the literature focusing on WNT/β-catenin signaling pathway involvement in adrenocortical tumorigenesis is not very abundant, recent publications of animal models suggest that the WNT/β-catenin pathway may also be activated in mouse models of adrenocortical tumorigenesis [93, 94]. PPNAD is a bilateral form of benign multiple ACA that can be observed in patients with Carney

Table 16.2 Different *CTNNB1* mutations reported in adrenocortical tumors

Conn adenoma	ACA	ACC	PPNAD	H295R
	DinsS33S[a]			
		pTyr30X[c]		
	C37C[b]			
		T41A[a]	T41A[c,d]	
	S45F[a,b]	S45F[a]		
	S45P[a]	S45P[a]	S45P[c,d]	S45P[a,b]
	S45Y[a]			
		Del S45[a]		
		26993 del 489 bp[a]		
	26813 del 376 bp[a]			
	26943 del 55 pb[b]			
	27127 del 6 pb[b]			
26995 del 271 bp[b]				
			c.236_349-191 del 304[d]	

The table summarizes the *CTNNB1* mutations reported in Conn adenomas, adrenocortical adenomas (ACA), adrenocortical carcinomas (ACC), primary pigmented nodular adrenocortical diseases (PPNAD), and the adrenocortical cancer cell line (H295R)
[a]Tissier [92]; [b]Tadjine [90]; [c]Tadjine [91]; [d]Gaujoux [89]

complex. It is most often due to germline mutations of the regulatory subunit R1A of the protein kinase A (*PRKAR1A*) [95, 96]. *PRKAR1A* somatic mutations have also been occasionally observed in hormonally functional ACA [96]. PRKAR1A is a key component of the cAMP pathway, and the inactivating *PRKAR1A* mutations observed in Carney complex lead to stimulation of PKA activity [95, 97, 98].

Gene expression [99] and miRNA [100] profiling study in PPNAD suggest an abnormal activation of the Wnt/β-catenin pathway in PPNAD-associated tumorigenesis. This is consistent with the observation [89, 91] of β-catenin accumulation in the cytoplasm and nucleus of adrenal lesions in Carney complex, supporting activation of the WNT/β-catenin pathway in these bilateral benign adrenocortical tumors (Fig. 16.3). β-Catenin somatic activating mutations are in part responsible for this activation, and interestingly, these mutations are only found in macronodules (defined as >10 mm), whereas micronodules and contralateral adrenal glands do not harbor any mutation [89, 91]. These data suggest that this molecular alteration might be linked to the appearance of these unusually large nodules in PPNAD, and that progressive accumulation of genetic alterations would favor the development of macronodules in PPNAD, a type of tumor with a very low growth potential. In parallel to the canonical mechanism of WNT/β-catenin signaling, there are multiple alternative pathways that regulate the stability of β-catenin [101–103]. It is likely that cross talks between the cAMP and the WNT/β-catenin signaling pathways are in part responsible for β-catenin accumulation in cases of PPNAD without β-catenin mutation. Activation of the WNT/β-catenin pathway by PKA is supported by recent in vitro studies [104, 105]. Additionally, such cross talk is supported by the diffuse bilateral pattern of β-catenin accumulation observed in multiple macronodules as well as micronodules in PPNAD, regardless of β-catenin mutational status [89, 90]. The β-catenin accumulation observed in ACA with *PRKAR1A* somatic mutations also supports the involvement of PKA dysregulation in these specific tumors. Indeed, among the ACA showing β-catenin accumulation by immunohistochemistry, the nuclear and cytoplasmic accumulation of β-catenin appears stronger in the ACA with *PRKAR1A* mutation than in others [89, 90].

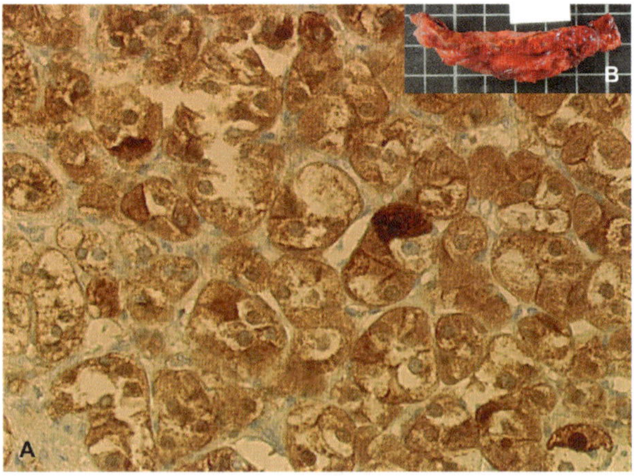

Fig. 16.3 β-Catenin immunohistochemistry in a case of primary pigmented nodular adrenocortical disease (PPNAD). Upper right panel: Gross pattern of PPNAD. Main panel: Immunohistochemical staining for β-catenin (X200): β-catenin accumulation in the cytoplasm and nucleus of nodules, supporting activation of the Wnt/β-catenin pathway

Adrenocortical Adenoma

The involvement of the WNT/β-catenin signaling pathway in ACA is now well documented. Tissier et al. [92] first reported the frequent involvement of WNT/β-catenin signaling pathways in ACA. In this study, immunohistochemistry revealed abnormal cytoplasmic and/or nuclear accumulation of β-catenin in 10 of 26 adrenocortical adenomas, and an activating somatic mutation of the β-catenin gene was shown in 7 of 26 ACA. Interestingly, these mutations were observed only in adrenocortical tumors with abnormal β-catenin accumulation (Fig. 16.4). In ACA, β-catenin alterations seem more frequent in nonfunctioning tumors, suggesting that β-catenin pathway activation might be mostly involved in the development of nonsecreting ACA. Nevertheless, this observation was not confirmed by Tadjine et al. [90]. Both point mutation and long deletions causing part or entire loss of exon 3 were found in ACT. All these mutations in exon 3 of CTNNB1 affected specific serine and threonine residues and amino acids adjacent to them, which are essential for the targeted degradation of β-catenin [106–108]. The observations were later confirmed by Tadjine et al. [90].

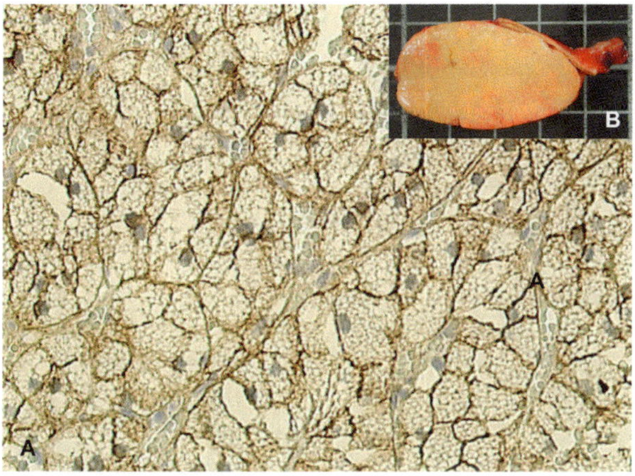

Fig. 16.4 β-Catenin immunohistochemistry in an adrenocortical adenoma. Upper right panel: Gross pattern of adrenocortical adenoma. Main panel: Immunohistochemical staining for β-catenin (X200): in this ACA, the β-catenin is located at the cell membrane. This corresponds to the localization in absence of the activation of the signaling pathway. This suggests in this adenoma the lack of abnormal activation of the Wnt/β-catenin pathway

ACTH-Independent Macronodular Hyperplasia

Previous large-scale cDNA microarray analysis of ACTH-independent macronodular hyperplasia (AIMAH) demonstrated the differential expression of several WNT/β-catenin signaling-related genes [109], suggesting the involvement of the WNT/β-catenin signaling in this tumorigenesis. Nevertheless, to date, no β-catenin activation mutations were found in the 13 cases analyzed by Tadjine et al. [90].

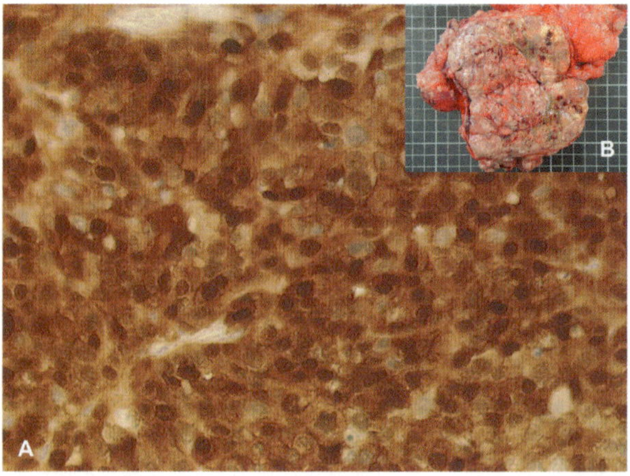

Fig.16.5 β-Catenin immunohistochemistry in an adrenocortical carcinoma. Upper right panel: Gross pattern of adrenocortical carcinoma. Main panel: Immunohistochemical staining for β-catenin (X200): β-catenin accumulation in the cytoplasm and nucleus of nodules, supporting activation of the Wnt/β-catenin pathway

16.4 The WNT Signaling Pathway in Adrenocortical Carcinoma

16.4.1 Activation of the WNT/β-Catenin Pathway and β-Catenin Mutations

Activation of the WNT signaling pathway in ACC has been suggested initially by gene profiling studies reporting overexpression of target genes of the WNT/β-catenin pathway in ACC [110]. Involvement of the WNT/β-catenin pathway in ACC has also been suggested by immunohistochemistry and genetic studies [92]. In a series of 13 ACC samples, immunohistochemistry revealed an abnormal cytoplasmic and/or nuclear accumulation of β-catenin in 11 ACC samples. Activating somatic mutations of *CTNNB1* were found in 4 of these 13 tumors, and they were associated with abnormal β-catenin accumulation (Fig. 16.5) [92]. Somatic activating mutations of *CTNNB1* are thus the first molecular defect to be reported with the same prevalence in both benign and malignant adrenocortical tumors. This is in contrast, for instance, to *TP53* mutations, which are exclusively found in ACC and *PRKAR1A* mutations that are exclusively observed in ACA. However, it is important to note that the pattern of β-catenin accumulation in ACC is more dramatic than in ACA. Indeed, β-catenin is more often detected in the nucleus in ACC than in ACA. Finally, the more diffuse pattern of β-catenin immunostaining in ACC vs. ACA may serve as a diagnostic/prognostic marker for malignancy in adrenocortical tumors. However, this diagnostic and prognostic value requires validation.

16.4.2 Role of β-Catenin Activation in Adrenocortical Tumor Development

The NCI-H295R cell line is currently the most widely used cell model of human adrenocortical carcinoma. Interestingly, the NCI-H295R cell line contains a naturally occurring activating Ser45 β-catenin mutation. In vitro experiments in this cell line have shown a constitutive activation of TCF-dependent transcription, using transfection of a TCF reporter gene (*pTOPFLASH*) [92]. This demonstrates that an activating mutation of β-catenin has nuclear effects on gene expression. Doghman et al. [111] have shown that the small molecule PKF115–584 that antagonizes the formation of the TCF/β-catenin complex inhibits proliferation of the NCI-H295R cell line. By flow cytometric analysis, PKF115–584 dose-dependently inhibits entry of NCI-H295R cells into the cell cycle and increases apoptosis. These observations support the importance of the WNT/β-catenin pathway in adrenocortical tumorigenesis. Activation of this pathway could increase cell proliferation and decrease apoptosis, leading to a more aggressive tumorigenesis.

A multistep process based on the progressive accumulation of multiple genetic and epigenetic alterations resulting in a transition from a benign to a malignant tumor is still under debate for adrenocortical tumorigenesis. Such a hypothesis is supported by the findings that β-catenin mutations appear to be one of the first molecular alteration identified in both ACA and ACC. Moreover, in some rare adrenocortical tumors, both malignant and a benign tumoral tissue are found within the same adrenal gland, consistent with this model [89, 112]. However, the high frequency of ACA, which is usually incidentally discovered, contrasts with the rarity of ACC, suggesting that this multistep progression from benign to malignant tumors might be very rare. Considering the high rate of benign and malignant adrenocortical tumors that harbor β-catenin alterations, activation of the WNT/β-catenin pathway is now considered the most prevalent defect identified in adrenocortical tumorigenesis. However, the observation that various types of adrenocortical tumors are associated with β-catenin somatic mutations demonstrates that this single event is not sufficient to induce a specific type of adrenal tumor (AIMAH, ACA, ACC). However, it is likely that this genetic defect does contribute to the development of a more aggressive tumor. Such hypothesis is supported by the observation of a heterogeneous tumor [89], in which a β-catenin mutation was restricted to the portion that was more aggressive (i.e., malignant component and its metastasis). Similarly, in PPNAD, somatic β-catenin mutations are found only in macronodules [89, 90]. Whether activation of the WNT/β-catenin pathway, as determined by β-catenin immunohistochemistry, is associated with a different clinical outcome in patients with ACC remains to be demonstrated.

16.4.3 Alternatives to CTNNB1 Mutation for WNT/β-Catenin Pathway Activation in Adrenocortical Carcinoma

Activation of the WNT/β-catenin pathway in ACC can currently be observed in about a quarter of the tumors by somatic β-catenin mutations. Considering the immunohistochemical and gene profiling studies, it is likely that activation of the pathway is more frequent in ACC, occurring in the majority of these neoplasms. Activation of β-catenin in ACC could be the result of cross talk with other signaling pathways, such as the IGF2 system which is almost always activated in these tumors [113]. Alternatively, other genetic defects that could activate the WNT/β-catenin signaling pathway are likely to be found in tumors that do not have a β-catenin mutation. Several genes that could be considered putative candidates for genetic alterations leading to activation of the WNT/β-catenin signaling pathway in adrenocortical tumors have already been identified in others tumor types [38, 114].

16.4.3.1 WTX, AXIN1, AXIN2, or GSK3β

To date, while no study has focused on *WTX*, *AXIN1*, *AXIN2*, or *GSK3β* mutations in ACC, such mutations could explain the gap between the frequency of WNT/β-catenin signaling pathway activation found by immunohistochemistry and mutational analysis of β-catenin. Epigenetic changes could also be involved in the activation of the pathway, as previously reported in other cancers, but no data are available at this time.

16.4.3.2 APC

Regarding *APC* involvement in ACC, available data are lacking with no large cohort having been screened for APC mutations in ACA or ACC. Nevertheless, it is well known that the incidence of ACA is increased in patients with FAP due to a germline mutation of *APC* [73, 76, 115]. In patients with FAP, the prevalence of adrenal masses has been reported from 7.4 to 13% vs. 0.6 to 3% in the general population [115, 116]. While these clinical studies suggest a possible role of *APC* in adrenocortical tumorigenesis, most evidence is observational [75, 117].

16.5 The WNT/β-Catenin Signaling Pathway: A Potential Target for Cancer Treatment

The frequent involvement of WNT/β-catenin signaling pathway in adrenocortical tumorigenesis suggests that targeting this pathway would have potential therapeutic applications. Recently, a high-throughput screening identified small molecules that antagonize the formation of the TCF/β-catenin complex and inhibit growth of colon, prostate cancer, and multiple myeloma cell lines [118, 119]. These compounds may be very useful in the treatment of a variety of cancers. Doghman et al. recently showed that one of these TCF/β-catenin antagonists, PKF115–584, inhibits proliferation of the NCI-H295R cell line, which harbors a β-catenin mutation along with mutation in the *TP53* gene [120]. Moreover, PKF115–584 can overcome the proliferative effects of increased SF1 levels in NCI-H295R ACC cells [120]. In the near future, inhibitors of the TCF/β-catenin complex may prove useful in the treatment of adrenocortical tumors.

16.6 Conclusion

Although quite recently discovered, the involvement of the WNT/β-catenin signaling pathway in ACC seems to be of great significance, in keeping with previous studies in a broad spectrum of cancers. This pathway plays a major role in adrenal development. WNT/β-catenin activation and *IGF2* overexpression are frequently observed in ACC and are two examples of signaling pathways activated both in fetal adrenal organogenesis and in adrenal tumorigenesis. As for IGF2, it is tempting to speculate that new therapies targeting this signaling pathway might be of potential interest for future development in the treatment of ACC.

References

1. Bienz M (2005) Beta-catenin: a pivot between cell adhesion and Wnt signalling. Curr Biol 15(2):R64–67
2. Kemler R (1993) From cadherins to catenins: cytoplasmic protein interactions and regulation of cell adhesion. Trends Genet 9(9):317–321
3. Lilien J, Balsamo J (2005) The regulation of cadherin-mediated adhesion by tyrosine phosphorylation/dephosphorylation of beta-catenin. Curr Opin Cell Biol 17(5):459–465
4. Giles RH et al (2003) Caught up in a Wnt storm: Wnt signaling in cancer. Biochim Biophys Acta 1653(1):1–24
5. Logan CY, Nusse R (2004) The Wnt signaling pathway in development and disease. Annu Rev Cell Dev Biol 20:781–810
6. Nusse R (2005) Cell biology: relays at the membrane. Nature 438(7069):747–749
7. Polakis P (2000) Wnt signaling and cancer. Genes Dev 14(15):1837–1851
8. Huang H, He X (2008) Wnt/beta-catenin signaling: new (and old) players and new insights. Curr Opin Cell Biol 20(2):119–125
9. Liu C et al (2002) Control of beta-catenin phosphorylation/degradation by a dual-kinase mechanism. Cell 108(6):837–847
10. Aberle H et al (1997) Beta-catenin is a target for the ubiquitin-proteasome pathway. Embo J 16(13):3797–3804
11. Winston JT et al (1999) The SCFbeta-TRCP-ubiquitin ligase complex associates specifically with phosphorylated destruction motifs in IkappaBalpha and beta-catenin and stimulates IkappaBalpha ubiquitination in vitro. Genes Dev 13(3):270–283
12. Townsley FM et al (2004) Pygopus and Legless target Armadillo/beta-catenin to the nucleus to enable its transcriptional co-activator function. Nat Cell Biol 6(7):626–633
13. Clevers H, van de Wetering M (1997) TCF/LEF factor earn their wings. Trends Genet 13(12):485–489
14. Polakis P (1999) The oncogenic activation of beta-catenin. Curr Opin Genet Dev 9(1):515–21
15. Behrens J, Lustig B (2004) The Wnt connection to tumorigenesis. Int J Dev Biol 48 (5–6):477–487
16. Johnson ML et al (2004) LRP5 and Wnt signaling: a union made for bone. J Bone Miner Res 19(11):1749–1757
17. Li L et al (1999) Axin and Frat1 interact with dvl and GSK, bridging Dvl to GSK in Wnt-mediated regulation of LEF-1. Embo J 18(15):4233–4240
18. Kishida S et al (1999) DIX domains of Dvl and axin are necessary for protein interactions and their ability to regulate beta-catenin stability. Mol Cell Biol 19(6):4414–4422
19. Peifer M, Polakis P (2000) Wnt signaling in oncogenesis and embryogenesis–a look outside the nucleus. Science 287(5458):1606–1609

20. Aberle H et al (1994) Assembly of the cadherin–catenin complex in vitro with recombinant proteins. J Cell Sci 107(Pt 12):3655–3663
21. Hulsken J et al (1994) E-cadherin and APC compete for the interaction with beta-catenin and the cytoskeleton. J Cell Biol 127(6 Pt 2):2061–2069
22. Yost C et al (1996) The axis-inducing activity, stability, and subcellular distribution of beta-catenin is regulated in *Xenopus* embryos by glycogen synthase kinase 3. Genes Dev 10(12):1443–1454
23. Munemitsu S et al (1996) Deletion of an amino-terminal sequence beta-catenin in vivo and promotes hyperphosphorylation of the adenomatous polyposis coli tumor suppressor protein. Mol Cell Biol 16(8):4088–4094
24. Rubinfeld B et al (1995) The APC protein and E-cadherin form similar but independent complexes with alpha-catenin, beta-catenin, and plakoglobin. J Biol Chem 270(10):5549–5555
25. Behrens J et al (1996) Functional interaction of beta-catenin with the transcription factor LEF-1. Nature 382(6592):638–642
26. Aberle H et al (1996) Single amino acid substitutions in proteins of the armadillo gene family abolish their binding to alpha-catenin. J Biol Chem 271(3):1520–1526
27. Huber O et al (1996) Nuclear localization of beta-catenin by interaction with transcription factor LEF-1. Mech Dev 59(1):3–10
28. Molenaar M et al (1996) XTcf-3 transcription factor mediates betacatenin-induced axis formation in *Xenopus* embryos. Cell 86(3):391–399
29. van de Wetering M et al (1997) Armadillo coactivates transcription driven by the product of the *Drosophila* segment polarity gene dTCF. Cell 88(6):789–799
30. Kraus C et al (1994) Localization of the human beta-catenin gene (CTNNB1) to 3p21: a region implicated in tumor development. Genomics 23(1):272–274
31. van Hengel J et al (1995) Assignment of the human beta-catenin gene (CTNNB1) to 3p22–>p21.3 by fluorescence in situ hybridization. Cytogenet Cell Genet 70(1–2):68–70
32. Nollet F et al (1996) Genomic organization of the human beta-catenin gene (CTNNB1). Genomics 32(3):413–424
33. Zeng L et al (1997) The mouse fused locus encodes Axin, an inhibitor of the Wnt signaling pathway that regulates embryonic axis formation. Cell 90(1):181–192
34. Salahshor S, Woodgett JR (2005) The links between axin and carcinogenesis. J Clin Pathol 58(3):225–236
35. Fearnhead NS et al (2001) The ABC of APC. Hum Mol Genet 10(7):721–733
36. Hsu W et al (1999) Identification of a domain of Axin that binds to the serine/threonine protein phosphatase 2A and a self-binding domain. J Biol Chem 274(6):3439–3445
37. Zhang Y et al (2002) Casein kinase I and casein kinase II differentially regulate axin function in Wnt and JNK pathways. J Biol Chem 277(20):17706–17712
38. Satoh S, et al (2000) AXIN1 mutations in hepatocellular carcinomas, and growth suppression in cancer cells by virus-mediated transfer of AXIN1. Nat Genet 24(3):245–250
39. Dong X et al (2001) Genomic structure, chromosome mapping and expression analysis of the human AXIN2 gene. Cytogenet Cell Genet 93(1–2):26–28
40. Jho EH et al (2002) Wnt/beta-catenin/Tcf signaling induces the transcription of Axin2, a negative regulator of the signaling pathway. Mol Cell Biol 22(4):1172–1183
41. Lustig B et al (2002) Negative feedback loop of Wnt signaling through upregulation of conductin/axin2 in colorectal and liver tumors. Mol Cell Biol 22(4):1184–1193
42. Yan D et al (2001) Elevated expression of axin2 and hnkd mRNA provides evidence that Wnt/beta-catenin signaling is activated in human colon tumors. Proc Natl Acad Sci USA 98(26):14973–14978
43. Bienz M (2002) The subcellular destinations of APC proteins. Nat Rev Mol Cell Biol 3(5):328–338
44. Kinzler KW et al (1991) Identification of FAP locus genes from chromosome 5q21. Science 253(5020):661–665

45. Groden J et al (1991) Identification and characterization of the familial adenomatous polyposis coli gene. Cell 66(3):589–600
46. Rubinfeld B et al (1996) Binding of GSK3beta to the APC-beta-catenin complex and regulation of complex assembly. Science 272(5264):1023–1026
47. Yamamoto H et al (1999) Phosphorylation of axin, a Wnt signal negative regulator, by glycogen synthase kinase-3beta regulates its stability. J Biol Chem 274(16):10681–10684
48. Rivera MN et al (2007) An X chromosome gene, WTX, is commonly inactivated in Wilms tumor. Science 315(5812):642–645
49. Major MB et al (2007) Wilms tumor suppressor WTX negatively regulates WNT/beta-catenin signaling. Science 316(5827):1043–1046
50. Perotti D et al (2008) Functional inactivation of the WTX gene is not a frequent event in Wilms' tumors. Oncogene 27(33):4625–4632
51. Ruteshouser EC et al (2008) Wilms tumor genetics: mutations in WT1, WTX, and CTNNB1 account for only about one-third of tumors. Genes Chromosomes Cancer 47(6):461–470
52. Jenkins ZA et al (2009) Germline mutations in WTX cause a sclerosing skeletal dysplasia but do not predispose to tumorigenesis. Nat Genet 41(1):95–100
53. Grohmann A et al (2007) AMER1 regulates the distribution of the tumor suppressor APC between microtubules and the plasma membrane. J Cell Sci 120(Pt 21):3738–3747
54. Cavallo RA et al (1998) *Drosophila* Tcf and Groucho interact to repress Wingless signalling activity. Nature 395(6702):604–608
55. Roose J et al (1998) The *Xenopus* Wnt effector XTcf-3 interacts with Groucho-related transcriptional repressors. Nature 395(6702):608–612
56. Chen G et al (1999) A functional interaction between the histone deacetylase Rpd3 and the corepressor Groucho in *Drosophila* development. Genes Dev 13(17):2218–2230
57. Hecht A et al (2000) The p300/CBP acetyltransferases function as transcriptional coactivators of beta-catenin in vertebrates. Embo J 19(8):1839–1850
58. Levy L et al (2004) Acetylation of beta-catenin by p300 regulates beta-catenin-Tcf4 interaction. Mol Cell Biol 24(8):3404–3414
59. Wolf D et al (2002) Acetylation of beta-catenin by CREB-binding protein (CBP). J Biol Chem 277(28):25562–25567
60. Lammi L et al (2004) Mutations in AXIN2 cause familial tooth agenesis and predispose to colorectal cancer. Am J Hum Genet 74(5):1043–1050
61. Mostowska A et al (2006) Axis inhibition protein 2 (AXIN2) polymorphisms may be a risk factor for selective tooth agenesis. J Hum Genet 51(3):262–266
62. He TC et al (1998) A simplified system for generating recombinant adenoviruses. Proc Natl Acad Sci USA 95(5):2509–2514
63. Shtutman M et al (1999) The cyclin D1 gene is a target of the beta-catenin/LEF-1 pathway. Proc Natl Acad Sci USA 96(10):5522–5527
64. Tetsu O, McCormick F (1999) Beta-catenin regulates expression of cyclin D1 in colon carcinoma cells. Nature 398(6726):422–426
65. Zhang X et al (2001) Regulation of vascular endothelial growth factor by the Wnt and K-ras pathways in colonic neoplasia. Cancer Res 61(16):6050–6054
66. Brabletz T et al (1999) Beta-catenin regulates the expression of the matrix metalloproteinase-7 in human colorectal cancer. Am J Pathol 155(4):1033–1038
67. Conacci-Sorrell ME et al (2002) Nr-CAM is a target gene of the betacatenin/LEF-1 pathway in melanoma and colon cancer and its expression enhances motility and confers tumorigenesis. Genes Dev 16(16):2058–2072
68. Crawford HC et al (1999) The metalloproteinase matrilysin is a target of beta-catenin transactivation in intestinal tumors. Oncogene 18(18):2883–2891
69. Moon RT et al (2004) WNT and beta-catenin signalling: diseases and therapies. Nat Rev Genet 5(9):691–701
70. Chiang JM et al (2002) Nuclear beta-catenin expression is closely related to ulcerative growth of colorectal carcinoma. Br J Cancer 86(7):1124–1129

71. Clements WM et al (2002) Beta-catenin mutation is a frequent cause of Wnt pathway activation in gastric cancer. Cancer Res 62(12):3503–3506
72. Laurent-Puig P et al (2001) Genetic alterations associated with hepatocellular carcinomas define distinct pathways of hepatocarcinogenesis. Gastroenterology 120(7):1763–1773
73. Kartheuser A et al (1999) Familial adenomatous polyposis associated with multiple adrenal adenomas in a patient with a rare 3′ APC mutation. J Med Genet 36(1):65–67
74. Ono C et al (1991) A case of familial adenomatous polyposis complicated by thyroid carcinoma, carcinoma of the ampulla of vater and adrenocortical adenoma. Jpn J Surg 21(2):234–240
75. Seki M et al (1992) Loss of normal allele of the APC gene in an adrenocortical carcinoma from a patient with familial adenomatous polyposis. Hum Genet 89(3):298–300
76. Wakatsuki S et al (1998) Adrenocortical tumor in a patient with familial adenomatous polyposis: a case associated with a complete inactivating mutation of the APC gene and unusual histological features. Hum Pathol 29(3):302–306
77. Kim AC et al (2008) Targeted disruption of beta-catenin in Sf1-expressing cells impairs development and maintenance of the adrenal cortex. Development 135(15):2593–2602
78. Gummow BM et al (2003) Convergence of Wnt signaling and steroidogenic factor-1 (SF-1) on transcription of the rat inhibin alpha gene. J Biol Chem 278(29):26572–26579
79. Kim AC et al (2009) In search of adrenocortical stem and progenitor cells. Endocr Rev 30(3):241–263
80. Val P, Swain A (2010) Gene dosage effects and transcriptional regulation of early mammalian adrenal cortex development. Mol Cell Endocrinol 323(1):105–114
81. Beuschlein F et al (1994) Clonal composition of human adrenocortical neoplasms. Cancer Res 54(18):4927–4932
82. Gicquel C et al (1994) Clonal analysis of human adrenocortical carcinomas and secreting adenomas. Clin Endocrinol (Oxf) 40(4):465–477
83. Libe R et al (2007) Adrenocortical cancer: pathophysiology and clinical management. Endocr Relat Cancer 14(1):13–28
84. Reincke M et al (1994) p53 mutations in human adrenocortical neoplasms: immunohistochemical and molecular studies. J Clin Endocrinol Metab 78(3):790–794
85. Sidhu S et al (2002) Comparative genomic hybridization analysis of adrenocortical tumors. J Clin Endocrinol Metab 87(7):3467–3474
86. Kirschner LS et al (2000) Mutations of the gene encoding the protein kinase A type I-alpha regulatory subunit in patients with the Carney complex. Nat Genet 26(1):89–92
87. Boulle N et al (1998) Increased levels of insulin-like growth factor II (IGF-II) and IGF-binding protein-2 are associated with malignancy in sporadic adrenocortical tumors. J Clin Endocrinol Metab 83(5):1713–1720
88. Libe R, Bertherat J (2005) Molecular genetics of adrenocortical tumours, from familial to sporadic diseases. Eur J Endocrinol 153(4):477–487
89. Gaujoux S et al (2008) Wnt/beta-catenin and 3′,5′-cyclic adenosine 5′-monophosphate/protein kinase A signaling pathways alterations and somatic beta-catenin gene mutations in the progression of adrenocortical tumors. J Clin Endocrinol Metab 93(10):4135–4140
90. Tadjine M et al (2008) Frequent mutations of beta-catenin gene in sporadic secreting adrenocortical adenomas. Clin Endocrinol (Oxf) 68(2):264–270
91. Tadjine M et al (2008) Detection of somatic beta-catenin mutations in primary pigmented nodular adrenocortical disease (PPNAD). Clin Endocrinol (Oxf) 69(3):367–373
92. Tissier F et al (2005) Mutations of beta-catenin in adrenocortical tumors: activation of the Wnt signaling pathway is a frequent event in both benign and malignant adrenocortical tumors. Cancer Res 65(17):7622–7627
93. Bernichtein S et al (2008) Adrenal gland tumorigenesis after gonadectomy in mice is a complex genetic trait driven by epistatic loci. Endocrinology 149(2):651–661

94. Bielinska M et al (2005) Gonadotropin-induced adrenocortical neoplasia in NU/J nude mice. Endocrinology 146(9):3975–3984
95. Groussin L et al (2002) Mutations of the PRKAR1A gene in Cushing's syndrome due to sporadic primary pigmented nodular adrenocortical disease. J Clin Endocrinol Metab 87(9):4324–4329
96. Bertherat J et al (2003) Molecular and functional analysis of PRKAR1A and its locus (17q22-24) in sporadic adrenocortical tumors:17q losses, somatic mutations, and protein kinase A expression and activity. Cancer Res 63(17):5308–5319
97. Bossis I, Stratakis CA (2004) Minireview: PRKAR1A: normal and abnormal functions. Endocrinology 145(12):5452–5458
98. Horvath A et al (2008) Large deletions of the PRKAR1A gene in Carney complex. Clin Cancer Res 14(2):388–395
99. Horvath A et al (2006) Serial analysis of gene expression in adrenocortical hyperplasia caused by a germline PRKAR1A mutation. J Clin Endocrinol Metab 91(2):584–596
100. Iliopoulos D et al (2009) MicroRNA signature of primary pigmented nodular adrenocortical disease: clinical correlations and regulation of Wnt signaling. Cancer Res 69(8):3278–3282
101. Li G, Iyengar R (2002) Calpain as an effector of the Gq signaling pathway for inhibition of Wnt/beta-catenin-regulated cell proliferation. Proc Natl Acad Sci USA 99(20):13254–13259
102. Liu J et al (2001) Siah-1 mediates a novel beta-catenin degradation pathway linking p53 to the adenomatous polyposis coli protein. Mol Cell 7(5):927–936
103. Matsuzawa SI, Reed JC (2001) Siah-1, SIP, and Ebi collaborate in a novel pathway for beta-catenin degradation linked to p53 responses. Mol Cell 7(5):915–926
104. Hino S et al (2005) Phosphorylation of beta-catenin by cyclic AMP-dependent protein kinase stabilizes beta-catenin through inhibition of its ubiquitination. Mol Cell Biol 25(20):9063–9072
105. Taurin S et al (2006) Phosphorylation of beta-catenin by cyclic AMP-dependent protein kinase. J Biol Chem 281(15):9971–9976
106. Hagen T, Vidal-Puig A (2002) Characterisation of the phosphorylation of beta-catenin at the GSK3 priming site Ser45. Biochem Biophys Res Commun 294(2):324–328
107. Kikuchi A (2003) Tumor formation by genetic mutations in the components of the Wnt signaling pathway. Cancer Sci 94(3):225–229
108. Wu R et al (2001) Diverse mechanisms of beta-catenin deregulation in ovarian endometrioid adenocarcinomas. Cancer Res 61(22):8247–8255
109. Bourdeau I et al (2004) Gene array analysis of macronodular adrenal hyperplasia confirms clinical heterogeneity and identifies several candidate genes as molecular mediators. Oncogene 23(8):1575–1585
110. Giordano TJ et al (2003) Distinct transcriptional profiles of adrenocortical tumors uncovered by DNA microarray analysis. Am J Pathol 162(2):521–531
111. Doghman M et al (2008) The T cell factor/beta-catenin antagonist PKF115-584 inhibits proliferation of adrenocortical carcinoma cells. J Clin Endocrinol Metab 93(8):3222–3225
112. Bernard MH et al (2003) A case report in favor of a multistep adrenocortical tumorigenesis. J Clin Endocrinol Metab 88(3):998–1001
113. Gicquel C et al (2001) Molecular markers and long-term recurrences in a large cohort of patients with sporadic adrenocortical tumors. Cancer Res 61(18):6762–6767
114. Morin PJ et al (1997) Activation of beta-catenin-Tcf signaling in colon cancer by mutations in beta-catenin or APC. Science 275(5307):1787–1790
115. Smith TG et al (2000) Adrenal masses are associated with familial adenomatous polyposis. Dis Colon Rectum 43(12):1739–1742
116. Marchesa P et al (1997) Adrenal masses in patients with familial adenomatous polyposis. Dis Colon Rectum 40(9):1023–1028
117. Traill Z et al (1995) Adrenal carcinoma in a patient with Gardner's syndrome: imaging findings. AJR Am J Roentgenol 165(6):1460–1461

118. Lepourcelet M et al (2004) Small-molecule antagonists of the oncogenic Tcf/betacatenin protein complex. Cancer Cell 5(1):91–102
119. Sukhdeo K et al (2007) Targeting the beta-catenin/TCF transcriptional complex in the treatment of multiple myeloma. Proc Natl Acad Sci USA 104(18):7516–7521
120. Doghman M et al (2007) Increased steroidogenic factor-1 dosage triggers adrenocortical cell proliferation and cancer. Mol Endocrinol 21(12):2968–2987

Part VI
Models of Adrenocortical Cancer

Chapter 17
Adrenocortical Stem and Progenitor Cells: Implications for Cancer

Joanne H. Heaton and Gary D. Hammer

It is estimated that close to 1.5 million men and women will be diagnosed with cancer and over 500,000 will die of cancer in 2010 (http://seer.cancer.gov/). While scientific discovery has begun to uncover mechanisms of both tumor initiation and tumor maintenance, these discoveries have until recently been slow to be translated into effective treatments that significantly change cancer death statistics. Whereas non-transformed cells proliferate only in response to environmental signals in a limited window of their life history, cancer involves the acquisition of autonomous proliferative potential by these once normal cells. To develop more successful therapies for cancer patients as well as to establish effective preventive techniques, two broad fundamental issues must be addressed. First, how is cancer initiated and, more specifically, in what cell type(s) is cancer initiated? Second, once a cancer is established, how is it maintained? Specifically, do all cells in the tumor continue to proliferate or are there a few specific cells that maintain the proliferative capacity of the tumor while other cells differentiate?

While genetic profiling suggests that most cancers are clonal (i.e., derived from a single cell), the occurrence of additional "secondary" mutations in the daughter cells often yields significant heterogeneity within a given cancer, both in terms of differentiation state and proliferative capacity. Although the mechanism and importance of this heterogeneity remains to be determined, two models have been put forward [1]. The stochastic model predicts that all cells in a tumor are biologically equivalent with any heterogeneity based on extrinsic/environmental factors. In this model all cells in a tumor have the potential to proliferate and metastasize (Fig. 17.1). The "cancer stem cell" model posits that heterogeneity in a given tumor reflects tumor cells that are biologically different. In this model, a distinct, generally rare (<1%) subpopulation of tumor cells display stem-cell like potential that endows them with the ability both to self renew and to generate cells that differentiate into multiple different cells types within a cancer (Fig. 17.1) [2–5]. Only the cancer stem cells can maintain the cancer and, importantly, only these special cells can reinitiate tumor

J.H. Heaton (✉)
Department of Internal Medicine, Division of Metabolism, Endocrinology & Diabetes, University of Michigan Medical School, 109 Zina Pitcher Place, 1680 BSRB, Ann Arbor, MI 48109, USA
e-mail: heatonj@med.umich.edu

G.D. Hammer, T. Else (eds.), *Adrenocortical Carcinoma*,
DOI 10.1007/978-0-387-77236-3_17, © Springer Science+Business Media, LLC 2011

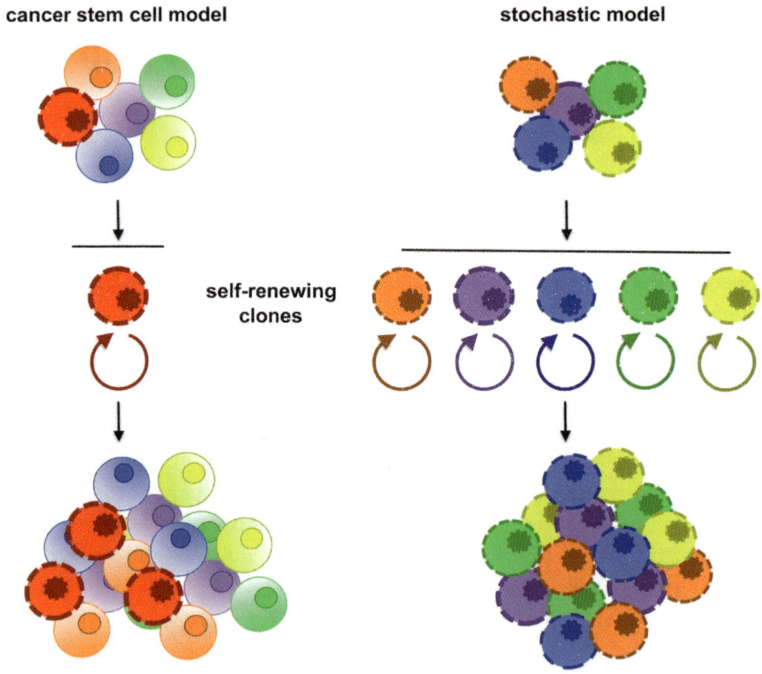

Fig. 17.1 Maintenance of cancer: stochastic/clonal evolution vs. cancer stem cell model. Stochastic/clonal evolution model: Cancer cells are heterogeneous. Multiple clones (cell lineages) are present in a given tumor, with each clone resulting from multiple different mutations. Moreover, most cells in each clone can proliferate and form new tumors. All clones must be killed to cure the cancer. Cancer stem cell model: Cancer cells are heterogeneous. Only cancer stem cells can proliferate and form new tumors. Selectively killing the cancer stem cells is necessary and sufficient for cure

growth in a metastatic lesion or in experimental models of cancer initiation. The other cells in the cancer are unable to support such growth. This is analogous to the subpopulation of adult/tissue stem cells in normal organs that are responsible for replenishing the differentiated cells as normal cells of that organ reach the natural end of their lifespan. While cancer stem cells with this unique ability have been identified in blood, breast, brain, colon, and pancreatic cancers, it is important to note that not all tumors have been shown to be driven by such rare cells [4, 6]. A recent study of human melanoma reported that as high as 27% of cells in the tumor were tumorigenic in xenografts [7]. However, it is distinctly possible that different cancers possess different percentages of cells endowed with stem cell characteristics; in some neoplasias, these cells may be rare and in others they may be more prevalent.

Historically, the goal of cancer therapeutics has been to eliminate the majority or totality of cells within a tumor, because all tumor cells were assumed to possess equal malignant potential. However, in addition to being the only cells within a tumor that can give rise to new tumor cells, cancer stem cells are also predicted to be the cells that are least responsive to standard chemotherapeutic protocols (see reference [3] and references therein). This concept is predicated on the understanding that, because cytotoxic chemotherapy best targets proliferating cells, it can eliminate rapidly amplifying progenitor cells, but it cannot easily kill the relatively quiescence (albeit self-renewing) cancer stem cells. In this setting, effective drug therapy might necessitate the specific targeting of this tumorigenic subpopulation of cancer stem cells.

Even in cases where cancer stem cells have been found, in general the origin of the cancer stem cell has not been determined. An adult tissue stem cell, a progenitor cell, or even a differentiated cell may acquire tumorigenic properties that currently define a cancer stem cell (Fig. 17.2).

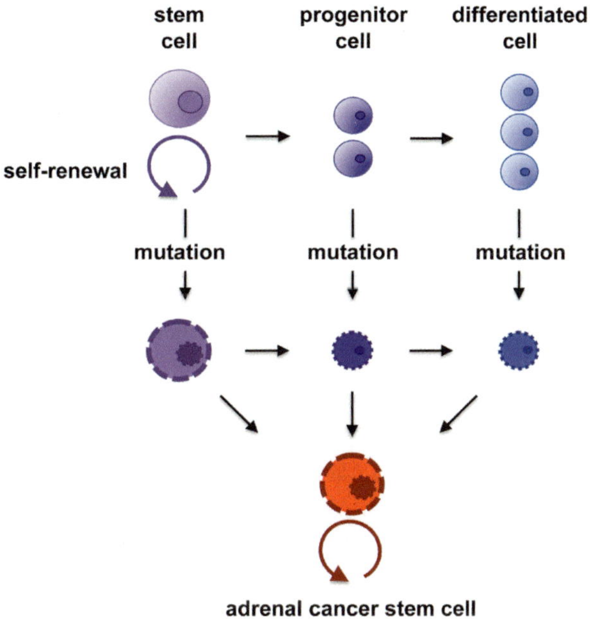

Fig. 17.2 Origins of cancer stem cells. Cancer stem cells might appear after mutations in specific tissue stem cells or progenitor cells derived from the organ-specific stem cell. Additionally, cancer stem cells may be derived from differentiated cells that activate stem cell-specific genetic programs that support the emergent stem cell characteristics

17.1 Adrenocortical Tumors

Benign adrenal tumors or adrenocortical adenomas (ACA) are fairly common, found in 3–7% of the population. In contrast, malignant adrenal tumors or adrenocortical carcinomas (ACCs) are extremely rare with the incidence ranging from 1 to 10 cases per million people per year [8, 9] (www.seer.cancer.gov) Moreover, patients with this rare cancer have an extremely poor prognosis as a consequence of metastasis or local invasion prior to diagnosis, and the overall 5-year survival rate in patients diagnosed with advanced disease is less than 10%. The only potentially curative option for ACC is complete operative resection. Currently, the only FDA-approved pharmacologic therapy for unresectable or metastatic ACC is the adrenolytic drug mitotane, which is often used in combination with cytotoxic chemotherapies. As cancer stem cells have not yet been identified in ACC, this chapter will focus on data that address ACC initiation and maintenance. It is predicted that future therapies for ACC will need to incorporate these emerging biological insights.

17.2 Normal Adrenal Adult Stem Cells

A chapter on ACC initiation in relation to the normal function of adrenocortical stem cells demands a discussion of adrenal development, structure, and cellular composition.

17.2.1 Adrenal Development and Structure

The adrenal gland is composed of two embryologically and functionally distinct organs. The inner adrenal medulla is derived from neural ectoderm and functions in the adult as a mediator of the acute stress response through secretion of catecholamines. The adrenal cortex is derived from intermediate mesoderm and in the adult is organized into three distinct concentric zones with three distinct functions. The outer zona glomerulosa synthesizes and secretes mineralocorticoids that function to maintain sodium balance and intravascular volume, the zona fasciculata synthesizes glucocorticoids that function to regulate energy storage, and the zona reticularis synthesizes sex-steroid precursors (Fig. 17.3) [10].

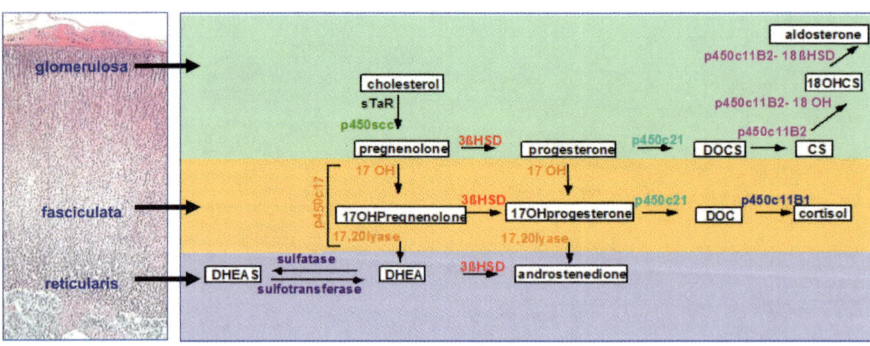

Fig. 17.3 Histologic organization of the adrenal cortex and steroidogenic pathways of each compartment

In humans and mice, adrenal gland organogenesis occurs via carefully orchestrated phases [10, 11]. The initial phase in the 4th week of human development, or the embryonic day 9.0 (E9.0) in mice, is marked by the proliferation of the mesoderm-derived, coelomic epithelia and underlying mesonephric mesenchymal cells of the primitive urogenital ridge and dorsal mesentery. Together these form the adrenogonadal primordium (AGP). Loss-of-function studies in mice have demonstrated that the transcription factor steroidogenic factor 1 (Sf1 or Ad4BP

Nuclear Receptor Subfamily 5, Group A, Member 1 [Nr5a1]) is essential for formation of the AGP [12]. Other transcription factors, including pre-B-cell leukemia homeobox 1 (Pbx1), odd-skipped related 1 (Odd1, Osr1), and polycomb group protein M33 participate in specification and/or expansion of the AGP [13–16]. In the 8th week in human gestation (E10.5 in the mouse) the AGP separates into the adrenal primordium and the gonadal primordium. This step appears to be initiated through the upregulation of *Sf1* expression by Wilm's tumor 1 (Wt1) and Cbp/p300-interacting transactivator, with Glu/Asp-rich carboxy-terminal domain, 2 (Cited2) [17]. When the adrenal primordium separates from the AGP, a different transcription complex, containing the homeobox protein PKNOX1 (Pknox1, Prep1), homeobox gene 9b (Hox9b), and Pbx1, is recruited to maintain fetal zone expression of Sf1 [18]. Later in development, Sf1 is able to activate its own expression in a feed forward manner. In the 8th and 9th weeks of gestation in humans (E11.5–12.5 in mice), the mesenchymal capsule forms around the fetal cortex and neural crest cells migrate and invade the cortex to establish the adrenal medulla [11, 19]. Once encapsulation is complete, the 3rd stage, the initiation of the definitive zone or adult cortex occurs (Fig. 17.4). Throughout life, peripheral cells in or just beneath the capsule proliferate and give rise to centripetally displaced cells that establish the adult cortex.

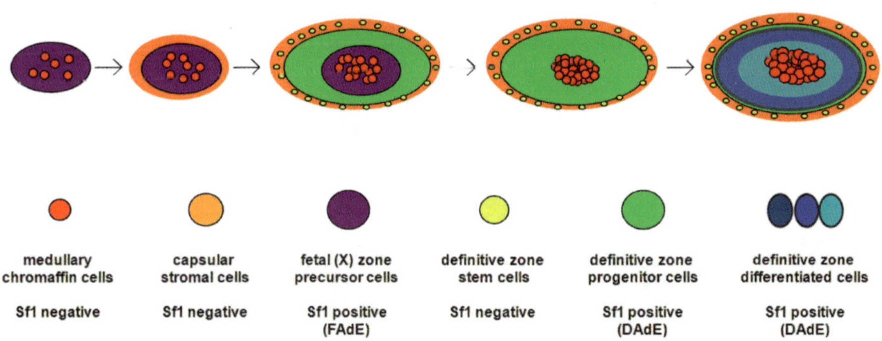

Fig. 17.4 Organogenesis of the adrenal cortex. Cell types are defined in lower panel of Figure

17.2.2 Where Do the Adrenal Adult Stem Cells Reside?

Following maturation of the gland, the adult organ maintains organ homeostasis by replenishment of the adrenocortical cells throughout the life of the organism. Cells of the adult adrenal cortex are continually renewed and centripetally displaced from the outer capsular/subcapsular region inward. This centripetal movement, together with PCNA immunochemical staining for proliferating cells, BrdU or H^3 pulse chase experiments and tissue remodeling studies, supports the current hypothesis that the stem and progenitor cells necessary for adult organ maintenance are located in and just under the capsule (Fig. 17.5) [20–22]. The stem/progenitor cells remain quiescent and relatively undifferentiated with the potential to self-renew or differentiate as dictated by the homeostatic needs of the adrenal cortex. As they

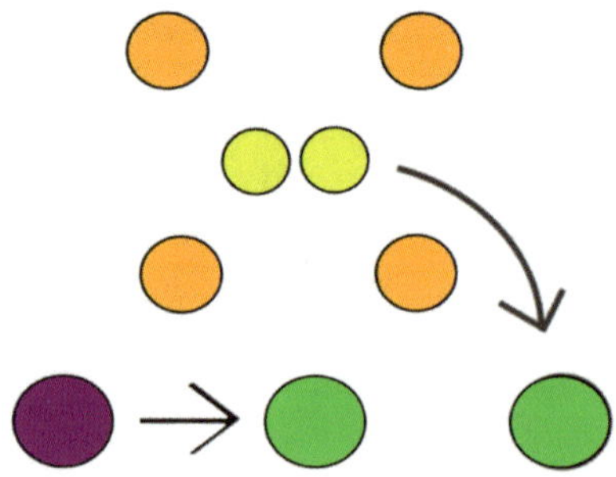

Fig. 17.5 Current models of establishment of capsular stem cell niche and definitive cortex. Depiction of two recent reports that provide data that the definitive cortex is derived from (**a**) Sf1-positive fetal cortex cells and/or (**b**) Sf1-negative cells in the capsule. Cell types are defined by color as detailed in Fig. 17.4

differentiate, they are centripetally displaced to sequentially populate the concentric steriodogenic zones of the adrenal cortex before undergoing apoptosis at the cortico-medullary boundary (Fig. 17.6).

17.2.3 Establishment of the Stem Cell Niche

As the adrenal cortex must continually renew itself throughout the life of the organism, any model of organogenesis must include the establishment of a homeostatic mechanism to support such a constant replenishment of dying cells (i.e., establishing a tissue stem cell pool and niche). The examination of cell lineages in the development of the adrenal cortex should provide clues to the residence of such stem and progenitor cells.

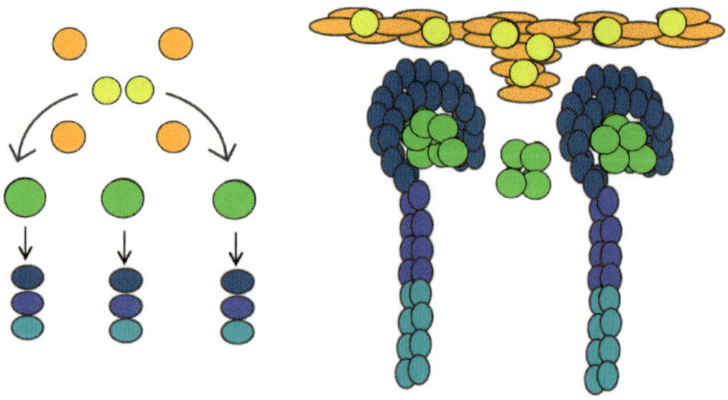

Fig. 17.6 Homeostatic model of adrenocortical growth. After the fetal zone has regressed, the definitive cortex is maintained by quiescent self-renewing Sf1-negative stem cells embedded in the capsule. The stem cells give rise to emerging subcapsular definitive cells that serve as rapidly amplifying progenitor cells which ultimately differentiate into the functional adrenocortical cells of the zona glomerulosa, zona fasciculata, and zona reticularis. Cells die at the cortico-medullary boundary. Cell types are defined by color as detailed in Fig. 17.4

17.2.3.1 Adrenal Precursor Cells in Fetal Zone

Zubair et al. carried out extensive cell lineage studies in mice and concluded that Sf1-positive cells of the fetal adrenal cortex give rise to all adult Sf1-positive adrenocortical cells [23]. These authors had previously demonstrated that a sequence found in intron 4 of the *Sf1* gene harbors a fetal adrenal enhancer (FAdE) that activates *Sf1* expression in the fetal adrenal primordium. Using a transgenic mouse with lacZ driven by a basal promoter and the FAdE sequence, they found that *Sf1* expression in the adrenal primordium/fetal cortex is activated initially by a Hox-Pbx-Prep1 protein complex and later by Sf1 protein itself, both interacting with the FAdE sequence. The fetal enhancer is not active in the adult cortex as evidenced by the temporal disappearance of LacZ as the fetal zone regresses [18]. Presumably, *Sf1* is regulated in the definitive/adult cortex through a yet to be defined definitive enhancer (DAdE).

Using a *Rosa26* mouse bred with a transgenic mouse harboring a *Cre-recombinase* gene driven by a basal *Sf1* promoter and FAdE enhancer, these investigators were able to follow the fate of the fetal adrenal cells as the gland developed. Because fetal cortex cells in which FAdE is active will permanently activate *Cre* (and because they had previously demonstrated that this enhancer is not active in the definitive cortex), any cells that exhibit LacZ are presumed to derive from the fetal cortex. Adult adrenal glands from these transgenic mice have a cortex that is almost entirely blue, whereas the capsule and the medulla do not show LacZ. Using a similar mouse in which the *FAdE-cre* gene is tamoxifen-inducible, they were able to carry out a temporal study. When tamoxifen is administered early in embryogenesis (E11.5–E12.5) and embryos examined 2 days later, LacZ is seen in most of the cortex. Sequentially later administration of tamoxifen resulted in an adult cortex in which the *LacZ*-expressing cells are sequentially restricted to more inner cortical cells. Their results suggest that the fetal cortex gives rise to the definitive/adult cortex and that this contribution is complete by about E14.5, after which time the proliferating definitive cortex expands and the fetal cortex regresses. When tamoxifen was administered after E14.5 or after birth, no LacZ-positive cells were observed, consistent with the absence of FAdE activity. Thus, these authors conclude that all definitive/adult cortical cells derive from the fetal cortex. They did not report any contribution to or from the capsule. Importantly, this model does not provide an explanation for the establishment of adrenocortical stem cells necessary to replenish the adult organ.

17.2.3.2 Stem/Progenitor Cells in Adrenal Capsule

A second model has been proposed as a result of studies on the role of the Hedgehog pathway in mouse adrenal organogenesis. The Hedgehog pathway (Hg) is important in vertebrate development and has been implicated in the regulation of both embryonic and adult stem cells [24–27]. The activation of this signaling pathway occurs through binding of one of the hedgehog ligands [Sonic hedgehog (Shh), Desert hedgehog (Dhh) or Indian hedgehog (Ihh)] to the cell surface receptor Patched-1 (Ptch1). Upon binding to ligands, Ptch1 releases inhibition of the

Smoothened (Smo) cell surface receptor and allows activation of the Gli transcription factors. Two clinical syndromes implicate the Hedgehog signaling pathway in normal human adrenocortical development. Adrenal hypoplasia/aplasia has been reported in Pallister-Hall syndrome due to loss-of-function GLI3 mutations and in Smith-Lemli-Opitz syndrome due to cholesterol synthetic defects that result in altered Hg signaling. Gli3 mutations in mice result in adrenal aplasia, supporting a role for the Hg signaling pathway in mouse adrenal development.

Recently, three laboratories [28–30] reported that tissue-specific (*Sf1-cre*-mediated) knock-out of *Shh* in mice results in marked adrenocortical hypoplasia, a thin adrenal capsule and fewer Ki67-positive (proliferating cells) in the capsule, further indicating a role for this pathway in adrenal maintenance. Using a *LacZ* knock-in mouse model, King et al. show that Shh is first detected at about E11.5, is expressed primarily in the periphery of the adrenal and co-localizes with Sf1, but does not co-localize with markers of differentiation, Cyp11B1 or Cyp11B2. They conclude that *Shh* is expressed in Sf1-positive, non-differentiated cells in the periphery of the cortex. Their embryonic cell lineage studies using transgenic mice harboring a *GFP* reporter and *cre-recombinase* under control of a tamoxifen-inducible *Shh* promoter (*Shh* creT2:R26 mR/mG) demonstrate that *Shh*-expressing (green) cells are initially (5 days after tamoxifen) found in the subcapsular region. A number of days after the tamoxifen pulse (28 day), descendants of these cells are found as radial stripes of GFP-positive cells in the cortex. Similar results were obtained when adults were administered tamoxifen and examined 13 days later. These results demonstrate that Shh-positive/Sf1-positive subcapsular cells proliferate and migrate centripetally to become differentiated (*Cyp11b1* or *Cyp11b2* expressing) cortex cells, and indicate that these subcapsular cells function as progenitor cells during adrenal development and in adult organ maintenance [28]. In this study the earliest tamoxifen treatment was at E14.5. Because this is the embryonic time when the FAdE is shut off, while not inconsistent with results from Zubair et al., these experiments do not address the fetal origin of the definitive cortex.

Huang et al. observed a similar decrease in size of the adrenal in *Sf1-cre/Shh*$^{flox/-}$ mice, which is evident at P5 [29]. The observation that this smaller adrenal gland displays normal zonation is used to hypothesize that Shh is not required for cell differentiation. As expected, conditional *Shh* knock-out results in significantly decreased Gli1 in the adrenal capsule. Utilizing TUNEL assays and inmmunohistochemistry for Ki67 expression, these investigators concluded that loss of Shh does not alter the rate of cell death but rather results in decreased proliferation specifically in the adrenal capsule. This is consistent with a model in which Shh from the cortex activates capsular *Gli1* to stimulate proliferation.

These same laboratories carried out similar cell lineage studies using the downstream activator of the Hg pathway, *Gli1*. In the adrenal gland *Gli1* is expressed primarily in the capsule although a few sporadic cortex cells are Gli1 positive [28, 30]. Using a tamoxifen-inducible *Cre-recombinase* under control of the *Gli1* promoter, and either a *GFP* or *lacZ* reporter, the authors show that during organogenesis capsular Sf1-negative cells give rise to radial stripes of differentiated cortical cells [28, 29]. Importantly, similar capsular to cortex lineage was observed when tamoxifen was administered to adult mice, arguing for residence of adult stem cells in the adrenal capsule.

Results from these publications suggest two different models of cell lineage in adrenal development. The results reported by Zubair et al. support a model in which the Sf1-positive fetal zone gives rise to all cells of the Sf1-positive definitive zone. King et al. posits a dual-lineage model in which the cortex is derived primarily from Shh-positive/Sf1-positive fetal adrenal cells. A secondary lineage, which is substantiated by the experiments of Huang et al., is from *Gli1*-expressing capsular cells. Similarly, in the adult gland, Shh-positive/Sf1-positive subcapsular cells can give rise to differentiated cells of the cortex. While it is probable that these cells are progenitor cells, their origin has not been confirmed. It is most interesting that both in the embryo and in the adult, Sf1-negative/Gli1-positive capsular cells give rise to cortical cells. It is reasonable to propose that *Shh*-expressing subcapsular cells signal to *Gli1*-expressing capsular cells to activate these cells to replenish the cortex.

In summary, while the presence of stem cells and progenitor cells in the adrenal capsule and subcapsular region is being substantiated in lineage tracing experiments, more studies will be necessary to verify the homeostatic regulation of these cells in the adult gland.

17.3 What Factors Regulate Adrenal Adult Stem and Progenitor Cells?

17.3.1 Dax1

A number of factors have emerged as critical mediators of adrenocortical growth and differentiation and have been predicted to play a role in adrenocortical stem and progenitor cell biology. In the adult adrenal gland, Dax1 (Dosage-sensitive sex reversal-adrenal hypoplasia congenita critical region on X chromosome gene 1) is enriched in the subcapsular region [31, 32]. Human patients with DAX1 deficiency classically present with adrenal insufficiency due to histologic adrenal hypoplasia [33, 34]. However, there is some evidence that this presentation may be preceded by a period of hyperfunction [35, 36]. This paradoxical hyperfunction is also evident in mice lacking Dax1 in which the pronounced early adrenocortical hyperfunction is consistent with the Dax1-mediated repression of Sf1-dependent adrenocortical steroidogenesis (differentiation) [37]. *Dax1* transcription is activated by Sf1 in cooperation with Wnt signaling (peripheral adrenocortical cells) and glucocorticoids (differentiated steroidogenic cells of the fasciculata) [38, 39]. Parenthetically, the data from the Morohashi and Parker labs indicate that Dax1 may also be responsible for repressing the FAdE activity during the transition from fetal to adult cortex [23]. Taken together, these observations suggest that in the adrenal cortex Dax1 maintains multipotency of adrenal progenitor cells in part by suppressing Sf1-induced differentiation. This paradigm has recently been extended to the mouse embryonic stem (mES) cells in which *Dax1* is activated by LRH1 and subsequently expressed at high levels, and where knock-down of this gene results in increased differentiation, suggesting an important for Dax1 in maintenance of pluripotency [40, 41].

17.3.2 Shh

In the adult mouse, *Shh* is expressed primarily in the subcapsular region of the adrenal and *Gli1* is expressed primarily in the capsule [28–30]. As discussed above, results using temporal activation of *cre* and expression of *Shh-LacZ* or *Gli1-LacZ* demonstrate that in the adult adrenal both subcapsular (Shh) and capsular (Gli1) cells give rise to differentiated cells of the adrenal cortex [28, 29]. Targeted knock-out of *Shh* in *Sf1*-expressing cells of the mouse results in small adrenals with a thin capsule and cortex [28–30]. Because the adrenal forms in the absence of Shh, these results argue for a role of Shh in maintaining a pool of progenitor cells necessary to develop or maintain the normal architecture. It could be postulated that Shh in the subcapsular region signals to the capsule, activating Gli1 to stimulate stem cells to maintain the progenitor pool.

17.3.3 Wnt/β-Catenin

The Wnt/β-catenin signaling pathway has been shown to play a role in embryonic development, stem cell maintenance, and cell fate in a number of tissues [42, 43]. Activating mutations in β-catenin have been found in a number of cancers. (see Chapter 16) Activation of the canonical Wnt/β-catenin signaling pathway occurs upon binding of one of the Wnt ligands to the Frizzled (Fzd) cell surface receptor. In the absence of Wnt ligands, β-catenin is sequestered in a cytoplasmic complex with APC (adenomatous polyposis coli), Axin, and GSK3β, where it is maintained in a phosphorylated state and targeted for ubiquitin-mediated degradation. Upon activation of Frizzled receptor, the complex is disrupted and cellular levels of non-phosphorylated/activated β-catenin are increased. Increased cytoplasmic β-catenin results in increased nuclear β-catenin and target gene activation. Early in development of the wild-type mouse, β-catenin is expressed in the fetal cortex, but by day E18.5 it is restricted to the subcapsular region. Mice with knockout (KO) of β-catenin, directed specifically to *Sf1*-expressing cells, display adrenocortical aplasia [44]. Careful examination of embryonic stages of these KO mice revealed that *Sf1*-expressing cells and a developing adrenal are seen early in embryogenesis (E12.5) but disappear by E16.5. Histological analyses of E16.5 KO mice embryos show a very small adrenal gland composed of capsule and medulla with little or no cortex. These results indicate that β-catenin is essential for proper adrenal development and point to a critical role for this signaling pathway in sustaining subcapsular progenitor cell multipotency and/or the ability of cells to differentiate to functional cortex [44]. The direct transcriptional activation of *Dax1* by β-catenin and Sf1 suggests that Dax1 is a critical mediator of Wnt action in the adrenal cortex.

17.3.4 IGF2

Insulin-like growth factors 1 and 2 are mitogens that exert their effects by binding to the dimeric/heterodimeric cell surface insulin receptors (IR)/IGF 1 receptor (IGF1R). Ligand binding to the IGF1R results in autophosphorylation of the receptor and activation of two dominant downstream signaling pathways, Ras/MEK/ERK and PI3K/AKT, which in turn induce target genes resulting in cell cycle activation [45]. In general, IGF2 has been portrayed as a key growth factor employed during early fetal development, with IGF1 endorsed as a regulator of postnatal growth maintenance (see Chapter 15). Indeed, infusion of IGF2 during embryogenesis results in a marked increase in adrenocortical growth [46]. Although IGF2 expression is 25-fold higher in the fetal adrenal cortex (both definitive and fetal cortex through 20 weeks) compared to the adult gland [47], it is restricted to the adrenal capsule of the postnatal adrenal (www.genepaint.org), predicting a role in organ homeostasis. Specifically, because IGF ligands along with FGF have been reported to be critical mediators of stem cell niche, these data and observations support a role for IGF2 in stem/progenitor cell maintenance [48].

17.3.5 Telomerase

Telomeres are the single-stranded hexameric repeats at the ends of chromosomes and function to ensure complete replication and prevent loss of genetic material during cell division (see Chapter 13). Telomerase is a ribonucleoprotein that is responsible for adding these repeats at the end of the replication process. Telomerase activity is necessary in proliferating cells, but is absent in normal resting cells. In the adult human adrenal gland the RNA component of telomerase is exclusively expressed under the capsule (www.genepaint.org), consistent with this rapidly amplifying progenitor cell population. The requirement of telomerase for maintenance of stem cells is inferred by its role in maintaining cells in a proliferative state and preventing the onset of senescence or apoptosis.

17.4 How Do Normal Adrenal Cells Become Cancer Cells/or How Is Adrenocortical Carcinoma Initiated?

A few studies have examined the clonality of the human adrenocortical tumors by PCR-based analysis of X-chromosome inactivation in heterologous female tissue (see Chapter 9). While ACAs have been found to be of either monoclonal or polyclonal origin, carcinomas have uniformly been found to be monoclonal in origin (3 of 3 and 4 of 4 informative samples) [49, 50]. This strongly suggests that most, if not all, ACCs are initiated by a single mutation. Whether familial or sporadic, a single cell (after additional mutational events) acquires the ability to proliferate autonomously and ultimately undergo neoplastic transformation. However, there are no clear data that identify the origin of this initiating cell. As depicted in Fig. 17.2, such mutations might occur in adult stem cells, progenitor cells, or even differentiated cells. While stem or progenitor cells alone display active proliferation and would be predicted to acquire autonomous growth potential, differentiated cells would be expected to acquire multiple alterations before attaining the proliferative capacity and multipotency needed for tumor development.

It is reasonable to expect that mutations in genes involved in maintenance of stem cell properties are critical for the transformation process, and that these mutations may confer the autonomous proliferative capacity that results in tumorigenesis. Thus, to define the mutations that may initiate ACC, it is helpful to compare genes that exhibit robust expression in ACC with those that play significant roles in maintenance of multipotency of normal stem/progenitor cells.

17.4.1 Wnt/β-Catenin

Alterations in the Wnt/β-catenin signaling pathway have been implicated in a variety of cancers, including colon cancers, gastric cancer, hepatocarcinoma, medulloblastoma, melanoma, ovarian cancer, pancreatic cancer, and prostate cancer [51–53]. The most frequently observed alterations in this pathway are mutations in either β-catenin or one of its protein-binding partners, *Axin, APC* or *GSKβ3*. These mutations prevent phosphorylation or phosphorylation-dependent degradation of β-catenin, resulting in stabilization of β-catenin and thereby significantly higher expression. Familial adenomatous polyposis (FAP) is a hereditary disorder that is characterized by mutations in the APC gene, which result in a truncated and/or non-functional APC protein [54, 55]. Patients with this disorder typically present with multiple colonic polyps and ultimately develop colonic cancer [56]. These patients also have increased risks of other cancers including pancreatic and thyroid. In addition, there is an increased risk for the development of benign ACAs (see Chapters 10 and 16) [57, 58].

Predicated on the known role of APC in the regulation of the canonical Wnt signaling pathway in tissue development and homeostasis, a number of laboratories have analyzed the status of β-catenin in sporadic adrenocortical tumors. The Bertherat laboratory reported an increase in the nuclear/cytoplasmic ratio of β-catenin in sporadic ACC [59]. When examining a panel of ACC samples for stabilization of β-catenin, Giordano et al. observed a subset of carcinoma samples with strong nuclear accumulation of β-catenin indicative of active signaling. When compared to carcinomas with only membranous β-catenin staining, carcinomas with enhanced nuclear β-catenin staining have marked upregulation of classical β-catenin-mediated transcription targets. Because stabilizing β-catenin mutations are also observed in benign ACAs, such activation of Wnt signaling, while potentially an initiating mutation, is probably not sufficient to induce ACC [60].

To further test the hypothesis that active β-catenin signaling may initiate adrenocortical carcinogenesis, Berthon et al. generated transgenic mice with constitutively active β-catenin targeted specifically to adrenocortical cells [61]. By crossing mice that harbor the *Ctnnb1*$^{lox(ex3)}$ gene with mice that express cre-recombinase under control of an aldo-keto reductase promoter (*0.5 akr1b7;Cre*), they were able to express a truncated β-catenin restricted to the steroidogenic cells of the adrenal cortex. (The exon 3 truncated β-catenin protein lacks the serine/threonine targets of GSK3β phosphorylation and thereby avoids the degradation pathway and remains stable and active [62]). Heterozygous offspring of this cross express the truncated protein in the adrenal, but not in other tissues tested, and display elevated Axin2 levels, consistent with activated β-catenin. Whereas adrenal β-catenin is restricted to the subcapsular region in the wild-type mice, 5-month-old mutant mice have β-catenin scattered throughout the cortex and in clusters of cells at the cortical/medullary boundary. By 10 months of age larger areas of the cortex and most of the central adrenal express β-catenin. While the effects vary between animals and, curiously, are more dramatic in females than males, certain conclusions are clear. Mice expressing constitutively active β-catenin in the adrenals exhibit adrenal hyperplasia (hyperproliferation) and dysplasia, with aberrant cells and disruption of normal adrenal architecture. By 10 months of age, Sf1 expression is found in the region of the medulla. Adrenals from these mice also show decreased differentiation into fasciculata cells (assessed by *Akr1b7* expression) and increased differentiation of the zona glomerulosa (as assessed by *Cyp11b2* expression), with glomerulosa cells expanded into the fasciculata region. Most importantly, when compared with wild-type mice, both 5- and 10-month-old mutant mice exhibit increased Vegf expression and vascularization. By 17 months, 2 of 9 females examined had large masses with features of malignant tumors. Interestingly, one of the tumors had very low *Sf1* expression and was highly proliferative, prompting the authors to suggest it may derive from undifferentiated cells.

These results, taken together with the elevated nuclear β-catenin seen in many ACCs, suggest that canonical Wnt signaling regulates the proliferation and undifferentiated state of adrenocortical stem/progenitor cells.

17.4.2 IGF2

IGF2 is the most upregulated gene in most studies of human ACC (comparing malignant with benign adrenal tumors) [63–66]. As discussed above, in normal mouse adrenal, this mitogen is highly expressed in the fetal adrenal cortex, but in the adult adrenal expression is low and restricted to the capsule (see Chapter 15). Patients with Beckwith-Wiedemann Syndrome (BWS), a rare embryonic overgrowth disorder, have defects in imprinting of the 11p15.5 region, resulting in high levels of IGF2 and low levels of the cell cycle inhibitor p57 and the noncoding RNA, *H19* [64, 67]. One of the defining characteristics of BWS is an increase in a variety of childhood cancers including ACC (see Chapter 14). Mouse models have also confirmed that overexpression of the *IGF2* gene results in a BWS-like syndrome that includes adrenal hyperplasia and cytomegaly [68, 69]. Furthermore, Zac1, a transcription factor that regulates embryonic growth presumably through its coordination of imprinting of a number of genes including *IGF2* [70], is restricted to the adrenal capsule (www.genepaint.org). *ZAC1* is one of the most downregulated gene in pediatric ACC [65]. As emerging data support the loss of imprinting of the *IGF2* locus in stem cells as a critical event in cancer initiation, these observations support a role of capsular IGF2 in the etiology of ACC and point to the IGF signaling pathway as a viable target for ACC therapy. Indeed, recent preclinical and early phase I clinical trials indicate that monoclonal antibodies or small molecule inhibitors of the IGF1R are effective in blocking IGF signaling in ACC cells and effectively inhibits tumor growth in model systems and in select patients [71, 72].

17.4.3 Pod1

Pod1, also known as Tcf21, capsulin, and epicardin, is a basic HLH transcription factor involved in mesodermal development [73, 74]. Pod1 has been shown both in cell culture and in a mutant mouse model to suppress Sf1 action and is predicted to maintain the pool of Sf1-negative Leydig and adrenal stem/progenitor cells [75, 76]. Interestingly, a recently published expression data set of ACC tissue samples revealed a marked downregulation of POD1 at 6q23 in ACCs vs. benign ACAs and normal adrenal tissue [60]. A potential pathogenic role of *Pod1* loss is supported by recent observations that forced *Sf1* overexpression can induce adrenocortical subcapsular tumor formation in mice and that increased SF1 levels in pediatric ACC is correlated with a more aggressive tumor phenotype [77].

17.4.4 p53/Telomerase

Although discussed in detail in a different chapter in this book (see Chapter 13), it is important to discuss the telomere/telomerase system. The adrenocortical dysplasia mouse (*acd*) has been a valuable mouse model system to explore the involvement of telomere integrity in adrenocortical development and tumorigenesis. As the name implies, the *acd* mouse exhibits anatomic adrenal dysplasia and functional adrenal failure. The adrenal glands in the *acd* mutant mice display an abnormal morphology, often with no distinct boundary between cortex and medulla and are somewhat reminiscent of the adrenal gland of *DAX1* mutant human patients [78]. It can be speculated that cytomegaly and the other observed morphological changes may represent a common endpoint of stem cell failure, resulting in an inability to maintain organ homeostasis over the lifespan of the organism.

The gene responsible for the adrenal dysplasia mouse phenotype (and thus monikered acd) is the ortholog of the human *ACD/TPP1*, a gene that codes for a component of the telomere cap complex. As discussed earlier, telomeres, together with the telomere cap complex, are critical for protecting the ends of chromosomes and ensuring complete replication of the coding sequences. The ribonucleoprotein telomerase functions to maintain telomere length and integrity [79]. Normal cells lack active telomerase and with each successive division telomeres shorten, eventually leading to senescence or apoptosis. In contrast, telomerase is activated in 90%

of cancers, ensuring genomic stability of a malignant clone and gaining independence from telomere-induced crisis, senescence, or apoptosis [80]. As disruption of the telomere cap complex results in cellular programs (e.g., crisis, senescence, or apoptosis) that promote non-proliferative states, one can speculate that this may in fact be one cause of the abnormalities seen in the *acd* mutant mouse.

De-protected telomeres can be detected by the cellular DNA surveillance machinery. The tumor suppressor gene, *p53*, is a critical component of the DNA repair and senescence pathway. Crossing the *acd* mutant mouse with the *p53* null mouse resulted in rescue of adrenal senescence and overall dysplasia. Most interestingly, the *acd* mutation in combination with *p53* loss (when compared with *p53* loss alone) caused significant increase in tumor formation and decrease in tumor-free survival.

The clinical association between *p53* and ACC is found in Li-Fraumeni syndrome, a rare autosomal dominant condition that is characterized by early (<45 years) onset of any of a variety of malignancies. The most prominent cancers seen in affected families are breast, brain, acute leukemia soft tissue sarcomas, bone sarcomas, and ACC (refer to Chapter 11 and 12). Moreover, the majority of sporadic ACCs also display mutations in the tumor-suppressor gene, *p53*. However, mutations in or loss of *p53* is the most common mutation in all human cancer accounting for half of all sporadic cancer cases [81]. Nevertheless, taken together these data suggest that mutations that affect genes involved in telomere maintenance together with checkpoint deficiency, such as absence of p53, can be contributing events in adrenocortical tumorigenesis [82].

17.5 How Is Adrenocortical Carcinoma Maintained: Cancer Stem Cell or Stochastic Model?

To develop effective therapies for any cancer it will be helpful to know, for the particular cancer type, whether a cancer stem cell or stochastic model applies, or more precisely, the percentage of cells with proliferative potential (stem/progenitor cells) vs. differentiated and non-dividing cells in the tumor. If marked genetic heterogeneity within a tumor is prominent with multiple clones exhibiting proliferative potential, it would be predicted to be necessary to kill all cells of a tumor. If a neoplasia is sustained by rare cancer stem cells, only those rare cells might need to be targeted. Unfortunately, these cancer stem cells (quiescent and slowly self-renewing) are also predicted to be more resistant to standard chemotherapeutic protocols (that target rapidly amplifying "progenitor" cells) and will necessitate development of innovative target therapies [3]. Thus, for ACC, as for other malignancies, it will be valuable to discover whether all cells are endowed with the ability to self-renew or whether maintenance and metastasis depend on rare cancer stem cells. A third possibility is that both models are operative in different cancers and different patients.

Identification of cancer stems cells has taken advantage of the presence of unique cell surface makers present on cancer stem cells that allow the cells to be sorted (in vitro) and studied in xenograft models in immunocompromised mice (in vivo) [4, 83]. In the absence of known cell surface markers, investigators have employed a technique that capitalizes on the multidrug resistance characteristic of multipotent cells. Cells with this property are equipped with a membrane pump that can remove a foreign dye from their cytosol. In this method, cells are treated with Hoeschst dye 33342 followed by FACS (Fluorescence Activated Cell Sorting). Those cells that exclude the dye are considered to be progenitor cells with multidrug resistance and dubbed the "side population" [84, 85]. For example, this technique has been used to isolate a "side population" of neuroblastoma cells, which have enhanced tumorigenic potential [86]. Lichtenauer et al. have used this method to isolate distinct side populations of cells from ACA, ACC, and ACC cell lines in culture [87]. The side population was a rare population accounting for an extremely low percentage of the cells in the cancer (<1% in carcinomas and <3% in adenomas and tissue culture cell lines). Examination of the NCI-H295 side population confirmed that this subpopulation of cells expressed lower levels of adrenal differentiation markers and higher levels of the multidrug resistance gene. However, the NCI-H295 side population cells did not show differences in growth potential and resistance to cytotoxic drugs compared to the non-gated (non-side population) cells. Furthermore, after some time in culture, secondary FACS analyses resulted in a similar side population. While arguing against the existence of cancer stem cells in adrenocortical tumors, the study does not rule out the possibility. Most importantly, however, the data indicate that the side populations of the H295 cell lines do not constitute rare cells with proliferative potential [85]. As such studies have not been performed with cells isolated from ACC patients, it remains unclear if such a population is a major contributor to ACC initiation and or maintenance.

17.6 Summary

Much progress has been made in the past 10 years in defining the molecular development of the adrenal cortex and the role of various signaling pathways in the developmental lineage of the gland. Current data suggest that the capsular/subcapsular stem cells are critical components of the functional unit of the adrenal cortex. Perturbation of genetic pathways known to control this unit results in hypoplasia and cancer. Questions that remain include: What is the origin of Sf1-negative adrenocortical stem cells embedded within capsule? Does adrenal cancer originate from a normal stem cell, progenitor cell, or differentiated adrenocortical cell that assumes stem cell characteristics? Does ACC fit a cancer stem cell model, stochastic heterogeneous multiple clone model or both? Answers to these questions are predicted to glean new insights into the pathophysiology of ACC and lead to exciting new targets for therapy.

References

1. Dick JE (2003) Breast cancer stem cells revealed. Proc Natl Acad Sci U S A 100(7): 3547–3549
2. Reya T et al (2001) Stem cells, cancer, and cancer stem cells. Nature 414(6859):105–111
3. Dalerba P et al (2007) Cancer stem cells: models and concepts. Annu Rev Med 58:267–284
4. Lobo NA et al (2007) The biology of cancer stem cells. Annu Rev Cell Dev Biol 23:675–699
5. Shackleton M et al (2009) Heterogeneity in cancer: cancer stem cells versus clonal evolution. Cell 138(5):822–829
6. Ailles LE, Weissman IL (2007) Cancer stem cells in solid tumors. Curr Opin Biotechnol 18(5):460–466
7. Quintana E et al (2008) Efficient tumour formation by single human melanoma cells. Nature 456(7222):593–598
8. Libe R et al (2007) Adrenocortical cancer: pathophysiology and clinical management. Endocr Relat Cancer 14(1):13–28
9. Bertherat J, Bertagna X (2009) Pathogenesis of adrenocortical cancer. Best Pract Res Clin Endocrinol Metab 23(2):261–271
10. Keegan CE, Hammer GD (2002) Recent insights into organogenesis of the adrenal cortex. Trends Endocrinol Metab 13(5):200–208
11. Kim AC, Hammer GD (2007) Adrenocortical cells with stem/progenitor cell properties: recent advances. Mol Cell Endocrinol 265–266:10–16
12. Luo X et al (1994) A cell-specific nuclear receptor is essential for adrenal and gonadal development and sexual differentiation. Cell 77(4):481–490
13. Sadovsky Y et al (1995) Mice deficient in the orphan receptor steroidogenic factor 1 lack adrenal glands and gonads but express P450 side-chain-cleavage enzyme in the placenta and have normal embryonic serum levels of corticosteroids. Proc Natl Acad Sci U S A 92(24):10939–10943
14. Schnabel CA et al (2003) Pbx1 is essential for adrenal development and urogenital differentiation. Genesis 37(3):123–130
15. James RG et al (2006) Odd-skipped related 1 is required for development of the metanephric kidney and regulates formation and differentiation of kidney precursor cells. Development 133(15):2995–3004
16. Katoh-Fukui Y et al (2005) Mouse Polycomb M33 is required for splenic vascular and adrenal gland formation through regulating Ad4BP/SF1 expression. Blood 106(5):1612–1620
17. Val P et al (2007) Adrenal development is initiated by Cited2 and Wt1 through modulation of Sf-1 dosage. Development 134(12):2349–2358
18. Zubair M et al (2006) Two-step regulation of Ad4BP/SF-1 gene transcription during fetal adrenal development: initiation by a Hox-Pbx1-Prep1 complex and maintenance via autoregulation by Ad4BP/SF-1. Mol Cell Biol 26(11):4111–4121
19. Else T, Hammer GD (2005) Genetic analysis of adrenal absence: agenesis and aplasia. Trends Endocrinol Metab 16(10):458–468
20. Beuschlein F et al (2002) Steroidogenic factor-1 is essential for compensatory adrenal growth following unilateral adrenalectomy. Endocrinology 143(8):3122–3135
21. Pignatelli D et al (2002) Proliferation of capsular stem cells induced by ACTH in the rat adrenal cortex. Endocr Res 28(4):683–691
22. Ford JK, Young RW (1963) Cell proliferation and displacement in the adrenal cortex of young rats injected with tritiated thymidine. Anat Rec 146:125–137
23. Zubair M et al (2008) Developmental links between the fetal and adult zones of the adrenal cortex revealed by lineage tracing. Mol Cell Biol 28(23):7030–7040
24. Ingham PW, McMahon AP (2001) Hedgehog signaling in animal development: paradigms and principles. Genes Dev 15(23):3059–3087
25. Xie K, Abbruzzese JL (2003) Developmental biology informs cancer: the emerging role of the hedgehog signaling pathway in upper gastrointestinal cancers. Cancer Cell 4(4):245–247

26. Han YG et al (2008) Hedgehog signaling and primary cilia are required for the formation of adult neural stem cells. Nat Neurosci 11(3):277–284
27. Komada M et al (2008) Hedgehog signaling is involved in development of the neocortex. Development 135(16):2717–2727
28. King P et al (2009) Shh signaling regulates adrenocortical development and identifies progenitors of steroidogenic lineages. Proc Natl Acad Sci U S A 106(50):21185–21190
29. Huang CC et al (2010) Progenitor Cell Expansion and Organ Size of Mouse Adrenal Is Regulated by Sonic Hedgehog. Endocrinology 151(3):1119–1128
30. Ching S, Vilain E (2009) Targeted disruption of Sonic Hedgehog in the mouse adrenal leads to adrenocortical hypoplasia. Genesis 47(9):628–637
31. Muscatelli F et al (1994) Mutations in the DAX-1 gene give rise to both X-linked adrenal hypoplasia congenita and hypogonadotropic hypogonadism. Nature 372(6507):672–676
32. Kim AC et al (2009) In search of adrenocortical stem and progenitor cells. Endocr Rev 30(3):241–263
33. Phelan JK, McCabe ER (2001) Mutations in NR0B1 (DAX1) and NR5A1 (SF1) responsible for adrenal hypoplasia congenita. Hum Mutat 18(6):472–487
34. Zanaria E et al (1994) An unusual member of the nuclear hormone receptor superfamily responsible for X-linked adrenal hypoplasia congenita. Nature 372(6507):635–641
35. Peter M et al (1998) Congenital adrenal hypoplasia: clinical spectrum, experience with hormonal diagnosis, and report on new point mutations of the DAX-1 gene. J Clin Endocrinol Metab 83(8):2666–2674
36. Achermann JC et al (2000) Presymptomatic diagnosis of X-linked adrenal hypoplasia congenita by analysis of DAX1. J Pediatr 137(6):878–881
37. Babu PS et al (2002) Interaction between Dax-1 and steroidogenic factor-1 in vivo: increased adrenal responsiveness to ACTH in the absence of Dax-1. Endocrinology 143(2):665–673
38. Gummow BM et al (2003) Convergence of Wnt signaling and steroidogenic factor-1 (SF-1) on transcription of the rat inhibin alpha gene. J Biol Chem 278(29):26572–26579
39. Gummow BM et al (2006) Reciprocal regulation of a glucocorticoid receptor-steroidogenic factor-1 transcription complex on the Dax-1 promoter by glucocorticoids and adrenocorticotropic hormone in the adrenal cortex. Mol Endocrinol 20(11):2711–2723
40. Niakan KK et al (2006) Novel role for the orphan nuclear receptor Dax1 in embryogenesis, different from steroidogenesis. Mol Genet Metab 88(3):261–271
41. Khalfallah O et al (2009) Dax-1 knockdown in mouse embryonic stem cells induces loss of pluripotency and multilineage differentiation. Stem Cells 27(7):1529–1537
42. Logan CY, Nusse R (2004) The Wnt signaling pathway in development and disease. Annu Rev Cell Dev Biol 20:781–810
43. Blanpain C et al (2007) Epithelial stem cells: turning over new leaves. Cell 128(3):445–458
44. Kim AC et al (2008) Targeted disruption of beta-catenin in Sf1-expressing cells impairs development and maintenance of the adrenal cortex. Development 135(15):2593–2602
45. Samani AA et al (2007) The role of the IGF system in cancer growth and metastasis: overview and recent insights. Endocr Rev 28(1):20–47
46. Mesiano S et al (1993) Mitogenic action, regulation, and localization of insulin-like growth factors in the human fetal adrenal gland. J Clin Endocrinol Metab 76(4):968–976
47. Rainey WE et al (2002) The adrenal genetic puzzle: how do the fetal and adult pieces differ? Endocr Res 28(4):611–622
48. Bendall SC et al (2007) IGF and FGF cooperatively establish the regulatory stem cell niche of pluripotent human cells in vitro. Nature 448(7157):1015–1021
49. Beuschlein F et al (1994) Clonal composition of human adrenocortical neoplasms. Cancer Res 54(18):4927–4932
50. Gicquel C et al (1994) Clonal analysis of human adrenocortical carcinomas and secreting adenomas. Clin Endocrinol (Oxf) 40(4):465–477
51. Kikuchi A (2003) Tumor formation by genetic mutations in the components of the Wnt signaling pathway. Cancer Sci 94(3):225–229

52. Polakis P (2007) The many ways of Wnt in cancer. Curr Opin Genet Dev 17(1):45–51
53. Fodde R, Brabletz T (2007) Wnt/beta-catenin signaling in cancer stemness and malignant behavior. Curr Opin Cell Biol 19(2):150–158
54. Kinzler KW et al (1991) Identification of FAP locus genes from chromosome 5q21. Science 253(5020):661–665
55. Groden J et al (1991) Identification and characterization of the familial adenomatous polyposis coli gene. Cell 66(3):589–600
56. Fearnhead NS et al (2001) The ABC of APC. Hum Mol Genet 10(7):721–733
57. Naylor EW, Gardner EJ (1981) Adrenal adenomas in a patient with Gardner's syndrome. Clin Genet 20(1):67–73
58. Painter TA, Jagelman DG (1985) Adrenal adenomas and adrenal carcinomas in association with hereditary adenomatosis of the colon and rectum. Cancer 55(9):2001–2004
59. Tissier F et al (2005) Mutations of beta-catenin in adrenocortical tumors: activation of the Wnt signaling pathway is a frequent event in both benign and malignant adrenocortical tumors. Cancer Res 65(17):7622–7627
60. Giordano TJ et al (2009) Molecular classification and prognostication of adrenocortical tumors by transcriptome profiling. Clin Cancer Res 15(2):668–676
61. Berthon A et al (2010) Constitutive β-catenin activation induces adrenal hyperplasia and promotes adrenal cancer development. Hum Mol Genet 19(8):1561–1576
62. Harada N et al (1999) Intestinal polyposis in mice with a dominant stable mutation of the beta-catenin gene. EMBO J 18(21):5931–5942
63. Liu J et al (1995) H19 and insulin-like growth factor-II gene expression in adrenal tumors and cultured adrenal cells. J Clin Endocrinol Metab 80(2):492–496
64. Giordano TJ et al (2003) Distinct transcriptional profiles of adrenocortical tumors uncovered by DNA microarray analysis. Am J Pathol 162(2):521–531
65. West AN et al (2007) Gene expression profiling of childhood adrenocortical tumors. Cancer Res 67(2):600–608
66. Velazquez-Fernandez D et al (2005) Expression profiling of adrenocortical neoplasms suggests a molecular signature of malignancy. Surgery 138(6):1087–1094
67. Enklaar T et al (2006) Beckwith-Wiedemann syndrome: multiple molecular mechanisms. Expert Rev Mol Med 8(17):1–19
68. Sun FL et al (1997) Transactivation of Igf2 in a mouse model of Beckwith-Wiedemann syndrome. Nature 389(6653):809–815
69. Weber MM et al (1999) Postnatal overexpression of insulin-like growth factor II in transgenic mice is associated with adrenocortical hyperplasia and enhanced steroidogenesis. Endocrinology 140(4):1537–1543
70. Varrault A et al (2006) Zac1 regulates an imprinted gene network critically involved in the control of embryonic growth. Dev Cell 11(5):711–722
71. Barlaskar FM et al (2009) Preclinical targeting of the type I insulin-like growth factor receptor in adrenocortical carcinoma. J Clin Endocrinol Metab 94(1):204–212
72. Haluska P et al (2009) Safety, tolerability, and pharmacokinetics of the anti-IGF-1R monoclonal antibody figitumumab in patients with refractory adrenocortical carcinoma. Cancer Chemother Pharmacol 65(4):765–773
73. Lu J et al (1998) Capsulin: a novel bHLH transcription factor expressed in epicardial progenitors and mesenchyme of visceral organs. Mech Dev 73(1):23–32
74. Quaggin SE et al (1998) Pod-1, a mesoderm-specific basic-helix-loop-helix protein expressed in mesenchymal and glomerular epithelial cells in the developing kidney. Mech Dev 71(1–2):37–48
75. Cui S et al (2004) Disrupted gonadogenesis and male-to-female sex reversal in Pod1 knockout mice. Development 131(16):4095–4105
76. Tamura M et al (2001) Pod-1/Capsulin shows a sex- and stage-dependent expression pattern in the mouse gonad development and represses expression of Ad4BP/SF-1. Mech Dev 102 (1–2):135–144

77. Doghman M et al (2007) Increased steroidogenic factor-1 dosage triggers adrenocortical cell proliferation and cancer. Mol Endocrinol 21(12):2968–2987
78. Keegan CE et al (2005) Urogenital and caudal dysgenesis in adrenocortical dysplasia (acd) mice is caused by a splicing mutation in a novel telomeric regulator. Hum Mol Genet 14(1):113–123
79. Bianchi A, Shore D (2008) How telomerase reaches its end: mechanism of telomerase regulation by the telomeric complex. Mol Cell 31(2):153–165
80. Deng Y et al (2008) Telomere dysfunction and tumour suppression: the senescence connection. Nat Rev Cancer 8(6):450–458
81. Ljungman M (2000) Dial 9-1-1 for p53: mechanisms of p53 activation by cellular stress. Neoplasia 2(3):208–225
82. Else T (2009) Telomeres and telomerase in adrenocortical tissue maintenance, carcinogenesis, and aging. J Mol Endocrinol 43(4):131–141
83. Dick JE (2008) Stem cell concepts renew cancer research. Blood 112(13):4793–4807
84. Goodell MA et al (1996) Isolation and functional properties of murine hematopoietic stem cells that are replicating in vivo. J Exp Med 183(4):1797–1806
85. Lichtenauer UD, Beuschlein F (2009) The tumor stem cell concept-implications for endocrine tumors? Mol Cell Endocrinol 300(1–2):158–163
86. Hirschmann-Jax C et al (2004) A distinct "side population" of cells with high drug efflux capacity in human tumor cells. Proc Natl Acad Sci U S A 101(39):14228–14233
87. Lichtenauer UD et al (2008) Side population does not define stem cell-like cancer cells in the adrenocortical carcinoma cell line NCI h295R. Endocrinology 149(3):1314–1322

Chapter 18
Adrenocortical Cell Lines

Jeniel Parmar, Anita Kulharya, and William Rainey

Initially, primary cultures of adrenocortical cells have traditionally been utilized to study the mechanisms controlling adrenocortical steroidogenesis. However, the eventual onset of senescence in culture creates a recurring need for the costly and difficult isolation of fresh cultures, and subsequently increases the risk of contamination. For these reasons, the use of primary cultures has been increasingly replaced by immortalized cell lines. This chapter describes the major adrenocortical cell lines that are available for the study of physiologic and pathologic adrenocortical functions. Adrenocortical cell lines that have been derived from adrenal tumors which have developed spontaneously or experimentally from a variety of species will be discussed. These in vitro models have allowed a multitude of studies that have broadened our understanding of normal adrenocortical endocrine function as well as the properties of adrenal tumor cells.

The adrenal gland is an integral part of the endocrine system, as it regulates essential physiological functions in all vertebrates. It is noteworthy, however, that considerable variations exist with regard to the anatomical locations of the adrenal gland and its significance as an endocrine organ among different animals. In mammals, the adrenal gland is subdivided into two different compartments, the outermost cortex and the innermost medulla. This division does not exist in amphibians or fish; in fact, adrenal cells of some fish are found within the kidneys, where they are collectively termed the "intrarenal" gland. During mammalian embryonic adrenocortical development, the adrenocortical mesenchymal cells originate from the coelomic cavity near the urogenital ridge. These cells go on to form first the adrenogonadal primordium, which is the precursor of the adrenal cortex and the somatic cells of the gonads. Later, the adrenocortical primordium separates to form the fetal adrenal gland, which becomes encapsulated by surrounding mesenchymal cells. With ongoing development, adrenal medullary cells start to migrate into

W. Rainey (✉)
Department of Physiology, Medical College of Georgia, 1120 15th Street Room CA3094, Augusta, GA 30912, USA
e-mail: wrainey@mail.mcg.edu

G.D. Hammer, T. Else (eds.), *Adrenocortical Carcinoma*,
DOI 10.1007/978-0-387-77236-3_18, © Springer Science+Business Media, LLC 2011

the fetal adrenal gland, eventually forming the adrenal medulla. In a last step the adult adrenal cortex arises with its classical zonation and the fetal adrenal cortex regresses.

The histologic zonation of the cortex in three functionally distinct regions (zona glomerulosa, zona fasciculata, and zona reticularis) was first described by Arnold in 1866 [1]. For all adrenocortical steroidogenesis, the rate-limiting step is the translocation of cholesterol from the outer mitochondrial membrane into the mitochondrion for cholesterol side-chain cleavage by the cytochrome P450 CYP11A1, the first enzyme in the steroidogenic pathway (Fig. 18.1) [2].

In the zona glomerulosa cholesterol is used to synthesize mineralocorticoids in response to angiotensin II (ANG II) and potassium (K^+) stimulation (Fig. 18.1). In the zona fasciculata cholesterol is used for glucocorticoid synthesis under the regulation of ACTH. In humans, the zona reticularis metabolizes cholesterol to 19-carbon (C_{19}) steroids, including DHEA and DHEA-sulfate, a process that is regulated by ACTH and yet-to-be determined factors. There is no physical barrier separating the three different adrenocortical zones. The molecular mechanisms that cause the zone-specific expression pattern of these enzymes are yet to be resolved. However, it has been established that these regulatory mechanisms control the relative expression of

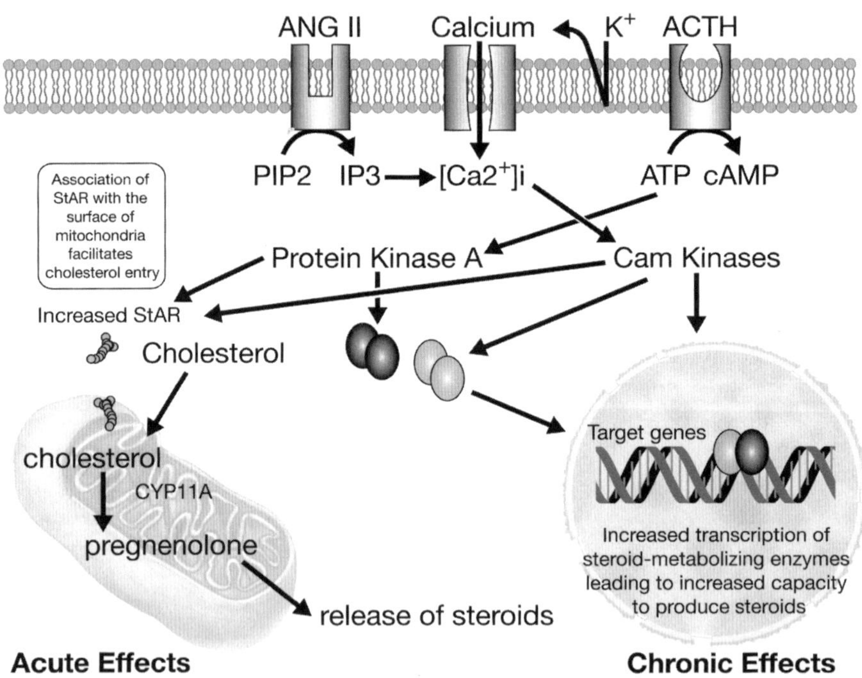

Fig. 18.1 Intracellular adrenocortical cell signaling and mechanisms leading to adrenocortical steroid synthesis upon stimulation with the physiological agonists Ang II, K^+, and ACTH

the enzymes required for steroidogenesis as well as the size and structural integrity of each of the zones.

There are still numerous molecular and cellular studies needed to better define the mechanisms regulating adrenal cell steroid production, prompting the need for further studies both in vivo and in vitro. Appropriate, well-characterized adrenal model systems are critical for these studies. Initially, primary cultures of adrenocortical cells proved useful for examining the mechanisms controlling many aspects of adrenal physiology. However, several issues limit the use of primary adrenal cell culture models, including cell growth in culture, responses to agonists and maintenance of steroidogenic capacity. It is well documented that the ability of primary adrenocortical cultures and cell lines to produce steroids and/or to respond to ACTH, ANG II, and K^+ can change over time. The expression of the enzymes involved in steroid hormone biosynthesis can also change under in vitro culture conditions. As a result, the steroids produced by cells in culture can be quite different from those produced in vivo. Perhaps, the most practical limitation to the use of primary adrenocortical cell cultures is the constant requirement for freshly acquired tissue and the difficulties associated with the isolation of cortical cells in the numbers needed to accomplish in vitro studies. Taken together the problems and limitations of primary cultures have caused many groups to attempt the use of adrenocortical tumors cells as model systems. Moreover, these cell lines can be used in xenotransplant models and in vitro studies to research adrenocortical carcinoma (ACC). A number of in vitro tumor cell models have been investigated, including cell suspensions from acutely dispersed adrenal tumors, [3, 4, 5], established cell lines from tumors [6, 7, 8, 9], and the isolation of immortalized cells from transgenic animals [10, 11, 12, 13]. Herein, we provide a summary of the adrenocortical cell lines and provide some information as to their development and utility.

18.1 Human Adrenocortical Cell Lines

18.1.1 The NCI-H295, NCI-H295R, and NCI-H295A Adrenocortical Carcinoma Cell Lines

18.1.1.1 Origin and Development

The NCI-H295 cell line was established from a female patient diagnosed with an ACC [6]. A large 14 × 13 × 11 cm adrenocortical invasive tumor was detected by CT imaging and was later reported to have metastasized to the lungs and liver. In the initial process of developing the original NCI-H295 cell line, the tumor tissue was finely minced, defragmented, and maintained in various serum-containing and serum-free culture media for a 1-year period [6]. Monoclonal cell lines were not established and, therefore, the NCI-H295 cell line represents a mixed population of tumor cells from the original ACC (Table 18.1).

Table 18.1 Summary of information on adrenocortical cell lines

Cell Line Name	Species	Ang II	K⁺	ACTH	cAMP	Steroids produced	References
NCI-H295		ND	ND	–	ND	Mineralocorticoids Glucocorticoids Adrenal Androgens	[6]
NCI-H295A	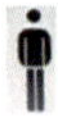	–	ND	–	+	Mineralocorticoids Glucocorticoids Adrenal Androgens	[14, 15]
NCI-H295R Strains	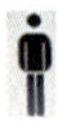	+	+	-/+	+	Mineralocorticoids Glucocorticoids Adrenal Androgens	[16–21]
RL-251	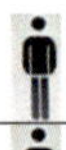	ND	ND	–	ND	None reported	[22]
ACT-1	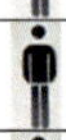	ND	ND	ND	ND	None reported	[23]
SW13	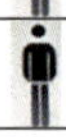	ND	ND	ND	ND	None reported	[24]
Pediatric adrenocortical adenoma derived cellline		ND	ND	ND	ND	Mineralocorticoids Glucocorticoids	[25]
Y1 and its mutant strains	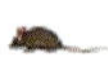	–	–	+	+	Progesterone metabolites	[26–30]
Rat adrenal cells: 2FASC and 7GLOM	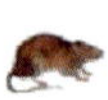	–	–	+	+	Progesterone metabolites	[13, 31]
Rat adrenocortical line: TRA	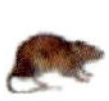	–	–	+	+	Progesterone metabolites	[32, 33]
Mouse adrenal cell-lines: ATC1 and ATC7-L	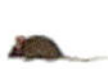	–	ND	+	+	Glucocorticoids	[34]
Immortalized mouse adrenal cell lines: AcA201, AcE60 and AcA101	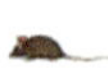	–	–	–	+	Progesterone metabolites	[12]

Table 18.1 (continued)

Immortalized mouse adrenal cell lines: ST2, ST5-R, and ST5-L	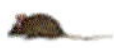	ND	ND	–	+	Progesterone metabolites	[11]
Immortalized mouse adrenal cell line ST5Lc	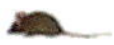	ND	ND	–	+	Progesterone metabolites and Glucocorticoids	[35]
SBAC and other Bovine Adrenocortical Cell Lines	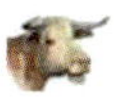	+	ND	–	+	None reported	[36]

Abbreviation: ND, Not determined

18.1.1.2 Cell Line Growth and Characterization

Since parental NCI-H295 cells sustained a slow rate of growth in the initially described culture media, alternative growth conditions were sought in order to segregate a population of cells with better attachment and growth. Initially, the cell culture medium growth supplement, Ultroser G, a relatively defined bovine-derived serum substitute, was used to increase cell growth rate. Previous assessments of this media supplement reported increased adrenal cell growth and retention of steroidogenic function [37, 38].

In an attempt to establish a superior cell model, the parental NCI-H295 cells were continuously flushed with fresh growth medium for a period of 3 months to deliberately remove the floating suspended cells and keep the viable attached subtype. The newly selected population of cells was subsequently designated as NCI-H295R to differentiate this strain from the original cells. NCI-H295R cells grow as an adherent monolayer. The population doubling time of the new NCI-H295R cells was approximately 2 days in comparison to the original parental NCI-H295 cell line, which grows in suspension and takes approximately 5 days to double in population. Unfortunately, the success of NCI-H295R was challenged by the limited availability of the Ultroser-G medium in select countries.

Consequently, a series of sera were tested in an attempt to develop a population of NCI-H295R cells that would grow in a relatively inexpensive commercial serum and retain ANG II and K^+ responsiveness. Growth of cells in DME/F12 medium supplemented with 5 % cosmic calf serum (CCS) (Hyclone, Logan, UT) was found to maintain cell growth and responsiveness to ANG II and K^+. Another strain of NCI-H295R cells was also selected to grow in commercially available Nu-Serum type I (10% – Collaborative Biomedical Products, Bedford, MA). This strain is available from the American Type Culture Collection as ATCC CRL-2128. These cells, however, have a decreased response to ANG II and K^+, though the cell doubling time is relatively similar to those grown in other sera. Since their first establishment, NCI-H295R cells have been cultured with variety of media in which they have shown a range of steroidogenic responses and adherent properties. As a result the agonist responses and growth characteristics of NCI-H295R cells vary depending on individual laboratory conditions.

As with NCI-H295R, a second population of the parental NCI-H295 cell line was selected to grow as a monolayer, yielding another strain of the original cell line [8], designated NCI-H295A. The method for isolation of the NCI-H295A strain was similar to that described for NCI-H295R, relying on the removal of non-attached cells with medium changes and, therefore, selecting a population of cells that grow as a monolayer.

18.1.1.3 Expression of Hormone Receptors and Hormonal Responsiveness

Although ANG II, K^+, and ACTH are the primary hormonal regulators of steroid hormone production in the human adrenal cortex (Fig. 18.1), there is no description of hormonal responsiveness in the original description of the NCI-H295 cells [6]. Subsequently, the responses to ANG II, K^+, and ACTH treatment, as well as expression of hormone receptors, were characterized for the NCI-H295R cell strain.

ANG II is the primary hormonal regulator within the renin-angiotensin-aldosterone system (RAAS); upon conversion from its precursor by angiotensin-converting enzyme, it acts on the adrenal glomerulosa by binding to type 1 ANG II (AT1) receptors to increase the production of aldosterone. NCI-H295R cells have proven to be a useful model to study ANG II-regulated aldosterone production. Only AT1 receptor antagonists have a significant inhibitory effect while type 2 ANG II (AT2) receptor antagonists have little impact on ANG II stimulation, demonstrating that NCI-H295R cells respond almost exclusively to the AT1 receptors [39, 40]. Subsequent studies also revealed AT1 receptor couple with phosphoinositidase C and increased production of inositol phosphates in NCI-H295R cells [16].

Circulating extracellular K^+ is the other major physiologic regulator of adrenal aldosterone production. An increase in intracellular calcium levels in response to elevated K^+ mediates an increase in aldosterone biosynthesis. In addition, there is evidence of an intra-adrenal renin/angiotensin system [41], in which K^+ stimulation increases the production of both ANG I and ANG II. The NCI-H295R cells are used by many laboratories as a model to study the mechanisms of K^+ regulation of adrenal steroid production [42–47].

ACTH is the primary hormonal regulator of adrenal cortisol production. The NCI-H295R cell line is only mildly responsive to ACTH, while most other adrenocortical cell lines are completely unresponsive [7]. ACTH treatment of NCI-H295R cells does cause an acute increase in aldosterone biosynthesis, though the cell line lacks long-term responsiveness [48]. The low response to ACTH is therefore a drawback of this cell model. Poor ACTH response is in part a reflection of low levels of ACTH receptor expression in the NCI-H295R cell, however, even after induction of receptor expression the cells still exhibit a poor response [49]. Since ACTH primarily regulates cortisol production through cAMP signaling, the addition of either forskolin (to activate adenylyl cyclase) or cAMP analogs [17, 20, 40, 50, 51] can be used to overcome this dilemma. An alternate strategy could involve the use of transgenic technology to reinstate ACTH receptor expression in the NCI-H295R cell line; however, attempts to do so have increased receptor expression but not response to ligand (unpublished observation). At present, investigations of ACTH responsiveness rely heavily on the mouse adrenal cell line Y1, which retains ACTH responsiveness [26].

18.1.1.4 Steroidogenesis

Most research focuses on adrenal production of aldosterone, cortisol, and DHEA for which the steroidogenic pathways are well defined (Fig. 18.2). After isolation and establishment of the parental NCI-H295, the cell line was found to produce an array of steroids, including those characteristic of the adrenal cortex and some unique to tumor cells. Primary assessment of steroidogenic capacity was performed using gas chromatography/mass spectroscopy (GCMS) and radioimmunoassay. Of a total of 30 different steroids reportedly synthesized and secreted by NCI-H295, approximately 20 were formally identified as known steroid hormones. The production of these steroids suggested the presence of all of the adrenocortical steroidogenic enzymes including CYP11A1, HSD3B2, CYP11B1, CYP21, CYP17, CYP11B2, and 3β-hydroxysulfotransferase. The NCI-H295R strain also maintains this steroidogenic profile; however, it is greatly influenced by serum conditions.

The ability of these cells to produce steroids that originate from multiple zones of the adrenal suggests that the NCI-H295R cell line remains pluripotent with regard to adrenocortical differentiation. These cells produce an array of steroids even under basal conditions [16, 51]. This is particularly important when one considers the difficulty in obtaining primary cultures of aldosterone-producing cells. It is noteworthy

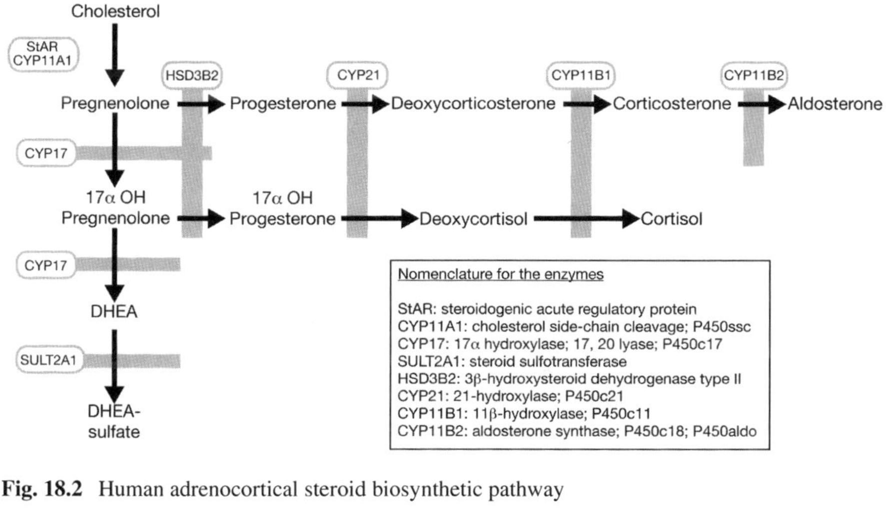

Fig. 18.2 Human adrenocortical steroid biosynthetic pathway

that treatment with agonists appears to selectively promote the synthesis of certain zone-specific steroid hormone groups in NCI-H295R [18, 39, 52]. For instance, production of aldosterone drastically increases following ANG II and K^+ stimulation, while treatment with forskolin induces cortisol, 11β-hydroxyandrostenedione, DHEA, DHEA-sulfate, corticosterone, 11-deoxycortisol, and androstenedione production [51]. While NCI-H295R cells do not represent a single zone of the adrenal cortex, the cell line provides ample flexibility for studies on adrenocortical steroidogenesis. As stated above, with a wide variety of effective agonists, a mosaic of unique steroid expression profiles are possible in NCI-H295R cells, thus making this cell line a potential model for steroid hormone biosynthesis in all adrenocortical zones [53–61].

18.1.1.5 Steroidogenic Enzyme Expression

The original NCI-H295 adrenocortical cells express all of the enzymes participating in normal human adrenal steroidogenesis [62–64]. Along with the parental NCI-H295, the NCI-H295R and NCI-H295A cell strains have also been used as genetic models for studying steroidogenic enzyme gene expression. Transcripts encoding *StAR*, as well as the five forms of cytochrome P450 known to be involved in normal adrenal steroidogenesis (*CYP11A1*, *CYP17*, *CYP21*, *CYP11B2*, and *CYP11B1*), are detectable in the NCI-H295R cell strains [16, 17, 19–21, 39, 40, 48, 50–52]. Moreover, as with primary cultures and other mammalian adrenal cells [65, 66], the levels of mRNA encoding *CYP17* and *HSD3B2* appear to be differentially regulated in NCI-H295R cells [16]. Furthermore, the transcripts encoding *CYP11B1* and *CYP11B2* enzymes are increased by treatment of NCI-H295R cells with activators of the protein kinase-A pathway, although the effect on *CYP11B1* mRNA levels is greater (Fig. 18.1). In addition, ANG II and K^+ cause a drastic increase in *CYP11B2* mRNA encoding aldosterone synthase [16, 21, 39, 67, 68].

The original NCI-H295 and its strains have proven to be useful models for defining the mechanisms controlling adrenocortical steroidogenesis. The basal promoter and enhancer elements of the genes encoding *CYP11B1*, *CYP11B2*, *CYP17*, and *HSD3B2* [8, 69, 70] together with the transcription factors mediating the expression of these genes have been studied in great detail using these cell lines [44, 57, 71–83].

18.1.1.6 NCI-H295 Cell Line As Adrenal Cancer Therapy Tool

In vitro cancer therapy screening represents an important mechanisms of drug testing [84]. The National Cancer Institute has made wide use of neoplasms and carcinoma cell lines for anticancer drug screening and drug discovery [85–88]. Below is a brief description of the use of the NCI-H295 and its substrains as model systems for the study cancer therapies.

NCI-H295 has been widely used as a model for screening anti-cancer drugs. Suramin, one of the first anti-cancer drugs tested in the NCI-H295 cells, reduced the production of glucocorticoids, mineralocorticoids, and adrenal androgens in this cell line [89]. Schteingart and colleagues screened mitotane and mitometh, two distinct anti-cancer drugs in NCI-H295. Mitotane strongly suppressed cell growth and mitometh was not effective [90]. Fallo et al. tested the cytotoxic/antiproliferation drugs, taxol and paclitaxel, which effectively exhibited dose-dependent inhibition of cellular growth and reduced steroidogenesis in NCI-H295 [91, 92]. Adrenostatic compounds aminoglutethimide, metyrapone, and etomidate were also tested in NCI-H295 for their antiproliferative property. Aminoglutethemide and etomidate inhibited cell proliferation and etomidate was much more potent [93]. Thiazolidinediones (TZDs) are specific peroxisome proliferator-activated receptor (PPAR)-gamma ligands. Examination in NCI-H295 suggest that TZDs might have favorable effects in the treatment of a variety of tumors as differentiation-inducing agents [94]. NCI-H295 cells have also been utilized to assess the role of certain interferons, chemokines, and growth factors in ACCs [22, 25 95]. Preclinical assessment of anticancer compounds with potent antiproliferative activity in NCI-295 cells is an essential first step before any clinical evaluation in phase I, II, and III programs could be commenced.

Recent studies have utilized NCI-H295 cells in cell culture and as a xenograft model to evaluate the efficacy of a variety of new potential targeted therapies. T-cell factor/β-catenin antagonists, PKF115-584 [96], and type I insulin-like growth factor receptor inhibitors have been recently tested in NCI-H295 [97]. These studies are aimed at a limited number of known genetic mutations in ACC that are present in the NCI-H295 cells.

18.1.2 Human Adrenocortical Carcinoma, Clone 15 (HAC15) Cell Line, and Related Clones

The above mentioned NCI-H295 cell line and its strains have proven useful due to the retention of ANG II-dependent aldosterone production. However, as previously discussed, they lack significant ACTH responsiveness. In addition, the NCI-H295 models are polyclonal, as they represent a mixture of cells isolated from primary cultures of the original tumor. In an attempt to develop a new human adrenocortical carcinoma (HAC) cell line, monoclonal populations of cells from an adrenal tumor were recently isolated [7]. Primary ACC cells were isolated and used to develop 47 discrete clones, six of which grew well enough for further characterization. Initially, the cells were maintained in DME/F12-based growth medium supplemented with 10% CCS, penicillin, streptomycin, gentamicin, and ITS+ Premix (a solution containing human recombinant insulin, human transferrin, selenious acid, BSA, and linoleic acid). Preliminary results suggested that ACTH stimulation increased cortisol production in two of the clones. The same clones also retained responsiveness to ANG II and K^+ through the production of aldosterone. Further analyses of these cells will judge whether they are an improvement over the currently available systems for the study of human adrenocortical steroid production.

18.1.3 Pediatric Adrenocortical Adenoma Derived Cell Line

18.1.3.1 Origin and Development

Primary ACA cells were isolated from a non-hemorrhagic region of a functional tumor from a 1-year-old female that presented with virilization and Cushing's syndrome [25]. This pediatric adrenocortical cell line was last reported to have sustained growth and viability after eight passages. Sections of tumor were initially fragmented and subjected to collagenase digestion. Fine tumor fragments were then segregated and plated in two different media; DMEM and Opti-MEM 1 (reduced serum medium of MEM) and supplemented with 10% and 2% fetal bovine serum (FBS) and 1% penicillin/streptomycin maintained under standard culture conditions (37°C in 95% air 5% CO_2).

18.1.3.2 Growth and Steroidogenesis

The cell line initially grew at a slow rate with a spindle-like morphology in both of the media. As with the HAC15 cell line, a flattened homogeneous morphology, characteristic of a single cell type origin was noted. Melan-A, a melanocytic differentiation marker, which is expressed in steroid hormone producing adrenal adenomas and carcinomas [98], was seen in all examined cells. All steroidogenic studies were performed during the fifth passage in medium from 5 day experiments. Biosynthesis of cortisol, aldosterone, androstenedione, and 17-OH progesterone were observed along with the expression of steroidogenic enzymes namely *HSD3B2, CYP11B1, and CYP21.*

Taking into consideration that this newly developed pediatric cell line has last reported to have only reached eight passages, the likelihood of the cell line's viability remains to be established. As these cells are part of a mixed tumor cell population, further clonal selection may be necessary.

18.1.4 The SW13 Human Adrenal Carcinoma Derived Cell Line

Although adrenal in origin, SW13 cells produce no steroids and it is unclear whether the cell line was derived from steroidogenic adrenal cells. These cells were derived from a human ACC [24] and are available from the American Type Culture Collection (CCL-105). The SW13 is an interesting cell culture model that has a mosaic pattern of vimentin expression and is deficient in the mammalian homologs of Brahma genes, *Brm* and *BRG1* [99]. Due to the lack of steroidogenesis, its usefulness as an adrenocortical model system is limited.

18.1.5 The ACT-1 Human Adrenal Carcinoma Derived Cell Line

Tumor cells were isolated from a 62-year-old male who was initially diagnosed with a left ACC. After surgical removal of tumor tissue, aggregated pieces were excised, minced, and passed through a cell strainer to dissociate the cells. Cells were supplemented with 10% FBS, insulin-transferrin-selenium solution and appropriate antibiotics maintained at 5% CO_2 and 95% air. In its initial description, ACT-1 cells were only shown to express *HSD3B2* genes and were devoid of any adrenocortical steroids [23]. Hence, ACT-1 has limited adrenocortical function and therefore serves a restricted role for normal adrenal function. However, these cells may prove useful to screen adrenocortical carcinoma therapies.

18.1.6 The RL-251 Human Adrenal Carcinoma Derived Cell Line

An adrenocortical carcinoma was identified by CT scan in a 75-year-old male who presented with high blood pressure (219/107 mm Hg) and multiple spells of chills, warmth, sweating, and flushing. A 5 × 6 × 7 cm right adrenal mass was removed by laparotomy and placed in cell suspension. Initially, tumor sample was treated with collagenase and plated in fibronectin-coated plastic with RPMI 1640 medium containing 10% FBS and fibroblast growth factors, with a population doubling time of 36 h. As with NCI-H295R and HAC15 cell lines, RL251 also exhibits abnormal karyotypic profile with diploid karyotype consisting of numerous deletions and translocations. Assessments of adrenocortical function showed atypical steroidogenesis and hormonal response with insignificant cortisol production and no ACTH stimulation [22]. To date, there is no description of any other corticosteroid production by the RL251 cell line. Intriguingly, in its initial report, RL251 cells expressed ample amounts of interleukin-8, epithelial cell-derived neutrophil-activating peptide 78, growth-regulated oncogene-α, *and* growth-regulated oncogene-y. These are CXC chemokine family cytokines that have potent angiogenic activity essential for tumor growth. It is speculated that these chemokines may play a role in enhancement of carcinoma growth and proliferation by an autocrine or paracrine manner. A lack of reported steroidogenesis and hormonal responses do not make these cells an appropriate model to study normal adrenocortical function; however, these cells may prove useful in identifying the role of chemokines in ACCs.

18.1.7 Human Adrenal Cell Lines from Viral Oncogenes

Simian virus 40 (SV40) T-antigen is a hexamer protein that is an oncogene which is capable of transforming many cell types. SV40 T-antigen was used by Hornsby and colleagues to transform human fetal adrenal cells [100]. The strategy yielded human fetal adrenal cell clones that responded to cAMP with an increase in both CYP17 and CYP11A, but no change in CYP21 and CYP11B1. Transformed cells were maintained in culture for 30–40 population doublings after isolation, but then entered "crisis" and stopped dividing. The cause of this late passage "senescence" is the result of telomere shortening that occurs with each population doubling and is normally not corrected by SV40 expression [101].

18.2 Rodent Adrenocortical Cell Lines

18.2.1 The Y1 Adrenal Cell Line

Presumably following exposure to radiation during nuclear weapon testing, an adult LAF_1 (C57L x A/HeJ) mouse developed an adrenal tumor [102]. Gordon Sato and colleagues [103] adapted the transplantable tumor to grow in vitro by alternately propagating dispersed tumor cells as monolayer cultures and as tumors in mice. The most robust clones developed from the mixed population of tumor cells was named Y1, and it was this clone that was deposited at the American Type Culture Collection (ATCC CCL-79) [9] (see Table 18.1).

It is noteworthy that the major steroid pathways present in cultured Y1 cells are unlike the normal physiologic mouse adrenocortical steroid pathway. For instance, Y1 cells in culture produces 20α-hydroxy-Δ^4-pregnen-3-one (20α-dihydroxyprogesterone) and 11β,20α-dihydroxy-Δ^4-pregnen-3-one (11β,20α-dihydroxyprogesterone) [80, 104] (Fig. 18.3). This abnormal steroid profile relates to the deficiency in 21-hydroxylase (Cyp21) [105] coupled with an increase in 20α-hydroxysteroid dehydrogenase activity [106].

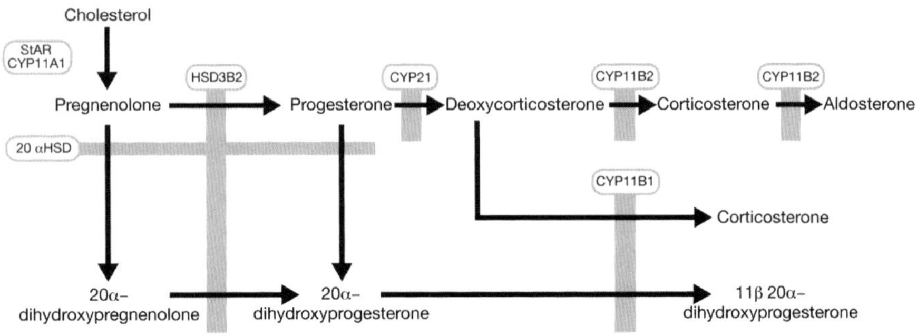

Fig. 18.3 Murine adrenocortical steroid biosynthetic pathway including modifications seen in some mouse cell lines

Y1 cells could be grown under a humidified atmosphere of 5% CO_2 and 95% air in a variety of growth media supplemented with serum. Doubling time for this cell line is merely 30–40 h [26, 107]. These cells grow in culture as flat, adherent cells with polyhedral shapes maintained by a network of stress fibers and focal adhesions near the cell surface. Upon stimulation with any of the cAMP-inducing agonists, Y1 cells retract their extended plasma membranes, become spherical with short processes, and detach easily from the substrate on which they are grown [9, 108–110].

The ability of ACTH to stimulate Y1 cell steroidogenic activity and enzymes is similar to that seen in primary mouse adrenal cells and other agents that raise intracellular levels of cAMP, for instance, genes encoding the ACTH receptor [49, 111], Cyp11a [112–115], Cyp11b1 [115–117], Star [114, 118, 119], adrenodoxin [112, 113], adrenodoxin reductase [112], and the HDL receptor (SR-BI) [120]. A wealth of information has been gained through studying this cell line and several of its subclones that have proved to be invaluable in assessing the roles of cAMP, protein kinase A, adenylyl cyclases, ACTH, and ACTH receptor in adrenocortical cell physiology. Y1 cells do not respond to ANG II, although transgene expression of the ANG II receptor in Y1 cells has been described [121].

18.2.2 Experimentally Induced Rodent Adrenal Cell Lines

Kirsten murine sarcoma virus (MSV) transforms cells resulting in reduced requirement for attachment, density and reliability of other cells in terms of growth and development. Auersperg et al. took primary cultures of rat adrenal cells in early passage and infected them with MSV and allowed them to overgrow the normal cell population [13, 32, 33, 122]. The clones exhibited little steroidogenic potential and only produced progesterone and 20α-dihydroxyprogesterone. Similarly, an adrenal cell line from rat zona glomerulosa cells [13] was created but found to produce negligible steroids (8 ng per 10^5 cells per 24 h), despite responsiveness to ACTH and cAMP agonists.

An SV40 T-antigen strategy was also attempted in the quest of developing immortal rodent cell lines. Several investigators established immortalized adrenal cell lines from adrenal tumors in mice carrying the Simian Virus 40 T-antigen as a transgene [11, 35, 123, 124]. Mellon et al. used a human *CYP11A* promoter to target expression of T-antigen to the adrenal cortex [11, 35] and generated adrenal tumors in female mice and used these tumors to establish cell lines. These cell lines were not responsive to either ANG II or ACTH and only produced progesterone following treatment with cAMP analogs. Progesterone was synthesized at a rate of 100 ng/μg of DNA per 24 h under stimulated conditions. Noteworthy, these cells reportedly produced renin-1 mRNA [35].

In terms of developing immortalized rodent adrenocortical cell lines, several others have utilized similar transgenic approaches such as the use of mouse inhibin α-subunit promoter to drive T-antigen expression to generate adrenal tumors [123, 124]. As with others, these cells only produced progesterone. Subsequently, another group used a strategy with mice bearing a transgene with a temperature-sensitive form of T-antigen under control of T-antigen promoter [12]. At the permissive temperatures, one group of cells expressed *Sf1, Cyp11a1, Star*, and *Cyp11b1*, suggesting that they were of fasciculata-reticularis origin. A second cell line expressed *Sf1, Cyp11a1*, and *Star* but not *Cyp11b1*, suggesting that they had lost differentiated function or were derived from an undifferentiated cell layer situated between the glomerulosa zone and the fasciculata zone. None of the cells were responsive to ACTH or ANG II and none of the cells expressed aldosterone synthase (*Cyp11b2*).

Perhaps, the most successful oncogene targeted mouse adrenocortical tumor cell lines are described and characterized by Ragazzon et al. [34]. Using genetically targeted oncogenesis, adrenocortical immortalized cell lines, ATC1 and ATC7-L, were developed. The *AKr1b7* gene promoter was used to drive the expression of SV40 T-antigen. The two cell lines were established from adrenal tumors of two transgenic mice harboring the large T-antigen of SV40. Both ATC1 and ATC7-L have retained a zona fasciculata phenotype, evident by their robust steroidogenic capacity, ACTH responsiveness, and expression profile of steroid-metabolizing genes. Both cell lines responded well to ACTH stimulation with a concentration-dependent increase in corticosterone production. Examination of hormone responsiveness revealed detectable levels of *Mc2r* and *Cyp21* mRNAs, but these transcripts were not responsive to ACTH in either cell line. By contrast, mRNA levels for *Srb1, Star, Cyp11a1, Cyp11b1*, and *Akr1b7* were strongly induced in a time-dependent manner by ACTH treatment, and these inductions were not abolished by the protein synthesis inhibitor, cycloheximide. The ATC cell lines represent novel in vitro models, maintaining differentiated endocrine functions of zona fasciculata. They may prove to be very useful in investigating the mechanisms of steroidogenic gene regulation in response to the physiological activator of glucocorticoid synthesis, ACTH.

18.3 Bovine Adrenocortical Cell Lines

In terms of primary cultures, due to the size and availability of bovine adrenals, bovine adrenocortical cells have remained a critical resource for the study of adrenocortical biology. Hornsby and colleagues have used SV40 to create a series of clonal bovine adrenal cell lines [36]. The introduction of SV40 greatly enhanced the lifespan of the cells in culture. A population of cells continued to respond to cAMP-related agonists by induction of *CYP17* and *CYP11A*. However, cellular expression of *CYP21* and *CYP11B* was found to require specialized growth conditions [125]. Subsequently, Hornsby et al. have combined expression of human telomerase reverse transcriptase with SV40 T-antigen and *ras* oncogene to immortalize bovine adrenocortical cells [126]. The immortalized bovine adrenal cells have been used in vivo to rescue adrenalectomized SCID (severe combined immunodeficient) mice from glucocorticoid deficiency through the production of cortisol (see Chapters 13 and 19) (see Table 18.1).

18.4 Summary

Adrenal cell lines represent a crucial tool for molecular and cellular studies that cannot practically be done in animal models. The murine Y1 and human NCI-H295 adrenocortical cell lines are currently the most widely used adrenal cell culture models. The Y1 adrenal cell line has long provided a unique experimental system to dissect the mechanisms of ACTH action on steroidogenesis, cell proliferation, morphology, and the factors that govern the expression of genes required for steroidogenesis. The additions of the human NCI-H295R ACC cells that produce mineralocorticoids, glucocorticoids, and C19 steroids have provided valuable models to study the processes involved in adrenocortical differentiation. However, both the human and murine adrenal model systems have limitations. The Y1 cell, due to the deficiency of 21-hydroxylase, cannot produce corticosteroids. On the other hand, the NCI-H295 cell models have low or no ACTH response. The recently described ACTH-responsive murine ATC1/ATC7-L cell lines offer new opportunities to study the regulation of adrenal steroid production. Together, they provide unique model systems to study both the molecular and biochemical characteristics of adrenal function.

References

1. Arnold J (1866) Ein Beitrag zu der feiner Struktur und dem Chemismus der Nebennieren. Virchows Arch 35:64–107
2. Simpson ER WM (1988) Regulation of the synthesis of steroidogenic enzymes in adrenal cortical cells by ACTH. Annu Rev Physiol 50:427–440
3. Cardoso CC et al (2009) New methods for investigating experimental human adrenal tumorigenesis. Mol Cell Endocrinol 300:175–179
4. Gospodarowicz D et al (1977) Control of bovine adrenal cortical cell proliferation by fibroblast growth factor. Lack of effect of epidermal growth factor. Endocrinology 100:1080–1089
5. O'Hare MJ, Neville AM (1973) Morphological responses to corticotrophin and cyclic AMP by adult rat adrenocortical cells in monolayer culture. J Endocrinol 56:529–536
6. Gazdar AF et al (1990) Establishment and characterization of a human adrenocortical carcinoma cell line that expresses multiple pathways of steroid biosynthesis. Cancer Res 50:5488–5496
7. Parmar J, Rainey WE (2009) Comparisons of adrenocortical cell lines as in vitro test systems. Adrenal toxicology, Chapter 8, pp. 183–204
8. Rogriquez H et al (1997) Transcription of the human genes for cytochrome P450scc and P450c17 is regulated differently in human adrenal NCI-H295 cells than in mouse adrenal Y1 cells. J Endocrinol Metab 82:365–371
9. Yasumura Y et al (1966) Clonal analysis of differentiated function in animal cell cultures. I. Possible correlated maintenance of differentiated function and the diploid karyotype. Cancer Res 26:529–535
10. Auersperg N et al (1990) V-K-ras transformation induces reversion to an earlier developmental form in adult rat adrenal cells. Differentiation 43:29–36
11. Mellon SH et al (1994) Steroidogenic adrenocortical cell lines produced by genetically targeted tumorigenesis in transgenic mice. Mol Endocrinol 8:97–108
12. Mukai K et al (2002) Conditionally immortalized adrenocortical cell lines at undifferentiated states exhibit inducible expression of glucocorticoid-synthesizing genes. Eur J Biochem 269:69–81
13. Pan J et al (1995) Influence of cell type on the steroidogenic potential and basal cyclic AMP levels of ras-oncogene-transformed rat cells. Differentiation 58:321–328
14. Huang N et al (2005) Regulation of cytochrome b5 gene transcription by Sp3, GATA-6, and steroidogenic factor 1 in human adrenal NCI-H295A cells. Mol Endocrinol 19:2020–2034
15. Samandari E et al (2007) Human adrenal corticocarcinoma NCI-H295R cells produce more androgens than NCI-H295A cells and differ in 3beta-hydroxysteroid dehydrogenase type 2 and 17,20 lyase activities. J Endocrinol 195:459–472
16. Bird IM et al (1993a). Human NCI-H295 adrenocortical carcinoma cells: a model for angiotensin-II-responsive aldosterone secretion. Endocrinology 133:1555–1561
17. Rainey WE et al (1994) The NCI-H295 cell line: a pluripotent model for human adrenocortical studies. Mol Cell Endocrinol 100:45–50
18. Clark BJ et al (1995) The steroidogenic acute regulatory protein is induced by angiotensin II and K+ in H295R adrenocortical cells. Mol Cell Endocrinol 115:215–219

19. Bird IM et al (1995b). Potassium negatively regulates angiotensin II type 1 receptor expression in human adrenocortical H295R cells. Hypertension 25:1129–1134
20. Bird IM et al (1996b). Differential control of 17 alpha-hydroxylase and 3 beta-hydroxysteroid dehydrogenase expression in human adrenocortical H295R cells. J Clin Endocrinol Metab 81:2171–2178
21. Denner K et al (1996) Differential regulation of 11 beta-hydroxylase and aldosterone synthase in human adrenocortical H295R cells. Mol Cell Endocrinol 121:87–91
22. Schteingart DE et al (2001) Overexpression of CXC chemokines by an adrenocortical carcinoma: a novel clinical syndrome. J Clin Endocrinol Metab 86:3968–3974
23. Ueno M et al (2001) Characterization of a newly established cell line derived from human adrenocortical carcinoma. Int J Urol 8:17–22
24. Leibovitz A et al (1973) New human cancer cell culture lines. I. SW-13, small-cell carcinoma of the adrenal cortex. J Natl Cancer Inst 51:691–697
25. Almeida MQ et al (2008) Expression of insulin-like growth factor-II and its receptor in pediatric and adult adrenocortical tumors. J Clin Endocrinol Metab 93:3524–3531
26. Schimmer BP (1979) Adrenocortical Y1 cells. Methods Enzymol 58:570–574
27. Schimmer BP, Zimmerman AE (1976) Steroidogenesis and extracellular cAMP accumulation in adrenal tumor cell cultures. Mol Cell Endocrinol 4:263–270
28. Havelock JC et al (2004) Ovarian granulosa cell lines. Mol Cell Endocrinol 228:67–78
29. Rainey WE et al (2004) Adrenocortical cell lines. Mol Cell Endocrinol 228:23–38
30. Rainey MD et al (2006) Analysing the DNA damage and replication checkpoints in DT40 cells. Subcell Biochem 40:107–117
31. Roskelly CD, Auersperg N (1995) Rapid ras-oncogene-mediated transformation maintains steroidogenic differentiation in adrenocortical parenchymal cells. Differentiation 59: 103–111
32. Auersperg N (1978) Effects of culture conditions on the growth and differentiation of transformed rat adrenocortical cells. Cancer Res 38:1872–1884
33. Auersperg N et al (1977) Transformation of cultured rat adrenocortical cells by Kirsten murine sarcoma virus (Ki-MSV). Int J Cancer 19:81–89
34. Ragazzon B et al (2006) Adrenocorticotropin-dependent changes in SF-1/DAX-1 ratio influence steroidogenic genes expression in a novel model of glucocorticoid-producing adrenocortical cell lines derived from targeted tumorigenesis. Endocrinology 147:1805–1818
35. Compagnone NA et al (1997) Characterization of adrenocortical cell lines produced by genetically targeted tumorigenesis in transgenic mice. Steroids 62: 238–243
36. Cheng CY, Hornsby PJ (1992) Expression of 11 beta-hydroxylase and 21-hydroxylase in long-term cultures of bovine adrenocortical cells requires extracellular matrix factors. Endocrinology 130:2883–2889
37. Hornsby PJ, McAllister JM (1991) Culturing steroidogenic cells. Methods Enzymol 206:371–380
38. McAllister JM et al (1994) The effects of growth factors and phorbol esters on steroid biosynthesis in isolated human theca interna and granulosa-lutein cells in long term culture. J Clin Endocrinol Metab 79:106–112
39. Bird IM et al (1993b). Angiotensin-II stimulates an increase in cAMP and expression of 17 alpha-hydroxylase cytochrome P450 in fetal bovine adrenocortical cells. Endocrinology 132:932–934
40. Bird IM et al (1994) Regulation of type 1 angiotensin II receptor messenger ribonucleic acid expression in human adrenocortical carcinoma H295 cells. Endocrinology 134:2468–2474
41. Hilbers U et al (1999) Local renin-angiotensin system is involved in K+-induced aldosterone secretion from human adrenocortical NCI-H295 cells. Hypertension 33:1025–1030
42. Inagaki K et al (2007) Regulatory expression of bone morphogenetic protein-6 system in aldosterone production by human adrenocortical cells. Regul Pept 138:133–140

43. Nogueira EF et al (2007) Angiotensin-II acute regulation of rapid response genes in human, bovine, and rat adrenocortical cells. J Mol Endocrinol 39:365–374
44. Nogueira EF et al (2009) Role of angiotensin II-induced rapid response genes in the regulation of enzymes needed for aldosterone synthesis. J Mol Endocrinol 42:319–330
45. Otani H et al (2008) Aldosterone breakthrough caused by chronic blockage of angiotensin II type 1 receptors in human adrenocortical cells: possible involvement of bone morphogenetic protein-6 actions. Endocrinology 149:2816–2825
46. Romero DG et al (2006a). RGS2 is regulated by angiotensin II and functions as a negative feedback of aldosterone production in H295R human adrenocortical cells. Endocrinology 147:3889–3897
47. Shah BH et al (2006) Mechanisms of endothelin-1-induced MAP kinase activation in adrenal glomerulosa cells. J Steroid Biochem Mol Biol 102:79–88
48. Hanley NA et al (1993) Parathyroid hormone and parathyroid hormone-related peptide stimulate aldosterone production in the human adrenocortical cell line, NCI-H295. Endocr J 1:447–450
49. Mountjoy KG et al (1994) ACTH induces up-regulation of ACTH receptor mRNA in mouse and human adrenocortical cell lines. Mol Cell Endocrinol 99:R17–20
50. Bird IM et al (1995a). Hormonal regulation of angiotensin II type 1 receptor expression and AT1-R mRNA levels in human adrenocortical cells. Endocr Res 21:169–182
51. Rainey WE et al (1993b). Regulation of human adrenal carcinoma cell (NCI-H295) production of C19 steroids. J Clin Endocrinol Metab 77:731–737
52. Rainey WE et al (1993a). Effect of angiotensin II on human luteinized granulosa cells. Fertil Steril 59:143–147
53. Kanczkowski W et al (2009) Differential expression and action of Toll-like receptors in human adrenocortical cells. Mol Cell Endocrinol 300:57–65
54. Lucki N, Sewer MB (2009) The cAMP-responsive element binding protein (CREB) regulates the expression of acid ceramidase (ASAH1) in H295R human adrenocortical cells. Biochim Biophys Acta 75:390–399
55. Noda M et al (2007) Mono-(2-ethylhexyl) phthalate (MEHP) induces nuclear receptor 4A subfamily in NCI-H295R cells: a possible mechanism of aromatase suppression by MEHP. Mol Cell Endocrinol 274:8–18
56. Romero DG et al (2006c). Angiotensin II-mediated protein kinase D activation stimulates aldosterone and cortisol secretion in H295R human adrenocortical cells. Endocrinology 147:6046–6055
57. Song R et al (2009) Cytotoxicity and gene expression profiling of two hydroxylated polybrominated diphenyl ethers in human H295R adrenocortical carcinoma cells. Toxicol Lett 185:23–31
58. Stigliano A et al (2008) Modulation of proteomic profile in H295R adrenocortical cell line induced by mitotane. Endocr Relat Cancer 15:1–10
59. Xing Y et al (2009) The farnesoid X receptor regulates transcription of 3beta-hydroxysteroid dehydrogenase type 2 in human adrenal cells. Mol Cell Endocrinol 299:153–162
60. Ye P et al (2009a). Differential effects of high and low steroidogenic factor-1 expression on CYP11B2 expression and aldosterone production in adrenocortical cells. Endocrinology 150:1303–1309
61. Ye P et al (2009b). Contrasting effects of eplerenone and spironolactone on adrenal cell steroidogenesis. Horm Metab Res 41:35–39
62. Deshpande N et al (1967) In vivo steroidogenesis by the human adrenal gland. Steroids 9:393–404
63. Lanman JT, Silverman LM (1957) In vitro steroidogenesis in the human neonatal adrenal gland, including observations on human adult and monkey adrenal glands. Endocrinology 60:433–445
64. Villee DB (1972) The development of steroidogenesis. Am J Med 53:533–544

65. McAllister JM, Hornsby PJ (1988) Dual regulation of 3 beta-hydroxysteroid dehydrogenase, 17 alpha- hydroxylase, and dehydroepiandrosterone sulfotransferase by adenosine 3′,5′-monophosphate and activators of protein kinase C in cultured human adrenocortical cells. Endocrinology 122:2012–2018
66. Rainey WE et al (1991) Regulation of 3 beta-hydroxysteroid dehydrogenase in adrenocortical cells: effects of angiotensin-II and transforming growth factor beta. Endocr Res 17:281–296
67. Holland OB et al (1993) Angiotensin increases aldosterone synthase mRNA levels in human NCI-H295 cells. Mol Cell Endocrinol 94:R9–13
68. Pezzi V et al (1997) Ca(2+)-regulated expression of aldosterone synthase is mediated by calmodulin and calmodulin-dependent protein kinases. Endocrinology 138:835–838
69. Clyne CD et al (1997) Angiotensin II and potassium regulate human CYP11B2 transcription through common cis-elements. Mol Endocrinol 11:638–649
70. Leers-Sucheta S et al (1997) Synergistic activation of the human type II 3á-hydroxysteroid dehydrogenase/delta 5 – delta 4 isomerase promoter by the transcription factor steroidogenic factor-1/adrenal 4-binding protein and phorbol ester. J Biol Chem 272:7960–7967
71. Bollag WB et al (2008) Phorbol ester increases mitochondrial cholesterol content in NCI H295R cells. Mol Cell Endocrinol 296:53–57
72. Brenner T, O'Shaughnessy KM (2008) Both TASK-3 and TREK-1 two-pore loop K channels are expressed in H295R cells and modulate their membrane potential and aldosterone secretion. Am J Physiol Endocrinol Metab 295:E1480–1486
73. Burton TJ et al (2009) Expression of the epithelial Na(+) channel and other components of an aldosterone response pathway in human adrenocortical cells. Eur J Pharmacol 61: 176–181
74. Gizard F et al (2002) The transcriptional regulating protein of 132 kDa (TReP-132) enhances P450scc gene transcription through interaction with steroidogenic factor-1 in human adrenal cells. J Biol Chem 277:39144–39155
75. Guo W et al (1995) Expression of DAX-1, the gene responsible for X-linked adrenal hypoplasia congenita and hypogonadotropic hypogonadism, in the hypothalamic-pituitary-adrenal/gonadal axis. Biochem Mol Med 56:8–13
76. Isaka T et al (2009) Azelnidipine inhibits aldosterone synthesis and secretion in human adrenocortical cell line NCI-H295R. Eur J Pharmacol 605:49–52
77. Kempna P et al (2007) Pioglitazone inhibits androgen production in NCI-H295R cells by regulating gene expression of CYP17 and HSD3B2. Mol Pharmacol 71:787–798
78. Lehoux JG, Lefebvre A (2007) Angiotensin II activates p44/42 MAP kinase partly through PKCepsilon in H295R cells. Mol Cell Endocrinol 265-266:121–125
79. Muller-Vieira U et al (2005) The adrenocortical tumor cell line NCI-H295R as an in vitro screening system for the evaluation of CYP11B2 (aldosterone synthase) and CYP11B1 (steroid-11beta-hydroxylase) inhibitors. J Steroid Biochem Mol Biol 96: 259–270
80. Qin H et al (2009) The Role of Calcium Influx Pathways in Phospholipase D Activation in Bovine Adrenal Glomerulosa Cells. J Endocrinol 202:77–86
81. Romero DG et al (2006b). Interleukin-8 synthesis, regulation, and steroidogenic role in H295R human adrenocortical cells. Endocrinology 147:891–898
82. Sugawara T et al (2006) CREM confers cAMP responsiveness in human steroidogenic acute regulatory protein expression in NCI-H295R cells rather than SF-1/Ad4BP. J Endocrinol 191:327–337
83. Vilain E et al (1997) DAX1 gene expression upregulated by steroidogenic factor 1 in an adrenocortical carcinoma cell line. Biochem Mol Med 61:1–8
84. Shoemaker RH (2006) The NCI60 human tumour cell line anticancer drug screen. Nat Rev Cancer 6:813–823
85. Bodrogi I. (1989) Third-line chemotherapy of resistant advanced testicular cancer. Prog Clin Biol Res 303:749–758

86. Fisher RI et al (1981) Adjuvant immunotherapy or chemotherapy for malignant melanoma. Preliminary report of the National Cancer Institute randomized clinical trial. Surg Clin North Am 61:1267–1277
87. Lopez Garcia N (1980) Contribution to the study of adenocarcinoma of the endometrium [Part I: Introduction. Part II: Material and methods]. Rev Esp Oncol 27:443–521 contd
88. Weiss RB et al (1980) m-AMSA: an exciting new drug in the National Cancer Institute Drug Development Program. Cancer Clin Trials 3:203–209
89. La Rocca RV et al (1990) Suramin in adrenal cancer: modulation of steroid hormone production, cytotoxicity in vitro, and clinical antitumor effect. J Clin Endocrinol Metab 71:497–504
90. Schteingart DE et al (1993) Comparison of the adrenalytic activity of mitotane and a methylated homolog on normal adrenal cortex and adrenal cortical carcinoma. Cancer Chemother Pharmacol 31:459–466
91. Fallo F et al (1996) Effects of taxol on the human NCI-H295 adrenocortical carcinoma cell line. Endocr Res 22:709–715
92. Fallo F et al (1998) Paclitaxel is an effective antiproliferative agent on the human NCI-H295 adrenocortical carcinoma cell line. Chemotherapy 44:129–134
93. Fassnacht M et al (2000) New mechanisms of adrenostatic compounds in a human adrenocortical cancer cell line. Eur J Clin Invest 30 Suppl 3:76–82
94. Betz MJ et al (2005) Peroxisome proliferator-activated receptor-gamma agonists suppress adrenocortical tumor cell proliferation and induce differentiation. J Clin Endocrinol Metab 90:3886–3896
95. van Koetsveld PM et al (2006) Potent inhibitory effects of type I interferons on human adrenocortical carcinoma cell growth. J Clin Endocrinol Metab 91:4537–4543
96. Doghman M et al (2008) The T cell factor/beta-catenin antagonist PKF115-584 inhibits proliferation of adrenocortical carcinoma cells. J Clin Endocrinol Metab 93:3222–3225
97. Barlaskar FM et al (2009) Preclinical targeting of the type I insulin-like growth factor receptor in adrenocortical carcinoma. J Clin Endocrinol Metab 94:204–212
98. Ghorab Z et al (2003) Melan A (A103) is expressed in adrenocortical neoplasms but not in renal cell and hepatocellular carcinomas. Appl Immunohistochem Mol Morphol 11: 330–333
99. Mizutani T et al (2002) Maintenance of integrated proviral gene expression requires Brm, a catalytic subunit of SWI/SNF complex. J Biol Chem 277:15859–15864
100. Hornsby PJ et al (1989) Replicative senescence and differentiated gene expression in cultured adrenocortical cells. Exp Gerontol 24:539–558
101. Cong YS et al (2002) Human telomerase and its regulation. Microbiol Mol Biol Rev 66: 407–425
102. Cohen AI et al (1957) In vitro response of experimental adrenal tumors to corticotropin (ACTH). Proc Soc Exp Biol Med 95:304–309
103. Buonassisi V et al (1962) Hormone-producing cultures of adrenal and pituitary tumor origin. Proc Natl Acad Sci U S A 48:1184–1190
104. Kowal J, Fiedler R (1968) Adrenal cells in tissue culture. I. Assay of steroid products; steroidogenic responses to peptide hormones. Arch Biochem Biophys 128:406–421
105. Parker KL et al (1985) Expression of murine 21-hydroxylase in mouse adrenal glands and in transfected Y1 adrenocortical tumor cells. Proc Natl Acad Sci U S A 82:7860–7864
106. Pierson RWJ (1967) Metabolism of steroid hormones in adrenal cortex tumor cultures. Endocrinology 81:693–707
107. Schimmer BP (1985) Isolation of ACTH-resistant Y1 adrenal tumor cells. Methods Enzymol 109:350–356
108. Cuprak LJ et al (1977) Scanning electron microscopy of induced cell rounding of mouse adrenal cortex tumor cells in culture. Tissue Cell 9:667–680
109. Mattson P, Kowal J (1978) The ultrastructure of functional mouse adrenal cortical tumor cells in vitro. Differentiation 11:75–88

110. Voorhees H et al (1984) Rounding and steroidogenesis of enzyme- and ACTH-treated Y-1 mouse adrenal tumor cells. Cell Biol Intl 8:483–497
111. Schimmer BP et al (1995) Adrenocorticotropin-resistant mutants of the Y1 adrenal cell line fail to express the adrenocorticotropin receptor. J Cell Physiol 163:164–171
112. Black SM et al (1993) Regulation of proteins in the cholesterol side-chain cleavage system in JEG-3 and Y-1 cells. Endocrinology 132:539–545
113. Guo IC et al (1993) Differential regulation of the CYP11A1 (P450scc) and ferredoxin genes in adrenal and placental cells. DNA Cell Biol 12:849–860
114. Lin X et al (2001) Salt-inducible kinase is involved in the ACTH/cAMP-dependent protein kinase signaling in Y1 mouse adrenocortical tumor cells. Mol Endocrinol 15:1264–1276
115. Wong M et al (1989) The roles of cAMP and cAMP-dependent protein kinase in the expression of cholesterol side chain cleavage and steroid 11 beta-hydroxylase genes in mouse adrenocortical tumor cells. J Biol Chem 264:12867–12871
116. Mitani F et al (1998) Localization of replicating cells in rat adrenal cortex during the late gestational and early postnatal stages. Endocr Res 24:983–986
117. Rice DA et al (1989) A cAMP-responsive element regulates expression of the mouse steroid 11 beta-hydroxylase gene. J Biol Chem 264:14011–14015
118. Lin D et al (1995) Role of steroidogenic acute regulatory protein in adrenal and gonadal steroidogenesis. Science 267:1828–1831
119. Lopez D et al (2001) Effects of mutating different steroidogenic factor-1 protein regions on gene regulation. Endocrine 14:353–362
120. Temel RE et al (1997) Scavenger receptor class B, type I (SR-BI) is the major route for the delivery of high density lipoprotein cholesterol to the steroidogenic pathway in cultured mouse adrenocortical cells. Proc Natl Acad Sci U S A 94:13600–13605
121. Endoh A et al (1996) The zona reticularis is the site of biosynthesis of dehydroepiandrosterone and dehydroepiandrosterone sulfate in the adult human adrenal cortex resulting from its low expression of 3 beta-hydroxysteroid dehydrogenase. J Clin Endocrinol Metabo 81:3558–3565
122. Auersperg N et al (1981) Morphological and functional differentiation of Kirsten murine sarcoma virus-transformed rat adrenocortical cell lines. Cancer Res 41:1763–1771
123. Kananen K et al (1996) Gonadectomy permits adrenocortical tumorigenesis in mice transgenic for the mouse inhibin alpha-subunit promoter/simian virus 40 T-antigen fusion gene: evidence for negative autoregulation of the inhibin alpha-subunit gene. Mol Endocrinol 10:1667
124. Rilianawati et al (1998) Direct luteinizing hormone action triggers adrenocortical tumorigenesis in castrated mice transgenic for the murine inhibin alpha-subunit promoter/simian virus 40 T-antigen fusion gene. Mol Endocrinol 12:801–809
125. Chang CW et al (1991) The response of 21-hydroxylase messenger ribonucleic acid levels to adenosine 3′,5′-monophosphate and 12-O-tetradecanoylphorbol-13-acetate in bovine adrenocortical cells is dependent on culture conditions. Endocrinology 128:604–610
126. Thomas M et al (2002) Cooperation of hTERT, SV40 T antigen and oncogenic Ras in tumorigenesis: a cell transplantation model using bovine adrenocortical cells. Neoplasia 4:493–500

Chapter 19
Mouse Models of Adrenal Tumorigenesis

Felix Beuschlein

Over the past decade, a number of high-throughput techniques have emerged as powerful tools for molecular and functional characterization of cancer cells. These techniques allow for genetic or epigenetic analysis of DNA, determination of RNA expression pattern, proteomic profiling, or characterization of posttranslational modification. Despite these technical advances that aid thorough molecular characterization of surgical tumor material, most of the functional properties of biological molecules are still unpredictable from pure expression and sequence analysis. For functional studies of gene products, mouse models continue to be intensively utilized as an experimental system due to the similarity to humans with respect to genome organization, development, and physiology. Incidental discovery of adrenal tumors in genetically modified animals can provide clues on pathways involved in adrenal tumorigenesis that would not have been predicted on the basis of structural analysis or in vitro exploration. Mouse models can also be used to verify functional significance of a given gene for adrenal growth and function in vivo through targeted genetic modification. Furthermore, high incidence of adrenal tumors in inbred mouse strains can serve as the starting point for genetic approaches to identify underlying genetic mechanism. Similarly, chemically or radiation-based mutagenesis can be utilized to create informative mouse models, referred to as forward (phenotype-driven) genetics. Finally, well-defined tumor models have been successfully used for preclinical intervention trials to screen for novel therapeutic approaches.

An overview of rodent models that have been described to either have adrenocortical tumors as part of their phenotype or have been utilized for therapeutic screens will be provided.

F. Beuschlein (✉)
Department of Medicine, Endocrine Research, University Hospital Innenstadt, Ziemssenstr. 1, 80336 Munich, Germany
e-mail: felix.beuschlein@med.uni-muenchen.de

G.D. Hammer, T. Else (eds.), *Adrenocortical Carcinoma*,
DOI 10.1007/978-0-387-77236-3_19,

19.1 Mouse Models with Spontaneous or Induced Adrenal Tumor Growth

As reported by Cohen and co-worker, in 1951 a group of inbred mice of the LAF1 strain was exposed to the irradiation of a test atomic bomb explosion (Operation Greenhouse). In less than 1% of animals development of adrenal tumors was observed although it remained uncertain whether the incidence of adrenal tumors was in fact induced by the irradiation or arose spontaneously. One male animal had a tumor in the right adrenal cortex measuring 12 by 20 mm while the left adrenal gland was atrophic. Necropsy of the mouse revealed numerous small metastases of the lung as proof of a malignant phenotype of this adrenocortical tumor [1]. The tumor was excised and implanted intramuscularly in the thigh of male and female LAF1 from which it was maintained as a transplantable tumor. While during early propagation through transplantation metastatic spread was noted on a regular basis in host animals, upon later passages the tumors lost their metastatic properties [2]. Histological and laboratory evidence of steroid secretion by the tumor were noted including thymic involution and adrenal atrophy, increase in serum sodium and decrease of serum potassium, as well as eosinopenia and lymphopenia [1]. Tumor-bearing animals were used to assay ACTH bioactivity from transplanted corticotroph tumors [3]. Consequently, a clone of steroid-producing tumor cells was established by Yasamura and colleagues as a continuous cell line named Y1 [4], which has since been widely used by the scientific community [5].

In addition to an adrenal tumor phenotype induced by radiation, one of the earliest documented observation of adrenal tumorigenesis in the mouse has been reported by Wooley and Little as part of the phenotypic characterization of the inbred mouse strain CE which was described to display a high incidence of adrenocortical tumor development after surgical gonadectomy [6]. These early observations could be reproduced not only in the CE/J strain [7] but also in other inbred mouse strains including DBA/2 J [8], C3H, BALB/c [9], and NU/J animals [10], while other strains such as C57BL/6 J [11] and FVB/N [8] were found to be resistant to tumor formation. As both surgical gonadectomy and xenografting of hCG producing tumors [10] were able to induce adrenocortical tumor growth in the described mouse strains, these experimental designs suggested that chronic elevation of gonadotropins represents a major determinant of adrenocortical tumorigenesis.

Gonadectomy-induced adrenal tumors in susceptible mouse strains have been characterized in detail. During the initial morphological characterization, parts of the adrenal tumors have been described to be reminiscent of seminiferous tubules of the testis or follicular structures similar to that found in the cortex of the ovary [6]. Furthermore, the occurrence of these tumors, also when transplanted into littermates [12], was accompanied by morphological changes in hormone-responsive organs such as the uterus or the mammary glands indicative of sex steroid production [13]. These tumors are of a benign or semi-malignant phenotype as metastases are usually not present. In accordance with early morphological findings, later functional and molecular studies revealed that the adrenal tumors indeed express markers which are otherwise restricted to the gonad including receptors for LH (*Lhr*) and Mullerian inhibiting substance (*Mis*) as well as steroidogenic enzymes such as *P450cyp17* and *P450cyp19* [7, 8, 10]. Accordingly, these tumors have adapted the gonad's ability to secret sex steroids [7]. This functional change is also accompanied by a switch in the expression of the transcription factor *Gata6* to that of *Gata4* [7, 8, 10]. Gata4 has been implicated in the regulation of tissue-specific gene expression and cellular proliferation in the gonad [14, 15]. Moreover, overexpression of *Gata4* is sufficient to induce the expression of gonadal markers in adrenocortical tumor cells in vitro [16]. Thus, these findings provide indirect evidence that induction of *Gata4* expression is linked to the phenotypic shift observed in gonadectomy-induced adrenal tumors (Fig. 19.1).

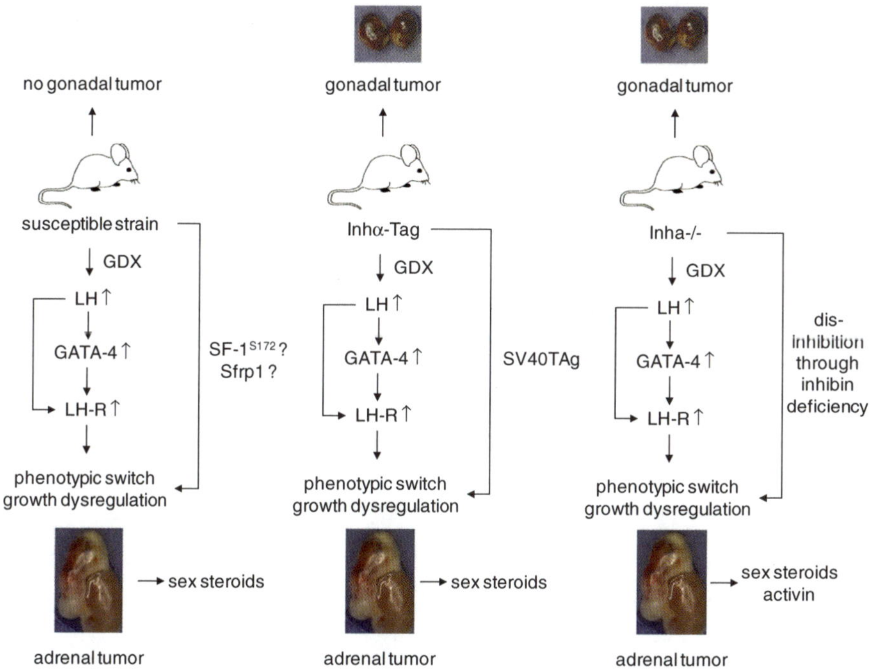

Fig. 19.1 Schematic overview on adrenal and ovarian phenotype and molecular pathways involved in mouse models of adrenal tumorigenesis

To identify genetic markers that are associated with gonadectomy-induced adrenal tumorigenesis, Bernichtein and colleagues performed a genome-wide association study in non-susceptible C57BL/6 J and susceptible DBA/2 J animals [17]. Linkage analysis identified a major locus on chromosome 8, which spans approximately a 10 cM region and contains 31 candidate genes. Among these genes *Sfrp1*, a dominant negative regulator of the Wnt signalling pathway which is downregulated in a number of tumor entities through epigenetic modifications, was highlighted as a promising candidate [17]. However, the exact contribution of the genes identified on the basis of genetic association studies remains to be determined. In addition, it has been recognized that mouse strains with high tumor susceptibility have in common a polymorphism in steroidogenic factor-1 (*Sf1*), a transcription factor necessary for proper development and function of the adrenal cortex [18]. This polymorphism, which results in a substitution from alanine to serine at residue 172 of the protein, appears to influence steroidogenic capacity of adrenocortical cells [19]. Since *Sf1* dosage has been described as a relevant trigger of adrenocortical tumor growth in childhood adrenocortical carcinoma (ACC) [20] as well as in a transgenic mouse model [21], it is possible that the polymorphism could be associated with higher baseline *Sf1* expression levels, thus predisposing the development of adrenocortical tumor growth.

As adrenal cortices and gonads are derived from the same embryological primordium, the morphological, functional, and molecular changes are observed in adrenal tumors of susceptible strains. The presence of pluripotent progenitor cells in the adrenal cortex has been proposed, which can be driven towards a gonadal phenotype [22]. Accordingly, adrenal tumor growth that requires chronic stimulation by pituitary gonadotropins has been interpreted as a result of adrenocortical stem cell misspecification during oncogenic transformation.

19.2 Mouse Models Utilizing Transplanted Adrenal Tumor Cells

Tumor transplantation models represent well-established tools that can be used to answer specific questions of tumor pathogenesis or can be applied for preclinical screening of anticancer treatments. As only very few instances of successful engraftment of primary adrenocortical tumor material have been reported in the literature [23], the number of available adrenal tumor models is limited by the number of

Table 19. 1 Cell lines used for transplantation models of ACC

Cell line	Origin	Host	Purpose of Model	Reference
NCI H295	Hormonally active human ACC	Immunocompromised mouse	– Intervention trials	[24, 25, 28]
SW13	Nonsecreting "small cell" human ACC	Immunocompromised mouse	– Intervention trials	[26, 29]
RL251	Chemokine-secreting human ACC	Immunocompromised mouse	– Studies of pathophysiology – Intervention trials	[27, 28]
Y1 and Y6 cells	Murine cell lines derived from transplantable adrenocortical tumors	Syngenic mouse model (LAF1 strain)	– Studies of pathophysiology – Intervention trials	[4, 30]
Bovine and human adrenocortical cells	Transgenic expression of oncogenes	Immunocompromised mouse	– Studies of pathophysiology	[36, 38, 73]

well-characterized ACC cell lines (see Chapter 18) (Table 19.1). One example is the subcutaneous transplantation of the human ACC cell line NCI-H295 in immunocompromised animals. Upon subcutaneous injection of 6×10^6 cells in nude mice tumor take rate has been reported in the range of 90% with a medium doubling time of 12 days [24]. The NCI-H295 cell line which had been established from a patient with hormonally active ACC has been demonstrated to retain its ability to produce all of the major adrenal steroids [25]. Accordingly, adrenal androgens among others have been shown to be elevated in nude mice bearing subcutaneous NCI-H295 tumors [24]. Moreover, the tumors were characterized by dysregulation of the insulin- like growth factor system such as high expression of *IGF2* and IGF-binding protein-2 similar to that observed in primary human tumor specimens. Similarly, adrenocortical SW13 cells, which had been established in the 1970s from a nonsecreting "small cell" ACC [26], and RL251 cells from a chemokine-secreting adrenal tumor [27, 28] have also been demonstrated to engraft in immunocompromised animals [29].

Adrenal tumor cells can also be maintained in immune competent mice as long as the strain is chosen from which the particular cell line had been derived. Accordingly, Y1 cells, which had been established from LAF1 mice as described above, can be re-transplanted in this strain of animals (see Chapter 18). A potential use of this model in the investigation of tumor relevant regulatory pathways is to genetically alter these cells and assay for tumor growth behavior in vivo. Following this approach the human ACTH receptor was introduced in an ACTH unresponsive subclone of Y1 cells (Y6 cells; [19]). These cells upon transplantation into LAF1 animals could have been demonstrated to have a lower proliferative potential in comparison to wild-type Y6 cells under baseline conditions and after ACTH stimulation (Fig. 19.2) [30]. Thus, these studies supported clinical evidence that ACTH receptor expression in ACC is associated with a less aggressive adrenal tumor phenotype [31] and demonstrated that ACTH-dependent antiproliferative effects can be amplified through stimulation with physiological doses of ACTH.

Genetic modification have also been applied on primary cultures of normal human and bovine adrenocortical cells to recapitulate molecular alterations found in the course of tumorigenesis in vivo and to define those to be required and sufficient to induce malignant tumor growth in transplanted animals. Following this approach, Hornsby and colleagues have developed a model in which a suspension of adrenocortical cells is introduced under the kidney capsule [32]. Once implanted at this location. cells rapidly aggregate followed by invasion by host endothelial cells, formation of a vascular system, and the subsequent survival, growth and function of the transplant tissue [32]. As structure and function of the transplant are dependent on circulating pituitary hormones from the host, transplantation experiments are usually performed in adrenalectomized animals [33]. Utilizing this transplantation model in a number of experiments, Thomas and colleagues could demonstrate that introduction of telomerase reverse transcriptase (*TERT*) into bovine adrenocortical cells resulted in a tissue phenotype similar to that of untransfected cells [34]. In contrast, forced expression of SV40 large T antigen (*SV40 TAg*), oncogenic Ras^{G12V} together with *TERT* were sufficient to induce a malignant phenotype of the

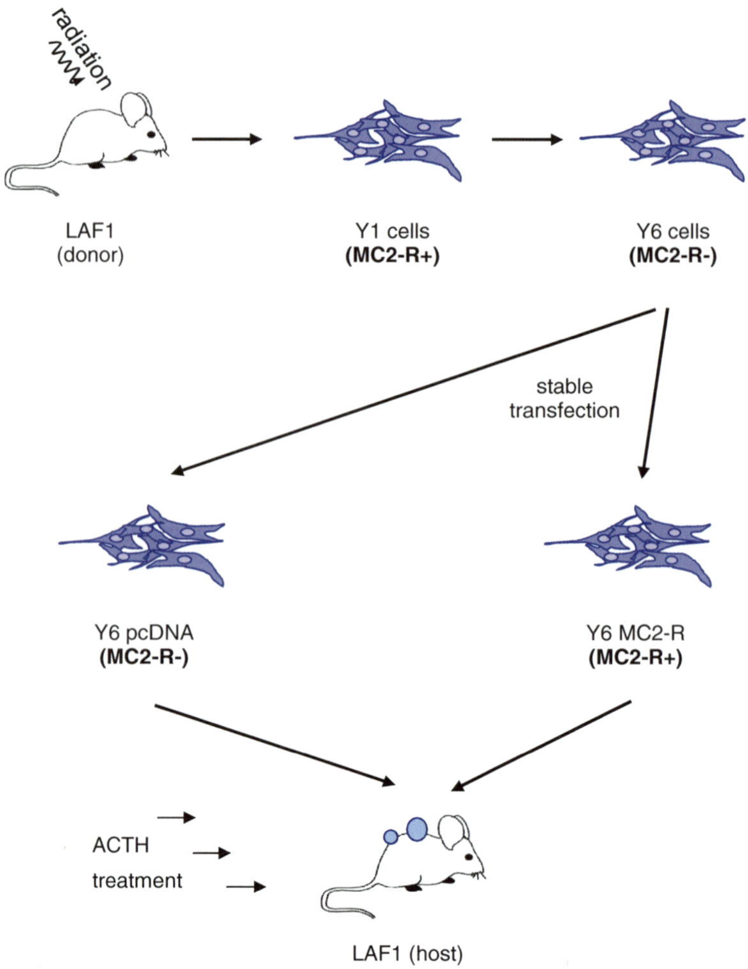

Fig. 19.2 Generation and experimental utilization of different clones of mouse adrenocortical cell lines

transgenic tissue that gave rise to a tumor resembling many features of ACC [35]. Consequently, even in the absence of *TERT, SV40 Tag* and Ras^{G12V} alone were demonstrated to be sufficient to induce a malignant phenotype in bovine and human adrenocortical cells [36]. However, these tumors displayed a reduction in growth rate after several consecutive rounds of transplantation, which was accompanied with the progressive entry of cells into crisis (see Chapter 13). These changes could be reversed after transduction with *TERT*, thus restoring tumorigenicity of the cells [36]. Interestingly, *TERT* was also required to form tumors when cells were injected subcutaneously. Taken together, the described experiments performed in a well-defined in vivo setting allowed to pinpoint molecular alterations that could well be of pathophysiological relevance also in ACC patients and, thus, provide the framework for further interventional approaches.

A similar experimental design was chosen to investigate the role of illicit receptor expression, which has been identified as the cause of ACTH-independent hypercortisolism in bilateral adrenal macronodular hyperplasia as well as adrenocortical tumors [37]. Bovine adrenal cells upon transduction with the receptor for the gastric inhibitory polypeptide (*Gipr*) [38] or the luteinizing hormone receptor (*Lhr*) [39] in both instances developed into hyperproliferative adenomatous, but not overtly malignant tissue when transplanted under the kidney capsule and resulted in a mild ACTH-independent hypercortisolism in the host animal. Thus, while it remained uncertain whether the ectopic expression of G protein-coupled receptors in human patients reflects a cause or a consequence of hyperplastic or adenomatous adrenocortical growth, the mouse modeling informs that the expression of the *Gipr* or the *Lhr* each is sufficient to induce a phenotype similar to those defining the clinical entity.

An ideal animal model that could be utilized for intervention trials of ACC should be simple and reproducible, and it should allow for reliable follow-up examination (Table 19.2). At present these requirements are most closely matched by transplantation models and only recently experiments using mouse

Table 19. 2 Overview on basic characteristics of animal models of adrenocortical tumorigenesis

Characteristics	Transplantation	Susceptible strains	Inhibinα-Tag	Sf1 transgenic	Inhibinα knockout	MEN1 knockout
• Reproducibility:						
– Penetrance	+	+/–	+	+	+	–
– Time of onset	+	–	+	–	–	–
– Growth kinetics	+	–	+	–	+/–	–
• Simplicity:						
– Spontaneous tumor growth	–	–	–	+	–	+
– Inducible tumor growth	+	+	+	–	+	–
• Specificity:						
– Adrenal as only tumor manifestation	ν.α.	+	–	+	–	–
• Biological significance:						
– Eutopic/ndogenous tumor model	–	+	+	+	+	+
– Alteration of pathways involved in human tumorigenesis	+/–+	+/?	–	+	(+)	+
• Follow-up						
– Quantification of tumor size	+/–	–	–	–	–	–
– Tumor marker	+	(+)	+	?	+	?

models of ACC have been published to assess therapeutic options in a preclinical setting.

An immune-competent host is required for transplanted tumor cells, when endpoints of immune function are assessed. To create an experimental system with clearly defined antigenic targets, genetically modified non-adrenal tumor cells expressing adrenal specific antigens have been generated. Following this approach it could be shown that immunization using DNA vaccination followed by vaccinia virus boosting is sufficient to break immune tolerance against the adrenal StAR antigen and to raise an immune response strong enough to inhibit transplanted tumor growth [40]. It remains to be determined whether it is possible, using this protocol, to raise an immune response potent enough to efficiently target established tumors.

Utilizing SW13 cells grown as subcutaneous tumors in immunodeficient mice, Wolkersdörfer and colleagues provided the first evidence for the usefulness of gene transfer of a HSV thymidine kinase expressing adenoviral shuttle as part of a therapeutic approach. Gancyclovir treatment induced oncolytic effects. Upon this therapeutic approach, oncolytic effects through replicating adenoviral vectors could be demonstrated, which was followed by tumor reduction and significant increase in animal survival [29].

As insulin-like growth factors have been defined as major contributors of adrenocortical tumor growth [41, 42] targeting of type I insulin-like growth factor receptor (IGF1R)-dependent pathways represents a promising approach to modulate the proliferative phenotype of ACC cells (see Chapter 15). In accordance with this notion Barlaskar and colleagues could demonstrate that treatment of animals bearing NCI-H295-derived subcutaneous tumors with IGF1R antagonistic compounds resulted in a significant amelioration of tumor growth and increase in survival time [28].

It is foreseeable that the standardization of these described tumor models will play an increasing role in preclinical feasibility studies necessary for early clinical trials in patients with ACC. However, further improvement of the described tumor models is being sought. Utilizing the subcutaneous transplantation site, these models allow for close evaluation of time-dependent tumor growth kinetics. However, from a clinical perspective the subcutaneous tumor niche represents an "unphysiological" manifestation of ACC. More relevant metastatic sites would include local lymph nodes, liver, lung, and bones. Although these manifestations could be mimicked in the mouse model through local or intravenous administration of tumor cells, these models would have the disadvantage of hindered follow-up examination. To further improve suitability of such a model, ACC cells stably expressing GFP or luciferase could allow in vivo imaging approaches in the future. Additionally, adrenocortical tumor models could be used for therapeutic testing in the context of personalized medicine. For example, tumor material from patients that could be maintained in xenograft models would provide the opportunity to specifically test for the suitability of a specific compound for an individual patient. However, development of techniques that allow for reproducible experimental conditions will be required before such personalized models could be further investigated in a preclinical setting.

19.3 Genetically Modified Mouse Models with an Adrenal Tumor Phenotype

Mice that have been designed to harbor specific genetic modifications through transgenic techniques or knockout approaches have been instructive for the identification of molecular mechanisms involved in adrenocortical tumorigenesis. These models can be utilized to provide information of the functional significance of a specific gene or downstream pathway that might have been identified by in vitro experiments, through expression studies from surgical tumor samples, or on the basis of clinical information from patients with rare genetic syndromes. Furthermore, careful phenotypic characterization of available mouse models in which an adrenal phenotype had been discovered can serve as a starting point for further functional analysis.

19.4 Mouse Models with Transgenic Expression of an Oncogene-Inducing Adrenal Tumor

The Simian virus 40 large T-antigen (SV40) represents a commonly used oncogene that can be expressed in the adrenal cortex upon transgenic introduction under the control of a tissue-specific promoter sequence. Promoters that have been used to target the adrenal cortex include 5′-flanking sequences from the human *CYP11A* gene [43], the aldose reductase-like (*Akr1b7*) gene [44], as well as the inhibin alpha promoter [45]. While the former two models have been mainly used to generate cell lines for further in vitro analyses [46], the alpha inhibin promoter-driven transgenic animal (*Inhα/Tag*) has been phenotypically characterized in great detail.

While originally developed to study the role of inhibin in the gonad [47], it became soon clear that surgical gonadectomy not only rescued the animals from gonadal tumor associated death but also uncovered another phenotypic facet of inhibin action. Upon gonadectomy, all mice developed adrenocortical tumors [45]. The biological behavior of these tumors is mainly confined to a benign or semi-malignant phenotype. While these tumors exhibit a significant local growth, a frankly metastatic phenotype can usually not be observed. Inhibin, a member of the TGFβ family of growth factors, is composed of a unique alpha subunit and a beta subunit shared with activin. Inhibin is mainly expressed in the gonad and the adrenal cortex [48]. As such, the distribution of tumors in *Inhα/Tag* follows the resembles the expression pattern of the endogenous inhibin α subunit. However, further molecular studies revealed that the adrenal tumor phenotype was very similar to that of inbred mouse strains susceptible for gonadectomy-induced adrenal tumorigenesis. Thus, the *Inhα/Tag* model has provided valuable insights in more general mechanisms of adrenal tumorigenesis importantly accruing without the introduction of a viral oncogene. By induction of a hypogonadic state through pharmacological treatment with a GnRH antagonist or long-term testosterone treatment or by cross-breeding the mice into the hypogonadotropic *hpg* background, development of both gonadal and adrenal tumors could be prevented [49, 50]. Moreover, the proliferation rate of an adrenal tumor cell line derived from a gonadectomized *Inhα/Tag* animal could be increased by in vitro treatment with the LH receptor ligand hCG [51]. Taken together, these findings indicated that pituitary gonadotropins play an important role for the induction of the adrenal tumor phenotype in this mouse model. Interestingly, chronic elevation of LH levels results in upregulation of adrenal *Lhr* expression required to induce further LH-dependent functional changes. Gata4 has been identified as an important contributor to the interrelation of LH and its receptor. Gata4 and LH are coincidentally upregulated in this tumor model [52]. In addition, in vitro [52] and in vivo studies [53] suggested an LH-dependent increase in adrenal *Gata4* expression levels. Furthermore, a Gata-responsive element in the *Lhr* promoter was identified and Gata4-dependent transcriptional activation of the *Lhr* gene could be demonstrated using in vitro promoter experiments [52]. Overall, these findings describe a feed forward pathway, where chronically elevated LH levels induce *Gata4* expression, which in turn increases expression of the adrenal *Lhr*, which provides an important molecular switch in the initiation of adrenal tumorigenesis in this model (Fig. 19.1) [54].

Upon this detailed molecular characterization, gonadectomized *Inhα/Tag* animals were further utilized as a model of Lhr targeted therapy. Using a lytic peptide (hecate), which was conjugated to a fragment of the hCG beta chain (hecate-hCGbeta), treatment of animals with established adrenal tumors induced a significant reduction in adrenal tumor size in male animals. As hecate–hCGbeta conjugate treatment seemed not to affect normal adrenocortical function, this finding argued for a cell-specific effect that only targeted *Lhr*-expressing tumor cells [55]. While the conjugate was ineffective in female mice, these animals could successfully be treated with a GnRH antagonist or estradiol administration [56]. Although preliminary in its nature, these efforts provide the rationale to further explore the treatment modalities directly or indirectly targeting *Lhr*-expressing adrenal tumors.

Another example for a transgenic mouse model characterized by adrenal tumor growth has recently been reported in an animal harboring multiple copies of a yeast artificial chromosome including the *Sf1* genetic locus [21]. The gain in *Sf1* copy number, which resulted in an increase in adrenal Sf1 protein levels, was associated with the development of macronodular adrenocortical disease that further progressed into adrenal tumors in an age-dependent manner. Interestingly, tumors of *Sf1* transgenic animals displayed a similar expression pattern in comparison to those of inbred susceptible mouse strains including upregulation of *Gata4* and *Mis*, while adrenocortical markers including P450scc were absent [21]. Further gene expression profiling revealed that genes involved in cell adhesion and the immune response and transcription factor signal transducer and activator of transcription-3 (*Stat3*) were differentially expressed in *Sf1* transgenic mouse adrenals in comparison to wild-type littermates. Together with clinical findings from childhood ACC in which the *Sf1* is amplified and overexpressed this model presents further evidence that gene dosage of *Sf1* can contribute to the phenotype of adrenocortical tumors. As specific Sf1 inverse agonists have been developed and proved to be effective in in vitro adrenocortical systems [57], the transgenic in vivo model might aid in further preclinical testing of these compounds.

19.5 Mouse Models with Targeted Deletions Inducing Adrenal Tumors

In addition to susceptible inbred mouse strains and the *Inhα/Tag* transgenic model, animals with a targeted deletion of the inhibin alpha subunit (*Inha*$^{-/-}$) have also been characterized by the phenotype of gonadectomy-induced adrenal tumorigenesis. This animal model, which was originally introduced by Matzuk and colleagues in 1992, [58] has since been subjected to an in-depth phenotypic and molecular characterization. As introduction of a transgenic background with chronic elevation of pituitary LH secretion enhances adrenal tumor growth in gonadectomized *Inha*$^{-/-}$ animals, LH appears to also act as an adrenal growth factor in the context of inhibin deficiency. Very similar to what had been described in *Inhα/Tag* animals, adrenal tumors in *Inha*$^{-/-}$ mice are characterized by a switch from *Gata6* to *Gata4* [16] and a further change in expression pattern towards a gonadal phenotype (Fig. 19.1) [59]. Spatial analysis of *Gata4* expression revealed localization of Gata4-positive cells to the subcapsular region of the adrenal gland, which contains undifferentiated progenitor cells that continuously populate the adrenocortical zones. Thus, these data provide indirect evidence that *Inha*$^{-/-}$ adrenocortical tumors cells could be derived from pluripotent adrenocortical progenitor cells which adopt a gonadal fate due to the convergent loss of inhibin and chronic exposure to elevated gonadotropins. Interestingly, morphological characterization of intermediate stage adrenal tumors in *Inha*$^{-/-}$ allowed further subspecification of cells with a theca-cell-like and a granulosa-cell-like phenotype as indicated by Lhr and Mis positive staining, respectively. These tissue characteristics reminiscent of normal ovaries, however, is lost at later stages of tumor development [59].

One aspect that is not shared by other gonadectomy-dependent tumor models is the secretion of high levels of activin both by gonadal and by adrenal tumors in *Inha*$^{-/-}$ animals, which are associated with the development of cancer cachexia-like syndrome [60]. Interestingly, activin secreted by gonadal tumors has direct functional and morphological consequences on the adrenal cortex, which might contribute to the inhibition of adrenal tumor growth before gonadectomy is performed [59]. However, genetic removal of *Smad3*, which is required for activin signaling from *Inha*$^{-/-}$ mice, which attenuated adrenal tumor progression by uncoupling extracellular mitogenic signals from the cell cycle machinery including cyclin D2 [61]. These findings are endorsed by studies on gonadectomized *Inha*$^{-/-}$ animals, which had been cross-bred to generate double knockouts for *p27* or *cyclin D2*, respectively. Interestingly, while loss of *p27* had little effect on adrenal cortical tumor progression, in the absence of inhibin the loss of *cyclin D2* prolonged the lifespan of double knockouts animals [62].

Familial ACC occurs in the context of genetic/epigenetic predisposition, such as observed in Li-Fraumeni syndrome due to specific *TP53* mutations [63]. p53 acts as a cell cycle check point to regulate DNA repair or induce growth arrest or apoptosis in response to DNA damage, and its loss of function has been demonstrated to affect a large array of tumor entities [64]. However, only very recently has its role as a tumor suppressor gene in ACC has been highlighted in a mouse model of telomere dysfunction in which animals with *p53* haploinsufficiency developed ACC in 5% of cases [65]. While these tumors exhibited locally invasive growth and a malignant histology, no metastasis have been reported (see Chapter 13).

In patients with multiple endocrine neoplasia type 1 (MEN1) in addition to parathyroid adenomas, pancreatic islets tumors and pituitary adenomas, development of adrenocortical tumors has been described in up to 40% of patients [66]. Accordingly, animals with targeted deletion of the menin gene resembled the clinical features of MEN1 including that of development of adrenocortical nodular disease, which progressed into adrenal tumors [67–69]. Adrenocortical lesions described as microadenomas or tumors developed in 6% of heterozygous animals within the first year of life, and in up to 30% in a cohort of roughly 2-year-old animals [69]. In addition to these small lesions, adrenal tumors with a more aggressive growth behavior have been reported with an incidence after 18 months of up to 46% of heterozygous animals [68]. Notably, other MEN1-defining tumors including pancreatic islet cell tumors and pituitary adenomas developed at an earlier time point and with higher penetrance [67, 69]. As homozygous menin knockout animals die in utero, only heterozygous mice were phenotypically characterized. However, in accordance with a two hit model of a tumor suppressor gene, the remaining wild-type *Menin* allele could be demonstrated to be lost in somatic tumor cells [67–69]. This is in striking contrast to human adrenal lesions as part of MEN1, where LOH does not seem to be a dominant tumorigenic mechanism (see Chapter 10).

In addition to the summarized mouse models defined by an adrenal tumor phenotype, mouse models displaying a growth defect of the adrenal cortex either during embryogenesis or in the adult animal can often provide useful information about genes involved in normal growth and development that (by inference) may play a role in cancer. This concept is highlighted by Sf1, which had originally been identified as a transcription factor that, when absent, results in adrenal agenesis. As described above, however, *Sf1*, when overexpressed or excessively active, can be associated with an adrenal growth defect contributing to adrenal tumor growth. Other examples include animal models exploring transcription factors such as Pbx1 [70] or signaling pathways, such as Wnt/β-catenin [71] or sonic hedgehog (see Chapters 16 and 17) [72]. It is likely that in the future other mouse models with adrenal growth defects will provide novel insights in the pathogenesis of unrestricted growth as observed in ACC.

References

1. Cohen AI et al (1957) Histologic and physiologic characteristics of hormone-secreting transplantable adrenal tumors in mice and rats. Am J Pathol 33:631–651
2. Humphreys SR et al (1965) Transplantation characteristics and response to chemotherapy of a murine adrenal tumor. Eur J Cancer 1:125–133
3. Cohen AI, Furth J (1959) Corticotropin assay with transplantable adrenocortical tumor slices: application to the assay of adrenotropic pituitary tumors. Cancer Res 19:72–78
4. Yasumura Y et al (1966) Clonal analysis of differentiated function in animal cell cultures. I. Possible correlated maintenance of differentiated function and the diploid karyotype. Cancer Res 26:529–535

5. Rainey WE et al (2004) Adrenocortical cell lines. Mol Cell Endocrinol 228:23–38
6. Woolley GW, Little CC (1945) The incidence of adrenal cortical carcinoma in gonadectomized female mice of the extreme dilution strain. I Observation on the adrenal cortex. Cancer Res 5:193–202
7. Johnsen IK et al (2006) Gonadectomy in mice of the inbred strain CE/J induces proliferation of sub-capsular adrenal cells expressing gonadal marker genes. J Endocrinol 190:47–57
8. Bielinska M et al (2003) Mouse strain susceptibility to gonadectomy-induced adrenocortical tumor formation correlates with the expression of GATA-4 and luteinizing hormone receptor. Endocrinology 144:4123–4133.
9. Murthy AS et al (1970) Postcastrational adrenal tumors in two strains of mice: morphologic, histochemical, and chromatographic studies. J Natl Cancer Inst 45:1211–1222
10. Bielinska M et al (2005) Gonadotropin-induced adrenocortical neoplasia in NU/J nude mice. Endocrinology 146:3975–3984
11. Russfield AB (1975) Experimental endocrinopathies. Methods Achiev Exp Pathol 7:132–148
12. Woolley GW, Little CC (1946) Transplantation of an adrenal cortical carcinoma. Cancer Res 6:712–717
13. Woolley GW, Little CC (1945) The incidence of adrenal cortical carcinoma in gonadectomized female mice of the extreme dilution strain. II. Observation on the accessory sex organs. Cancer Res 5:203–210
14. Tremblay JJ, Viger RS (2001) GATA factors differentially activate multiple gonadal promoters through conserved GATA regulatory elements. Endocrinology 142:977–986
15. Laitinen MP et al (2000) Transcription factors GATA-4 and GATA-6 and a GATA family cofactor, FOG-2, are expressed in human ovary and sex cord-derived ovarian tumors. J Clin Endocrinol Metab 85:3476–3483
16. Looyenga BD, Hammer GD (2006) Origin and identity of adrenocortical tumors in inhibin knockout mice: implications for cellular plasticity in the adrenal cortex. Mol Endocrinol 20:2848–2863
17. Bernichtein S et al (2008) Adrenal gland tumorigenesis after gonadectomy in mice is a complex genetic trait driven by epistatic loci. Endocrinology 149:651–661
18. Luo X et al (1994) A cell-specific nuclear receptor is essential for adrenal and gonadal development and sexual differentiation. Cell 77:481–490
19. Frigeri C et al (2002) A polymorphic form of steroidogenic factor-1 is associated with adrenocorticotropin resistance in y1 mouse adrenocortical tumor cell mutants. Endocrinology 143:4031–4037
20. Figueiredo BC et al (2005) Amplification of the steroidogenic factor 1 gene in childhood adrenocortical tumors. J Clin Endocrinol Metab 90:615–619
21. Doghman M et al (2007) Increased steroidogenic factor-1 dosage triggers adrenocortical cell proliferation and cancer. Mol Endocrinol 21:2968–2987
22. Kim AC et al (2009) In search of adrenocortical stem and progenitor cells. Endocr Rev 30:241–263
23. Yamazaki H et al (1998) Establishment of an adrenocortical carcinoma xenograft with normotensive hyperaldosteronism in vivo. Apmis 106:1056–1060
24. Logie A et al (2000) Establishment and characterization of a human adrenocortical carcinoma xenograft model. Endocrinology 141:3165–3171
25. Gazdar AF et al (1990) Establishment and characterization of a human adrenocortical carcinoma cell line that expresses multiple pathways of steroid biosynthesis. Cancer Res 50:5488–5496
26. Leibovitz A et al (1973) New human cancer cell culture lines. I. SW-13, small-cell carcinoma of the adrenal cortex. J Natl Cancer Inst 51:691–697
27. Schteingart DE et al (2001) Overexpression of CXC chemokines by an adrenocortical carcinoma: a novel clinical syndrome. J Clin Endocrinol Metab 86:3968–3974
28. Barlaskar FM et al (2009) Preclinical targeting of the type I insulin-like growth factor receptor in adrenocortical carcinoma. J Clin Endocrinol Metab 94:204–212

29. Wolkersdorfer GW et al (2002) A novel approach using transcomplementing adenoviral vectors for gene therapy of adrenocortical cancerACC. Horm Metab Res 34: 279–287
30. Zwermann O et al (2005) ACTH 1-24 inhibits proliferation of adrenocortical tumors in vivo. Eur J Endocrinol 153:435–444
31. Reincke M et al (1997) Deletion of the adrenocorticotropin receptor gene in human adrenocortical tumors: implications for tumorigenesis. J Clin Endocrinol Metab 82:3054–3058
32. Hornsby PJ (2001) Transplantation of adrenocortical cells. Rev Endocr Metab Disord 2: 313–321
33. Thomas M et al (2003) Adrenocortical cell transplantation in scid mice: the role of the host animals' adrenal glands. J Steroid Biochem Mol Biol 85:285–290
34. Thomas M et al (2000) Formation of functional tissue from transplanted adrenocortical cells expressing telomerase reverse transcriptase. Nat Biotechnol 18: 39–42
35. Thomas M et al (2002) Cooperation of TERT, SV40 T antigen and oncogenic Ras in tumorigenesis: a cell transplantation model using bovine adrenocortical cells. Neoplasia 4:493–500
36. Sun B et al (2004) Progressive loss of malignant behavior in telomerase-negative tumorigenic adrenocortical cells and restoration of tumorigenicity by human telomerase reverse transcriptase. Cancer Res 64:6144–6151
37. Lacroix A et al (2004) Cushing's syndrome variants secondary to aberrant hormone receptors. Trends Endocrinol Metab 15:375–382
38. Mazzuco TL et al (2006) Ectopic expression of the gastric inhibitory polypeptide receptor gene is a sufficient genetic event to induce benign adrenocortical tumor in a xenotransplantation model. Endocrinology 147:782–790
39. Mazzuco TL et al (2006) Aberrant expression of human luteinizing hormone receptor by adrenocortical cells is sufficient to provoke both hyperplasia and Cushing's syndrome features. J Clin Endocrinol Metab 91:196–203
40. Ortmann D et al (2004) Steroidogenic acute regulatory (StAR)-directed immunotherapy protects against tumor growth of StAR-expressing Sp2-0 cells in a rodent adrenocortical carcinoma model. Endocrinology 145:1760–1766
41. Giordano TJ et al (2003) Distinct transcriptional profiles of adrenocortical tumors uncovered by DNA microarray analysis. Am J Pathol 162:521–531
42. Weber MM et al (1997) Insulin-like growth factor receptors in normal and tumorous adult human adrenocortical glands. Eur J Endocrinol 136:296–303
43. Compagnone NA et al (1997) Characterization of adrenocortical cell lines produced by genetically targeted tumorigenesis in transgenic mice. Steroids 62:238–243
44. Sahut-Barnola I et al (2000) Adrenal tumorigenesis targeted by the corticotropin-regulated promoter of the aldo-keto reductase AKR1B7 gene in transgenic mice. Endocr Res 26: 885–898
45. Kananen K et al (1996) Gonadectomy permits adrenocortical tumorigenesis in mice transgenic for the mouse inhibin alpha-subunit promoter/simian virus 40 T-antigen fusion gene: evidence for negative autoregulation of the inhibin alpha- subunit gene. Mol Endocrinol 10:1667–1677
46. Ragazzon B et al (2006) Adrenocorticotropin-dependent changes in SF-1/DAX-1 ratio influence steroidogenic genes expression in a novel model of glucocorticoid-producing adrenocortical cell lines derived from targeted tumorigenesis. Endocrinology 147: 1805–1818
47. Kananen K et al (1995) Gonadal tumorigenesis in transgenic mice bearing the mouse inhibin alpha-subunit promoter/simian virus T-antigen fusion gene: characterization of ovarian tumors and establishment of gonadotropin-responsive granulosa cell lines. Mol Endocrinol 9: 616–627
48. Roberts VJ et al (1991) Expression of inhibin/activin subunit messenger ribonucleic acids during rat embryogenesis. Endocrinology 128:3122–3129

49. Kananen K et al (1997) Suppression of gonadotropins inhibits gonadal tumorigenesis in mice transgenic for the mouse inhibin alpha-subunit promoter/simian virus 40 T-antigen fusion gene. Endocrinology 138:3521–3531
50. Rilianawati et al (1998) Direct luteinizing hormone action triggers adrenocortical tumorigenesis in castrated mice transgenic for the murine inhibin alpha-subunit promoter/simian virus 40 T-antigen fusion gene. Mol Endocrinol 12:801–809
51. Rilianawati et al (2000) Long-term testosterone treatment prevents gonadal and adrenal tumorigenesis of mice transgenic for the mouse inhibin-alpha subunit promoter/simian virus 40 T-antigen fusion gene. J Endocrinol 166:77–85
52. Rahman NA et al (2004) Adrenocortical tumorigenesis in transgenic mice expressing the inhibin alpha-subunit promoter/simian virus 40 T-antigen transgene: relationship between ectopic expression of luteinizing hormone receptor and transcription factor GATA-4. Mol Endocrinol 18:2553–2569
53. Mikola M et al (2003) High levels of luteinizing hormone analog stimulate gonadal and adrenal tumorigenesis in mice transgenic for the mouse inhibin-alpha-subunit promoter/Simian virus 40 T-antigen fusion gene. Oncogene 22:3269–3278
54. Vuorenoja S et al (2007) Adrenocortical tumorigenesis, luteinizing hormone receptor and transcription factors GATA-4 and GATA-6. Mol Cell Endocrinol 269:38–45
55. Vuorenoja S et al (2008) Targeted therapy for adrenocortical tumors in transgenic mice through their LH receptor by Hecate-human chorionic gonadotropin beta conjugate. Endocr Relat Cancer 15:635–648
56. Vuorenoja S et al (2009) Hecate-CG{beta} conjugate and gonadotropin suppression shows two distinct mechanisms of action in the treatment of adrenocortical tumors in transgenic mice expressing Simian Virus 40 T antigen under inhibin-{alpha} promoter. Endocr Relat Cancer 16:549–564
57. Doghman M et al (2009) Inhibition of adrenocortical carcinoma cell proliferation by steroidogenic factor-1 inverse agonists. J Clin Endocrinol Metab 94:2178–2183
58. Matzuk MM et al (1992) Alpha-inhibin is a tumour-suppressor gene with gonadal specificity in mice. Nature 360:313–319
59. Beuschlein F et al (2003) Activin Induces x-Zone Apoptosis That Inhibits Luteinizing Hormone-Dependent Adrenocortical Tumor Formation in Inhibin-Deficient Mice. Mol Cell Biol 23:3951–3964.
60. Matzuk MM et al (1994) Development of cancer cachexia-like syndrome and adrenal tumors in inhibin-deficient mice. Proc Natl Acad Sci U S A 91:8817–8821
61. Looyenga BD, Hammer GD (2007) Genetic removal of Smad3 from inhibin-null mice attenuates tumor progression by uncoupling extracellular mitogenic signals from the cell cycle machinery. Mol Endocrinol 21:2440–2457
62. Burns KH et al (2003) Cyclin D2 and p27 are tissue-specific regulators of tumorigenesis in inhibin alpha knockout mice. Mol Endocrinol 17:2053–2069
63. West AN et al (2006) Identification of a novel germ line variant hotspot mutant p53-R175L in pediatric adrenal cortical carcinoma. Cancer Res 66:5056–5062
64. Chari NS et al (2009) The p53 tumor suppressor network in cancer and the therapeutic modulation of cell death. Apoptosis 14:336–347
65. Else T et al (2009) Genetic p53 deficiency partially rescues the adrenocortical dysplasia phenotype at the expense of increased tumorigenesis. Cancer Cell 15:465–476
66. Skogseid B et al (1992) Clinical and genetic features of adrenocortical lesions in multiple endocrine neoplasia type 1. J Clin Endocrinol Metab 75:76–81
67. Crabtree JS et al (2001) A mouse model of multiple endocrine neoplasia, type 1, develops multiple endocrine tumors. Proc Natl Acad Sci U S A 98:1118–1123
68. Bertolino P et al (2003) Heterozygous Men1 mutant mice develop a range of endocrine tumors mimicking multiple endocrine neoplasia type 1. Mol Endocrinol 17:1880–1892
69. Loffler KA et al (2007) Broad tumor spectrum in a mouse model of multiple endocrine neoplasia type 1. Int J Cancer 120:259–267

70. Lichtenauer UD et al (2007) Pre-B-cell transcription factor 1 and steroidogenic factor 1 synergistically regulate adrenocortical growth and steroidogenesis. Endocrinology 148:693–704
71. Kim AC et al (2008) Targeted disruption of beta-catenin in Sf1-expressing cells impairs development and maintenance of the adrenal cortex. Development 135:2593–2602
72. Bose J et al (2002) Pallister-Hall syndrome phenotype in mice mutant for Gli3. Hum Mol Genet 11:1129–1135
73. Cardoso CC et al (2009) New methods for investigating experimental human adrenal tumorigenesis. Mol Cell Endocrinol 300:175–179

Part VII
Therapies

Chapter 20
Overview of Treatment Options for Adrenocortical Carcinoma

Gary D. Hammer

Complete surgical excision is the only treatment option for adrenocortical carcinoma (ACC), which provides the potential for cure. Nonetheless, the 5-year survival of patients following intent-to-cure surgery ranges between 32 and 48% [1–4]. For incidentally identified lesions that are suspected of being ACC, careful surgical judgment must be applied regarding the operative approach (laparoscopic vs. open exploration) [5].

Because of high rates of local recurrence and intraperitoneal dissemination, laparoscopic resection is reserved for patients with small (<3 cm), functional, presumed benign tumors or tumors with borderline malignancy risk and for the patients requiring adrenalectomy for metastatic disease [6–8]. Any difficulty in the laparoscopic approach requires immediate conversion to an open resection.

A transabdominal approach is considered standard of care to facilitate total gross removal of the tumor without capsular breach or tumor spillage. Resection of adjacent structures including liver kidney, spleen, pancreas, colon, or stomach is sometimes indicated due to tumor invasion in patients with stage III. Aggressive removal of tumor that has invaded the vena cava should be considered [9].

Regional recurrence and isolated distant metastases are sometimes treated surgically if complete resection can be achieved in a patient with excellent performance status. For patients with a symptomatic recurrence due to local mass effects or hormone excess, partial resection can relieve pain or control hormone excess [10–12, 13–16]. However, results are variable [17, 18]. Tumor involvement of the celiac axis and superior mesenteric artery are contraindications for surgery. [6]. See the Chapters 2 and 24 for more detailed discussion.

G.D. Hammer (✉)
Endocrine Oncology Program – Comprehensive Cancer Center, Department of Internal Medicine – Division of Metabolism, Endocrinology & Diabetes, Department of Molecular & Integrative Physiology, Department of Cell & Developmental Biology, University of Michigan, 1528 BSRB, 109 Zina Pitcher Pl., Ann Arbor, MI 48109-2200, USA
e-mail: ghammer@med.umich.edu

G.D. Hammer, T. Else (eds.), *Adrenocortical Carcinoma*,
DOI 10.1007/978-0-387-77236-3_20, © Springer Science+Business Media, LLC 2011

20.1 Adjuvant Treatment

The risk of recurrence in ACC remains significant even in stage 1 disease (tumor size < 5 cm) – particularly if the tumor is of high grade (Ki67 > 10%). For this reason, most ACC specialists support adjuvant therapy to prevent gross recurrence of disease – including systemic mitotane and/or local radiation therapy to the operative bed (see Chapters 22 and 25 for more detail).

Mitotane (Lysodren, o,p'-DDD; HRA Pharma, Paris; Bristol Meyer Squibb, New York) remains the only FDA-approved drug for the treatment of ACC. Developed in 1960 as a derivative of the pesticide DDT, mitotane is both an inhibitor of steroidogenesis and an adrenolytic agent that causes degeneration of the fascicula and reticularis cell, with relative sparing of the zona glomerulosa. Mechanistically, it directly inhibits 11β-hydroxylase and cholesterol side-chain cleavage (SCC) together with antagonizing chemotherapy drug efflux (MDR) [19–22].

Mitotane has a narrow therapeutic index with antitumor activity achieved at a plasma concentration of 14 mg/L, but significant side effects with levels over 20 mg/L, which include the gastrointestinal system or the central nervous system. Patients on mitotane must have close surveillance of the blood level of mitotane, adrenal function, and side effects. Unless patients present with active Cushing's syndrome, noncurrent administration of glucocorticoids is necessary as is the administration of stress dose steroids in the setting of acute illness.

In the adjuvant setting, mitotane has been used after curative or complete surgical resection [23–27]. In a recent study of 177 patients with resected ACC (stages I–III) treated with adjuvant mitotane in Italy and Germany [28, 29], nearly half received adjuvant mitotane (47/102 patients) at doses ranging from 1 to 5 grams daily. With a median duration of 29 months, both disease-free survival and overall survival were increased in the mitotane-treated patients. This work has raised both controversy and motivation on the utility of a prospective study on the benefits of adjuvant mitotane (see Chapter 22).

As detailed in Chapter 25, while radiotherapy has been considered by some to be ineffective in ACC [14, 30, 31], most ACC investigators view XRT as a valuable adjuvant regimen for the treatment of residual disease of tumor spillage following initial surgery of curative intent. Although no improvement in disease-free or overall survival was observed, Fassnacht et al. [32] reported a delay in disease-free recurrence in patients receiving adjuvant radiotherapy (79% vs. 12%, $P < 0.01$).

20.2 Treatment of Metastatic Disease

Most ACC patients present with metastatic or unresectable disease. Moreover, despite initial complete resection of ACC, 70–80% of patients ultimately develop recurrent or metastatic disease [33–35] and require medical therapy with chemotherapy with or without steroidogenic inhibition (see Chapters 21, 22 and 23).

Despite the lack of randomized prospective trials in patients with metastastic unresectable ACC, mitotane has been used for over 50 years, with objective radiographic response rates observed in approximately 25% of patients [1, 14, 17, 19–21, 23, 33, 36–41].

Cytotoxic chemotherapies have been mostly disappointing with response rates of only 15% [38, 42–46]. However, regimens utilizing cisplatin-based chemotherapy have reported response rates of approximately 20–30% [42–44, 47, 48,]. Using the combination of mitotane (4 g daily) with cisplatin, etoposide, and doxorubicin (M-EAP), Berutti and colleagues observed a response rate of 49% (by WHO criteria) and a concomitant decrease in hormone overproduction in 9 of 16 patients [49]. Another regimen that has gained popularity due to a lower side-effect profile is a

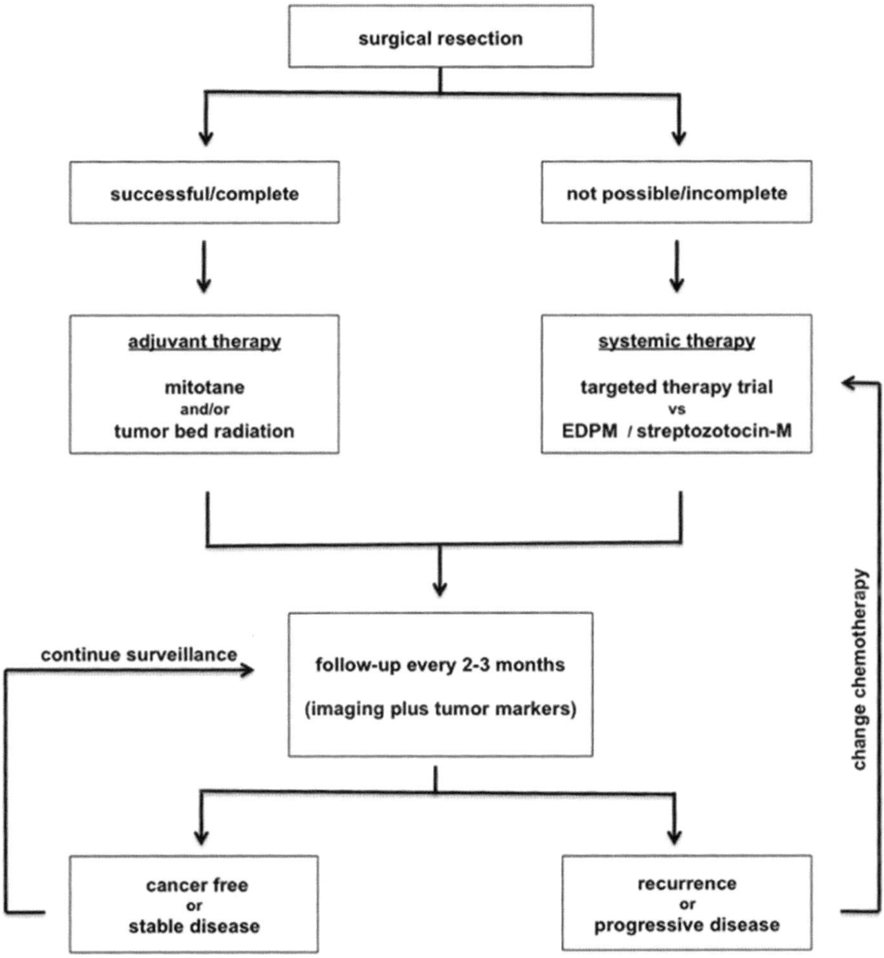

Fig. 20.1 Flow chart of therapeutic options for adrenocortical carcinoma

combination of mitotane–streptozotocin (M-S). Khan and colleagues [50] observed a response rate of 36% in patients with metastatic disease. Other small trials of various chemotherapy regimens combined with mitotane have reported response rate of about 32% [50–52, 47, 48].

Current efforts focus on the development and implementation of an international cooperative group to coordinate trial design and implementation. The FIRM-ACT (First International Randomized trial on locally advanced and Metastatic Adrenocortical Carcinoma Treatment) is the first of these effects. Patients with advanced ACC are treated either with M-EAP or M-S as front-line therapy (http://www.firm-act.org/) [53].

Additional treatment modalities that are used for isolated metastatic ACC include surgery, radiation therapy, cryotherapy, and chemo-embolization. These modalities are usually reserved to relieve symptomatic hormone excess, pain, or impending organ damage resulting from metastatic ACC.

See flow chart of therapeutic options in Fig. 20.1.

20.3 Medical Treatment of Adrenocortical Carcinoma Steroidogenic Hormone Excess

Patients with metastatic ACC that exhibits autonomous steroid secretion should be treated with steroidogenic inhibitors to ameliorate the effects of excessive mineralocorticoids (hypertension and hypokalemia), glucocorticoids (hypertension, hyperglycemia, hypokalemia, and muscle atrophy), and sex steroids (gynecomastia, virilization, erectile dysfunction, and menstrual irregularities). In addition to mitotane, inhibitors include ketoconazole, metyrapone, aminoglutethimide, and etomidate. While these agents have measurable benefits in benign adrenal disease, it is extremely difficult to control the extreme hormone excess in patients with ACC (Chapter 23).

20.4 Emerging Therapies

The modest effects of current chemotherapeutic regimens for metastatic ACC highlight the need for new therapeutic modalities to impact life expectancy in ACC. As the genetics of ACC is studied by international cooperative groups, it is becoming clear that common genetic alterations together with multiple rare secondary and tertiary events contribute to ACC. Preclinical and early clinical trials that target common signaling and transcription pathways shown to be important in ACC such as the IGF and Wnt pathways and the nuclear receptor SF1 have shown promise with NIH and industry sponsored trials emerging (Chapter 31).

References

1. Crucitti F et al (1996) The Italian Registry for Adrenal Cortical Carcinoma: analysis of a multiinstitutional series of 129 patients. The ACC Italian Registry Study Group. Surgery 119(2):161–170
2. Lee JE et al (1995) Surgical management, DNA content, and patient survival in adrenal cortical carcinoma. Surgery 118(6):1090–1098
3. Icard P et al (1992) Adrenocortical carcinoma in surgically treated patients: a retrospective study on 156 cases by the French Association of Endocrine Surgery. Surgery 112(6):972–979 [discussion: 979–980]
4. Zografos GC et al (1994) Adrenal adenocarcinoma: a review of 53 cases. J Surg Oncol 55(3):160–164
5. Saunders BD, Doherty GM (2004) Laparoscopic adrenalectomy for malignant disease. Lancet Oncology 5(12):718–726
6. Dackiw AP et al (2001) Adrenal cortical carcinoma. World J Surg 25(7): 914–26
7. Cobb WS et al (2005) Laparoscopic adrenalectomy for malignancy. Am J Surg 189(4): 405–411
8. Gonzalez RJ et al (2005) Laparoscopic resection of adrenal cortical carcinoma: a cautionary note. Surgery 138(6):1078–1085 [discussion: 1085–6]
9. Harrison LE et al (1999) Pathologic features of prognostic significance for adrenocortical carcinoma after curative resection. Arch Surg 134(2):181–185
10. Allolio B, Fassnacht M (2006) Clinical review: Adrenocortical carcinoma: clinical update. J Clin Endocrinol Metab 91(6):2027–2037
11. Ng L, Libertino JM (2003) Adrenocortical carcinoma: diagnosis, evaluation and treatment. J Urol 169(1):5–11
12. Schteingart DE et al (2005) Management of patients with adrenal cancer: recommendations of an international consensus conference. Endocr Relat Cancer 12(3):667–680
13. Icard P et al (2001) Adrenocortical carcinomas: surgical trends and results of a 253-patient series from the French Association of Endocrine Surgeons study group. World J Surg 25(7):891–897
14. Luton JP et al (1990) Clinical features of adrenocortical carcinoma, prognostic factors, and the effect of mitotane therapy. N Engl J Med 322(17):1195–201
15. Macfarlane DA (1958) Cancer of the adrenal cortex; the natural history, prognosis and treatment in a study of fifty-five cases. Ann R Coll Surg Engl 23(3):155–186
16. Grondal S et al (1990) Adrenocortical carcinoma. A retrospective study of a rare tumor with a poor prognosis. Eur J Surg Oncol 16(6):500–506
17. Wajchenberg BL et al (2000) Adrenocortical carcinoma: clinical and laboratory observations. Cancer 88(4):711–736
18. Hogan TF et al (1980) A clinical and pathological study of adrenocortical carcinoma: therapeutic implications. Cancer 45(11):2880–2883
19. Haak HR et al (1994) Optimal treatment of adrenocortical carcinoma with mitotane: results in a consecutive series of 96 patients. Br J Cancer 69(5):947–951
20. Baudin E et al (2001) Impact of monitoring plasma 1,1-dichlorodiphenildichloroethane (o,p'DDD) levels on the treatment of patients with adrenocortical carcinoma. Cancer 92(6):1385–1392
21. van Slooten H et al (1984) The treatment of adrenocortical carcinoma with o,p'-DDD: prognostic implications of serum level monitoring. Eur J Cancer Clin Oncol 20(1):47–53
22. Heilmann P et al (2001) Therapy of the adrenocortical carcinoma with Lysodren (o,p'-DDD): Therapeutic management by monitoring o,p'-DDD blood levels. Med Klin (Munich) 96(7):371–377
23. Venkatesh S et al (1989) Adrenal cortical carcinoma. Cancer 64(3): 765–769
24. Schteingart DF et al (1982) Treatment of adrenal carcinomas. Arch Surg 117(9): 1142–1146

25. Berruli A et al (2005) Adjuvant mitotane therapy for adreno-cortical carcinoma (abstract). J Clin Oncol 23(16S, part 1):4570
26. Dickstein G et al (1998) Is there a role for low doses of mitotane (o,p'- DDD) as adjuvant therapy in adrenocortical carcinoma? J Clin Endocrinol Metab 83(9): 3100–3103
27. Vassilopoulou-Sellin R et al (1993) Impact of adjuvant mitotane on the clinical course of patients with adrenocortical cancer. Cancer 71(10):3119–3123
28. Zhao J, Speel EJ et al (1999) Analysis of genomic alterations in sporadic adrenocortical lesions. Gain of chromosome 17 is an early event in adrenocortical tumorigenesis. Am J Pathol 155(4):1039–1045
29. Kjellman M et al (1996) Genetic aberrations in adrenocortical tumors detected using comparative genomic hybridization correlate with tumor size and malignancy. Cancer Res 56(18):4219–4223
30. Hutter AM Jr, Kayhoe DE (1996) Adrenal cortical carcinoma. Clinical features of 138 patients. Am J Med 41(4):572–580
31. Schulick RD, Brennan MF (1999) Long-term survival after complete resection and repeat resection in patients with adrenocortical carcinoma. Ann Surg Oncol 6(8):719–726
32. Fassnacht M et al (2006) Efficacy of adjuvant radiotherapy of the tumor bed on local recurrence of adrenocortical carcinoma. J Clin Endocrinol Metab 91(11):4501–4504
33. Pommier RF, Brennan MF (1992) An eleven-year experience with adrenocortical carcinoma. Surgery 112(6):963–970 [discussion: 970–971]
34. Bertagna C, Orth DN (1981) Clinical and laboratory findings and results of therapy in 58 patients with adrenocortical tumors admitted to a single medical center (1951 to 1978). Am J Med 71(5):855–875
35. Stojadinovic A et al (2002) Adrenocortical carcinoma: clinical, morphologic, and molecular characterization. J Clin Oncol 20(4):941–950
36. Hutter AM Jr, Kayhoe DE (1996) Adrenal cortical carcinoma. Results of treatment with o,p'DDD in 138 patients. Am J Med 41(4):581–592.
37. Lubitz JA et al (1973) Mitotane use in inoperable adrenal cortical carcinoma. JAMA 223(10):1109–1112
38. Decker RA et al (1991) Eastern Cooperative Oncology Group study 1879: mitotane and Adriamycin in patients with advanced adrenocortical carcinoma. Surgery 110(6): 1006–1013
39. Haak HR et al (1991) Prolonged bleeding time due to mitotane therapy. Eur J Cancer 27(5):638–641
40. Henley DJ et al (1983) Adrenal cortical carcinoma—a continuing challenge. Surgery 94(6):926–931
41. Kasperlik-Zaluska AA (2000) Clinical results of the use of mitotane for adrenocortical carcinoma. Braz J Med Biol Res 33(10):1191–1196
42. Schlumberger M et al (1991) 5-Fluorouracil, doxorubicin, and cisplatin as treatment for adrenal cortical carcinoma. Cancer 67(12):2997–3000
43. van Slooten H, van Oosterom AT (1983) CAP (cyclophosphamide, doxorubicin, and cisplatin) regimen in adrenal cortical carcinoma. Cancer Treat Rep 67(4):377–379
44. Williamson SK et al (2000) Phase II evaluation of cisplatin and etoposide followed by mitotane at disease progression in patients with locally advanced or metastatic adrenocortical carcinoma: a Southwest Oncology Group Study. Cancer 88(5):1159–1165
45. Baudin E et al (2002) Use of a topoisomerase I inhibitor (irinotecan, CPT-11) in metastatic adrenocortical carcinoma. Ann Oncol 13(11):1806–1809
46. La Rocca RV et al (1990) Suramin in adrenal cancer: modulation of steroid hormone production, cytotoxicity in vitro, and clinical antitumor effect. J Clin Endocrinol Metab 71(2):497–504
47. Bonacci R et al (1998) Cytotoxic therapy with etoposide and cisplatin in advanced adrenocortical carcinoma. Reseau Comete INSERM. Br J Cancer 78(4):546–549

48. Bukowski RM et al (1993) Phase II trial of mitotane and cisplatin in patients with adrenal carcinoma: a Southwest Oncology Group study. J Clin Oncol 11(1): 161–165
49. Berruti A et al (2005) Etoposide, doxorubicin and cisplatin plus mitotane in the treatment of advanced adrenocortical carcinoma: a large prospective phase II trial. Endocr Relat Cancer 12(3):657–666
50. Khan TS et al (2000) Streptozocin and o,p'DDD in the treatment of adrenocortical cancer patients: long-term survival in its adjuvant use. Ann Oncol 11(10): 1281–1287
51. Abraham J et al (2002) A phase II trial of combination chemotherapy and surgical resection for the treatment of metastatic adrenocortical carcinoma: continuous infusion doxorubicin, vincristine, and etoposide with daily mitotane as a P-glycoprotein antagonist. Cancer 94(9):2333–2343
52. Berruti A et al (1998) Mitotane associated with etoposide, doxorubicin, and cisplatin in the treatment of advanced adrenocortical carcinoma. Italian Group for the Study of Adrenal Cancer. Cancer 83(10):2194–2200
53. Koschker AC et al (2006) Adrenocortical carcinoma – improving patient care by establishing new structures. Exp Clin Endocrinol Diabetes 114(2):45–51

Chapter 21
Chemotherapy

Alfredo Berruti, Paola Sperone, Paola Perotti, Anna Ferrero, Luigi Dogliotti, and Massimo Terzolo

The extreme rarity of adrenocortical carcinoma (ACC) has hampered the conduction of well-designed high-powered prospective studies testing the efficacy of systemic therapy. This limitation notwithstanding, there is evidence that chemotherapy has some activity in advanced ACC. Patients considered eligible for chemotherapy are generally patients with advanced/inoperable disease progressing with mitotane treatment or patients with ACC demonstrating a rapid pattern of tumor growth. Cisplatin-containing regimens plus mitotane seem to be the most active chemotherapy schemes. Whether such combination schemes are more efficacious than non-cisplatin-containing regimens is being addressed by a currently ongoing large multicenter multinational randomized prospective study that compares the efficacy of etoposide, doxorubicin, and cisplatin (EDP) plus mitotane vs. streptozotocin plus mitotane (FIRM-ACT study).

Although only a minority of advanced ACC patients are expected to respond to chemotherapy, treatment response is often durable particularly if the residual disease becomes amenable to surgery with radical intent. These data suggest that chemotherapy may be efficacious in a subset of patients. Unfortunately, no predictive factors for chemotherapy efficacy in advanced ACC are actually available for the routine use.

Chemotherapy could be a reasonable option for ACC patients with advanced or metastatic disease not suitable for surgery with radical intent. The activity of cytotoxic drugs in this setting has been repeatedly tested over the past three decades. However, to date only phase II trials have been published, most of them recruiting a small number of patients. In the absence of prospective randomized clinical trials, there has been little demonstration that chemotherapy is able to change the natural history of the disease.

A. Berruti (✉)
Oncologia Medica, Azienda Ospedaliero Universitaria San Luigi, Regione Gonzole, 10, 10043 Orbassano, Italy
e-mail: alfredo.berruti@gmail.com

G.D. Hammer, T. Else (eds.), *Adrenocortical Carcinoma*,
DOI 10.1007/978-0-387-77236-3_21,

ACCs have strong expression of the multidrug-resistance gene *MDR1* [1], resulting in production of P-glycoprotein, which facilitates the efflux of cytotoxic agents. In addition, ACCs show defects in p53 signaling pathways [2], which prevent ACC cells to undergo apoptosis in response to damage induced by cytotoxic drugs. These features hamper the efficacy of cytotoxic drugs in this disease. ACC, therefore, represents an ideal disease for testing the drugs able to circumvent the chemotherapy resistance.

These issues notwithstanding, longlasting disease responses have been obtained with cytotoxic therapy in advanced patients. These data suggest that chemotherapy might be efficacious in a subset of patients. This chapter reviews the data currently available on the activity of chemotherapy in this rare disease.

21.1 Single-Agent Chemotherapy

Few chemotherapy drugs have been tested as single agents in ACC patients. Most papers have included only a few cases or were case reports. The most significant data are depicted in Table 21.1. Responses have been obtained with adriamycin, alkylating agents, and cisplatin.

Table 21.1 Activity of single-agent chemotherapeutic drugs

1st Author (year)	Drug	No patients	Responses
Haq (1980)	BCNU	2	0
Haq (1980)	Peptichemio	4	1
Haq (1980)	AMSA	2	0
Haq (1980)	Adriamycin	4	1
Decker (1991)	Adriamycin	16	3
Pommier (1992)	Adriamycin	4	2
Tattersall (1980)	Cisplatin	4	4
Grapski (1983)	Cisplatin	4	3
Chun (1983)	Cisplatin	5	0
Baudin (2002)	CPT-11	12	0
La Rocca (1990b)	Suramin	17	2
Arit (1994)	Suramin	9	3
Flack (1993)	Gossypol	21	3

In a phase II study conducted by the Eastern Cooperative Oncology Group (ECOG) from November 1979 to July 1986, 52 patients with advanced ACC received either mitotane treatment or adriamycin [3]. Thirty-six patients with well-differentiated or functional tumors received mitotane, 6 g daily; 16 patients with poorly differentiated tumors received adriamycin (60 mg/m^2 every 3 weeks). Eight patients (22%) responded to mitotane and three (19%) responded to adriamycin. Fifteen patients for whom mitotane failed were crossed over to treatment with adriamycin but no response was noted. The authors concluded that mitotane or adriamycin used initially can induce tumor regression in selected patients.

However, adriamycin was ineffective as second-line chemotherapy for patients with well-differentiated or functioning tumors for whom mitotane was ineffective.

Cisplatin is the compound that has shown the greatest activity. In a total of 13 patients recruited in three different small series [4–6], seven responses were recorded.

CPT-11, a topoisomerase-1 inhibitor, was tested against advanced ACC in a single institution study [9]. Twelve patients entered the study with progressive disease following prior treatment; two of them following mitotane alone, one following chemotherapy (cisplatin and etoposide) and eight after receiving mitotane followed by cytotoxic chemotherapy with cisplatin-containing schemes. CPT-11 (250 mg/m^2) was administered intravenously on day 1 in a 2-h infusion, every 14 days. No disease responses according to conventional WHO criteria were observed. Three patients achieved disease stabilization lasting from 1.5 to 4 months. The authors' conclusions were that CPT-11 is not active in heavily pretreated ACC patients.

Suramin is a polyanionic compound originally synthesized for use as an antiparasitic agent. Suramin has repeatedly shown to have adrenocorticolytic activity in humans [10]. The antitumor activity of suramin is based on the drug's ability to bind and inactivate growth factor and enzyme systems critical for cellular homeostasis and proliferation. The cytotoxic activity of suramin against ACC was observed in ACC cell lines in vitro. The clinical activity of suramin was tested in 17 patients with metastatic ACC [11]. Two patients achieved a partial response, two had a minor response, and five remained with stable disease for periods ranging from 3 to 10 months. Of the seven patients with excessive steroid hormone production at baseline conditions, one achieved a partial and one a complete normalization of steroid levels for the duration of suramin therapy. The antineoplastic activity of suramin in ACC patients was confirmed in a subsequent small phase II study in which three partial responses have been obtained out of 9 patients consecutively enrolled [12]. The responses obtained in this trial, however, were only transient and the toxicity (coagulopathy, thrombocytopenia, polyneuropathy) was remarkable. On the basis of these results the authors did not recommend suramin as the first-line treatment for metastatic ACC.

Gossypol, a spermatotoxin derived from crude cottonseed oil, inhibits the growth of human adrenocortical tumors in nude mice [13]. In a phase II study, 21 patients with metastatic adrenal cancer received oral gossypol at doses of 30–70 mg/day. Three of these patients, whose tumors were refractory to other chemotherapeutic agents, had partial tumor responses (>50% decrease in tumor volume) that lasted from several months to over 1 year. One patient had a minor response followed by resection of her remaining disease, one patient had stable disease, and thirteen patients had disease progression. Gossypol is currently being tested in a prospective phase II trial for efficacy in ACC patients.

The effects on the growth and survival of SW13 human ACC cells in culture of several established drugs, such as mitotane, cisplatin, etoposide, 5-fluorouracil, and suramin, have been tested in a recently published in vitro study [14]. The most potent chemotherapeutic agent in this system was paclitaxel. Cisplatin, etoposide, and mitotane required higher doses than paclitaxel to attain a cytotoxic effect.

The cytotoxic effect of paclitaxel has been also demonstrated against the human steroid-secreting NCI-H295 adrenocarcinoma cell line in a previous in vitro study [15]. These data suggest that paclitaxel might be a chemotherapeutic drug with promising activity in ACC. In contrast, the efficacy of paclitaxel in ACC patients has been scarcely explored. In unpublished experiences performed in a number of centers, paclitaxel administered at a conventional schedule (175–200 mg on day 1 every 21 days) did not show relevant activity in advanced ACC patients. Preclinical data, however, suggested that duration of exposures is an important factor in the cytotoxic activity of paclitaxel [16]. Prolonged exposure to relatively low concentrations of paclitaxel has been shown to induce apoptosis in several different cell lines and also demonstrated antiangiogenetic properties [17]. One strategy to produce extended cumulative drug exposures in vivo is the frequent, repetitive administration (metronomic schedule). A weekly paclitaxel schedule has been found to be more effective than an every 3-week schedule in a phase III trial involving advanced breast cancer patients [18]. Weekly paclitaxel has produced a partial response of lung metastases in one ACC patient with disease resistant to EDP plus mitotane regimen [19], while a minimal response was obtained with weekly paclitaxel plus interferon in a phase I study [20]. On these bases weekly paclitaxel deserves to be reconsidered for a prospective trial in advanced ACC.

Nab-paclitaxel, which combines a protein-conjugate with the chemotherapy agent in particle form, can increase intratumoral concentration of the paclitaxel by a receptor-mediated transport process across the endothelial cell wall, thereby breaching the blood/tumor interface [21]. Nab-paclitaxel, exhibits in vitro growth inhibition of ACC cells, NCI-H295R and SW13, at IC_{50} concentrations of 0.35 μM and 0.0087 μM, respectively, which are comparable to those obtained with paclitaxel. Interestingly, immunohistochemical staining of treated xenograft tumors showed no induction of MDR1 with Nab-paclitaxel treatment [22].

Nab-paclitaxel offers the additional advantages of delivery of a relatively higher dose of paclitaxel, the avoidance of the cremophor EL medium, and ease of administration. A more favorable toxicity profile would also be anticipated in comparison with either paclitaxel or docetaxel. Nab-paclitaxel has demonstrated a high degree of activity in metastatic breast and lung cancer [23, 24]. On these bases there is rationale of testing Nab-paclitaxel in advanced ACC patients.

21.2 Combination Chemotherapy

The activity of combination chemotherapy in advanced ACC has been explored in five small phase II studies. As outlined in Table 21.2, all these regimens contained cisplatin that was combined with etoposide, gemcitabine, or doxorubicin plus either 5-fluorouracil or cyclophosphamide. The overall response rate ranged between 11 and 45% with 95% confidence intervals largely overlapping. Disease response was in some cases durable. The cumulative response rate was 18% (95% CI: 10–24%). A complete clinical response was observed in only one case out of 99 cumulatively treated.

Table 21.2 Combination regimens without mitotane

1st Author (year)	Cytotoxic regimens	*n*	CR (*n*)	PR (*n*)	Overall Response rate (95% CI)	Response duration	Clinical benefit response + stable disease
Burgess (1993)	Cisplatin Etoposide	11	–	6	46% (16–76%)	Median 9 months	
Williamson (2000)	Cisplatin Etoposide	45	–	5	11% (4–24%)	n.r.	
Schlumberger (1991)	Cisplatin Doxorubicin 5-Fluorouracil	13	1	2	23% (5–54%)	42, 11, 6 months	6 (46%)
Van Slooten (1983)	Cisplatin, Doxorubicin, Cyclophosphamide	11	–	2	18% (0–41%)	18+, 23 months	8 (73%)
Menefee (2006)	Cisplatin Gemcitabine	18	–	2	11% (0–26%)	n.r.	5 (28%)
	TOTAL	98	1	17	17% (10–24%)		

The rationale of combining cisplatin and doxorubicin derived from the activity that these two drugs have demonstrated antineoplastic activity as single agents in ACC patients. Etoposide was employed in association with cisplatin due to the demonstrated synergistic activity of these two drugs in animal models [25] and the well-known efficacy of this combination in small cell lung cancer patients as well as patients with germ cell carcinoma. The combination of cisplatin plus etoposide obtained encouraging results in case report studies [26, 27] and in a small single institution experience from the MD Anderson Cancer Center in Houston (USA). The latter one showing a disease response in 6 out of 11 consecutive patients (46%) [28]. This was the rationale for a prospective phase II trial sponsored by the South West Oncology Group in the United States [29]. Forty-five patients with advanced, unresectable, or metastatic ACC received chemotherapy with cisplatin plus etoposide. Thirty-six of them were naive from systemic treatments, while nine had previously received mitotane therapy. At the time of disease progression, patients who had not previously received mitotane received the drug at 1000 mg orally four times a day. Even in a large cooperative group, this trial took 6.5 years to recruit the planned number of patients. Five patients attained only a partial disease response, and three additional patients attained a disease response that was not confirmed by a re-evaluation performed 4 weeks later. The authors did not report whether disease response was confined to treatment naive patients or was also observed in patients previously treated with mitotane. Interestingly, in this trial 24-h urine collections for determination of 17-ketosteroids and 17-hydroxycorticosteroids were performed before therapy and repeated every 3 weeks if initially abnormal. Fifteen patients had elevated hormone levels and nine of them attained a $\geq$50% reduction of baseline levels. Since chemotherapy is expected to have no influence on hormonal hypersecretion and none of these patients received concomitant mitotane treatment, in patients in whom hormonal response was associated with disease progression these results can be attributed to the achievement of an undifferentiated phenotype of cancer cells; but in case of disease stabilization or minimal response, an antineoplastic effect of chemotherapy can be reasonably taken into account. Such data can be used to underlines the importance of disease stabilization as a part of a clinical benefit in the context of a disease that usually shows an aggressive behavior. The proportion of patients attaining a disease stabilization in this trial was not reported, but the best treatment result was obtained in one patient who had no response but whose disease remained stable after 20 cycles. The patient survived 61 months from the date of the initiation of treatment and 46 months from the time of treatment withdrawal. Of the 36 patients did not receive mitotane therapy prior to protocol cytotoxic therapy. 17 of these patients were started on mitotane following progression of disease with cisplatin and etoposide therapy. Two of 16 evaluable patients in this group attained a partial response, suggesting some extent of anti-cancer activity of mitotane independent of cytotoxic chemotherapy.

The activity of the combination of cisplatin and doxorubicin was tested in two phase II trials. 5-Fluorouracil was added to this combination in one study, cyclophosphamide was added in the second one. In a single institution experience, the activity of the combination of cisplatin doxorubicin and 5-fluorouracil (FAP) was tested in 14 patients with advanced ACC recruited between 1983 and 1989 [30]. According to the WHO criteria one patient attained a complete response lasting 42 months, three patients a partial response lasting 6, 6 and 11 months. The overall response rate according to an intent to treat analysis was 28.5%, but one patient was excluded because mitotane was added to the FAP regimen. One patient attained a minimal response lasting 22 months and two patients had disease stabilization lasting 4 and 6 months, respectively. A clinical benefit (disease response plus stabilization) was obtained in 50% of cases (46% in the eligible ones).

Cisplatin, doxorubicin, and cyclophosphamide combination regimen was administered to 11 ACC patients with advanced disease in a single institution experience [31]. Two of them attained a partial response lasting 18+ and 23 months respectively, and six patients had disease stabilization so that an overall clinical benefit was observed in 73% of cases.

More recently, the results of the association of cisplatin and gemcitabine were reported as a meeting abstract [32]. Eighteen ACC patients with metastatic disease were recruited in a single institution. Five patients were treated at initial presentation, while thirteen were treated after disease progression or following a previous chemotherapy regimen. The partial response rate was 11%, with an additional 16% of patients demonstrating cytoreduction that did not meet the criteria for a partial response. Response duration was not reported.

The activity of combination chemotherapy in the management of advanced ACC patients was overall modest. However, disease responses and disease stabilizations were in some cases longlasting, suggesting that this treatment modality might be efficacious in a subset of patients.

21.3 Chemotherapy Plus Mitotane

Multidrug resistance (MDR) is a major cause of chemotherapy failure in cancer treatment. Surveys of human tumors have found very high levels of multidrug resistance 1 (*MDR1, ABCB1*) expression in a majority of ACC cases [33, 34]. Susan Bates and coworkers [1] showed that mitotane in vitro can increase drug accumulation by decreasing drug efflux, resulting in enhanced cytotoxicity. This effect was observed in cell lines expressing *MDR1*, suggesting that mitotane interferes with MDR1 function. Similar results have been obtained in a subsequent in vitro study [35]. These observations provided the rationale of combining cytotoxic therapy with mitotane.

The combination of mitotane with chemotherapy has been tested in six phase II studies involving a total of 232 patients. In two of them single agents, cisplatin or streptozotocin, were tested, two studies employed cisplatin containing regimens, while regimens without cisplatin were tested in the remaining two studies (Table 21.3).

The activity of cisplatin plus mitotane was assessed in 42 patients with advanced ACC consecutively enrolled in a phase II trial of the SouthWest Oncology Group

Table 21.3 Combination regimens with mitotane

Author (year)	Cytotoxic regimens	*n*	CR (*n*)	PR (*n*)	Overall Response rate (95% CI)	Response duration	Clinical benefit response + stable disease	Radical surgery of residual disease
Bukowsky (1993)	Cisplatin	37	-	11	30% (16–50%)	Median 7.9 months (range: 1.4–36.1)	nr	0
Bonacci (1998)	Cisplatin Etoposide	18	3	3	33% (11–55%)	Median 11 months (range: 9–26)	8 (44%)	0
Khan (2000)	Streptozotocyn	23	1	6	30% (11–49%)	Median 7 months (range 3–13.5)	11 (48%)	4 (17%)
Berruti (1998 and 2000)	Etoposide Doxorubicin Cisplatin	72	5	30	48% (37–60%)	Median 18 months	52 (78%)	10 (14%)
Abraham (2002)	Doxorubicin Vincristine Etoposide	36	1	4	14% (4–24%)	Median: 12.4 months	8 (22%)	4 (14%)
Menefee (2008)	Doxorubicin Vincristine Etoposide Tariquidar	46	2	2	9%	Complete response > 3 years; partial response mean 15 weeks	29 (66%)	6 (13%)
	TOTAL	232	13 (6%)	60 (26%)	31% (95% CI 25–37%)			

(SWOG) in the United States [36]. These patients were divided in good-risk and poor-risk categories, the former received cisplatin at 75 mg/m^2 the latter 100 mg/m^2. Thirty-seven were fully assessable while five were judged ineligible. Six patients had been previously treated with mitotane, two with chemotherapy not containing cisplatin. Objective responses were reported in 11 of 37 eligible patients (one complete and ten partial responses) for an overall response rate of 30% when considering evaluable patients and 26% according to the intent to treat analysis. Two of 11 responding patients had previously received mitotane therapy. Median duration of disease response was 8 months (range 1–36).

In a Swedish experience, the combination of streptozotocin plus mitotane was tested in 23 advanced ACC patients, 11 of them were previously radically operated patients who received this treatment only when local recurrences or metastases had developed, while the remaining 12 patients were in advanced stage in which surgery could not be curative [37]. Seven of these patients attained a disease response, one complete and six partial responses lasting 7 months on average. Four of these patients underwent radical surgery leading to long-term disease-free intervals and one of them was disease-free for 36 months and the remaining three were disease-free for 3, 10, and 18 years, respectively.

In a phase II study conducted at the Institut Gustave Roussy in Paris from 1993 to 1997 [38], 18 patients with progressive metastatic or residual ACC in whom complete surgical removal of the disease was not possible were treated with the combination of cisplatin, etoposide, and mitotane. All patients had progressive disease to previous mitotane therapy, six of them attaining serum drug levels in the therapeutic range (>14 mg/L). A complete response was observed in three cases lasting 26+, 15, and 11 months, respectively; a partial response was reported in three cases, lasting 9, 11, and 9+ months, for an overall response rate of 33%. Two further patients obtained a disease stabilization lasting 12 and 8 months, for an overall clinical benefit of 44%.

The largest prospective study published to date is a multicenter Italian phase II study, which recruited 72 consecutive locally advanced or metastatic ACC patients from 26 Institutions in 10 years [39, 40]. All patients had never been treated with systemic therapy for advanced disease, 13 patients had previously received mitotane in adjuvant setting. Thirty-five patients in this series (48%) attained an objective response (5 complete and 30 partial) lasting 18 months on average; 20 patients had a disease stabilization. A clinical benefit was therefore obtained in 78% of patients. Ten responding patients underwent radical surgery of residual disease and became disease-free. In one of them no neoplastic cells were observed at residual histology [41]. Patients attaining a disease-free status (complete or partial response followed by radical surgery) had significantly prolonged disease-free survival and overall survival than patients with partial response and no response.

In an interesting phase II trial conducted at the US National Cancer Institute [42], doxorubicin, vincristine, and etoposide, three natural products that can be transported out of cells by MDR1, were administered in association with mitotane (MAVE scheme) in 36 ACC patients with recurrent or metastatic disease. Mitotane was administered aggressively, seeking to achieve a serum level of 10–15 mg/L.

Thirteen patients (36%) had been previously submitted to chemotherapy and 12 patients (33%) had received mitotane therapy without success. Surgery with radical intent was attempted in responding patients. An objective response was documented in 5 of 36 evaluable patients (14%) with one complete response (3%), four partial responses (11%). In addition three minor responses were obtained leading to a clinical benefit obtained in 8 patients (8%). The mean duration of response exceeded 12.4 months. Of the responding patients, four went on to have surgical resections performed and were radically operated. Although the overall response rate was not high, patients who responded to therapy appeared to benefit a lot from the treatment regimen, since their overall survival after response was significantly higher than that of non-responders.

Tariquidar is a potent, specific, non-competitive inhibitor of MDR1 that inhibits the ATPase activity of MDR1. In clinical trials, tariquidar is tolerable and does not have significant pharmacokinetic interaction with chemotherapy [43]. The activity of the addition of tariquidar to the MAVE scheme was tested at the National Cancer Institute in the United States [44]. Forty-six patients with advanced ACC were enrolled. The overall response rate was modest, 9%, but complete responses were durable (>3 years). By contrast this scheme achieved a high rate of disease stabilization leading to a clinical benefit obtained in 66% of patients. Six patients underwent radical surgery of residual disease and eventually became disease-free. In these patients the in vivo MDR1 inhibition was tested using a surrogate assay that employs rhodamine accumulation in circulating CD56 positive cells and by [^{99m}Tc]-sestamibi scan. [^{99m}Tc]-sestamibi scans demonstrated inhibition of functional MDR1 with a median increased accumulation of [^{99m}Tc]-sestamibi of 133% (range 10–240%) and 179% (range 38–424%) in metatstatic ACC lesions and normal liver, respectively. Rhodamine efflux from CD56+ cells was blocked with a median inhibition of 92% at 24 h and 81% at 48 h, demonstrating excellent *MDR1* inhibition in vivo.

The low response rate obtained in this study despite the activity of tariquidar plus mitotane in inhibiting the MDR1 efflux pump suggests that MDR1 inhibition has only a limited effect in improving the chemotherapy efficacy. *MDR1* gene expression, therefore, is only one of the mechanisms involved in the chemotherapy resistance of ACC. Further efforts are needed to explain mechanisms of chemotherapy sensitivity and resistance of this disease. On the other hand, the proportion of patients attaining a stable disease in this trial was noteworthy. Even though disease stabilization might be a consequence of an indolent disease course in some cases, it remains plausible that the beneficial aspects are attributable to treatment efficacy in other cases.

The MAVE tested at the NCI in two subsequent studies led to an overall response rate that seems to be much lower than that obtained with cisplatin-containing regimens. These data suggest that cisplatin is a reference drug for ACC and should be included in the combination regimens employed in the management of this disease.

Taken together the overall cumulative activity of chemotherapy plus mitotane schemes seems to be higher than that obtained with chemotherapy without mitotane. Responses obtained can be longlasting particularly if surgery of residual disease is performed.

21.4 Chemotherapy Plus Target Therapy

Chemotherapy resistance in ACC (and other tumors as well) is a multi-factorial phenomenon. Therefore perturbing apoptotic pathways (e.g., p53), survival pathways (e.g., EGFR, PI3K/AKT, MAPK) and angiogenesis by specific molecular target therapies can increase the efficacy of cytotoxic agents (see Chapter 31). As mentioned elsewhere in this book, overexpression of the *IGF2* gene is the most frequent genetic alteration (see Chapter 29). Transduction of signals through IGF1R leads to multiple intracellular phosphorylation events and the activation of several signaling pathways. The two predominant effectors for this are the PI3K/Akt and MAPK pathways [45]. In addition, the expression of EGFR has been found to be present in the vast majority of ACCs [47, 46]. Growing evidence suggests that EGFR activation mediates resistance to chemotherapy and radiation therapy. Preclinical and clinical data show that inhibition of EGFR, together with enhanced induction of apoptosis, may counteract resistance to chemotherapy [48]. Cetuximab is a chimeric IgG1 monoclonal antibody that binds to EGFR with high specificity. In a prospective randomized phase III trial, the addition of cetuximab to irinotecan was able to reinstate sensitivity to this drug in advanced colon cancer patients whose disease had progressed during or within months after treatment with an irinotecan-based regimen [49].

In a multicenter German experience, patients registered with the German ACC Registry with progressive ACC after two to four previous systemic therapies were offered treatment with erlotinib, a small molecule targeting EGFR, and gemcitabine [50]. Ten patients were treated, eight of them had progressive disease at the first restaging and only one experienced a minor response lasting 8 months. Median overall survival of this case series was 5.5 months. The authors' conclusions were that salvage chemotherapy using erlotinib plus gemcitabine has very limited to no activity in heavily pretreated ACC patients with very advanced disease. Although this study cannot exclude that better results could have been obtained if patients were recruited at an earlier phase of the natural history of the disease. The results do not warrant further testing of this combination in the treatment of ACC.

Angiogenesis is a critical component, necessary for all tumor growth. Therefore, agents that can diminish or prevent tumor angiogenesis are likely to increase the cytotoxicity of chemotherapy. The combination of traditional chemotherapeutic drugs with agents that inhibit angiogenesis had obtained a significant improvement of time to progression and survival as opposed to chemotherapy alone in metastatic colorectal cancer patients [51].

Interestingly, chemotherapy alone can consistently increase its antiangiogenic activity simply by changing the schedule of administration. Clinically, this is achieved through the so-called metronomic schedule [52]. Metronomic chemotherapy is the frequent administration of cytotoxic drugs at doses that are low enough to avoid myelosuppression and other dose-limiting side effects that otherwise necessitate a rest period. This treatment modality may not target tumor cells directly (as is the aim of approaches that seek to determine the maximum tolerated dose), but indirectly inhibiting angiogenesis and vasculogenesis by continuously exposing the more slowly proliferating tumor endothelial cells to the damaging action of the cytotoxic therapy. Low-dose metronomic chemotherapy may offer several advantages over the maximum tolerated dose (MTD) approach, including reduced toxicity and treatment response irrespective of the resistance profile of the tumor cell population. Theoretically, a metronomic schedule is the best way to introduce a cytotoxic drug in cancer patients with disease resistant to cytotoxic therapy, and this schedule may have a synergistic effect with antiangiogenetic drugs [52]. A European trial, currently open for accrual in Italy, is testing the activity of the association of sorafenib to weekly metronomic paclitaxel. Sorafenib is an orally available multitarget serine/tyrosine kinase inhibitor that inhibits RAF1, a key enzyme in the RAS/RAF/MEK/ERK signaling pathway leading to cell proliferation, and VEGFR2 and PDGFRβ involved in angiogenesis [53]. The results of this trial are expected soon.

21.5 The FIRM-ACT Study

One of the most important problems in the management of patients with advanced ACC is the absence of a standard treatment. The international consensus conference on adrenal cancer, held in Ann Arbor, the United States in September 2003, recommended both etoposide, doxorubicin, and cisplatin in combination with mitotane and streptozotocin in combination with mitotane, as therapeutic options in advanced ACC [54]. However, it is not known which approach is the more efficacious regimen. To address this issue, the Collaborative Group for Adrenocortical Cancer (COACT) has set up a large international study: FIRM-ACT (First International Randomised Trial in Locally Advanced and Metastatic Adrenocortical Carcinoma Treatment) (www.firm-act.com). FIRMACT is a phase III, randomized, open-label, crossover trial involving Australia, France, Germany, Italy, The Netherlands, Sweden, the United Kingdom, and the United States. This trial compares the efficacy of etoposide, doxorubicin, cisplatin, and mitotane (EDP/M) with streptozotocin and mitotane (Sz/M) (Fig. 21.1). In total, 300 patients will be randomized in approximately 5 years.

The final results of this trial are expected in 2011. The main eligibility criteria are histological diagnosis of ACC and stage III–IV disease. Difference in survival between the two treatment arms is the primary aim of the study. Secondary end points are disease response, response duration, quality of life, and time to progression. Any correlation between plasma levels of mitotane and overall survival will be determined for both treatment groups. In case of unacceptable toxicity or progression of underlying disease, patients will be treated according to the treatment regimen of the other group, so that second-line treatment data will become available for both treatment regimens. This trial clearly demonstrates that relatively large prospective randomized clinical trials never previously attempted are feasible with multinational cooperation.

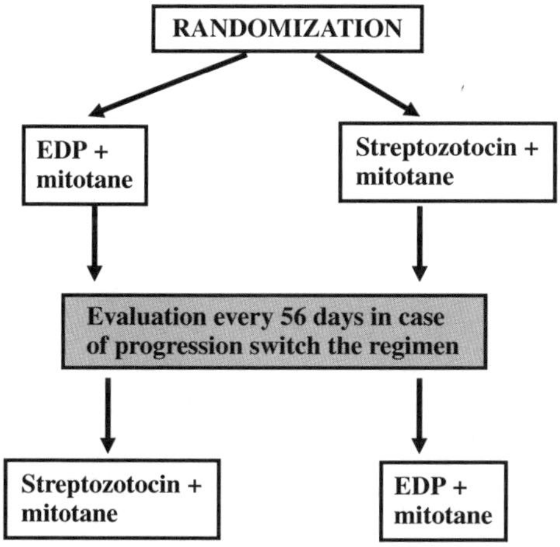

Fig. 21.1 FIRM-ACT trial design

21.6 Prognostic and Predictive Factors of Response to Chemotherapy in Advanced Patients

As previously mentioned, chemotherapy plus/minus mitotane has a modest activity in advanced ACC patients. However, in cases where disease response is obtained, the response is frequently durable, particularly if radical surgery of residual disease is performed. Occasionally, pathological complete responses can be obtained [42]. All these data suggest that a small subset of patients can obtain a great benefit from the therapy.

The identification of factors that predict drug efficacy is therefore of paramount importance in the management of ACC patients, since it allows treatment to be tailored to suit individual patients and avoid unhelpful toxicity to those whose disease is expected to be unresponsive to chemotherapy. Few data are available on prognostic and predictive factors in ACC patients. In a study testing the activity of cisplatin plus mitotane, the following factors were examined for their relation to response: risk status, functional status of the tumor, prior therapy, surgical status, and performance status [35]. None of these were associated with response. Prior surgical removal of the primary tumor or bulky disease and patient performance status were independent factors predictive for improved survival as a result of the multivariate analysis.

In a series of advanced ACC patients uniformly treated with etoposide, doxorubicin, and cisplatin, an Italian cooperative group showed that tumors secreting androgens or precursors alone have a better time to progression and overall survival than tumors secreting cortisol alone or with androgens [39]. The prognostic role of secretion was maintained in multivariate analysis, after adjustment for commonly recognized prognostic factors such as disease extent, disease-free survival, and patient performance status.

In the previously mentioned trial testing the activity of the MAVE combination regimen plus mitotane [40], patient outcome was correlated with gender, mitotane levels, and functional status. Among these variables, only the functional status of the tumor was related to overall survival. Patients with nonfunctional tumors exhibited increased survival as measured from on-study date. In this study the type of secretion was not considered separately. However, a negative prognostic role of cortisol hypersecretion was observed in a French series involving 202 consecutive ACC patients at various stages of disease treated with mitotane [55].

The prognostic role of several clinical and histology parameters have been tested in two separate series of patients with advanced disease recruited in two different reference institutions in Paris. This study had the merit of considering the role of histological parameters together with clinical parameters. The number of organs with metastasis and a high mitotic rate, but not the functional status, were found to be independently associated with overall survival.

To summarize, several indicators have been identified as prognostic factors in patients with ACC. However, it is impossible from the currently available data to identify predictive factors that can guide physicians to make the most appropriate treatment choice. In none of these studies, in fact were potentially predictive factors tested in a population of patients treated with chemotherapy vs. a patient population not receiving chemotherapy. This would be regarded a prerequisite for defining such a predictive factor. Predictive factors of treatment efficacy of epirubicin, docetaxel, and cisplatin plus mitotane or streptozotocin plus mitotane will be obtained from the FIRM-ACT study once final results are available.

It is known that cisplatin, the most widely used and one of the most active drug in ACC, works by binding to DNA and forming DNA adducts leading to intrastrand or interstrand cross-links that disrupt the structure of the DNA molecule, leading to steric changes in the double helix [56]. However, DNA repair mechanisms, in particular nucleotide excision repair and mismatch repair, can counteract these effects leading to platinum resistance in cancer patients. The excision repair cross-complementation group 1 (ERCC1) protein plays a key role in nucleotide excision repair. A negative correlation between *ERCC1* mRNA or protein expression and response to platinum-containing drugs has been observed in several retrospective clinical studies in different cancer types [56]. ERCC1 protein was recently assessed by immunohistochemistry in a large number of ACCs included in the German Adrenal Cancer Registry, and the expression was correlated with objective response to platinum-based chemotherapy. In this series disease response to platinum compounds was higher in patients with low *ERCC1* expression as opposed to those with high expression [57]. More interestingly, *ERCC1* expression was strongly correlated with overall survival after platinum treatment, but it did not correlate with survival in patients not receiving platinum compounds. These data demonstrated that efficacy of cisplatin containing regimens in advanced ACC patients can be predicted by the assessment of ERCC1 status. This important study opens the door to a pharmacogenomic approach of ACC, in particular the selection of chemotherapeutic agents best suited to the individual patient based on the identification of molecular markers that are predictive of drug sensitivity.

21.7 Conclusion

Chemotherapy has modest activity in advanced ACC, but few patients can obtain a significant benefit from this treatment modality. The greatest advantage is obtained in patients in whom tumor shrinkage obtained by chemotherapy leads to radical operation of residual disease. Cisplatin-containing schemes plus mitotane seemed the most active regimens in advanced ACC patients. The randomized FIRM-ACT trial currently being conducted in several countries will identify a standard regimen soon. Patients considered eligible for chemotherapy are generally patients with advanced/inoperable disease, progressing under mitotane treatment or patients with ACC demonstrating a rapid pattern of tumor growth. In the latter cases it is assumed that chemotherapy offers a more aggressive and perhaps more efficacious approach than mitotane alone.

While studies trying to circumvent chemotherapy resistance of ACC have led to unsatisfactory results, several trials testing the combination of cytotoxic drugs with molecular targeted therapies are ongoing.

In addition to the mentioned neo-adjuvant setting, the future of chemotherapy lies in the adjuvant setting. Chemotherapy regimens showing a modest activity in advanced disease can be more efficacious if employed post operatively in disease-free patients to prevent disease recurrence. A trial testing adjuvant chemotherapy plus mitotane vs. mitotane in high-risk radically resected patients is expected to start in the near future.

References

1. Bates SE et al (1991) Mitotane enhances cytotoxicity of chemotherapy in cell lines expressing a multidrug resistance gene (mdr-1/P-glycoprotein) which is also expressed by adrenocortical carcinomas. J Clin Endocrinol Metab 73:18–29
2. Volante M et al (2008) Pathological and molecular features of adrenocortical carcinoma:an update. J Clin Pathol 61:787–793
3. Decker RA et al (1991) Eastern Cooperative Oncology Group study 1879:mitotane and adriamycin in patients with advanced adrenocortical carcinoma. Surgery 110:1006-1013
4. Chun HG et al (1983) Cisplatin for adrenal cortical carcinoma Cancer Treat Rep 67:513–514
5. Tattersall MH et al (1980) Cis-platinum treatment of metastatic adrenal carcinoma. Med J Aust 1:419–4121
6. Grapski RT et al (1983) Cisplatin chemotherapy for adrenocortical carcinoma. Proc Am Soc Clin Oncol 2:232
7. Haq MM et al (1980) Cytotoxic chemotherapy in adrenal cortical cancer. Cancer Treat Rep 64:909–913

8. Pommier RF, Brennan MF (1992) An eleven year experience with adrenocortical carcinoma. Surgery 112:963–971
9. Baudin E et al (2002) Use of a topoisomerase I inhibitor (irinotecan, CPT-11) in metastatic adrenocortical carcinoma. Ann Oncol 13:1806–1809
10. La Rocca RV et al (1990a) Suramin, a novel antitumor compound. J Steroid Biochem Mol Biol 37:893–898
11. La Rocca RV et al (1990b) Suramin in adrenal cancer: modulation of steroid hormone production, cytotoxicity in vitro, and clinical antitumor effect. J Clin Endocrinol Metab 71:497–504
12. Arlt W et al (1994) Suramin in adrenocortical cancer: limited efficacy and serious toxicity. Clin Endocrinol 41:299–307
13. Flack MR et al (1993) Oral gossypol in the treatment of metastatic adrenal cancer. J Clin Endocrinol Metab 76:1019–1024
14. Montoya M et al (2008) Comparative effects of chemotherapeutic agents on the growth and survival of human adrenal carcinoma cells in culture. Horm Metab Res 40:302–305
15. Fallo F et al (1998) Paclitaxel is an effective antiproliferative agent on the human NCI-H295 adrenocortical carcinoma cell line. Chemotherapy 44:129–134
16. Lopes NM et al (1993) Cell kinetics and cell cycles effects of Taxol on human and hamster cell lines. Cancer Chemother Pharmacol 32:235–242
17. Klauber N et al (1997) Inhibition of angiogenesis and breast cancer in mice by the microtubule inhibitors 2-methoxyestradiol and Taxol. Cancer Res 57:81–86
18. Seidman AD et al (2008) Randomized phase III trial of weekly compared with every-3-weeks paclitaxel for metastatic breast cancer, with trastuzumab for all HER-2 overexpressors and random assignment to trastuzumab or not in HER-2 non overexpressors: final results of Cancer and Leukemia Group B protocol 9840. J Clin Oncol. 26:1642–1649
19. Sisani M et al (2008) Lung metastases from adrenocortical carcinoma, partial response after weekly docetaxel in patient unresponsive to Etoposide, Doxorubicin, Cisplatin and mitotane. XV national congress of the Italian Society of Urological Oncology, meeting abstract
20. Schneider B et al (2007) A phase I, pharmacokinetic and pharmacodynamic dose escalation trial of weekly paclitaxel with interferon-alpha2b in patients with solid tumors. Cancer Chemother Pharmacol 59:261–268
21. Desai N et al (2006) Increased antitumor activity, intratumor paclitaxel concentrations, and endothelial cell transport of cremophorfree, albumin-bound paclitaxel, ABI-007, compared with cremophor-based paclitaxel. Clin Cancer Res 12:1317–1324
22. Demeure MJ et al (2008) Pre-clinical evidence for nab-paclitaxel efficacy in the treatment of adrenocortical cancer. J Clin Oncol 26(May 20 suppl); abstr 22070
23. Blum JL et al (2007) Phase II study of weekly albumin-bound paclitaxel for patients with metastatic breast cancer heavily pretreated with taxanes. Clin Breast Cancer 7:850–856
24. Rizvi NA et al (2008) Phase I/II trial of weekly intravenous 130-nm albumin-bound paclitaxel as initial chemotherapy in patients with stage IV non–small-cell lung cancer. J Clin Oncol 26:639–643
25. Schabel FM Jr et al (1979) cis-Dichlorodiammineplatinum(II) combination chemotherapy and cross-resistance studies with tumors of mice. Cancer Treat Rep 63:1459–1473
26. Johnson DH, Greco FA (1986) Treatment of metastatic adrenal cortical carcinoma with cisplatin and etoposide (VP-16). Cancer 58:2198–2202
27. Zidan J et al (1996) Treatment of Metastatic Adrenal Cortical Carcinoma with Etoposide (VP-16) and Cisplatin After Failure with o,p'DDD: Clinical Case Reports. Am J Clin Oncol 19:229–231
28. Burgess MA et al (1993) Chemotherapy with cisplatinum and etoposide (VP16) for patients with advanced adrenal cortical carcinoma (ACC). Proc Ann Soc Clin Oncol 12 :abstr 188
29. Williamson SK et al (2000) Phase II evaluation of cisplatin and etoposide followed by mitotane at disease progression in patients with locally advanced or metastatic adrenocortical carcinoma: a Southwest Oncology Group Study. Cancer 88: 1159–1165

30. Schlumberger M et al (1991) 5-Fluorouracil, doxorubicin, and cisplatin as treatment for adrenal cortical carcinoma. Cancer 67:2997–3000
31. van Slooten H, van Oosterom AT (1983) CAP (cyclophosphamide, doxorubicin, and cisplatin) regimen in adrenal cortical carcinoma. Cancer Treat Rep 67:377–379
32. Menefee M et al (2006) The efficacy of combination chemotherapy with cisplatin and gemcitabine in patients with advanced adrenal cortical carcinoma (ACC). J Clin Oncol, 24 (June 20 Suppl): abstr 12033
33. Flynn SD et al (1992) P-glycoprotein expression and multidrug resistance in adrenocortical carcinoma. Surgery 112:981–986
34. Haak HR et al (1993) Expression of P-glycoprotein in relation to clinical manifestation, treatment and prognosis of adrenocortical cancer. Eur J Cancer 29A:1036–1038
35. Villa R et al (1999) Modulation of cytotoxic drug activity by mitotane and lonidamine in human adrenocortical carcinoma cells. Int J Oncol 14:133–138
36. Bukowski RM et al (1993) Phase II trial of mitotane and cisplatin in patients with adrenal carcinoma:a Southwest Oncology Group study. J Clin Oncol 11:161–165
37. Khan TS et al (2000) Streptozocin and o,p'DDD in the treatment of adrenocortical cancer patients:long-term survival in its adjuvant use. Ann Oncol 11:1281–1287
38. Bonacci R et al (1998) Cytotoxic therapy with etoposide and cisplatin in advanced adrenocortical carcinoma. Br J Cancer 78:546–549
39. Berruti A et al (1998) Mitotane associated with etoposide, doxorubicin, and cisplatin in the treatment of advanced adrenocortical carcinoma. Italian Group for the Study of Adrenal Cancer. Cancer 83:2194–2200
40. Berruti A et al (2005) Etoposide, doxorubicin and cisplatin plus mitotane in the treatment of advanced adrenocortical carcinoma:a large prospective phase II trial. Endocr Relat Cancer 12:657–666
41. Sperone P et al (2006) Long-term disease free survival in a patient with metastatic adrenocortical carcinoma after complete pathological response to chemotherapy plus mitotane. J Endocrinol Invest 29:560–562
42. Abraham JS et al (2002) A phase II trial of combination chemotherapy and surgical resection for the treatment of metastatic adrenocortical carcinoma: continuous infusion doxorubicin, vincristine, and etoposide with daily mitotane as a P-glycoprotein antagonist. Cancer 94:2333–2343
43. Fox E, Bates SE (2007) Tariquidar (XR9576) a P-glycoprotein drug efflux pump inhibitor. Expert Rev Anticancer Ther 7:447–459
44. Menefee ME et al (2008) Effects of the P-glycoprotein (*MDR1*) antagonist tariquidar (XR-9576; TQD) on *MDR1* function as well as the toxicity and efficacy of combined chemotherapy in patients with metastatic adrenocortical cancer (mACC). Proc Am Soc Clin Oncol J Clin Oncol 26 (May 20 suppl): abstr 2543
45. Barlaskar FM, Hammer GD (2007) The molecular genetics of adrenocortical carcinoma. Rev Endocr Metab Disord 8:343–348
46. Edgren M et al (1997) Biological characteristics of adrenocortical carcinoma: a study of p53, IGF, EGF-r, Ki-67 and PCNA in 17 adrenocortical carcinomas. Anticancer Res 17:1303–1309
47. Kamio T et al (1990) Immunohistochemical expression of epidermal growth factor receptors in human adrenocortical carcinoma. Hum Pathol 21:277–282
48. Goel S et al (2007) EGFR inhibitor-mediated apoptosis in solid tumors. J Exp Ther Oncol 6:305–320
49. Cunningham D et al (2004) Cetuximab monotherapy and cetuximab plus irinotecan in irinotecan-refractory metastatic colorectal cancer. N Eng J Med 351:337–345
50. Quinkler M et al (2008) Treatment of advanced adrenocortical carcinoma with erlotinib plus gemcitabine. J Clin Endocrinol Metab 93:2057–2062
51. Giantonio BJ et al (2007) Bevacizumab in combination with oxaliplatin, fluorouracil, and leucovorin (FOLFOX4) for previously treated metastatic colorectal cancer: results from the Eastern Cooperative Oncology Group Study E3200. J Clin Oncol 25:1539–1544

52. Kerbel RS, Kamen BA (2004) The anti-angiogenic basis of metronomic chemotherapy. Nat Rev Cancer 4:423–436
53. Adnane L et al (2006) Sorafenib (BAY 43–9006, Nexavar), a dual-action inhibitor that targets RAF/MEK/ERK pathway in tumor cells and tyrosine kinases VEGFR/PDGFR in tumor vasculature Methods Enzymol 407:597–612
54. Schteingart DE et al (2005) Management of patients with adrenal cancer: recommendation of an international consensus conference. Endocr Relat Cancer 12:667–680
55. Abiven G et al (2006) Clinical and biological features in the prognosis of adrenocortical cancer: poor outcome of cortisol-secreting tumors in a series of 202 consecutive patients. J Clin Endocrinol Metab 91:2650–2655
56. Rabik CA, DolanME (2007) Molecular mechanisms of resistance and toxicity associated with platinating agents. Cancer Treat Rev 33:9–23
57. Ronchi C et al (2009) Expression of excision repair cross complementing group 1 and prognosis in adrenocortical carcinoma patients treated with platinum-based chemotherapy Endocr Relat Cancer 16:907–918

Chapter 22
Mitotane

Massimo Terzolo, Arianna Ardito, Barbara Zaggia, Silvia De Francia, and Fulvia Daffara

Mitotane (o,p'-DDD), an analog of the insecticide DDT, has been used for the treatment of advanced adrenocortical carcinoma (ACC) since the 1960s. Its use as an adjunctive postoperative measure remained more controversial. Despite being in use for many years, the rarity of ACC precluded the organization of randomized trials; thus many areas of uncertainty and controversy remain regarding the role of this old drug in the clinical management of patients with ACC. The purpose of this chapter is to review the current evidence on two areas: (i) adjunctive mitotane treatment in patients with ACC after complete surgical resection; (ii) mitotane treatment as monotherapy in patients with advanced disease. The treatment strategy involving the combination of mitotane with cytotoxic agents is covered in Chapter 21.

22.1 Pharmacokinetics

Mitotane (o,p'-DDD) is an isomer of the insecticide o,p'-DDD and a chemical congener of the insecticide DDT (Chapter 1, Figs. 1.3 and 1.4). It is the only antineoplastic agent specifically indicated for the treatment of advanced ACC and specifically approved for this use by the Food and Drug Agency and the European Medicine Executive Agency [1, 2]. Mitotane acts as an adrenocortical suppressant and a steroid synthesis inhibitor and is commercially available (Lysodren®, Bristol Myers Squibb and HRA Pharma) as 500 mg tablets that may be stored at room temperature. Mitotane is a white crystalline powder with a slight aromatic odor, practically insoluble in water, soluble in alcohol and in ether, 10% soluble in oil or fat. Mitotane pure powder must be stored in airtight containers, protected from light [3].

Regarding the pharmacokinetics of the compound, up to 40% of a mitotane dose is absorbed from the gastrointestinal tract; absorption increases with food

M. Terzolo (✉)
Department of Clinical and Biological Sciences, Medicina Interna 1, AOU San Luigi Gonzaga, University of Turin, Regione Gonzole, 10, 10043 Orbassano, Italy
e-mail: terzolo@usa.net

G.D. Hammer, T. Else (eds.), *Adrenocortical Carcinoma*,
DOI 10.1007/978-0-387-77236-3_22,

Table 22.1 Summary of the pharmacologic characteristics of mitotane

Mitotane (o,p'-DDD)
Chemical name: (1,1-dichloro-2-(2-chlorophenyl)-2-(4-chlorophenyl)ethane) **Molecular formula**: C14H10Cl4 **Molecular weight**: 320.0 **Bioavailability after oral intake**: ~40% **Distribution**: fatty tissues **Metabolism**: liver **Renal excretion**: 10–25%

and there is a significant distribution of mitotane and its metabolites in fatty tissue (Table 22.1). After daily doses of 5–15 g, concentration of umetabolized drug in the blood of 7–90 mg/l and 29–54 mg/l of metabolites have been reported. Mitotane has been detected in the blood up to 6–9 weeks after stopping treatment, mainly metabolized in the liver with metabolites excreted in urine and bile. The elimination half-life of the parent compounds ranges between 18 and 159 days [3]. Patients treated for several years may take many months to clear mitotane from the circulation (Terzolo, unpublished observation). The therapeutic activity of mitotane depends on the metabolic transformation of the drug by the mitochondria, where it is hydroxylated at the β-carbon moiety and further transformed into an acyl-chloride. It has been reported that the active metabolites (o,p'-DDE and p,p'-DDA) (Chapter 1, Figs. 1.3 and 1.4) cause toxicity by oxygen activation with superoxide formation or by covalent binding to specific proteins [4]. Mitotane affects steroidogenesis by inhibiting the cytochrome cholesterol side-chain cleavage enzyme (P450scc), which converts cholesterol to pregnenolone [4]. Mitotane also inhibits other cytochrome P450-dependent enzymes, such as 11-hydroxylase and 18-β-hydroxylase, as well as P450-independent enzymes, e.g., 3-β hydroxysteroid-dehydrogenase [5]. However, despite these observations the molecular mechanisms of actions of mitotane are still not fully understood.

22.2 Historical Background

Nelson and Woodard in 1949 demonstrated that the insecticide DDD caused selective atrophy of the adrenal cortex in a dog. Subsequently, it was found that the majority of adrenolytic activity resided in a contaminant of the crude DDD preparation, 1,1-dichloro-2-(*o*-chlorophenyl)-2-(*p*-chlorophenyl)-ethane, the o,p' isomer of DDD [6, 7, 8]. Most of the early pharmacology studies of mitotane were done in dogs where degeneration of mitochondria was detected as early as 12 h after mitotane administration. The atrophic changes were most prominent in the zona fasciculata and zona reticularis and were associated with unresponsiveness to ACTH administration, whereas changes in the zona glomerulosa were relatively modest

[1, 9]. With prolonged treatment, most of the cells of the zona fasciculata and zona reticularis were destroyed. Dogs treated with mitotane for 2 days showed a diminished cortisol secretion [10].

Following the demonstration of the adrenotoxic effect in dogs, mitotane was used in humans in the late 1950s. In 1960, Bergenstal and colleagues [11] reported significant tumor regression and reduced corticosteroid secretion in 7 out of 18 ACC patients treated with o,p'-DDD. In 1966, Hutter and Kayhoe [12] observed reduced steroid levels and improvement of symptoms (pain, weakness, anorexia) in about half of 59 ACC patients. Of these patients, treated with mitotane and measurable disease, 20 patients (34%) showed objective tumor regression of a median duration of 7 months at a daily mitotane dose of 8–10 g. During the early 1970s, Lubitz and colleagues [13] investigated 115 patients with inoperable ACC using increasing doses of mitotane until side effects occurred. Most patients were treated with 5–10 g daily, but the maintenance dose varied greatly (0.5–20 g daily). Of 75 patients with measurable disease, 46 (61%) showed tumor regression and the survival in this series of mitotane treated patients was twice as high as reported in historical controls. In the same period, Hoffman and colleagues [14] reported a series of 19 patients who were given mitotane at variable doses (1–10 g daily) for a period ranging from 15 weeks to 19 months, but observed a much less convincing antiproliferative effects accompanied by substantial toxicity. These reports concluded that treatment with mitotane is justified in unoperable patients and in the event of severe steroid hypersecretion. The enthusiasm for mitotane peaked during the mid-1980s when Boven and colleagues [15] reported a patient with a histologically proven complete response and identified seven similar cases in the literature. Subsequent experience was less encouraging. Most reports described a partial and transient response only in a small proportion of the patients. In 1993, in an extensive review of the previous English literature, Wooten and King [16] analyzed more than 500 patients who received o,p'-DDD and found that 35% of them showed a response, which was most often partial and transient.

In summary, mitotane has been widely employed for medical treatment of advanced ACC for more than 40 years, but it is difficult to critically appraise the evidence of its efficacy due to several limitations of the published reports, particularly early studies that were performed before the era of modern imaging techniques. In such studies, assessment of tumor response did not utilize standard criteria [17], and in some reports the only marker of response was the decrease of steroid levels. More recent developments will be addressed in the following sections.

22.3 Mitotane in Advanced Adrenocortical Carcinoma

Mitotane has been used in advanced ACC as a monotherapy and also in combination with other cytotoxic agents. A meaningful comparison of results of early studies is not readily feasible because of the variability in the criteria used to assess response [16, 18, 19]. Because hormonal amelioration was initially used as a surrogate for response, it has been difficult to document a survival advantage in the series reporting a high percentage of remission [19, 20]. Another confounding variable is the fact that most studies were retrospective and employed variable dosages of mitotane, ranging from 3 to 20 g daily using two different formulations: Lysodren® (o,p'-DDD alone) and the so-called French mitotane (o,p'-DDD mixed with enteric gastroresistant coated granules of cellulose acetylphthalate), respectively.

Studies published before the 1980s showed considerable efficacy of mitotane in controlling hormone hypersecretion (response rate, 73–85% of treated patients), while the effect on tumor mass was less evident (34–61% of complete or partial remissions) [12–14, 21–25]. In more recent studies a limited antineoplastic activity was attributed to mitotane, with a rate of objective remissions of only 20–24% [5, 21, 25–29]; moreover, these responses were usually short-lasting [5, 10, 27–30]. Williamson and colleagues [31] used mitotane prospectively as a second-line treatment at disease progression after treatment with cisplatin and etoposide, and the observed response rate was only 13%.

Haak and colleagues [32] reported a response rate of 27% in 55 patients with advanced ACC (complete remission in eight patients and partial response in seven patients with duration of response of 2–190 months). Interestingly, a tumor response was seen only in patients who showed high maintenance mitotane serum levels; actually, the response rate was 55% among patients with elevated mitotane concentrations. This pivotal study introduced the concept of a therapeutic impact of mitotane concentrations after the preliminary observation by van Slooten and colleagues [33], even if the threshold of 14 mg/l was established retrospectively and was not used for clinical decision-making.

In a prospective study, Baudin and colleagues [34] included 13 patients with metastatic ACC showing an objective tumor response in four of them (31%). One response was complete and three were partial, lasting between 10 and 48 months. In this study the responses were observed only among the six patients who achieved plasma mitotane levels greater than 14 mg/l. In contrast, no response was observed among the seven patients with persistently low plasma mitotane concentrations. Interestingly, the authors reported that the four patients who initially responded to mitotane had mitotane levels less than 14 mg/l at the time of disease progression. Thus, in the only two studies employing monitoring of serum mitotane concentration, objective responses were observed only among patients whose serum mitotane concentrations were higher than 14 mg/l [32, 34]. However, Seki and colleagues [35] have reported a patient who attained complete remission of a local recurrence and lung metastases even though plasma mitotane levels were never above 10 mg/l.

Table 22.2 summarizes the outcome of mitotane monotherapy in advanced ACC as it was reported in studies of more than 10 patients published in the English literature over the past 20 years. Notwithstanding the great heterogeneity of these studies, mitotane appears to have some activity in inducing objective tumor regressions of variable duration (2–190 months); overall, the median response rate was about 24% (range, 13–33%). Moreover, mitotane treatment was able to control hormone secretion in most patients with functioning ACC [36]. Although a complete response in

Table 22.2 Outcome of mitotane treatment in advanced ACC

Author; study type	Dose g/day	Patients n.	Response n., (%)	Duration months
Venkatesh, 89; retrospective	NR	72	21 PRs (29)	NR
Luton, 90; retrospective	3–20	37	5 PRs (13)	5–25
Decker, 91; prospective	6	36	2 CRs, 6 PRs (22)	3–82
Pommier, 92; retrospective	NA	29	7 PRs (24)	NR
Haak, 94; retrospective	4–8	55	8 CRs, 7 PRs (27)	2–190
Barzon, 97; retrospective	4–8	11	2 PRs (18)	40–64
Williamson, 99; II line, prospective	4–10	16	2 PRs (13)	NR
Baudin, 01; prospective	6–12	13	1 CR, 3 PRs (33)	10–48
Summary		Tot. 269	Median, 24%	

NR not reported, *PR* partial remission, *CR* complete remission

patients with advanced ACC is infrequent and duration of response is extremely variable, long-term survival has been reported [36].

Mitotane has been used together with conventional cytotoxic agents in many series. The rationale for combining mitotane with classic cytotoxic drugs is based on the finding that the drug is able to reverse the multidrug resistance mediated by P-glycoprotein expression in vitro, thus enhancing the effects of doxorubicin, vincristine, and etoposide [37, 38]. However, such an effect could not be demonstrated in vivo [39].

The details of mitotane in combination with cytotoxic agents will be addressed elsewhere (see Chapter 21).

22.4 Toxicity and Dosage

The toxicity of mitotane and the fact that it appears to have only a narrow therapeutic range have been major hurdles for its clinical application [18, 28]. Limited studies have correlated mitotane activity and toxicity with drug blood concentration [32, 34], showing that the most severe adverse effects become manifest for blood levels greater than 20 mg/l, while disease response is mainly confined to patients achieving blood levels greater than 14 mg/dl [32, 34]. Although the threshold mitotane concentration of 14 mg/l was defined arbitrarily and retrospectively by van Slooten and colleagues [33], the therapeutic impact of such concentrations has been confirmed in a further prospective study [34].

The optimal mitotane schedule still remains matter of controversy. High mitotane doses may achieve the therapeutic range rapidly at the price of a substantial toxicity [34, 40]. While low doses are better tolerated but usually achieve the therapeutic range after some months, this time lag may pose a problem when treating patients with a rapidly progressive disease [41]. It is actually not clear how many patients are able to attain and maintain consistently over time mitotane levels in the therapeutic range. In a French experience, using the so-called French mitotane, elevated concentrations were reached in about 50% of patients [34], while in an Italian series

100% of the patients who were given Lysodren® reached the therapeutic levels after 3–5 months [41]. Both experiences, however, are too small for any generalization of these results.

The most common unwanted effects are gastrointestinal manifestations (nausea, vomiting, diarrhea, anorexia) that occur early in the course of treatment and are partially independent from mitotane levels [40, 42]. Interestingly, gastrointestinal symptoms are particularly evident at any increment in mitotane dose. However, well-informed and motivated patients are able to cope with side effects without discontinuing mitotane permanently, proven that expert care and careful counseling are provided [36, 42]. The application of temporary dose reduction or discontinuation is useful because patients may gradually develop tolerance to the unwanted effects of mitotane and then be able to resume treatment and to attain elevated drug levels without new episodes of toxicity [1, 42].

Typical adverse effects due to mitotane administration include elevation of liver enzymes and neurological toxicity (depression, lethargy, somnolence, ataxia, dizziness, confusion, vertigo). Almost universal is the elevation of GGT and alkaline phosphatase that, however, rarely assumes clinical relevance [42]. However, severe hepatotoxicity has also been described [36]. Neurologic effects of mitotane seem to be related to the plasma levels of the drug, and rarely occur when the plasma o,p'-DDD level is below 20 mg/l. These manifestations are always transient and disappear after the drug is discontinued for several days.

Theoretically, every patient on chronic mitotane treatment will develop adrenal insufficiency (if ACC is nonfunctional or mitotane is given in an adjuvant setting) requiring a high-dose glucocorticoid replacement (often reaching doses up to 50 mg-100 mg/day) due to increased metabolic clearance of glucocorticoids and remarkable induction of cortisol-binding globulin, leading to impaired bioavailability of free cortisol [36, 42, 43]. Inadequately treated adrenal insufficiency enhances mitotane induced side effects and reduces tolerance [44]. Conversely, mineralocorticoid supplementation is not mandatory in all patients because aldosterone production is relatively spared. Hypogonadism and gynecomastia may develop in the long term needing testosterone replacement in some patients, because testicular steroidogenesis is also affected by mitotane whereas synthesis of sex hormone-binding globulin is increased, thereby reducing free testosterone concentration [42]. In some patients, also free thyroid hormone concentrations also increase and thyroxin replacement may become necessary [36, 42]. The weak estrogen-like action of mitotane may contribute to sexual dysfunction in men while women are less affected [45]. Leukopenia, prolonged bleeding times, increase in cholesterol and triglycerides may also occur [36].

In this context, the monitoring of circulating mitotane levels may be useful to tailor individually the therapy and limit side-effects, thus attaining better compliance to treatment. The implementation of blood mitotane monitoring, through a service provided by the company distributing Lysodren® in Europe (Lysosafe, www.lysodren-europe.com), has rendered the use of this drug more feasible in the clinical practice because it is possible to anticipate and prevent toxicity. European experience with a monitored mitotane regimen is very promising and supports the measurement of circulating mitotane concentration as a standard practice guideline in the management of patients with ACC.

22.5 Mitotane in Adjuvant Setting

Since ACC has a high propensity to recur even after apparent complete resection, many investigators have considered the use of adjuvant therapy. Mitotane has been widely employed with this aim [18, 20, 46], but its efficacy remains a matter of debate. In fact, the literature reports conflicting results that may likely be explained by several reasons.

First, most studies have limited statistical power. Only three series included more than 20 patients [30, 44, 47, 48]. In the study of Luton and colleagues [27], 23 patients received mitotane after apparently curative surgery. However, the results of mitotane treatment in these patients were analyzed together with results in advanced disease, thus preventing a specific evaluation of the efficacy of adjuvant mitotane. Second, some studies did not include a concomitant control group of untreated patients with comparable baseline characteristics [25, 44, 47–50]. Third, a number of patients in these studies underwent multiple adjuvant treatments, making it difficult to appraise the specific effect of mitotane [28, 47]. Fourth, all studies but one [34] were retrospective and have employed variable doses of mitotane, ranging from 3 to 20 g daily, which were given for variable time periods. Table 22.3 reports the outcome of adjuvant mitotane treatment in the published studies.

Schteingart and colleagues [50] were the first to suggest that an adjunctive low-dose mitotane regimen was beneficial immediately after tumor resection in a small uncontrolled study. Additional data supporting the efficacy of adjuvant mitotane was provided by Venkatesh et al. [25], who reported that 6 out of 7 patients on adjuvant mitotane were alive 1 to 4 years after surgery, and by Dickstein and colleagues [49], who reported that a low-dose mitotane treatment started soon after surgical removal of ACC had a positive influence on survival in 4 patients. Furthermore, Kasperlik-Zaluska and colleagues [44, 48] reported that 18 out of 32 patients treated with mitotane immediately after surgery were alive at the last follow-up as compared to 6 out of 27 patients who had started treatment 2 to 15 months after surgery, versus 1 out of 8 untreated patients. However, a formal survival analysis was not performed and precise data on the proportion of patients who underwent complete resection were not reported.

On the other hand, Bodie and colleagues [30] did not demonstrate any difference in the overall survival between patients with localized disease treated with surgery alone or with surgery followed by adjuvant mitotane. Nevertheless, the authors argued that selected patients appeared to have some beneficial effects from adjuvant mitotane. Pommier and Brennan [28] likewise did not observe any positive effects of adjuvant mitotane on disease-free survival as compared with untreated patients. Moreover Vassilopoulou-Sellin and colleagues [19] did not observe any significant

Table 22.3 Outcome of mitotane treatment in an adjuvant setting

Author, year	Treatment groups	Dose g/day	Patients n.	RFS	Notes
Schteingart, 1982	Mitotane –	6	4	NR	Survival was 74 ± 33 months.
Venkatesh, 1989	Mitotane –	NR	7	NR	6/7 pts were alive at last F-U.
Bodie, 1989	Mitotane Control	NR	21 25	NR	No difference between groups.
Pommier, 1992	Mitotane Control	NR	10 43	2.4 years vs. 2.5 years	RT was also used in 3 pts.
Vassilopoulu-Sellin, 1993	Mitotane Control	4–6	8 6	10 mos vs. 23 mos	Treatment was discontinued early for toxicity in 5 pts.
Haak, 1994	Mitotane Control	4–8	11 15	NR	Survival was 51 vs. 61 mos. No impact of MIT levels on relapse.
Barzon, 1997	Mitotane Control	4–8	7 11	8 mos vs. 13 mos	71% pts in the MIT group are NED vs. 27% of controls.
Kasperlik-Zaluska, 2000	Mitotane –	4–5	55 –	18–68 mos	At the last F-U, 56% of pts treated earlier are alive vs. 22% of pts treated later and 12% of untreated pts.
Icard, 2001	Mitotane –	3–8	83 –	NR	MIT had no independent effect on survival.
Baudin, 2001	Mitotane –	6–12	11 –	72% of pts recurred in 1 year	No impact of MIT levels on relapse.
Terzolo, 2007	Mitotane Control Control	1–5	47 55 75	42 mos in the MIT group vs. 10 and 25 mos in control groups	MIT had an independent effect on survival ($p<0.001$).
Dickstein, 2007	Mitotane –	1.5–3	14 –	NR	5-year survival 75%
Bertherat, 2007	Mitotane Control	NR	86 80	No difference between groups	Trend for benefit of MIT in cortisol-secreting ACCs

Abbreviations are as follows, *NR* not reported, *mos* months, *pts* patients, *F-U* follow-up, *RT* radiotherapy, *MIT* mitotane, *NED* no evidence of disease, *ACCs* adrenocortical cancer

difference in the survival of eight patients who received adjuvant mitotane treatment and six patients who received no postoperative treatment. However, five of the patients on adjuvant mitotane discontinued the drug early because of toxicity. In the study of Barzon and colleagues [51, 52], seven patients treated with adjuvant mitotane showed a median disease-free survival of 8 months compared to 13 months in 11 untreated patients. However, 5 of 7 patients in the mitotane group were without any evidence of disease at the last follow-up, in contrast to 3 out of 11 patients in the control group.

Further evidence of the ineffectiveness of adjuvant mitotane came from the French multicentric study of Icard and colleagues [47, 53], who did not observe an independent effect of mitotane survival after apparent curative surgery in multivariate analysis. However, it was not reported whether the patients treated with mitotane had prognostic factors comparable to those of the untreated patients. Haak and colleagues [32] demonstrated that mitotane was ineffective as adjuvant therapy in 11 patients. In the experience of Baudin and colleagues [34] mitotane did not significantly influence disease-free recurrence and relapse rate in 8 out of 11 patients within 1 year. Even though these two groups [32, 34] employed the monitoring of serum mitotane concentrations, they did not find any association between elevated mitotane concentrations and outcome in an adjuvant setting.

Given its recognized toxicity and the lack of a clear evidence of efficacy, mitotane use as an adjunctive treatment had declined in recent years, and no recommendation regarding adjuvant treatment was made at a 2003 consensus conference on ACC held in Ann Arbor, MI, USA [2].

More recently, the results of a retrospective analysis involving a large cohort of patients with ACC, who were followed for up to 10 years at different institutions in Italy and Germany, have been published [54]. Adjuvant mitotane treatment was administered to 47 Italian patients after radical surgery, and recurrence-free survival in these patients (the primary outcome of the study) was compared with that of two independent groups of 55 Italian and 75 German patients whose surgery was not followed by mitotane. Recurrence-free survival was significantly prolonged in the mitotane group, as compared with the two groups of untreated patients (median recurrence-free survival, 42 months vs. 10 months in the Italian control group and 25 months in the German control group). The patients who were left untreated after radical resection of ACC had a significantly higher risk of recurrence than those receiving mitotane. Although the study was retrospective, the mitotane group and the Italian control group were highly comparable for the clinical characteristics known to affect outcome, while the control group from Germany had even better prognostic factors making mitotane effects more impressive. Indeed, multivariate analysis confirmed that mitotane treatment resulted in a significant advantage for recurrence-free survival. Similarly, overall survival appeared to be longer in patients receiving adjuvant mitotane, even if the difference between the mitotane group and untreated patients was less apparent.

The two major advantages of this study compared to previous ones are the large series, and the fact that mitotane was given adjuvantly to all patients in some centers while in other centers no treatment was recommended according to a predefined protocol and not on the basis of selected patient or tumor characteristics. Thus, the study included concomitant cohorts of patients with similar baseline characteristics and statistical analysis was intention-to-treat. Moreover, similar work-up protocols were used at the different centres and almost all histological diagnoses were reviewed centrally. The possibility of an unknown factor that may have contributed to the better outcome of the mitotane-treated patients can not be excluded. However, the study appears free of major biases, as long as this can be true for a retrospective study. Another important finding is that favorable outcomes were achieved with low doses of mitotane (1–5 g per day), thus explaining why treatment was associated with acceptable adverse event rates [54]. However, it may be argued that side effects have been likely underestimated due to the retrospective nature of the study. Conversely, severe and disabling toxicity was observed in the studies where high, rapidly increasing, daily doses of mitotane were employed [19, 28].

In contrast to this experience, Bertherat and colleagues [55] found that adjuvant mitotane was ineffective in a cohort of 166 patients who underwent complete tumor removal. In their series, mitotane use was not associated with any improvement in disease-free survival; however, they found a tendency for benefit of adjuvant mitotane in patients with cortisol-secreting ACCs. Bertherat and colleagues [55] raised the question whether the efficacy of mitotane may be influenced by the secretory activity of ACC. It is biologically plausible that hypercortisolism may portend to an unfavorable prognosis in patients with advanced ACC as previously reported by the same group [56]; in disease-free patients, however, its antisecretory activity may be less a factor to determine outcome. Because mitotane was administered to only half of the patients in this cohort, it is plausible that treated patients may have been selected for unfavorable prognostic factors [57].

In practice, after ACC is completely removed, physicians are challenged with dilemma of instituting adjuvant therapy or simply follow patients without initiating treatment. Schteingart [58] concluded that the study of Terzolo and colleagues [54] provided a compelling rationale for the use of low-dose mitotane as adjuvant therapy in patients presenting with stages I to III ACC whose surgical resection has been macroscopically complete [58]; controversy regarding mitotane as adjuvant therapy, however, may continue [55, 59].

Many areas of controversy remain concerning adjunctive mitotane therapy beyond the issue of efficacy can only be addressed by prospective studies. First, what is the optimal dose regimen? At some centers the use of a low-dose regimen appears to be better tolerated. However, even if all patients are able to attain elevated mitotane concentrations, the time needed to achieve a therapeutic levels is very long. This conflicts with the rationale of an adjuvant therapy, that aims to treat as close to surgery as possible. Conversely a high-dose regimen is able to provide elevated concentration more rapidly, but is fraught with increased side effects [40]. A solution to this dilemma may be the initiation of therapy before surgery with a loading dose and to proceed with maintenance doses as soon as therapeutic levels are achieved.

Second, which is the optimal duration of therapy? The time to first recurrence after complete tumor resection is highly variable ranging from a few months to more than 10 years, but most recurrences occur within 2 years after primary surgery [18, 20, 28, 46, 60]. In the multicenter series collected by Terzolo and colleagues [54, 57], approximately 70% of relapses took place in the first 2 years of follow-up, while the frequency of late (>5 year) relapses was less than 1%. The currently best approach to this dilemma is to discuss risks and benefits of mitotane therapy with the patient. The clinician can then accommodate patient preferences between a range of possibilities (2, 5 or even more years of therapy) in a shared decision-making depending on tumor and patient characteristics.

In conclusion, there is evidence that adjuvant mitotane treatment may benefit a proportion of patients with ACC, even if the retrospective nature of the recent study warrants caution in the interpretation of the results [51, 52]. A better understanding of which factors can influence prognosis and response to treatment will help stratifying patients according to their risk of relapse, with the aim to identify subgroups of patient for whom the benefits of adjunctive mitotane are maximal. The only way to answer these open questions is to perform randomized trials. Therefore, a trial for patients at low–intermediate risk of recurrence who are randomized to mitotane vs. observation only (ADIUVO trial, http://www.epiclin.cpo.it/adiuvo) has been initiated under the endorsement of the European Network for the Study of Adrenal Tumors. However, until results from this and other randomized trials are available, clinicians will be challenged by this uncertainty. In the meantime, clinical judgment and personal experience will be the main basis for decision-making regarding mitotane treatment of patients with ACC.

References

1. Hahner S, Fassnacht M (2005) Mitotane for adrenocortical carcinoma treatment. Curr Opin Investig Drugs 6(4):386–394
2. Schteingart DE et al (2005) Management of patients with adrenal cancer: recommendations of an international consensus conference. Endocr Relat Cancer 667–680
3. MICROMEDEX® Healthcare Series, Copyright © 1974–2009, Thomson Reuters
4. Schteingart DE (2000) Conventional and novel strategies in the treatment of adrenocortical cancer. Brazilian J Med Biol Res 33:1197–1200
5. Hart MM et al (1973) The effect of isomers of DDD on the ACTH-induced steroid output, histology and ultrastructure of the dog adrenal cortex. Toxicol Appl Pharmacol 24: 127–159
6. Cueto C, Brown JH (1958) The chemical fractionation of an adrenocorticolytic drug. Endocrinology 62:326–333
7. Nelson AA, Woodard G (1949) Severe adrenal cortical atrophy (cytotoxic) and hepatic damage produced in dogs by feeding 2,2-bis(parachlorophenyl)-1,1-dichloroethane (DDD or TDE). Arch Pathol (Chic) 48:387–394
8. Nichols J, Hennigar G (1957) Studies on DDD, 2,2-bis (parachlorophenyl)-1,1-dichloroethane. Exp Med Surg 15:310–316
9. Kaminsky N et al (1962) Ultrastructure of adrenal cortex of the dog during treatment with DDD. J Natl Cancer Inst 29:127–159
10. Vilar O, Tullner WW (1959) Effects of o,p'DDD on histology and 17-hydroxycorticosteroid output of the dog adrenal cortex. Endocrinology 65:80–86
11. Bergenstal DM et al (1960) Chemotherapy of adrenocortical cancer with o,p'DDD. Ann Intern Med 53:672
12. Hutter AM Jr, Kayhoe DE (1966) Adrenal cortical carcinoma: clinical features in 138 patients. Am J Med 41:572–580
13. Lubitz JA et al (1973 Mar 5) Mitotane use in inoperable adrenal cortical carcinoma. JAMA. 223(10):1109–1112
14. Hoffman DL, Mattox VR (1972 Jul) Treatment of adrenocortical carcinoma with o,p'-DDD. Med Clin North Am 56(4):999–1012

15. Boven E et al (1984) Complete response of metastatized adrenal cortical carcinoma with op'-DDD. Case report and literature review. Cancer 53: 26–29
16. Wooten MD, King DK (1993) Adrenal cortical carcinoma. Epidemiology and treatment with mitotane and a review of the literature. Cancer 72(11): 3145–3155
17. WHO handbook for reporting results of cancer treatment WHO Offset Publication No 48. Geneva, 1979
18. Dackiw AP et al (2001) Adrenal cortical carcinoma. World J Surg 25:914–926
19. Vassilopoulou-Sellin R et al (1993) Impact of adjuvant mitotane on the clinical course of patients with adrenocortical cancer. Cancer 71(10): 3119–3123
20. Wajchenberg B et al (2000) Adrenocortical carcinoma: clinical and laboratory observations. Cancer 88:711–736
21. Decker RA et al (1991) Eastern Cooperative Oncology Group study 1879: mitotane and adriamycin in patients with advanced adrenocortical carcinoma. Surgery 110(6):1006–1013
22. Hajiar RA et al (1975) Adrenal cortical carcinoma: a study of 32 patients. Cancer 35: 549–554
23. Haq MM et al (1980) Cytotoxic chemotherapy in adrenal cortical carcinoma. Cancer Treat Rep 64: 909–913
24. Hogan TF et al (1978) op',DDD (mitotane) therapy for adrenal cortical carcinoma: observation on drug dosage, toxicity, and steroid replacement. Cancer 42: 2177–2181
25. Venkatesh S et al (1989) Adrenal cortical carcinoma. Cancer 64: 765–769
26. Grapski RT et al (1983) Cisplatin chemotherapy of adrenocortical carcinoma. Proc Am Soc Clin Oncol 2: 232
27. Luton JP et al (1990) Clinical features of adrenocortical carcinoma, prognostic factors, and the effect of mitotane therapy. N Engl J Med 322:1195–2001
28. Pommier RF, Brennan MF (1992) An eleven-year experience with adrenocortical carcinoma. Surgery 112: 963–970
29. Tattersall MH et al (1980) Cis-platinum treatment of metastatic adrenal carcinoma. Med J Aust 1:419–421
30. Bodie B et al (1989) The Cleveland Clinic experience with adrenal cortical carcinoma. J Urol 141:257–260
31. Williamson SK et al (2000) Phase II evaluation of cisplatin and etoposide followed by mitotane at disease progression in patients with locally advanced or metastatic adrenocortical carcinoma: a Southwest Oncology Group Study. Cancer 88(5): 1159–1165
32. Haak HR et al (1994) Optimal treatment of adrenocortical carcinoma with mitotane: results in a consecutive series of 96 patients. Br J Cancer 69:947–951
33. Van Slooten H et al (1984) The treatment of adrenocortical carcinoma with o,p'-DDD: prognostic implications of serum level monitoring. Eur J Cancer Clin Oncol 20:47–53
34. Baudin E et al (2001) Impact of monitoring plasma 1,1-dichlorodiphenildichloroethane (o,p'DDD) levels on the treatment of patients with adrenocortical carcinoma. Cancer 92:1385–1392
35. Seki M et al (1999) Changes in neoplastic cell features and sensitivity to mitotane during mitotane-induced remission in a patient with recurrent, metastatic adrenocortical carcinoma. Endocr Relat Cancer 6:529–533
36. Allolio B, Fassnacht M (2006) Adrenocortical carcinoma: clinical update. J Clin Endocrinol Metab 91:2027–2037
37. Bates SE et al (1991) Mitotane enhances cytotoxicity of chemotherapy in cell lines expressing a multidrug resistance gene (mdr-1/Pglycoprotein) which is also expressed by adrenocortical carcinomas. J Clin Endocrinol Metab 73(1): 18–29
38. Villa R et al (1999) Modulation of cytotoxic drug activity by mitotane and lonidamine in human adrenocortical carcinoma cells. Int J Oncol 14(1):133–138
39. Abraham J et al (2002) A phase II trial of combination chemotherapy and surgical resection for the treatment of metastatic adrenocortical carcinoma: continuous infusion doxorubicin, vincristine, and etoposide with daily mitotane as a P-glycoprotein antagonist. Cancer 94(9): 2333–2343

40. Faggiano A et al (2006) Rapidly progressing high o,p'DDD doses shorten the time required to reach the therapeutic threshold with an acceptable tolerance: preliminary results. Clin Endocrinol 64:110–113
41. Terzolo M et al (2000) Low-dose monitored mitotane treatment achieves the therapeutic range with manageable side effects in patients with adrenocortical cancer J Clin Endocrin Metab 86 (6): 2234–2238
42. Daffara F et al (2008) Prospective evaluation of mitotane toxicity in adrenocortical cancer patients treated adjuvantly. Endocr Relat Cancer 15:1043–1053
43. Hague RV et al (1989) Hepatic microsomal enzyme induction and adrenal crisis due to o,p'DDD therapy for metastatic adrenocortical carcinoma. Clin Endocrinol 31:51–57
44. Kasperlik-Zaluska AA (2000) Clinical results of the use of mitotane for adrenocortical carcinoma. Brazilian J Med Biol Res 33:1191–1196
45. Nader N et al (2006) Mitotane has an estrogenic effect on sex hormone-binding globulin and corticosteroid-binding globulin in humans. J Clin Endocrinol Metab 91:2165–2170
46. Allolio B et al (2004) Management of adrenocortical carcinoma. Clin Endocrinol 60:273–287
47. Icard P et al (1992) Adrenocortical carcinoma in surgically treated patients: a retrospective study on 156 cases by the French Association of Endocrine Surgery. Surgery 112: 972–980
48. Kasperlik-Zaluska AA et al (1995) Adrenocortical carcinoma. A clinical study and treatment results of 52 patients. Cancer 75: 2587–2591
49. Dickstein G et al (1998) Is there a role for low doses of mitotane (o,p'-DDD) as adjuvant therapy in adrenocortical carcinoma? J Clin Endocrinol Metab 83:3100–3103
50. Schteingart DE et al (1982 Sep) Treatment of adrenal carcinomas. Arch Surg 117(9): 1142–1146
51. Barzon L et al (1999 Apr) Comment – Is there a role for low doses of mitotane (o,p'-DDD) as adjuvant therapy in adrenocortical carcinoma? J Clin Endocrinol Metab 84(4):1488–1489
52. Barzon L et al (1997 Nov–Dec) Adrenocortical carcinoma: experience in 45 patients. Oncology 54(6):490–496
53. Icard P et al (2001) Adrenocortical carcinomas: surgical trends and results of a 253-patient series from the French Association of Endocrine Surgeons study group. World J Surg 25: 891–897
54. Terzolo M (2007) Adjuvant mitotane treatment for adrenocortical carcinoma. N Engl J Med 356:2372–2380
55. Bertherat J et al (2007) Adjuvant mitotane in adrenocortical carcinoma. Letter to the Editor. N Engl J Med 357:1256–1257
56. Abiven G et al (2006) Clinical and biological features in the prognosis of adrenocortical cancer: poor outcome of cortisol-secreting tumors in a series of 202 consecutive patients. J Clin Endocrinol Metab 91:2650–2655
57. Terzolo M et al (2007) Adjuvant mitotane in adrenocortical carcinoma. Letter to the editor. N Engl J Med 357:1259
58. Schteingart DE (2007) Adjuvant Mitotane Therapy of Adrenal Cancer – Use and Controversy. N Engl J Med 356:2415–2418
59. Lee JE (2007) Adjuvant mitotane in adrenocortical carcinoma. Letter to the Editor. N Engl J Med 357:1256–1258
60. Stojadinovic A et al (2002) Adrenocortical carcinoma: clinical, morphologic, and molecular characterization. J Clin Oncol 20:941–950
61. Dickstein G et al (2007) Adjuvant Mitotane in Adrenocortical Carcinoma. Letter to the Editor. N Engl J Med 357(12):1257

Chapter 23
Pharmacotherapy for Hormone Excess in Adrenocortical Carcinoma

Richard J. Auchus

The morbidity caused by adrenocortical carcinoma (ACC) derives both from the spread of malignant cells into other organs and from the consequences of hormone excess. Consequently, the goals of treatment in ACC include both control of tumor growth and mitigation of the effects derived from hormone excess. Unlike benign hormone excess syndromes, ACC often presents with excessive production of multiple steroid hormones, which complicates management. Particularly with the advent of novel therapeutic strategies to control the growth and spread of ACC, the need to control hormone excess and thus optimize performance status looms large. This chapter will review current approaches to treatment of mineralocorticoid, glucocorticoid, and androgen excess due to ACC, as well as agents that are currently in development.

23.1 Adrenal Steroid Biosynthesis

23.1.1 Basics of Adrenal Steroidogenesis and Zonation

In the normal adrenal cortex, the binding of adrenocorticotropin (ACTH) to its receptor (melanocortin receptor type 2, MC2R) in the zonae fasciculata and reticularis or the binding of angiotensin II (Ang II) to its receptor on cells in the zona glomerulosa stimulate steroid biosynthesis. In the zona glomerulosa, high potassium levels also stimulate steroidogenesis. Each zone of the adrenal cortex expresses a specific repertoire of enzymes, which enables these cells to effectively complete the biosynthesis of their characteristic steroids: aldosterone for the zona glomerulosa, cortisol for the zona fasciculata, and dehydroepiandrosterone sulfate (DHEAS) for the zona reticularis (Fig. 23.1). Note that all of the steps contained in complex and complete pathway diagrams as often shown in textbooks and reviews do not all

R.J. Auchus (✉)
Division of Endocrinology and Metabolism, Department of Internal Medicine, UT Southwestern Medical Center Dallas, 5323 Harry Hines Boulevard, Dallas, TX 75390, USA
e-mail: richard.auchus@utsouthwestern.edu

G.D. Hammer, T. Else (eds.), *Adrenocortical Carcinoma*,
DOI 10.1007/978-0-387-77236-3_23, © Springer Science+Business Media, LLC 2011

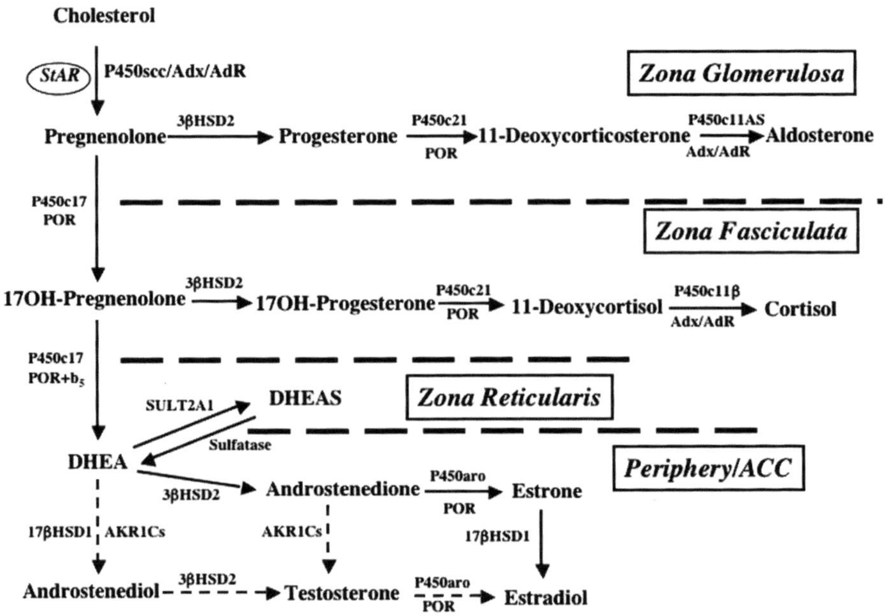

Fig. 23.1 Zones of the adrenal gland and the enzymatic machinery of each zone. Major enzymes and pathways are shown. The additional metabolism of DHEA(S) to androgens and estrogens in the periphery and ACC is demonstrated in the bottom section

normally occur in any one cell of the adrenal gland as discussed next. In contrast, steroidogenesis in ACC is more promiscuous and unpredictable.

The entire process of steroid hormone production can be dissected into five arbitrary components or characteristics for conceptual clarity.

1. *The conversion of cholesterol to pregnenolone*. All steroidogenesis begins with the conversion of 27-carbon cholesterol to 21-carbon pregnenolone, and this step is therefore tightly and acutely regulated. The only cells capable of synthesizing pregnenolone from cholesterol are the testicular Leydig cells, placental trophoblast cells, ovarian theca and corpus luteum cells, and of course the cells of the adrenal cortex. The cholesterol, which resides in a mobile pool on the outer mitochondrial membrane, is translocated to the inner mitochondrial membrane by the steroidogenic acute regulatory protein (StAR) [1, 2]. The cholesterol side-chain enzyme system (CYP11A1, P450scc) resides on the inner mitochondrial matrix and executes this first enzymatic step common to all cells that synthesize steroids. In this first step, steroidogenesis is *quantitatively* regulated, determining the amount of steroid produced at a given time.
2. *Downstream metabolism of pregnenolone to specific steroid products*. The end products of a specific steroidogenic cell are determined by the enzymes present in that cell, which metabolize nascent pregnenolone. In the adrenal gland, the

zonae glomerulosa, fasciculata, and reticularis convert pregnenolone into aldosterone, cortisol, and DHEAS, respectively. The efficiency of cortisol biosynthesis from pregnenolone, which requires four additional enzymes, is evidenced by circulating concentrations of the intermediates, which are generally 2–3 orders of magnitude lower than those of cortisol.

3. *Peripheral and target organ metabolism*. Whereas only a few cells convert cholesterol to pregnenolone and subsequent steroids, many tissues metabolize circulating steroids. Cortisol is inactivated to cortisone in the kidney, while DHEAS is converted into testosterone in peripheral tissues, and testosterone is activated to dihydrotestosterone (DHT) in the prostate gland.
4. *Redundant pathways and multiple layers of regulation*. Although the pathways to key steroids in the adrenal and gonads are very uniform and consistent, peripheral and secondary pathways are less clearly defined. Several enzymes and pathways to each steroid exist, and the contributions of each vary with age, gender, and genetic polymorphisms. The exact route(s) to testosterone in women remains enigmatic and likely varies day to day and person to person due to fluctuations in the regulation of each component of the axes as well as peripheral metabolism.
5. *Catabolic reactions*. The daily production rates of cortisol and testosterone for an adult man are roughly 15 and 5 mg/day, respectively, yet only micrograms of these compounds are excreted via the kidneys each day. Steroids undergo extensive metabolism, primarily by the liver, via 5α- and 5β-reductions, oxidation of hydroxyl groups, and oxygenations by nonsteroidogenic cytochromes P450. Androgens are primarily excreted as androsterone and etiocholanolone, accounting for >90% of the metabolites or up to 8 mg/day for an adult man.

23.1.2 Steroidogenic Enzymes

The two families of enzymes shown to catalyze most of the reactions in steroid biosynthesis are the cytochromes P450 and the hydroxysteroid dehydrogenases (HSDs). The P450-mediated reactions are mechanistically and functionally irreversible, whereas the HSDs catalyze bidirectional pseudoequilibria, which show a strong directional preference in intact cells [3, 4]. Consequently, steroid flux in a given steroidogenic cell is highly directional and efficient.

The cytochromes P450 use molecular oxygen and electrons from nicotinamide adenine dinucleotide phosphate (the reduced form, NADPH) to activate molecular oxygen to a highly reactive oxidizing agent. The remarkably selective chemistry of the steroidogenic P450s are due to the requirement of substrate binding to commence the catalytic cycle and the proximity of the steroid substrate to the heme–oxygen complex, which restricts the reaction to one region of the molecule. The P450 reactions are limited to hydroxylations or "oxygen insertions" according to the equation below, and occasionally carbon–carbon bond cleavage reactions.

$$\text{R-H} + O_2 + \text{NADPH} + H^+ \rightarrow \text{R-OH} + H_2O + \text{NADP}^+$$

Cytochromes P450 are classified as either type I or type II enzymes. Type I enzymes are found in bacteria and in eukaryotic mitochondria. Type I P450s accept electrons from NADPH via transfer first to ferredoxin reductase, a membrane-bound flavoprotein, and then to ferredoxin, a small, soluble iron-sulfur (Fe_2S_2) protein, which finally reduces the P450 complex. Of the 57 P450 enzymes encoded by the human genome [5], only a few are type I P450s, including CYP11A1, CYP11B1 (P450c11β, steroid 11-hydroxylase), CYP11B2 (P450c11AS, aldosterone synthase), and a few enzymes involved in vitamin D and bile acid metabolism. The remaining majority are type II P450s, which reside in the smooth endoplasmic reticulum and accept electrons from NADPH via cytochrome P450-oxidoreductase (POR), a membrane-bound protein containing two flavins. Steroidogenic type II enzymes are CYP17A1 (P450c17, steroid 17-hydroxylase/17,20-lyase), CYP21A2 (P450c21, steroid 21-hydroxylase), and CYP19A1 (P450aro, aromatase). All of these P450 enzymes, except aromatase, are normally present in the adrenal cortex in high abundance.

The other major class of steroidogenic enzymes is the HSDs, which catalyze the following two half-reactions.

$$R = O + NAD(P)H + H^+ \rightarrow R\text{-}OH + NAD(P)^+$$

$$R\text{-}OH + NAD(P)^+ \rightarrow R = O + NAD(P)H + H^+$$

HSDs exist in multiple isoforms encoded by separate genes, each with tissue-specific expression and regulation, many of which are found in peripheral tissues. Consequently, the HSDs regulate the fraction of a ketosteroid and its cognate hydroxysteroid in a given cell or in the circulation. Because the ketosteroid and corresponding hydroxysteroid have radically different biological potencies (i.e., estrone vs. estradiol, cortisol vs. cortisone), these enzymes profoundly modify steroid hormone action. In general, HSDs favoring ketosteroid reduction in intact cells bind NADP(H) with high affinity, whereas those that preferentially oxidize hydroxysteroids have poor affinity for NADP(H) and use NAD^+ as their primary electron acceptor, as exemplified by the human 17βHSDs types 1 and 2 [6]. The reason that this biochemical nuance translates in to directional preference is that cofactor concentrations in the cytoplasm of intact, well-fed cells show marked gradients, such that concentrations of NADPH exceed those of $NADP^+$ by roughly 700, and concentrations of NAD^+ similarly dwarf those of NADH. Consequently, mass action coupled to regeneration of cofactor gradients drives hydroxysteroid oxidation for "oxidative" enzymes such as 17βHSD2, despite the energetic preference for NADP(H) oxidation [3].

HSDs sort into two structural families, the short-chain dehydrogenase/reductases (SDRs) [7] or aldo-keto reductases (AKRs) [8]. The SDR enzymes have a beta-alpha-beta motif, where parallel beta strands form the center of the molecule with alpha helices draped on both sides, also called a Rossman fold. The AKR enzymes have beta-barrel or TIM-barrel fold motif, named after triosephosphate isomerase, the prototypical enzyme. In these proteins, eight obliquely oriented beta strands form the center of a "barrel", with alpha helices connecting the parallel beta strands on the outside. Key tyrosine and lysine residues drive proton transfers during catalysis for both oxidation and reduction. In the SDR enzymes, these residues reside on adjacent turns of an alpha helix, whereas in the AKR enzymes the residues are found at the tip of sequential beta strands, distant in linear sequence yet still adjacent in space.

The two major variations on the HSD theme are the 5α- and 5β-reductases, in which the enzyme uses NADPH to reduce a carbon–carbon double bond, and the 3βHSD isoenzymes, which also catalyze isomerization of the delta-5 double bond to the delta-4 configuration. The 5α-reductases are extremely hydrophobic enzymes with no close structural homologs in mammalian genomes, so little is known about their structure and biochemistry despite their great importance in androgen biology. The only human 5β-reductase is AKR1D1, which is critical for bile acid synthesis, but also catabolizes steroids. Human beings have 3βHSD/isomerase enzymes, the type 1 enzyme found in the liver, skin, placenta, and other peripheral tissues [9], and the type 2 enzyme, the major isoform in the adrenal cortex and gonads [10]. The only major and essential HSD in the adrenal cortex is 3βHSD2, although other enzymes are found in certain zones, such as AKR1C3 (17βHSD5), which likely accounts for the small amount of testosterone produced directly by the zona reticularis [11].

23.1.3 Steroidogenic Pathways in the Adrenal Gland

To simplify the seemingly complex array of steroid biosynthetic pathways, it is useful to consider each zone of the adrenal cortex, its end product, and the enzymes present in that zone. In addition, it is helpful to consider CYP17A1 as the qualitative regulator of adrenal steroidogenesis (Fig. 23.1) [12]. CYP17A1 17-hydroxylates pregnenolone and progesterone in the zona fasciculata and cleaves 17-hydroxypregnenolone to DHEA as well in the zona reticularis. In the absence of CYP17A1, the zona glomerulosa converts pregnenolone to progesterone via the enzyme 3βHSD2, and CYP21A2 metabolizes progesterone to 11-deoxycorticosterone (DOC). CYP11B2 then performs three sequential oxygenations on DOC, affording aldosterone. In the zona fasiculata, CYP17A1 and 3βHSD2 convert pregnenolone to 17-hydroxyprogesterone, the preferred substrate for CYP21A2. CYP21A2 produces 11-deoxycortisol, which is converted to cortisol by CYP11B1. The 17,20-lyase activity of CYP17A1 in the zona reticularis is activated by the presence of cytochrome b_5 [13], and the absence of 3βHSD2 limits steroidogenesis to DHEA, which is exported after sulfation by SULT2A1 [14]. DHEAS is desulfated in peripheral tissues, although the contribution of this pathway to the circulating pool of DHEA is controversial [15]. The liver, skin, and other peripheral tissues metabolize a small fraction of DHEA sequentially to weak and potent androgens and estrogens (Fig. 23.1).

23.1.4 Acute and Chronic Regulation of Adrenal Steroidogenesis and Dysregulation in Adrenocortical Carcinoma

Within minutes, ACTH, signaling via MC2R, stimulates a profound rise in steroidogenesis from the adrenal gland, an observation used clinically in the cosyntropin stimulation test. Although the presence of ACTH is required for chronic maintenance of steroidogenesis and adrenal cortex integrity, the time course of this acute rise is much too fast to derive from augmented expression of CYP11A1. The acute effect of ACTH is mediated by activation of the StAR protein [1, 2]. StAR, a 37 kDa protein, is cleaved to a 30 kDa form upon entering the mitochondria [16] and moves hundreds of cholesterol molecules before inactivation [17]. StAR contains a START domain, a hydrophobic beta-sheet pocket shared by other sterol-binding proteins, which stoichiometrically binds one molecule of cholesterol [18] and might participate in cholesterol mobilization. The precise details of how StAR mediates cholesterol transport and the roles of StAR phosphorylation and degradation have received intense study but remain controversial.

Chronically, ACTH stimulates cAMP generation, which induces adrenal cell hypertrophy via production of basic fibroblast growth factor [19], epidermal growth factor [20], and IGF2 [21]. In parallel, ACTH maintains transcription of genes encoding steroidogenic enzymes and the electron transfer proteins via activation of the cAMP-dependent protein kinase A (PKA). ACTH alone is insufficient for continued steroid production, and other transcription factors act in concert with PKA to maintain steroidogenesis. Among these factors, GATA4 and GATA6 (named for the GATA nucleotide motif targeted by these proteins), specific transcription factors 1 and 3 (SP1, SP3), and most importantly, steroidogenic factor1 (SF1, NR5A1) are known to be critical for adrenal function. SF1, an orphan nuclear receptor, not only regulates the coordination expression of steroidogenic enzymes [22] but also remains essential for the development of the adrenals and gonads, as well as specific cells in the pituitary and hypothalamus [23]. Consequently, regular tropic stimulation is required to maintain normal adrenal steroidogenesis, which faithfully yields the same products of each zone.

In ACC, however, steroidogenesis becomes independent of the tropic stimuli, and several steroids are produced in abundance. The combination of a large adrenal tumor with both aldosterone and cortisol excess, or androgens plus mineralocorticoids, is highly suspicious for ACC. Urinary profiling of steroid metabolites is particularly helpful in identifying ACCs [24]. In ACC cells, the normal restricted expression of zone-specific enzymes often does not occur. These cells may coexpress *CYP17A1*, *3βHSD2*, and cytochrome b_5 [25], enabling the direct production of androstenedione and possibly testosterone from a single cell, analogous to the Leydig cell. Coexpression of *CYP11B1* and *CYP11B2* allows production of cortisol and aldosterone. Consequently, although the general rules and discrete enzymatic steps remain the same, the major pathways operating in ACC vary amongst tumors and do not necessarily reflect any particular zone of the normal adrenal gland. The NCI-H295 cell line, derived from an ACC tumor, produces a variety of steroids and expresses multiple enzymes, illustrating the complex biosynthetic potential of ACC cells [26].

23.2 Approach to the Adrenocortical Carcinoma Patient

23.2.1 Clinical Manifestations of Adrenal Steroid Excess

Given the mixture of hormones typically produced by ACCs, the clinical manifestations are diverse and multiple. The aldosterone excess causes hypertension and hypokalemia, and in ACC, other precursors such as DOC often contribute. Cortisol excess, which is a form of the Cushing's syndrome, also causes hypertension and hypokalemia, but the catabolic effects of cortisol dominate the clinical syndrome. These consequences are both physical, including proximal muscle weakness, osteoporosis, fragile skin and blood vessels, fat redistribution, and metabolic, leading to dyslipidemia and glucose intolerance (see Table 23.1). Androgen excess rarely causes manifestations in men, because ACC cells do not normally make strong androgens such as testosterone (T) and dihydrotestosterone (DHT) directly, but rather primarily make precursors DHEA(S) and also androstenedione. These precursors are metabolized to T and DHT in peripheral tissues, yet the contribution is typically small compared to the T made by the testes. In contrast, women with ACC often show manifestations of androgen excess, primarily hirsutism and acne, but in more severe states voice deepening, clitoromegaly, increased aggression, and increased upper body muscle mass. Estrogen excess, which occurs when *CYP19A1* (P450aro, aromatase) is expressed, is extremely rare, and men with this complication develop gynecomastia, impotence, and neuropsychiatric changes.

Consequently, the clinical manifestations of steroid excess in ACC derive not only on the mix of hormones produced by the tumor but also vary with age, gender, and comorbidities of the specific patient. Consequences of each hormone that is overproduced must be addressed in the context of an overall strategy to manage the needs of the patient.

Table 23.1 Cushing's Syndrome: signs and symptoms

Specific signs and symptoms	Non-specific signs and symptoms
Plethora	Hypertrichosis
Supraclavicular and cervical fat pads	Acne
Central obesity	Libidinal dysfunction/impotence
Proximal muscle weakness	Menstrual irregularity/infertility
Skin thinning	Fungal infections
Ecchymosis	Poor wound healing
	Neuropsychiatric disorders
In children	Spinal epidural lipomatosis
Premature or delayed puberty	Nephrolithiasis /polyuria
Growth retardation	Hypertension

23.2.2 Therapeutic Strategies

Conceptually, several approaches can be used to treat overproduction of each adrenocortical steroid hormone (Table 23.2). First, enzyme inhibitors reduce the flux of precursors across specific steps in the pathways. The more distal the enzyme is located in a multistep pathway, the more selectively the agent will reduce the production of one hormone. The more proximal the enzyme is in steroidogenesis, the more versatile the agent, having the capacity to inhibit the production of several hormones simultaneously. For example, aromatase inhibitors have become first-line therapy for breast cancer [27], due to their ability to block one of the terminal steps of estradiol synthesis without blocking other steroidogenesis pathways. Conversely, trilostane inhibits 3βHSD2 and thus simultaneously impairs the synthesis of mineralocorticoids, glucocorticoids, androgens, and estrogens. Additional considerations include the accumulation of precursor steroids – which may themselves have biological activity – prior to the block, and simultaneous inhibition of gonadal steroidogenesis. Abiraterone acetate, for instance, is a selective inhibitor of CYP17A1 under development for the treatment of prostate cancer by inhibiting both testicular and adrenal 19-carbon synthesis [28]. One consequence of abiraterone therapy is the accumulation of DOC, which can cause hypertension and hypokalemia [29] as occurs in genetic forms of 17-hydroxylase deficiency due to inactivating *CYP17A1* mutations [30].

Table 23.2 Approaches to the management of hormone excess in ACC

Mechanism	Advantages	Disadvantages
Synthesis inhibitor	Rational design	Intermediates accumulate
	Potential specificity	Off-target inhibition
		Limited development
Receptor antagonist	Reliable efficacy	Difficulty titrating dose
	Several drugs available	Often mixed agonist–antagonists
Treat comorbidities	Many drugs available	Empiric
	Broad experience	Resistance to conventional drugs

A second approach is to employ nuclear hormone receptor antagonists to block the action of the hormone on its cognate receptor. This approach works well for androgen and mineralocorticoid excess. Several agents are commercially available to antagonize the mineralocorticoid and androgen receptors (MR and AR, respectively); and an increase in hormone production from relief of feedback inhibition, as occurs in normal physiology, does not happen, given the autonomous nature of steroid production by ACC. Glucocorticoid receptor antagonists are under development, but their use is complicated by the diverse actions of glucocorticoids in almost all tissues of the body. A further complication is the property inherent in many of these drugs is that, rather than pure antagonists or inverse agonists, most of these drugs are "selective receptor modulators." Tamoxifen, an "anti-estrogen," is a human estrogen receptor agonist in endometrium, an antagonist in breast, and a mixed agonist–antagonist in other tissues [31].

A third approach is to use nonspecific treatments of the comorbidities. The hypertension may be treated with conventional antihypertensive drugs, although mineralocorticoid-mediated hypertension tends to be resistant to treatment with most typical drugs [32]. The dyslipidemia, glucose intolerance, and cardiovascular risk may be managed with statins and other lipid-lowering agents, hypoglycemic drugs, and aspirin, respectively. These treatments are largely empiric and reviewed briefly in this section.

Because the adrenal does not store pre-formed hormones, drugs that block hormone secretion for other disorders, such as somatostatin analogs and dopamine receptor type 2 agonists, are not an option in ACC. The closest analogy would be an inhibitor of cholesterol transport or StAR action; however, no such agents are currently available.

23.3 Specific Treatments

23.3.1 Mineralocorticoid Excess

The goals of treatment of mineralocorticoid excess in ACC are to control blood pressure and, more importantly, to correct hypokalemia. Treatments are summarized in Table 23.3.

Table 23.3 Drugs for the treatment of mineralocorticoid excess in ACC

Mechanism	Drugs[a]	Comments
Synthesis inhibitor	*FAD286*	
	Aminoglutethimide	Broadly inhibits steroidogenesis
Receptor antagonist	**Spironolactone**	Also blocks androgens
	Eplerenone	Selective antagonist
Nonspecific therapies	**Triamterine, amiloride**	Controls potassium well
	Other antihypertensives	Empiric

[a]Agents shown in *italics* are not commercially available or not generally used; first-line agents are shown in **bold** type

23.3.1.1 Inhibitors of Mineralocorticoid Synthesis

A selective inhibitor of CYP11B2 would be a "magic bullet" to inhibit the synthesis of aldosterone, since this enzyme catalyzes the last three steps of aldosterone biosynthesis but participates in no other steroidogenic pathways. CYP11B2 inhibitors, such as FAD286, are being developed [33], but their utility in ACC is likely to be limited by the co-production of other mineralocorticoids such as DOC [34], which do not require CYP11B2 activity. Nevertheless, some ACC patients with tumors that have high flux of precursor to aldosterone might benefit from this type of treatment.

Trilostane, ketoconazole, and aminoglutethimide are each inhibitors of one or more enzymes in several steroidogenic pathways. Trilostane inhibits 3βHSD types 1 and 2 and would reduce aldosterone production, and trilostane also blocks cortisol and androgen synthesis. Similarly, aminoglutethimide primarily inhibits CYP11A1 and thus block synthesis of all steroids. Ketoconazole, in contrast, primarily inhibits CYP17A1. The use of these agents will be described in detail under the section on glucocorticoid excess.

23.3.1.2 Mineralocorticoid Receptor Antagonists

Antagonists of the MR are first-line medical treatments of mineralocorticoid excess of any etiology, including ACC. Spironolactone is an effective and high-affinity MR antagonist, and its primary metabolite, canrenone, is also a potent antagonist with a much longer half-life than spironolactone. Spironolactone and canrenone contain a spirolactone attached to the D-ring, and the hydrolysis product, potassium canrenoate, is used as an intravenous preparation and is metabolized to canrenone in vivo.

The main drawback of spironolactone is its lack of specificity. Spironolactone also antagonizes the progesterone and androgen receptors at doses used clinically. The main side effects in menstruating women include midcycle spotting and breast tenderness; in postmenopausal women, such problems usually do not occur. In males, the anti-androgen properties may cause gynecomastia and erectile dysfunction. The gynecomastia is reversible during the first 6 months and somewhat dose-dependent, but it is not possible to predict which men will develop this problem. The anti-androgen properties are advantageous in treating women with ACC if both mineralocorticoids and androgens are elevated (see below).

Spironolactone is administered orally, starting at about 25 mg a day and gradually advanced to achieve the therapeutic effect. Total daily doses above 50 mg/day may be divided twice daily and advanced up to 200 mg twice a day. The kaliuresis responds immediately to treatment, and this response can be monitored with urinary electrolyte measurements. Since most potassium is distributed intracellularly, however, many patients with hypokalemia from mineralocorticoid excess are severely depleted in total body potassium, so serum potassium responds more slowly than kaliuresis and requires exogenous (dietary or otherwise) potassium to replace the deficit. Potassium should be replaced cautiously, and serum potassium should be monitored at least weekly to guard against hyperkalemia. The primary risk factor for developing hyperkalemia during spironolactone treatment is renal insufficiency, while age and depressed cardiac output are additional factors [35]. The blood pressure response is much slower than the restoration of normokalemia and may take 2–4 weeks to reach maximal, and further more gradual reductions in blood pressure can occur for many weeks later [36]. A good response to the prescribed dose is documented by normalization of plasma renin activity as well as potassium and blood pressure. Intramenstrual spotting can be treated by co-administration of an oral contraceptive or depot medroxyprogesterone acetate. All women of childbearing age should use contraception while taking spironolactone, although the risk of genital malformation to a male fetus from spironolactone exposure is more theoretical than substantiated clinically. If gynecomastia develops, dose reduction may minimize the problem, but often therapy must be changed to another agent such as eplerenone.

Eplerenone is a selective MR antagonist that is used in hypertension at doses of 50 mg once or twice daily [37]. The general impression has been that eplerenone is less potent than spironolactone, but this bias may be in large part due to the conservative dosage limitations on the package insert, although published studies have used doses as high as 200 mg/day [38]. Eplerenone lacks many of the "off-target" side effects of spironolactone such as gynecomastia in men and vaginal spotting in women, and the same risk factors for hyperkalemia apply as for spironolactone. Clinical experience with eplerenone is more limited than for spironolactone, and the cost of eplerenone is significantly higher. Spironolactone and eplerenone should be considered the cornerstone of treatment for the mineralocorticoid excess of ACC.

23.3.1.3 Nonspecific Treatment of Hypertension and Hypokalemia

Amiloride and triamterene are potassium-sparing diuretics that compete with sodium ion for binding to the epithelial sodium channel (ENaC) in the tubular lumen, and these drugs are quite effective in ameliorating the hypokalemia of mineralocorticoid excess states. Amiloride is started at 5 mg once daily and advanced every 1–2 weeks. More than 10 mg/day is given as divided doses up to a maximum of 20 mg/day. Triamterene is typically used in preparations containing a thiazide, but triamterine may be used as monotherapy at 25–100 mg/day. Empirically, these drugs are not as effective as spironolactone and eplerenone in reducing blood pressure, so additional agents must be used in combination. Calcium channel blockers and other vasodilators, adrenergic blocking agents, and angiotensin receptor blockers or converting enzyme inhibitors are examples of such add-on agents, and the reader is referred to general texts on hypertension for more details of their use. Diuretics such as thiazides and furosemide must be used with caution, as these agents tend to worsen hypokalemia. Oral potassium supplements are added as necessary to balance potassium homeostasis.

23.3.2 Glucocorticoid Excess

The medical management of glucocorticoid excess states is one of the most difficult problems in endocrinology [39]. In ACTH-dependent Cushing's syndrome, bilateral adrenalectomy remains an option that is usually exercised when all other options fail, as typically occurs when the source of ACTH cannot be removed surgically. In ACC, metastatic and unresectable adrenal tissue precludes this option. Note that glucocorticoids such as cortisol and corticosterone both act as mineralocorticoids, particularly at high circulating concentrations. Ordinarily, these 11-hydroxysteroids are inactivated in the kidney by 11βHSD2 [40]; however, the enzyme cannot

up to 1440 mg/day found no reproducible reduction in cortisol or accumulation of delta-5 precursors [52]. Use of this drug has fallen out of favor, and no commercial preparation has become available.

23.3.2.2 Glucocorticoid Receptor Antagonists

Unlike the case for mineralocorticoid excess, no selective inhibitors of the glucocorticoid receptor are available for clinical use. Some agents, such as RU-43044 and 21-succinoyloxy-6,10-epoxyprogesterone, show promise as selective antagonists [53], but these compounds have not been studied in human beings. Mifepristone (RU-486) has been studied extensively as a progesterone antagonist and abortifactant, but mifepristone is also an antagonist of the glucocorticoid receptor. Small studies have suggested efficacy in the treatment of depression [54] and psychosis [55] associated with Cushing's syndrome. At least two trials are currently ongoing to evaluate mifepristone in the treatment of hypercortisolism, including ACC. These studies are assessing multiple measures of efficacy, including metabolic, cardiovascular, and neuropsychiatric, and this drug may be available for treatment of ACC in the future.

23.3.2.3 Nonspecific Treatment of Cardiovascular and Metabolic Consequences

The many disorders caused by the hypercortisolism of ACC are all ameliorated but often not reversed to normal with normalization of cortisol production, and many require concurrent or subsequent treatments. Only the special features of this vast topic in the context of ACC will be covered here. Diabetes rarely resolves completely with treatment of the cortisol excess. Short-acting insulin should be used with caution when advancing the dose of nauseating drugs such as metyrapone and aminoglutethimide. Dyslipidemia is common, but the dose of statins must be reduced substantially when using ketoconazole. Aggressive treatment should be considered in the context of life expectancy. Hypertriglyceridemia >500 mg/dL can cause pancreatitis and should be treated. Drugs like niacin and fibrates can exacerbate the hepatotoxicity of ketoconazole, and omega-3 fatty acid esters might be a safer choice. Bone loss requires attention, and infusional bisphosphonates are generally better tolerated than oral agents in the context of multi-drug regimens.

23.3.3 Androgen Excess

Of all the hormonal consequences with ACC, androgen excess is the least life-threatening but can be the most disfiguring. Although males rarely require treatment, given that testicular production dominates as a source of testosterone, women will suffer hirsutism, acne, breast atrophy, menstrual irregularity, voice deepening, clitoromegaly, and neuropsychiatric changes that can be devastating physically and emotionally if not treated specifically. Treatments are summarized in Table 23.5.

Table 23.5 Drugs for the treatment of androgen excess in ACC

Mechanism	Drugs[a]	Comments
Synthesis inhibitor	**Aminoglutethimide**	Broadly inhibits steroidogenesis
	Ketoconazole	Monitor transaminases
	Abiraterone acetate	Mineralocorticoids accumulate
	Finasteride, dutasteride	Limited data
Receptor antagonist	**Spironolactone**	Also blocks mineralocorticoids
	Flutamide	Gastrointestinal and liver toxicity
	Bicalutamide, nilutamide	Limited data
Nonspecific therapies	Topical eflornithine	Effective for small areas

[a]Agents shown in *italics* are not commercially available or not generally used; first-line agents are shown in **bold** type

23.3.3.1 Inhibitors of Androgen Synthesis

As discussed above, ketoconazole is a good inhibitor of CYP17A1, which generally reduces androgen production to a greater degree than cortisol production. Aminoglutethimide, which inhibits CYP11A1, will also lower androgen production when used to block cortisol synthesis. Metyrapone and etomidate, which primarily inhibit CYP11B1, will worsen androgen excess and should be avoided if androgens are a significant problem.

Abiraterone acetate is a selective CYP17A1 inhibitor that is under development for the treatment of castrate-resistant prostate cancer [28]. At doses of 250–1000 mg daily, serum androgen concentrations are reduced to virtually undetectable in most patients [29]. The drug has not been approved for use by regulatory agencies in any country at the present time, and the drug has not been studied in ACC, but this agent is likely to be extremely effective for the androgen excess of ACC. One problem with the drug in the context of ACC is that 17-deoxysteroids such as DOC accumulate above the block and can worsen hypertension and hypokalemia [29].

Finasteride and dutasteride are inhibitors of the 5α-reductase enzymes, limiting the conversion of testosterone and other precursors to the most potent androgen, dihydrotestosterone. Dutasteride inhibits both types 1 and 2 enzymes, and is therefore theoretically preferable over finasteride, which only inhibits the type 1 enzyme. Finasteride is used at 1–5 mg/day, and dutasteride is dosed at 0.5 mg/d. Limited data exist on the use of finasteride in the treatment of hirsutism [56], and nothing is known about the use of these drugs in ACC. These agents are likely to be helpful only as add-on therapy when testosterone production is not controlled by other means.

23.3.3.2 Androgen Receptor Antagonists

Several AR antagonists have been developed for the treatment of prostate cancer, and others have evolved out of efforts to develop synthetic progestins for oral contraceptives. Spironolactone is an attractive agent for the treatment of androgen excess due to ACC, since this drug will also treat the mineralocorticoid excess. Doses to treat androgen excess, particularly when severe, tend to be high (200–400 mg/day), so treatment is individualized. Titration is problematic, since hirsutism takes 3–6 months to improve, and biomarkers of androgen blockade are not available for women. Consequently, the dose is generally titrated upwards based primarily on blood pressure and potassium, with subsequent assessment of androgen blockade clinically. The potential of spironolactone to impair the efficacy of mitotane was discussed above and should be considered before starting treatment. The published literature on the use of these agents in ACC is scant, and most recommendations derive from studies of idiopathic hirsutism or polycystic ovary syndrome. In general, all agents are effective to varying degrees [57, 58], but the choice of drugs is based largely on which fit best and safest in the overall therapeutic plan.

Cyproterone acetate is a mixed progestin-antiandrogen, which is used alone or, more commonly, in combination with ethinyl estradiol as an oral contraceptive pill. When used alone, the dose is 25–100 mg/day depending on the severity of the hyperandrogenism. The dose is 2 mg/day when used in the fixed combination dose oral contraceptive with 35 mcg of ethinyl estradiol, but this low dose is unlikely to be very beneficial when the androgen excess is severe.

Flutamide is a nonsteroidal anti-androgen, which often lowers androgen synthesis slightly. Doses as low as 62.5 mg/day have been used in adolescents with ovarian hyperandrogenemia [59], but higher doses are usually needed to treat the androgen excess of ACC. Doses up to 500 mg/day can be used, but gastrointestinal side effects (nausea, diarrhea) often limit dose escalation. The drug can cause liver damage, and transaminases should be monitored, particularly when used in combination with ketoconazole.

Bicalutamide is another nonsteroidal anti-androgen that has had limited use in treatment of androgen excess. The dose is 25–50 mg/day, with hepatotoxicity reported above doses of 50 mg/day. Nilutimide is a third nonsteroidal anti-androgen developed for use in prostate cancer, but little or no information is available for its use in women. The dose is 150–300 mg/day, and this drug also has been implicated in causing liver damage.

23.3.3.3 Nonspecific Treatment of Androgen Excess

Only some of the consequences derived from androgen excess in women can be treated with non-endocrine therapies. Hirsutism can be managed with mechanical methods, including shaving, waxing, plucking, electrolysis, and laser hair removal. Small problem areas may be treated with eflornithine hydrochloride (14%) cream twice daily [57]. Acne will respond to retinoids such as tretinoin, but retinoids should be used with caution, given that their influence on tumor growth not known.

23.3.4 Treatment of Estrogen Excess

Estrogen-producing ACCs are extremely rare, and the prognosis is very poor [60]. Almost no data are available on pharmacotherapy of estrogen excess in men with

ACC, so this topic will be covered briefly. Estrogen antagonists, such as tamoxifen (20–40 mg daily), raloxefine (60 mg twice daily), and fulvestrant (250 mg intramuscular injection monthly) may be used to ameliorate gynecomastia. The main side effect of these agents is deep venous thrombosis, with a risk approaching 1% per year. Potent and selective aromatase inhibitors are now available [61], including anastrozole (1 mg/day), letrozole (2.5 mg/day), and exemestane (25 mg/day). Aminoglutethimide will inhibit aromatase as well as the synthesis of precursors, but may not be sufficiently potent to normalize estrogen concentrations. Other agents that block synthesis of precursors, such as ketoconazole, will also limit estrogen synthesis. Bone loss and nausea are common side effects of these agents. Surgical mastectomy may be necessary as a palliative measure.

23.4 Conclusions

Pharmacotherapy of steroid excess in ACC is a complex process that requires attention to the production of several classes of steroids and their consequences. Limited data exist on the use of specific agents, and the potential for drug–drug interactions with the available agents is significant. Priority should be given to the most pressing problem in each patient, and therapy should be tailored to combine the maximal benefits with the fewest agents. Many of the currently available drugs were developed for other purposes and exploited for their unintended properties. Better agents are in development for specific targets, but inhibition of cortisol biosynthesis in ACC remains a challenge that is unlikely to be met in the near future. Mifepristone holds promise as a more selective and reliable agent for treating the consequences of cortisol excess, and studies are ongoing. Until therapies that will reliably treat the tumor itself are developed, however, endocrinologists will have to address the hormonal disturbances of ACC with whatever tools are at our disposal.

References

1. Clark BJ et al (1994) The purification, cloning and expression of a novel luteinizing hormone-induced mitochondrial protein in MA-10 mouse Leydig tumor cells. Characterization of the steroidogenic acute regulatory protein (StAR). J Biol Chem 269:28314–28322
2. Stocco DM, Clark BJ (1996) Regulation of the acute production of steroids in steroidogenic cells. Endocr Rev 17:221–244
3. Sherbet DP et al (2007) Cofactors, redox state, and directional preferences of hydroxysteroid dehydrogenases. Mol Cell Endocrinol 265–266:83–88
4. Mizrachi D, Auchus RJ (2009) Androgens, estrogens, and hydroxysteroid dehydrogenases. Mol Cell Endocrinol 301:37–42
5. Nelson DR et al (1993) The P450 superfamily: update on new sequences, gene mapping, accession numbers, early trivial names of enzymes, and nomenclature. DNA Cell Biol 12:1–51
6. Sherbet DP et al (2009) Biochemical factors governing the steady-state estrone/estradiol ratios catalyzed by human 17beta-hydroxysteroid dehydrogenases types 1 and 2 in HEK-293 cells. Endocrinology 150:4154–4162

7. Jornvall H et al (1995) Short-chain dehydrogenases/reductases (SDR). Biochemistry 34:6003–6013
8. Jez JM, Penning TM (2001) The aldo-keto reductase (AKR) superfamily: an update. Chem Biol Interact 130–132:499–525.
9. Lorence MC et al (1990) Human 3β-hydroxysteroid dehydrogenase/$\Delta^5 \rightarrow \Delta^4$ isomerase from placenta: expression in nonsteroidogenic cells of a protein that catalyzes the dehydrogenation/isomerization of C21 and C19 steroids. Endocrinology 126:2493–2498
10. Rhéaume E et al (1991) Structure and expression of a new complementary DNA encoding the almost exclusive 3β-hydroxysteroid dehydrogenase/Δ^5-Δ^4-isomerase in human adrenals and gonads. Mol Endocrinol 5:1147–1157
11. Nakamura Y et al (2009) Type 5 17β-hydroxysteroid dehydrogenase (AKR1C3) contributes to testosterone production in the adrenal reticularis. J Clin Endocrinol Metab 94:2192–2198
12. Miller WL (1988) Molecular biology of steroid hormone synthesis. Endocr Rev 9:295–318
13. Auchus RJ et al (1998) Cytochrome b_5 augments the 17,20 lyase activity of human P450c17 without direct electron transfer. J Biol Chem 273:3158–3165
14. Auchus RJ, Rainey WE (2004) Adrenarche – physiology, biochemistry and human disease. Clin Endocrinol (Oxf) 60:288–296
15. Hammer F et al (2005) No evidence for hepatic conversion of dehydroepiandrosterone (DHEA) sulfate to DHEA: in vivo and in vitro studies. J Clin Endocrinol Metab 90:3600–3605
16. Bose H et al (2002) Rapid regulation of steroidogenesis by mitochondrial protein import. Nature 417:87–91
17. Artemenko IP et al (2001) Mitochondrial processing of newly synthesized steroidogenic acute regulatory protein (StAR), but not total StAR, mediates cholesterol transfer to cytochrome P450 side chain cleavage enzyme in adrenal cells. J Biol Chem 276:46583–46596
18. Tsujishita Y, Hurley JH (2000) Structure and lipid transport mechanism of a StAR-related domain. Nat Struct Biol 7:408–414
19. Gospodarowicz D et al (1977) Control of bovine adrenal cortical cell proliferation by fibroblast growth factor. Lack of effect of epidermal growth factor. Endocrinology 100:1080–1089
20. Hornsby PJ et al (1987) Loss of expression of a differentiated function gene steroid 17α-hydroxylase, as adrenocortical cells senesce in culture. Proc Natl Acad Sci USA 84:1580–1584
21. Voutilainen R, Miller WL (1987) Coordinate tropic hormone regulation of mRNAs for insulin-like growth factor II and the cholesterol side-chain cleavage enzyme, P450scc, in human steroidogenic tissues. Proc Natl Acad Sci USA 84:1590–1594
22. Parker KL, Schimmer BP (1997) Steroidogenic factor 1: a key determinant of endocrine development and function. Endocr Rev 18:361–377
23. Luo X et al (1994) A cell-specific nuclear receptor is essential for adrenal and gonadal development and sexual differentiation. Cell 77:481–490
24. Grondal S et al (1990) Steroid profile in urine: a useful tool in the diagnosis and follow up of adrenocortical carcinoma. Acta Endocrinol (Copenh) 122:656–663
25. Sakai Y et al (1994) Mechanism of abnormal production of adrenal androgens in patients with adrenocortical adenomas and carcinomas. J Clin Endocrinol Metab 78:36–40
26. Samandari E et al (2007) Human adrenal corticocarcinoma NCI-H295R cells produce more androgens than NCI-H295A cells and differ in 3β-hydroxysteroid dehydrogenase type 2 and 17,20 lyase activities. J Endocrinol 195:459–472
27. Osborne CK, Schiff R (2005) Estrogen-receptor biology: continuing progress and therapeutic implications. J Clin Oncol 23:1616–1622
28. O'Donnell A et al (2004) Hormonal impact of the 17α-hydroxylase/C(17,20)-lyase inhibitor abiraterone acetate (CB7630) in patients with prostate cancer. Br J Cancer 90:2317–2325
29. Attard G et al (2008) Phase I Clinical Trial of a Selective Inhibitor of CYP17, Abiraterone Acetate, Confirms That Castration-Resistant Prostate Cancer Commonly Remains Hormone Driven. J Clin Oncol 26:463–4571
30. Auchus RJ (2001) The genetics, pathophysiology, and management of human deficiencies of P450c17. Endocrinol Metab Clin North Am 30:101–119

31. Osborne CK (1998) Tamoxifen in the treatment of breast cancer. N Engl J Med 339: 1609–1618
32. Nishizaka MK et al (2003) Efficacy of low-dose spironolactone in subjects with resistant hypertension. Am J Hypertens 16:925–930
33. Fiebeler A et al (2005) Aldosterone synthase inhibitor ameliorates angiotensin II-induced organ damage. Circulation 111:3087–3094
34. Irony I et al (1987) Pathophysiology of deoxycorticosterone-secreting adrenal tumors. J Clin Endocrinol Metab 65:836–840
35. Palmer BF (2004) Managing hyperkalemia caused by inhibitors of the renin-angiotensin-aldosterone system. N Engl J Med 351:585–592
36. Laragh J (2001) Laragh's lessons in pathophysiology and clinical pearls for treating hypertension. Am J Hypertens 14:84–89
37. Burgess E (2004) Eplerenone in hypertension. Expert Opin Pharmacother 5:2573–2581
38. Levy DG et al (2004) Distinguishing the antihypertensive and electrolyte effects of eplerenone. J Clin Endocrinol Metab 89:2736–2740
39. Miller JW, Crapo L (1993) The medical treatment of Cushing's syndrome. Endocr Rev 14:443–458
40. White PC et al (1997) 11β-hydroxysteroid dehydrogenase and the syndrome of apparent mineralocorticoid excess. Endocr Rev 18:135–156
41. Stewart PM et al (1995) 11β-Hydroxysteroid dehydrogenase activity in Cushing's syndrome: explaining the mineralocorticoid excess state of the ectopic adrenocorticotropin syndrome. J Clin Endocrinol Metab 80:3617–3620
42. Wortsman J, Soler NG (1977) Mitotane. Spironolactone antagonism in Cushing's syndrome. JAMA 238:2527
43. Feldman D (1986) Ketoconazole and other imidazole derivatives as inhibitors of steroidogenesis. Endocr Rev 7:409–420
44. Small EJ et al (2004) Antiandrogen withdrawal alone or in combination with ketoconazole in androgen-independent prostate cancer patients: a phase III trial (CALGB 9583). J Clin Oncol 22:1025–1033
45. Santen RJ, Misbin RI (1981) Aminoglutethimide: review of pharmacology and clinical use. Pharmacotherapy 1:95–120
46. Santen RJ et al (1977) Adrenal suppression with aminoglutethimide. I. Differential e-fects of aminoglutethimide on glucocorticoid metabolism as a rationale for use of hydrocortisone. J Clin Endocrinol Metab 45:469–479
47. Hartzband PI et al (1988) Assessment of hypothalamic-pituitary-adrenal (HPA) axis dysfunction: comparison of ACTH stimulation, insulin-hypoglycemia and metyrapone. J Endocrinol Invest 11:769–776
48. Orth DN (1978) Metyrapone is useful only as adjunctive therapy in Cushing's disease. Ann Intern Med 89:128–130
49. Drake WM et al (1998) Emergency and prolonged use of intravenous etomidate to control hypercortisolemia in a patient with Cushing's syndrome and peritonitis. J Clin Endocrinol Metab 83:3542–3544
50. Schulte HM et al (1990) Infusion of low dose etomidate: correction of hypercortisolemia in patients with Cushing's syndrome and dose-response relationship in normal subjects. J Clin Endocrinol Metab 70:1426–1430
51. Allolio B et al (1988) Nonhypnotic low-dose etomidate for rapid correction of hypercortisolaemia in Cushing's syndrome. Klin Wochenschr 66:361–364
52. Dewis P et al (1983) Experience with trilostane in the treatment of Cushing's syndrome. Clin Endocrinol (Oxf) 18:533–540
53. Clark RD (2008) Glucocorticoid receptor antagonists. Curr Top Med Chem 8:813–838
54. Nieman LK et al (1985) Successful treatment of Cushing's syndrome with the glucocorticoid antagonist RU 486. J Clin Endocrinol Metab 61:536–540
55. van der Lely AJ et al (1991) Rapid reversal of acute psychosis in the Cushing syndrome with the cortisol-receptor antagonist mifepristone (RU 486). Ann Intern Med 114:143–144

56. Swiglo BA et al (2008) Clinical review: antiandrogens for the treatment of hirsutism: a systematic review and metaanalyses of randomized controlled trials. J Clin Endocrinol Metab 93:1153–1160
57. Blume-Peytavi U, Hahn S (2008) Medical treatment of hirsutism. Dermatol Ther 21:329–339
58. Venturoli S et al (1999) A prospective randomized trial comparing low dose flutamide, finasteride, ketoconazole, and cyproterone acetate-estrogen regimens in the treatment of hirsutism. J Clin Endocrinol Metab 84:1304–1310
59. Ibanez L et al (2000) Treatment of hirsutism, hyperandrogenism, oligomenorrhea, dyslipidemia, and hyperinsulinism in nonobese, adolescent girls: effect of flutamide. J Clin Endocrinol Metab 85:3251–3255
60. Moreno S et al (2006) Feminizing adreno-cortical carcinomas in male adults. A dire prognosis. Three cases in a series of 801 adrenalectomies and review of the literature. Ann Endocrinol (Paris) 67:32–38
61. Rugo HS (2008) The breast cancer continuum in hormone-receptor-positive breast cancer in postmenopausal women: evolving management options focusing on aromatase inhibitors. Ann Oncol 19:16–27

Chapter 24
Surgery for Adrenocortical Carcinoma

James T. Broome, Barbra S. Miller, Paul G. Gauger, and Gerard M. Doherty

Surgery is the mainstay of therapy for adrenocortical carcinoma (ACC). It is thought that the first technically successful resection of an ACC was performed in 1889 by Thornton [1]. Although reported as a sarcoma, it is likely this was an ACC based on the description of size (>20 pounds), accompanying hirsutism, and recurrence of disease with death 2 years later. The development of the technique for adrenalectomy has slowly evolved since the first early descriptions in the 1880s. Initially, using a T-shaped incision and incisions low in the abdomen, the incision site was progressively moved superiorly to allow better access to the adrenal glands [2–4]. Further refinements in technique and approaches involved resection of the lower ribs. A posterior approach to adrenal resection was also developed [5], but presently does not have much utility in resections for ACC. In the early 1990s, a laparoscopic approach to adrenalectomy was first described [6, 7] and a number of other laparoscopic techniques and approaches have subsequently been described (transperitoneal, retroperitoneal, posterior retroperitoneal). While laparoscopic adrenalectomy has become the gold standard for resection of benign masses, its use is not recommended for resection of primary ACCs.

A recent study [8] revealed that in the past 20 years no significant progress has been made with regard to the treatment of ACC, and 5-year survival outcomes remain static. In the United States, 45% of adrenalectomies for ACC are performed in community hospitals, 30% in academic centers, and only 15% in National Cancer Institute designated cancer centers [9]. Despite increased utilization of imaging studies, ACC is not identified at earlier stages in the United States; however, at select quarternary referral centers, it does appear that there may be some progress in terms of treatment [10, 11]. The majority of patients with ACC present with stage III or IV disease.

Complete surgical resection of all tumor currently provides the only opportunity for cure or long-term survival from ACC. Appropriate preoperative evaluation and planning are of utmost importance in these patients to assure optimal outcome.

J.T. Broome (✉)
Vanderbilt Endocrine Surgery Center, Vanderbilt University, 597 Preston Research Building, 2220 Pierce Ave, Nashville, TN, USA
e-mail: james.broome@vanderbilt.edu

G.D. Hammer, T. Else (eds.), *Adrenocortical Carcinoma*,
DOI 10.1007/978-0-387-77236-3_24, © Springer Science+Business Media, LLC 2011

However, resection with curative intent is not the only indication for surgical intervention in the patient diagnosed with ACC. Adrenal surgical anatomy, the potential complications of surgical intervention, expected outcomes including the tempo of recovery, and the various options for intervention are all important considerations with regard to the beneficial application of surgical management strategies for patients with ACC.

24.1 Surgical Adrenal Anatomy

An intimate knowledge of adrenal anatomy is paramount to successful surgical planning and execution. The adrenals are paired, goldenrod-yellow colored glands that are situated superior and medial to each kidney in the retroperitoneum (Fig. 24.1). A review of the vascular supply and regional anatomy creates the foundation upon which to discuss decisions about operative management and anticipate potential intraoperative challenges.

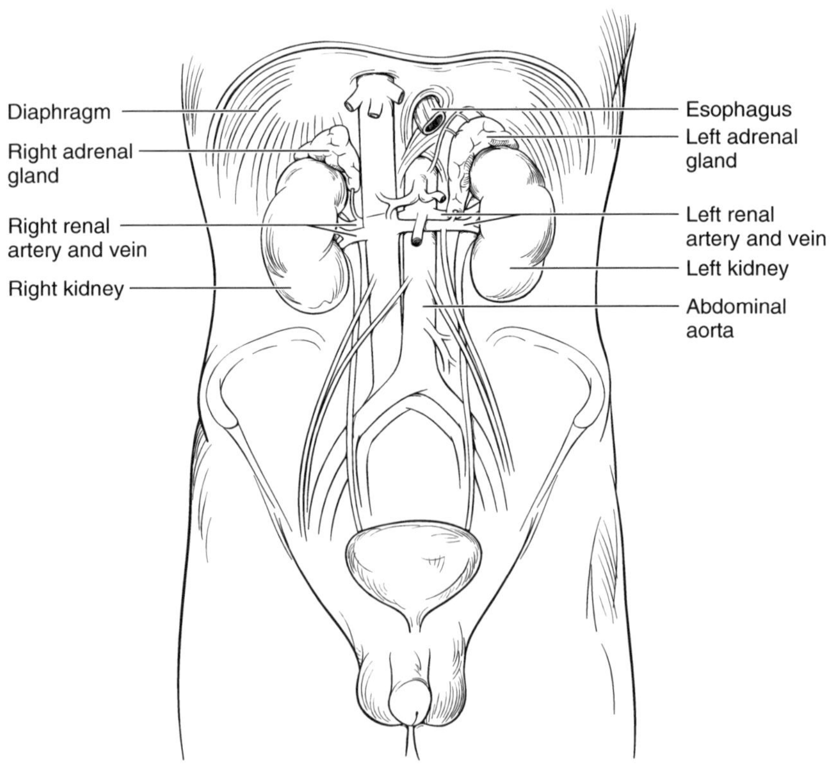

Fig. 24.1 The adrenal glands and surrounding retroperitoneal structures

24.1.1 Arterial Supply

Both the right and left adrenal glands receive their arterial supply (Fig. 24.2) from multiple small branches. Most of the arterial supply is oriented on the medial side of the gland, eventually flowing to the lateral aspect of the gland. The superomedial aspect of the gland is supplied by the superior suprarenal arteries, which originate from the inferior phrenic artery. The middle suprarenal artery and its branches originate directly from the lateral aspect of the aorta. The branches of the inferior suprarenal artery supply the inferior aspect of the adrenal gland and originate from the renal artery. The surgeon should pay specific attention to arterial anomalies involving the blood supply to the kidneys to avoid ligation of any aberrant arteries to the kidney that may compromise renal function. Lumbar arteries should be avoided during dissection or appropriately ligated and divided if necessary. Inadvertent transection can result in retraction of the vessel and significant bleeding as vascular control can be difficult. The left lateral aspect of the aorta is commonly used as a dissection plane for resection of large left-sided adrenal tumors. Some ACCs may partially or completely encase the celiac axis and origin of the superior mesenteric artery. The splenic artery may be directly invaded by tumor on the left side as it directly overlies the left adrenal gland. Careful attention to preoperative imaging is necessary to anticipate these situations.

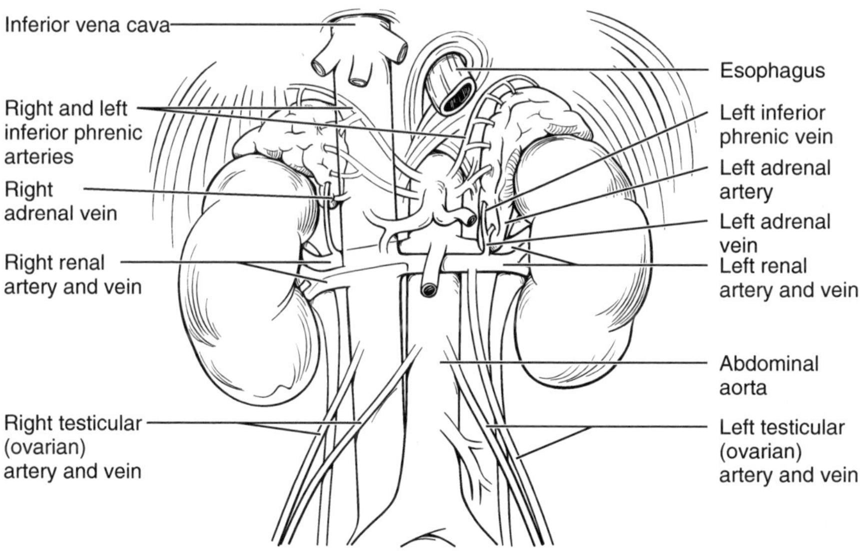

Fig. 24.2 Arterial supply to and venous outflow from the adrenal glands

24.1.2 Venous Drainage

Each adrenal gland is drained by a single *central* adrenal vein (Fig. 24.2). The right adrenal vein is shorter than the left adrenal vein and drains directly into the posterolateral aspect of the inferior vena cava. The short length of the central adrenal vein on the right makes careful dissection imperative to prevent lacerations of the vein or the inferior vena cava, which can result in large-volume blood loss. Aberrant venous drainage to the right hepatic vein is infrequent but dangerous if not appreciated. The proximity of the right adrenal gland and direct drainage of the short right adrenal vein to the inferior vena cava accounts for the increased rate of direct venous invasion and extension of intracaval tumor thrombus observed in right-sided ACC.

The left adrenal vein takes an oblique lateral to medial course draining into the superior aspect of the left renal vein just lateral to the left lateral wall of the aorta. There is often a venous communication from the inferior phrenic vein present on both the right and the left sides requiring ligation and division during dissection. Other small draining veins originating from the adrenal gland itself rarely cause significant bleeding. Lumbar veins may also cause troublesome bleeding and should be carefully ligated and divided when necessary. Failure to recognize the variations in venous or arterial anatomy can complicate operations from any approach. The surgeon should pay specific attention to anomalies in venous drainage from the kidneys to avoid ligation of main draining veins that may compromise renal function. Obstruction of draining veins may cause collateralization and formation of engorged veins in the area of the adrenal gland and adjacent organs, necessitating careful dissection in order to prevent significant bleeding.

24.1.3 Lymphatics

Lymphatic drainage of the adrenal glands follows a fairly orderly route, with lymph traveling to the lateral aortic, pre-aortic (celiac and superior mesenteric), and phrenic nodes bilaterally, ascending through the lumbar trunks ultimately to the cisterna chyli and then to the thoracic duct. Dissection especially along the right side of the aorta and posterior to the cava, but also along the left side of the aorta, should proceed carefully making sure to ligate tissue in order to prevent a chyle leak. The thoracic duct and posterior mediastinal nodes may also be encountered in the thorax during the course of dissection depending on whether or not the thoracic and mediastinal cavities are entered.

24.1.4 Adjacent Structures

Given the locally aggressive nature of ACC, knowledge of the anatomic structures adjacent to the adrenal glands is important for understanding the potential structures that may be involved by ACC and for anticipating potential intraoperative challenges and postoperative complications that may arise related to surgical extirpation. Both adrenal glands are surrounded by retroperitoneal fat, and are intimately associated with the superomedial surface of the kidneys. The anterior surface of the right adrenal gland is separated by the posterior peritoneum from the overlying liver. Aggressive ACCs often invade through the overlying peritoneum and may invade structures within the peritoneal cavity. Additionally, tumor may directly invade the liver in the retroperitoneum at a posteromedial point without intervening peritoneum. The posterior aspect of the right lobe of the liver overlies the right adrenal gland and the diaphragm is situated superior and posteriorly to the adrenal gland (Fig. 24.3). The posterior portion of the gland is situated within a variable amount of retroperitoneal fat. From medial to lateral on both sides of the body, the crura of the diaphragm, psoas major, psoas minor, quadratus lumborum, and transverses abdominus musculature form the posterior border of the retroperitoneum. Tumor frequently lies directly on the musculature, and despite appearing grossly negative at the time of completion of adrenalectomy, microscopic tumor deposits may remain. Inferiorly, the anteromedial surface of the right adrenal gland can be bordered by the duodenum while the medial border lies along and slightly posterior to the inferior vena cava. The lateral border of the right adrenal gland is surrounded by retroperitoneal fat. If the tumor is large enough and extends inferiorly, it may involve the hepatic flexure of the colon or duodenum.

The anterior surface of the left adrenal gland lies posterior to the body and tail of the pancreas and the medial portion of the spleen (Fig. 24.4). The inferior portion of

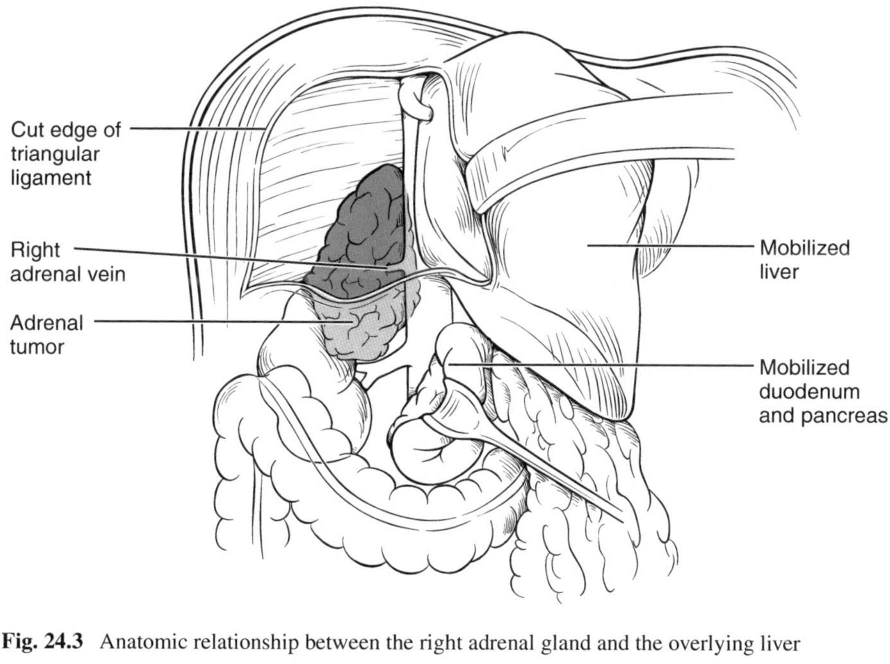

Fig. 24.3 Anatomic relationship between the right adrenal gland and the overlying liver

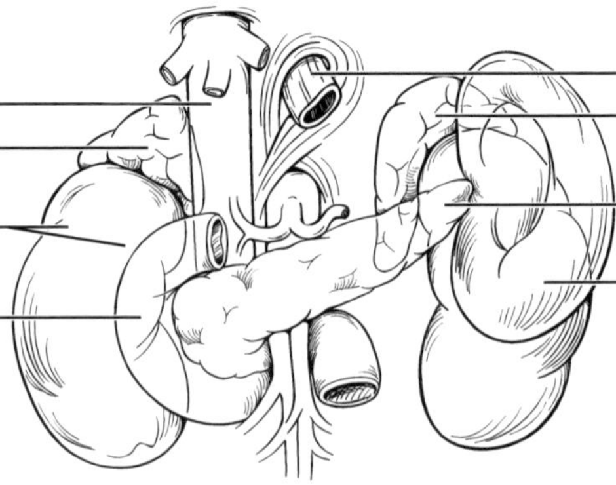

Fig. 24.4 Anatomic relationship between the left adrenal gland and the overlying pancreas and spleen

the left adrenal gland is bordered by the left renal vein; the upper pole of the kidney and Gerota's fascia are contiguous with the inferolateral aspect of the adrenal gland. The proximity of the left renal vessels frequently mandates resection of the left kidney for left adrenal malignancies, as direct involvement of the upper pole can be managed by partial nephrectomy; but renal parenchyma can rarely be spared in the presence of direct invasion or encasement of the left renal pedicle. Anterosuperiorly, the stomach overlies the adrenal gland, and directly superior is the diaphragm, which courses inferiorly and posterior to an enlarged adrenal tumor. The aorta borders the medial aspect of the left adrenal gland. The celiac axis and origin of the superior mesenteric artery are nearby and may be intimately involved with or encased by tumor. Anteroinferior and lateral to the left adrenal gland is the transverse and splenic flexure of the colon. The colon may be invaded by large aggressive ACCs.

24.2 Perioperative Considerations

Perioperative evaluation for patients with ACC is similar to other major abdominal procedures in terms of cardiac, pulmonary, and nutritional evaluation.

24.2.1 Preoperative

Standard preoperative screening for significant cardiac and pulmonary disease should begin with a thorough history and physical followed by appropriate supplemental testing as indicated. Beta-adrenergic blockade should be initiated preoperatively if patients are found to be at risk for perioperative coronary events. Preoperative assessment of renal function is important to judge the effect of possible nephrectomy. The past surgical history, particularly prior abdominal procedures, helps the surgeon anticipate difficulties that may be encountered during surgery related to adhesions or obliteration of the usual anatomic planes. ACC patients are in the highest risk group for venous thromboembolic disease and require prophylaxis with subcutaneous heparin. Patients should receive perioperative antibiotics to decrease the risk of wound infection. Antibiotics should be given and continued for no more than 24 h unless there is spillage of enteric contents or other direct contamination. If splenectomy is anticipated, patients should receive vaccination against encapsulated bacteria (*Neisseria meningococcus, Haemophilus influenzae*, and *Streptococcus pneumoniae*) at least 2 weeks prior to operation.

High-quality preoperative imaging should be obtained to evaluate for tumor invasion of surrounding anatomic structures and can guide the surgeon as to the expected extent of operation. Careful attention should be paid to adjacent organs, the adrenal and renal veins, the inferior vena cava, and the aorta, including the takeoff of the celiac and superior mesenteric arteries (Figs. 24.5 and 24.6). Computed tomography is sufficient in many cases, though magnetic resonance imaging provides better evaluation of intravascular tumor thrombus, vascular invasion, or invasion of tumor into adjacent structures. Imaging should be obtained within several weeks of the anticipated date of surgery as many high-grade and aggressive ACCs grow quickly and involvement of adjacent structures by the tumor may change, thereby altering the operative plan. Intravascular ultrasound or venography may also complement other imaging studies to determine the extent of tumor involvement.

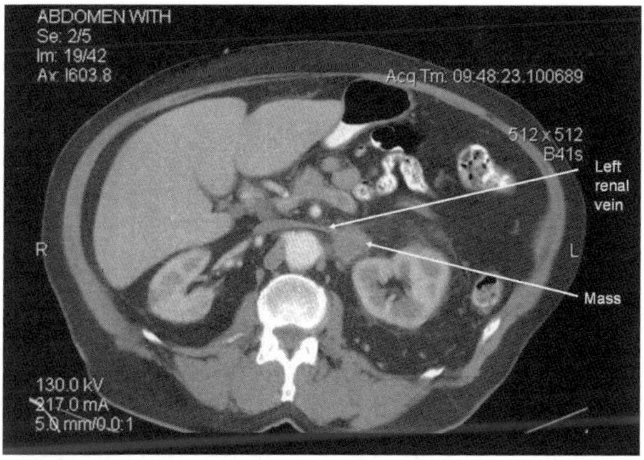

Fig. 24.5 CT scan showing invasion of left renal vein by inferior aspect of left-sided ACC

Specific risks related to hormone excess should be considered for each patient. Cushing's syndrome is the most common hormone syndrome manifested in patients with ACC and increases the risk of suffering from a variety of complications including wound infection, hernia formation, post-operative adrenal insufficiency, and hemorrhage from thin-walled vessels. Glucocorticoid insufficiency should be anticipated in patients who have cortisol excess noted preoperatively, and adequate supplementation initiated after resection of the tumor (see Chapter 4). The recovery time for people who have complete tumor resection, a normal contralateral adrenal gland, a normal pituitary gland, and a normal hypothalamus varies, but is a minimum of 6 months [12].

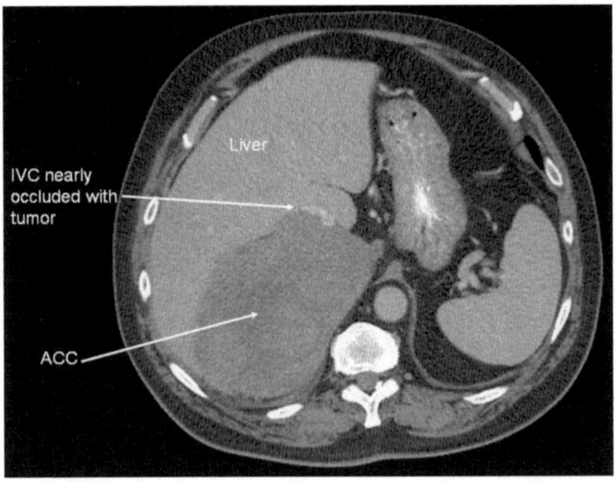

Fig. 24.6 CT scan showing invasion of liver and inferior vena cava

Hyperaldosteronism leading to severe hypokalemia must be corrected prior to anesthetic induction either by use of aldosterone receptor antagonists, other potassium-sparing diuretics, or supplementation with potassium chloride. A potassium level should be checked on the day of surgery in the preoperative area to ensure normokalemia.

24.2.2 Intraoperative

Perioperative intravenous glucocorticoid stress-dose therapy for adults is 80–100 mg every 8 h. Dosing can then be tapered postoperatively over 1–2 weeks. The goal of the taper should be replacement therapy with hydrocortisone 12.5 mg/m^2 or an equivalent dose of other steroid preparation. This dose should support normal nonstressed function. In certain situations it is desirable to understand the presence or amount of residual or even excess corticosteroid production depending on the indication for operation. Hydrocortisone is detected as free cortisol in the urinary free cortisol assay, but supplemental therapy with dexamethasone is not; therefore, temporary use of dexamethasone allows interpretable 24-h urine-free cortisol measurement. In those patients with no endogenous cortisol production, a mineralocorticoid such as fludrocortisone is also usually required.

Consideration should be given to having blood products immediately available during the operation. While the majority of patients with adrenal tumors undergoing resection do not require blood products intraoperatively or postoperatively, those with imaging suggestive of the need for resection of adjacent structures or involvement of major vasculature should certainly have blood products available.

The choice of an appropriate retractor system can be vital to adequate exposure. The Bookwalter, Omni-tract, Thompson, and Rochard retractor systems all have advantages and disadvantages. Surgeons should be familiar with all of the available retractor systems and these should be specifically chosen with regard to the operative approach, planned incision, and requirements for exposing the tumor in the optimal fashion. The authors favor the Omni-tract or Thompson retractor when using a subcostal incision as this allows for excellent retraction of the costal margin.

24.2.3 Postoperative

Any adrenalectomy patient who develops hypotension, hyponatremia, hyperkalemia, hypoglycemia, or acidosis should be treated immediately with intravenous hydrocortisone. Patients must also be counseled regarding the dangers of corticosteroid insufficiency and Addisonian crisis in episodes of acute illness. Those who have undergone splenectomy should also be warned regarding the small chance of overwhelming post-splenectomy sepsis. Encouraging use of a medical identification bracelet or chain can be lifesaving. Primary care and referring physicians should also be counseled regarding issues faced by these patients. Hypotension can also denote severe postoperative bleeding and this should be quickly and carefully evaluated. Because of the proximity of surgery to the diaphragm, an occult pneumothorax should also be ruled out. The possibility of a pulmonary embolus should also be entertained since these patients are at higher risk for venous thromboembolism from a deep venous thrombosis or from tumor embolization. Loss of pulses in a lower extremity may result if the aorta has been clamped or manipulated during the course of the operation and atherosclerotic emboli have migrated to lower extremity vessels. Checking distal pulses by palpation or Doppler at the end of a difficult case is prudent.

24.3 Role of Surgery

24.3.1 Primary Therapy – Curative Intent

The goal of surgery in the management of ACC is the removal of all cancerous tissue. A careful and complete resection (R0) provides the best opportunity for long-term survival and potential cure. In those rare patients with stage I ACC ($\sim$3% of cases) [13, 14] (Table 24.1), adrenalectomy with the widest available margin of surrounding retroperitoneal fat and lymphatics is generally sufficient for removal. In patients with stage II and III ACC, complete removal of the tumor may require concomitant resection of the ipsilateral kidney, liver, spleen, pancreas, stomach, colon, or a portion of the vena cava. Removal of contiguous structures should be included if there is any question of involvement by the tumor, but only if this will allow complete resection of the tumor. Functional organs (such as the kidney) should typically not be included in the resection if the resection is incomplete in other areas. One should not attempt to “create” a plane between the tumor and adjacent tissue or organs, as this will potentially cause tumor fracture and intraperitoneal dissemination, increasing locoregional recurrence. This is a common reason for early recurrence involving the superior aspect of the kidney. Intraoperative imaging with

Table 24.1 ENSAT (European Network for the Study of Adrenal Tumors) Staging system of adrenocortical carcinoma: T1 = tumor ≤5 cm, T2 = tumor >5 cm; T3 = infiltration into surrounding tissue; T4 invasion into adjacent organs or venous tumor thrombus in vena cava or renal vein; N0 = no lymph node involvement; N1 = lymph node involvement; M0 = no distant metastases; M1 = distant metastases present

	ENSAT 2008		
Stage	T	N	M
I	1	0	0
II	2	0	0
III	1–2	1	0
	3–4	0–1	0
IV	1–4	0–1	1

ultrasound can be useful to define the extent of resection necessary prior to violating any tissue planes, particularly on the right side when the vena cava or liver may be involved by tumor. Tumor thrombus is not a contraindication to resection and is indicated when technically feasible. In rare circumstances veno-venous bypass may be useful. If the ability to maintain vascular control intraoperatively is a concern during the preoperative evaluation, placement of intravascular devices to maintain vascular control can be accomplished at the beginning of the case. Multiple retrospective studies [8, 15–18] suggest an association of complete surgical resection with survival advantage from ACC although there is selection bias involved in comparing patients who were able to undergo surgery to those who were not.

The difference in outcomes for surgical patients is highly dependent upon the completeness of operative dissection and the absence of penetration of the tumor capsule. ACC typically has a very thin pseudocapsule that can be easily ruptured during the course of dissection, thus spilling tumor (microscopic or macroscopic) into the surrounding field and elsewhere in the peritoneal cavity. Any capsular disruption should be considered a surgical failure due to increased locoregional recurrence. ACCs frequently invade through the tumor capsule, and every effort should be made to perform en bloc resection.

24.3.2 Recurrences

Unfortunately, even with pathologically documented complete resection of ACC, up to two thirds of patients have recurrence of tumor in a locoregional or distant site, or both. Individual markers of tumor biology such as histologic grade, length of disease-free interval, and slow progression of tumor can be used as a guide when considering re-operation. If a resectable local recurrence presents without evidence of distant metastases, re-operation is associated with an increased mean survival when compared to patients treated with chemotherapy alone [19], although in these types of series there is a greater selection bias than for those patients being considered for initial operation. The development of completely resectable recurrent

ACC usually implies a fundamentally favorable biology and certainly in some a suboptimal initial operation.

24.3.3 Palliation: Hormonal Control and Tumor Debulking

Surgery can be helpful for select patients with metastatic ACC (stage IV). Patients with limited metastatic disease may benefit from resection of all disease with an intent to cure (Fig. 24.7). Even patients whose disease cannot be completely resected may, in select situations, benefit from operation. This is particularly true in those patients suffering from biochemically active ACC and sequelae of excess hormone. If more than 90% of the tumor mass can be removed in patients with a slow tempo of disease during observation or systemic therapy, then operation should be considered although no definitive study exists to indicate what percentage of tumor must be removed for adequate results [20]. Once again, indirect markers of tumor biology should be used to guide the decision for operation in stage IV patients. Short-interval recurrences or patients with rapidly progressive disease may not have time to benefit from surgical intervention. In some institutions, mitotane and other chemotherapeutic regimens are given to patients with metastatic disease who are potential candidates for resection. If the areas of disease decrease in size or remain stable over a period of 3–6 months while on chemotherapy, then further surgery is considered. If there is evidence of disease progression while on chemotherapy, surgery is not pursued. Tumor grade is likely important in this subset of patients and studies are currently investigating this topic. Careful judgment must be used in this specific subset of patients. The preceding chapter discusses other therapies for excess hormone production by ACC in addition to potential surgical debulking of tumor mass.

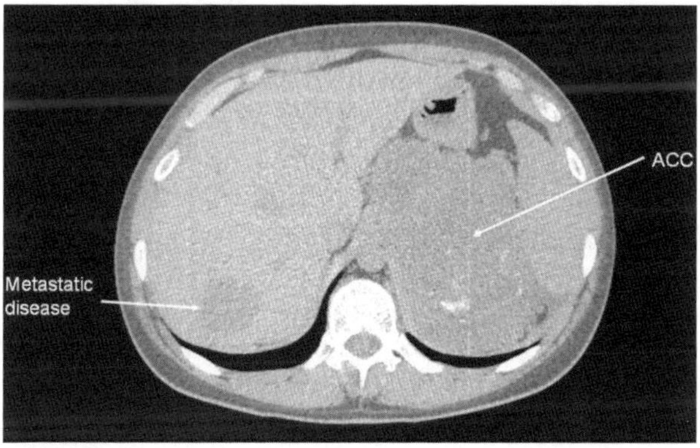

Fig. 24.7 A 23-year-old with stage IV cortisol-secreting ACC and severe Cushing's syndrome. Metastases were noted in the liver and a small amount of disease in the chest. A left adrenalectomy, distal pancreatectomy, splenectomy, and segment 7 liver resection were performed to help palliate symptoms of cortisol excess

24.4 Surgical Approaches to the Adrenal Glands

The choice of operative approach depends upon anatomic considerations with regard to the extent of tumor. While most clinicians advocate a laparoscopic approach for benign appearing adrenal lesions, suspicion or certainty of malignancy mandates an open resection. An open anterior transabdominal procedure allows for access to surrounding structures, thorough evaluation of the peritoneal cavity and, if needed, access to the thoracic cavity or mediastinum. The open posterior approach, although useful in some selected situations, does not allow access to the peritoneal cavity and should not be used in those patients with known or suspected ACC.

24.4.1 Anterior Transabdominal – Open

This classic approach to the adrenal glands allows the surgeon a complete view of the gland, its relationships to surrounding structures, and the overall condition of the abdominal cavity. The surgeon can choose either a subcostal or vertical midline incision. Both allow adequate exposure to the peritoneal cavity, although access to the lower abdomen and pelvis may be limited with subcostal approaches. Either incision allows superior extension and possible sternotomy to deal with unexpected diaphragmatic or retrohepatic venous involvement or bleeding from the vena cava or aorta.

Exposure of the right adrenal gland requires varying degrees of organ mobilization involving the liver (triangular, coronary, and falciform ligaments), hepatic flexure of the colon, duodenum, and retrohepatic vena cava dependent on tumor size and extension. Right medial visceral rotation of these structures (Cattell-Brasch maneuver) and dissection into the retroperitoneum provides exposure of the right adrenal gland and access to the relevant vasculature. The extent and precise technique of rotation depends on the size of the tumor and the ability to visualize critical structures. Involvement of the right lobe of the liver may require division of affected liver parenchyma in order to resect the involved area en bloc.

Exposure of the left adrenal gland can be accomplished by two main approaches. Small tumors of the left adrenal may be approached through the lesser sac in conjunction with retraction of the pancreas superiorly and the transverse colon and its mesentery inferiorly; however, this is rarely adequate exposure for a malignancy. A left medial visceral rotation (Mattox maneuver) of the spleen, pancreatic tail, and the splenic flexure of the colon affords excellent exposure of the retroperitoneum, renal vessels, aorta and diaphragm if the spleen and pancreas are not involved by tumor. Alternatively, if involved by tumor, the pancreas and splenic vessels can be divided anterior to the aorta, medial to the tumor, allowing for resection of the tumor, distal pancreas and spleen after division of the short gastric vessels to separate the stomach from the specimen.

24.4.2 Thoracoabdominal

A right thoracoabdominal incision (Fig. 24.8) provides extended direct exposure of the superior aspect of the right retrohepatic space. Although even very large right adrenal tumors can generally be removed using a subcostal incision with a midline extension and wide mobilization of the liver, there are some tumors with involvement of the upper abdominal vena cava, particularly in re-operative cases that are best performed using a thoracoabdominal approach. The patient is placed

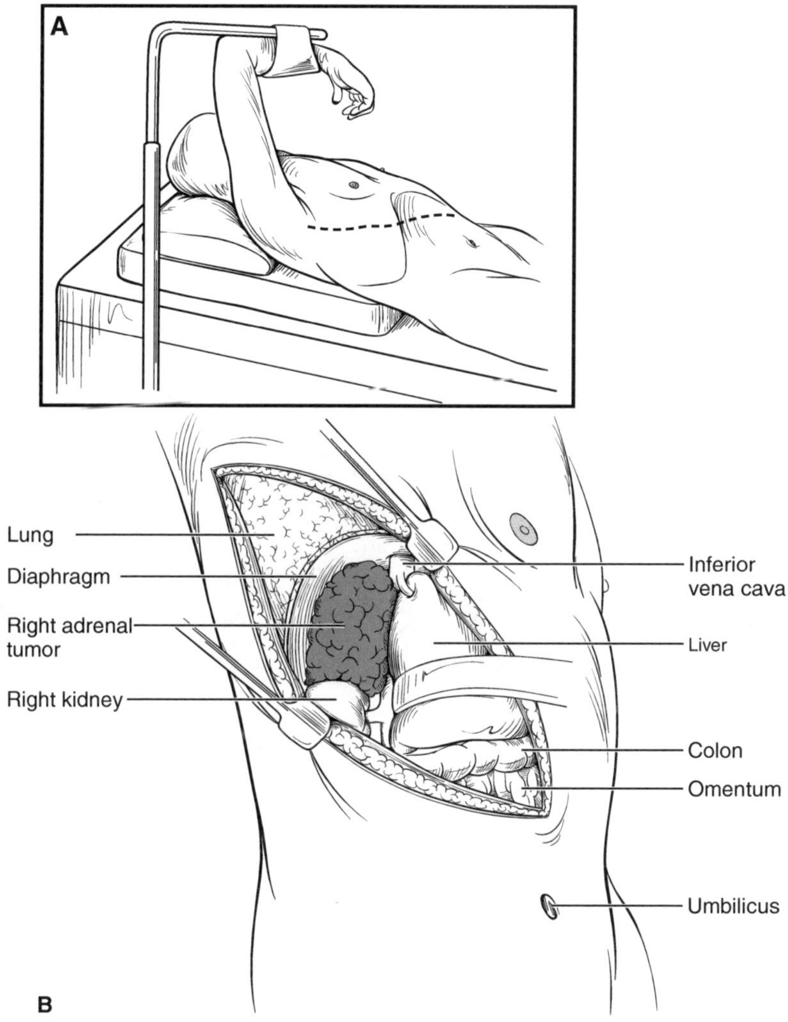

Fig. 24.8 Right thoracoabdominal incision and exposure of adrenal gland

in an intermediate position between supine and lateral decubitus orientation, with the operating room table extended slightly and the kidney rest elevated. The incision follows the ninth or tenth intercostal space and is extended down onto the anterior-lateral abdominal wall. The diaphragm is divided peripherally along its circumference approximately 2 cm from the lateral edge to minimize denervation of the muscle. Stay sutures can be placed on both sides of the cut edge to facilitate re-approximation at the end of the case. Vascular control of the mediastinal inferior vena cava is possible through the pericardium in the chest facilitating safe and complete resection of the tumor and surrounding structures. While providing excellent exposure for complex cases, complications are increased by entering two major body cavities in this approach. Denervation of abdominal musculature commonly occurs with damage to the motor nerves running across this incision. Pulmonary support and adequate analgesia are imperative to minimize risks during recovery.

24.4.3 Approaches to Difficult Resections

Extirpation of large ACCs can be extremely challenging for even the most experienced surgeon (Fig. 24.9a, b). Adequate visualization of the upper peritoneal cavity can be difficult to achieve, especially with fixed and extensively infiltrating masses.

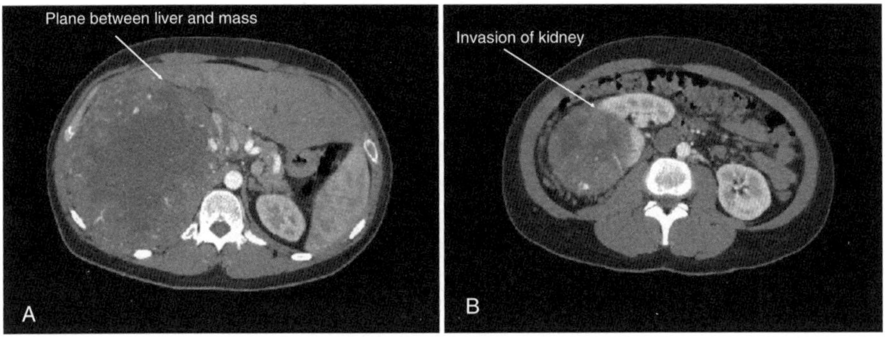

Fig. 24.9 (**a**) CT showing large right ACC invading the liver and compressing abdominal contents to the left side of the abdomen. (**b**) Tumor extends inferiorly to invade the right kidney. Patient underwent right adrenalectomy, nephrectomy, and partial hepatectomy

Liver. Partial hepatectomy may be required in some patients to achieve en bloc resection. In carefully selected patients with liver metastases, liver resection may also be helpful. Liver resection for those with infiltrating tumor is usually along non-anatomic planes, but in some cases right hepatic lobectomy or other anatomically guided resections may be performed. Anatomic resections can be performed in standard fashion. For those cases involving non-anatomic resections, in many cases development of a subcapsular plane of dissection can achieve negative margins. The area of adhesion may be dense inflammatory reaction rather than tumor that involves the liver capsule, but one should not assume this and should attempt to achieve an appropriate margin along this border. Many new alternative energy devices have been introduced (Ligasure, Harmonic, CUSA, Argon Beam Coagulator) to provide hemostasis and control of small bile ducts. Staplers, clips, hemostatic agents, and other more conventional approaches are certainly still appropriate.

Mobilization of the liver for patients with large ACCs on the right is crucial. Techniques used for liver transplantation can be extremely beneficial to the adrenal surgeon [21] (Fig. 24.10). If needed, the liver can be completely mobilized from the inferior vena cava, leaving the liver attached to the vena cava by only the hepatic veins, allowing the surgeon access to the full length of the retrohepatic inferior vena cava. Liver mobilization is begun in standard fashion by releasing the falciform, coronary, and triangular ligamentous attachments. The porta hepatis is encircled with a Rommel tourniquet so that a Pringle maneuver may be applied if needed. Vascular control of the IVC should be obtained superiorly (at the level of the diaphragm) and inferiorly (just above the renal veins). Vessels passing from the bare area of the liver to the diaphragm are ligated and divided as needed. The visceral peritoneum is incised to the right of the retrohepatic IVC. Small veins from the IVC to the caudate lobe of the liver can also be ligated and divided as needed, thereby leaving the liver attached only to the IVC by the three main hepatic veins. This affords superb visualization and allows full access to the IVC should partial resection and reconstruction be necessary or to facilitate removal of intravascular tumor thrombus.

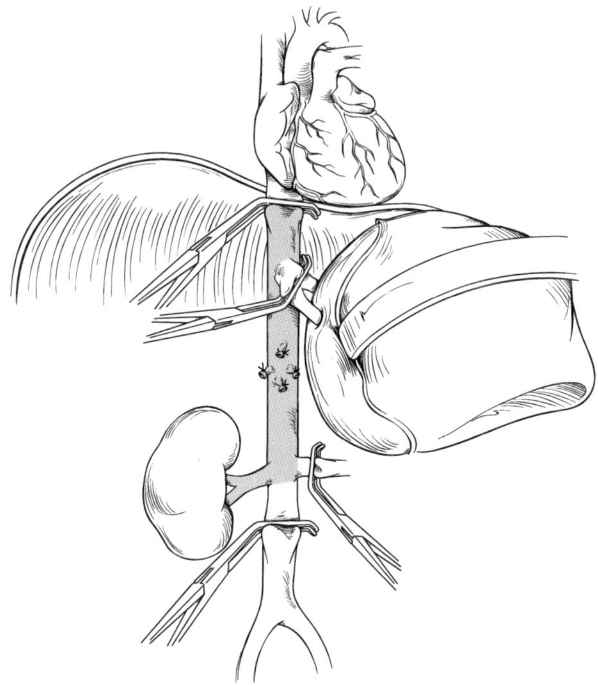

Fig. 24.10 (Fischer 7) Schematic showing full mobilization of the liver off of the upper abdominal vena cava with proximal and distal control of main venous tributaries to facilitate partial resection of IVC or extraction of intracaval tumor thrombus

24.4.3.1 Vascular Control and Resection

Vena Cava. A classification of tumor thrombus extending from ACCs into the vena cava has been described [22] (Fig. 24.11). With proximal and distal vascular control of the vena cava and application of a Pringle maneuver, a venotomy may be carried out in order to extract tumor thrombus. Vascular control of the vena cava can also be achieved in the chest using a median sternotomy or by a thoracoabdominal approach. Veno-venous bypass can also be useful but is rarely required. For thrombus extending into the right atrium, cardiopulmonary bypass can facilitate complete

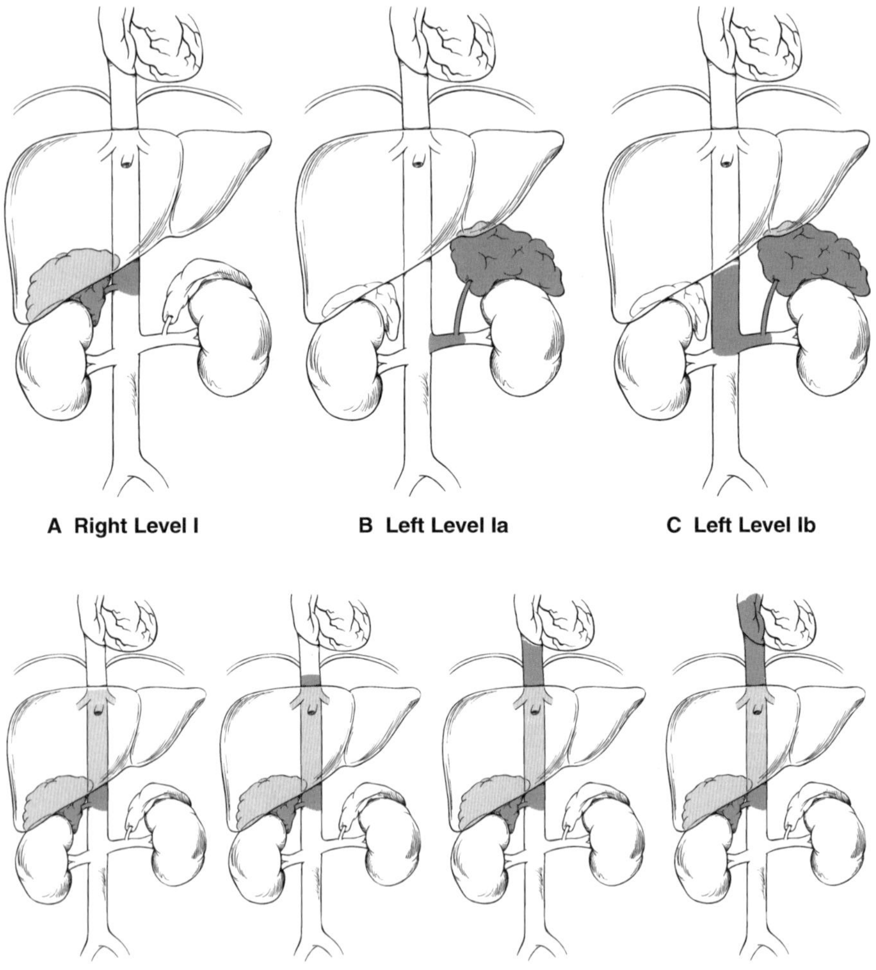

Fig. 24.11 (Fischer 8) Schematic for categorizing tumor thrombus within the renal veins and inferior vena cava

resection. Transesophagal echocardiography should be employed to help identify the level of thrombus extension if it extends into the thorax. In some cases, thrombus involving the thoracic portion of the inferior vena cava (IVC) can be gently fed back into the abdominal portion of the IVC inferior to the hepatic veins and a clamp placed superior to the thrombus. With proximal and distal vascular control of the vena cava, the Pringle maneuver can then be released to allow perfusion of the liver while removing the thrombus in a more standard fashion.

In most cases, venotomy and simple closure suffices for removal of tumor; however, in certain cases, resection of a portion of the vena cava may be required. If the diameter of the vena cava is not decreased by more than 50%, resection using a side-biting clamp and primary closure is adequate. For cases requiring larger segments of caval resection, autologous vein using saphenous, internal jugular, or superficial femoral vein can be used. Other types of prosthetic graft material may be used, but autologous tissue is preferred especially if bowel is also resected or entered during the operation.

Should bleeding from the vena cava be encountered, it can be voluminous but is low pressure and can be controlled proximally and distally using sponge sticks. Two fingers placed on either side of the cava occlude lumbar branches while the surgeon or assistant repairs any defects [23]. In dire situations, shunts placed within the cava may control bleeding and consist of atrio-caval [24] or Schrock shunts [25] using a modified endotracheal tube. More recently, devices have been introduced with catheter and balloon systems deployed from the femoral vein and positioned more superiorly to obtain proximal and distal control. Large Fogarty catheters or even small foley catheters with balloons may be inserted into the defect, inflated with saline and retracted to help control bleeding [23].

Aorta and arterial supply. Need for resection of portions of arteries or their branches is a general contraindication to surgery for ACC; however, the same general vascular principles apply in terms of obtaining proximal and distal control. Superb exposure of the aorta is attained with use of a Mattox maneuver (left medical visceral rotation). Extension into the chest and mediastinum can be accomplished by median sternotomy or left thoracoabdominal incision. It is not uncommon for the celiac axis and takeoff of the superior mesenteric artery to be partially encased with tumor. Because of the muscular walls of the aorta, injury is infrequent. If tumor involves a short segment of the celiac axis, it is possible to remove this short segment prior to its branching into end arteries. The gastroduodenal artery can supply the liver in a retrograde fashion via supply from the superior mesenteric artery; however, adequacy of this alternate pathway of hepatic perfusion should be tested first by palpating for a pulse or evaluating the proper hepatic artery with Doppler ultrasound after occluding the celiac axis. Watching for a change in the color of the liver is also important. The surgeon should be aware that large tumors on the left side tend to distract the celiac axis and superior mesenteric artery takeoff to the left side of the aorta, and one should be careful when dissecting in this area so as not inadvertently ligate and divide one of these structures.

Diaphragm. En bloc resection of tumor with an accompanying portion of the diaphragm may be required in order to achieve negative margins. Smaller diaphragmatic defects may be closed primarily using monofilament suture in a running locking or interrupted mattress fashion. A small suction catheter can be placed in the pleural cavity through the defect and removed at the time of forced ventilation as closure is completed and the knot is tied down, obviating a need for an intercostal chest tube. For larger defects, a number of prosthetic materials may be used for closure, including PTFE and prolene mesh.

24.4.4 Laparoscopic Surgery for Primary Adrenal Malignancy

Controversy surrounds the appropriateness of laparoscopic resection for patients with ACC. At this time, laparoscopic adrenalectomy (LA) is contraindicated in those patients in whom ACC is either diagnosed or suspected pre-operatively. Laparoscopic adrenalectomy has become the gold standard for resection of benign adrenal masses, and it has been shown to result in significantly lower morbidity, pain, shorter hospital stays and decreased overall time to recovery when compared to open resection. On occasion ACCs have been unknowingly resected using a laparoscopic approach. More recently, some surgeons have begun to advocate deliberate laparoscopic resection for ACCs despite a paucity of data on this topic. Most accounts of laparoscopically resected ACCs are part of series that cover LA mainly for benign disease, include only a few heterogeneous cases such as malignant pheochromocytomas or malignancies metastatic to the adrenal gland, and suffer from a lack of long-term oncologic follow-up. Because effective adjuncts to surgery for the treatment of ACC are extremely limited and uniformly unsuccessful, ensuring a complete, margin-negative tumor resection at the initial operation is critical. The rationale for avoiding LA are the inability to routinely achieve negative margins and the difficulty in retracting large tumors with laparoscopic instruments which may abrade the tumor, penetrate the tumor (grossly or microscopically), or tear the capsule of the tumor, leading to early local recurrence, peritoneal carcinomatosis and the potential for distant metastatic spread.

While some centers perform open adrenalectomy for all suspected or known ACCs [26], others perform laparoscopy initially to assess for evidence of intraperitoneal metastasis or invasion of the adrenal gland into other organs. Intraoperative laparoscopic ultrasound is helpful to evaluate for evidence of invasion. Some surgeons recommend removal of noninvasive ACCs laparoscopically, while the majority of surgeons prefer to convert to an open procedure if there is any indication that the tumor is malignant. The difficulty is knowing when to convert and doing this prior to penetrating the capsule of the adrenal gland or spreading tumor throughout the abdomen while applying traction/countertraction to the gland surface during the initial stages of the operation.

While tumors metastatic to the adrenal gland do not tend to invade beyond the capsule of the adrenal gland, ACCs do invade through the capsule. Since tumor is usually at the surface of the gland in ACC, application of laparoscopic instruments to the tumor can result in shedding of malignant cells that is undetectable to the operating surgeon. Tactile sensation is limited with laparoscopy compared to an open approach and is nonexistent with robotically performed procedures [27]. Some groups have used colorectal cancer data to support their practice of resection of ACCs by a laparoscopic approach. The authors believe this thought process is flawed, as the tumor biology and physical characteristics of ACC are substantially different and usually much more aggressive than colorectal cancer. The initially high rates of locoregional recurrence (laparoscopic and port site) of colorectal cancers operations performed laparoscopically decreased as techniques changed; however, it is not clear whether this benefit will ultimately be realized in similarly treated patients with ACC.

In a study [26] in which the patient population was referred after initial operation for evaluation and management of newly diagnosed ACC or recurrent ACC, overall recurrence rates were reported to be 86% in the open resection group (154 patients) and 100% in the LA group (6 patients). In the open approach group, 35% had local recurrence and 8% peritoneal recurrence. In the LA group, 50% had local recurrence as a component of initial failure and 83% ($p = 0.0001$) had peritoneal carcinomatosis. There were no port site recurrences. A subset of patients with relatively small ACCs which would have been technically amenable to LA (6 cm or less) but who underwent open resections did relatively well. Four of six were without disease at 21 months in contrast to the uniformly poor outcome of the LA group. The patients with isolated local recurrence after open resection who underwent reoperation experienced a relatively long overall survival duration (median 70 months), suggesting that local recurrence may be related more to inadequate primary operation than to particularly aggressive tumor biology.

Henry et al. [28] reported their experience with laparoscopic adrenalectomy for potentially malignant tumors. Six of the 19 tumors were proven to be ACC on final pathology (31.6%). Two of these patients underwent conversion to an open procedure based on intraoperative signs of invasion. Overall results are acceptable given five out of six of the ACC patients were without signs of disease with a follow-up of 8–83 months. One patient died 6 months after surgery of metastatic disease. However, closer scrutiny of these results reveals they are skewed by the fact that the study includes six patients with malignant pheochromocytomas.

A recent report by Miller et al. [29] retrospectively reviewed ACC patients referred to or treated at a tertiary medical center. Eighty-eight patients were included in the study, of which 17 underwent laparoscopic adrenalectomy (all performed at outside institutions prior to referral). Both the open and laparoscopic groups had high rates of recurrence (local and distant) at 59 and 58.8% respectively; however, the laparoscopic group had a significantly shorter interval to recurrence than the open group (9.2 months compared to 19.2 months). This was despite a significantly higher percentage of smaller tumors (stage I and II) in the laparoscopic group (7.0 cm vs. 12.3 cm). Finally, despite the significantly smaller size of tumors in the laparoscopic group, 29% in the laparoscopic group were identified as having either intraoperative tumor rupture/spill or positive pathologic margins as compared to 13% of patients in the open surgical resection group. These data strongly suggest that although laparoscopic resection may be technically feasible (even for large tumors [30, 31]), the use of laparoscopic adrenalectomy in ACC leads to a shorter disease-free interval and a higher incidence of incomplete and suboptimal resections.

Some surgeons argue that in "expert" hands, laparoscopic resection is appropriate. Without a consensus definition of adequate expertise – either in technical or experiential terms – this is not adequate justification. Guerrieri et al. [32] stated that the learning curve just to learn how to perform the laparoscopic adrenalectomy procedure itself requires 30–40 cases. Importantly, ACC is an extremely rare and aggressive disease demanding optimal surgical therapy, the number of patients able to undergo resection fewer, and the technique of resection more complex than a standard LA for a benign adrenal neoplasm. The overall number of patients studied undergoing laparoscopic adrenalectomy for ACC is still small and with limited evidence to support laparoscopic resection, this risk is difficult to justify at this time.

24.5 Surgical Complications

Complications, while generally infrequent, occur regardless of the operative approach utilized, and include some risks specific to adrenalectomy as well as risks associated with surgical procedures in general. Among those associated with surgery in general are wound infection, intra-abdominal abscess, bleeding, damage to surrounding structures, incisional hernia, cardiovascular and thromboembolic complications, anesthetic reactions, and tumor recurrence. Specific to complex adrenal resections, complications may include but are not limited to pneumothorax, pancreatitis or pancreatic leak, renal insufficiency or failure, and chyle leak. Some potential complications can be predicted and avoided. Surgical site infection is a significant risk in patients with hypercortisolism. The risk of infection is minimized by careful tissue dissection, minimizing blood loss and limiting dead space in the wound or organ space. Prophylactic antibiotics appropriate to the planned procedure are always indicated, and should include skin flora and enteric organism prophylaxis if there is a likelihood of opening the gastrointestinal tract. Bleeding is usually avoided with meticulous surgical technique, although significant hemorrhage may occur. This is a particular risk when the tumor has invaded major vascular structures such as the renal pedicle or vena cava or when liver resection is indicated for tumor removal.

Hernia formation is a potential complication from any abdominal incision and is even more likely to occur in the setting of hypercortisolism and infection. In those approaches that involve exposure and resection of a rib (e.g., thoracoabdominal approach), hernia formation must be differentiated from abdominal wall laxity due to muscle denervation.

Cardiac, pulmonary, and thromboembolic complications are infrequent but do occur and should be evaluated and treated promptly. Appropriate prophylaxis can minimize those risks although cancer is a known risk factor for thrombosis. The direct risks of anesthetic techniques are minimal.

Prevention of injury to structures surrounding the adrenal glands requires careful preoperative planning and application of appropriate operative technique. The surgical anatomy reviewed earlier gives an overview of the at-risk structures located near the adrenal glands. Although unusual, injuries to the pancreas, spleen, liver, diaphragm, kidneys, or vasculature can occur during adrenalectomy. Pancreatic leaks can occur after resection of or inadvertent injury to the tail of the pancreas during left adrenalectomy. Significant injury to the spleen may necessitate splenectomy. After unplanned splenectomy, patients should be vaccinated against encapsulated bacteria. Specific literature regarding overwhelming post-splenectomy sepsis should be provided to the patient and primary care or referring physician. Some practitioners provide a prescription for antibiotics for use in emergencies if patients become ill are unable to seek immediate medical attention. Rarely, inadvertent injury to the renal arteries or their branches may manifest as ongoing hypertension in the post-operative patient. Liver resection for tumor removal raises the possibility of biliary leak, hepatic insufficiency, or frank liver failure depending on the extent of resection. With violation of the thoracic cavity and diaphragmatic resection there is the possibility of emphysema, pneumonia, persistent air leak/pneumothorax, biliary-pleural fistula, or tumor seeding that may complicate the resection.

24.6 Conclusion

Surgery remains the mainstay of treatment for ACC. Given the impact on disease-free survival as well as overall survival, radical R0 resection including all surrounding structures involved should be the ultimate goal for all patients presenting with ACC. This impact on survival persists with re-resection of those tumors whose location of recurrence and tumor biology make them favorable for re-operative intervention. For those patients in whom there is no chance of curative resection, debulking (>90%) of tumor mass either for severe local symptoms or hormone excess may prove beneficial. Although the size of the tumor is not in and of itself a contraindication to surgical extirpation, the rate of ACC in tumors ≥6 cm even after careful pre-operative screening (25% or greater) is high enough to warrant open resection. The increased rate of incomplete resections and shorter intervals before recurrence with laparoscopy, in conjunction with the impact of R0 resection on survival, justify the use of an open approach for ACC. At this time, the use of laparoscopy is contraindicated for suspected or known ACCs.

References

1. Thornton JK (1890) Abdominal nephrectomy for large sarcoma of the left suprarenal capsule: recovery. Trans Clin Soc Lond 23:150–153
2. Mayo CH (1927) Paroxysmal hypertension with tumour of retroperitoneal nerve. JAMA 89:1047–1050

3. von Langenbuch C (1882) Ein Fall von Exstirpation der Gallenblase. Berlin Klin Wochenschr 19:725–727
4. Wellbourn RB (1990) The history of endocrine surgery. Praeger, London, p 151 [Quoted]
5. Young HH (1936) Technique for simultaneous exposure and operation on the adrenals. Surg Gynaecol Obstet 63:179–188
6. Gagner M et al (1992) Laparoscopic adrenalectomy in Cushing's syndrome and pheochromocytoma [letter]. N Engl J Med 327:1033
7. Gagner M et al (1993) Early experience with laparoscopic approach for adrenalectomy. Surgery 114:1120–1125
8. Bilimoria KY et al (2008) Adrenocortical carcinoma in the United States: treatment utilization and prognostic factors. Cancer 1/113(11):3130–3136
9. National Cancer Institute Cancer Center Programs. http://cancercenters.cancer.gov
10. Kendrick ML et al (2001) Adrenocortical carcinoma – surgical progress or status quo? Arch Surg 136:543–549
11. Vassiolopoulou-Sellin R, Schultz PN (2001) Adrenocortical carcinoma – clinical outcome at the end of the 20th century. Cancer 92(5):1113–1121
12. Doherty GM et al (1990 Dec) Time to recovery of the hypothalamic-pituitary-adrenal axis after curative resection of adrenal tumors in patients with Cushing's syndrome. Surgery 108(6):1085–1090
13. Fassnacht M et al (2009) Limited prognostic value of the 2004 international union against cancer staging classification for adrenocortical carcinoma – proposal for a revised TNM classification. Cancer 115(2):243–250
14. Paton BL et al (2006 Dec) Outcomes of adrenal cortical carcinoma in the United States. Surgery 140(6):914–920 [discussion 919–920]
15. Kendrick ML et al (2001 May) Adrenocortical carcinoma: surgical progress or status quo? Arch Surg 136(5):543–549
16. Dackiw AP et al (2001 Jul) Adrenal cortical carcinoma. World J Surg 25(7):914–926
17. Icard P et al (2001) Adrenocortical carcinomas: surgical trends and results of a 253-patient series from the French association of endocrine surgeons study group. World J Surg 25: 891–897
18. Schulick RD, Brennan MF (1999) Long-term survival after complete resection and repeat resection in patients with adrenocortical carcinoma. Ann Surg Oncol 6(8):719–726
19. Bellantone R et al (1997 Dec) Role of reoperation in recurrence of adrenal cortical carcinoma: results from 188 cases collected in the Italian National Registry for Adrenal Cortical Carcinoma. Surgery 122(6):1212–1218
20. Schteingart DE et al (2005) Management of patients with adrenal cancer: recommendations of an international consensus conference. Endoc Relat Cancer 12:667–680
21. Cianco G et al (2000) The use of liver transplant techniques to aid in the surgical management of urological tumors. J Urol 164:665–672
22. Ekici S, Ciancio G (2004) Surgical management of large adrenal masses with or without thrombus extending into the inferior vena cava. J Urol 172:2340–2343
23. Perry MO (2002) Injuries to the vena cava figure 25–4 and 25–8 pages 319 and 321. In: Thal ER et al (eds) Operative trauma management: an atlas, 2nd edn. McGraw Hill, Columbus, OH
24. Pachter HL (2002) Perihepatic venous injuries figure 20–5a, 5b, 5c page 253. In: Thal ER et al (eds) Operative trauma management: an atlas, 2nd edn. McGraw Hill, Columbus, OH
25. Schrock T et al (1968 May) Management of blunt trauma to the liver and hepatic veins. Arch Surg 96(5):698–704
26. Gonzalez RJ et al (2005) Laparoscopic resection of adrenal cortical carcinoma: a cautionary note. Surgery138:1078–1086
27. Zafar SS, Abaza R (2008) Robot-assisted laparoscopic adrenalectomy for adrenocortical carcinoma: initial report and review of the literature. J Endourol 22(5):985–989
28. Henry JF et al (2002) Results of laparoscopic adrenalectomy for large and potentially malignant tumors. World J Surg 26:1043–1047

29. Miller BS et al (2010) Laparoscopic resection is inappropriate in patients with known or suspected adrenocortical carcinoma. World J Surg 34(6):1380–1385
30. Castillo OA et al (2008) Laparoscopic adrenalectomy for adrenal masses: does size matter? Urology 71:1138–1141
31. Palazzo FF et al (2006) Long-term outcome following laparoscopic adrenalectomy for large solid adrenal cortex tumors. World J Surg 30:893–898
32. Guerrieri M et al (2008) The learning curve in laparoscopic adrenalectomy. J Endocrinol Invest 31:531–536

Chapter 25
Radiation Therapy for Adrenocortical Carcinoma

Aaron Sabolch and Edgar Ben-Josef

Radiotherapy has been historically considered ineffective in the management of ACC, despite the fact that the modality provides good palliation in unresectable tumors. Further, new research has shown that radiotherapy may also be effective in an adjuvant setting, though it remains underutilized in this regard.

This chapter examines the pattern of failure after surgical management of ACC, which provides the rationale for adjuvant radiotherapy. Data are presented that surgical resection is often incomplete, results in high rates of local (and distant) recurrence, and carries a poor prognosis even when combined with chemotherapy. Emerging evidence is reviewed, suggesting that radiotherapy is synergistic with mitotane therapy, effective in producing tumor regression, and successful in lowering rates of local recurrence. The chapter closes with several clinical cases, demonstrating the application of radiotherapy in various clinical settings.

Radiotherapy, until recently, has been considered an ineffective treatment for ACC. This notion started to change with the publication of Percarpio et al., documenting a good palliative response in 12 out of 12 evaluable patients, and occasional long-term control of unresectable tumors [1]. The authors suggested that doses of 30–40 Gy in 2–3 weeks are required for adequate palliation. Following this publication, a number of other groups have reported their limited experience, suggesting that palliative responses can be attained in 22–100% of patients [2–10]. Given the rarity of ACC, the paucity of data is understandable. However, the existing literature lacks in quality and cannot support a conclusion that radiotherapy is ineffective.

To design a rational strategy for adjuvant therapy, one needs to understand the pattern of failure after surgical management of ACC. Outcome data are presented that surgical resection is often incomplete, results in high rates of local (and distant) recurrence, and carries a poor prognosis even when combined with chemotherapy. Additional evidence will be outlined that points to the efficacy of radiotherapy in improving outcomes, presumably through improvement in local control.

E. Ben-Josef (✉)
Department of Radiation Oncology, University of Michigan Health System, University of Michigan, 1500 East Medical Center Drive, Room UHB2C490, Ann Arbor, MI 48109-0010, USA
e-mail: edgarb@med.umich.edu

G.D. Hammer, T. Else (eds.), *Adrenocortical Carcinoma*,
DOI 10.1007/978-0-387-77236-3_25,

25.1 Current Surgical and Adjuvant Management

ACC is a rare disease, with an annual incidence of 0.72 per million in the United States based on an analysis of the National Cancer Institute's Surveillance, Epidemiology, and End Results (SEER) database [11]. Individual studies have not included large numbers of patients, so it is particularly useful to examine such series in aggregate.

The majority of studies classify patients at their initial presentation according to a staging system that was first proposed by Macfarlane and later modified by Sullivan et al. [12–13]. Stage I is defined as a tumor less than or equal to 5 cm and stage II as a tumor greater than 5 cm. Stage III includes locally infiltrative tumors without positive lymph nodes and non-infiltrative tumors with positive lymph nodes. Stage IV includes metastatic disease, in addition to locally infiltrative tumors with positive lymph nodes, and any tumor that invades adjacent organs, regardless of nodal status. This staging system has been variously modified [14–15], and the most recently proposed revision would categorize all locally invasive tumors or those with positive lymph nodes as stage III, while stage IV would be reserved for metastatic disease [16]. Although such a reclassification would result in staging system with more prognostic significance [16], the Macfarlane-Sullivan system will be employed in this chapter, as it has been utilized by the majority of papers reviewed.

Only one half of patients are diagnosed with localized stage I or II disease (Table 25.1). Unfortunately, the advanced stage at which the other half of patients presents is much less amenable to surgical resection. Aggregate data from seven large series show that the majority of patients (54%) are diagnosed with stage III or IV disease [11, 15, 17–21]. Only 5% of patients are diagnosed with ACC in its most localized stage [11, 15, 17–21]. Furthermore, the ability to detect ACC in its earliest stages may not be improving with time. In a study that included data on 545 staged patients, Kebebew et al. showed that the initial presentation of ACC has not significantly changed between 1973 and 2000 despite advances in imaging and diagnostic techniques [11]. Similarly, a study by Bilimoria et al. on 3982 patients

Table 25.1 Cancer stage at diagnosis

	Stage I Number of patients (% of staged patients)	Stage II	Stage III	Stage IV
Bellantone [18][a]	24 (13%)	68 (36%)	65 (35%)	30 (16%)
Schulick [21][a]	5 (4%)	52 (46%)	12 (11%)	44 (39%)
Icard [15][a]	16 (6)	126 (50%)	57 (23%)	54 (21%)
Abiven [17]	12 (6%)	103 (51%)	38 (19%)	49 (24%)
Kebebew [11]	16 (3%)	157 (29%)	120 (22%)	252 (46%)
Paton [20]	20 (4%)	218 (40%)	122 (22%)	189 (34%)
Gonzalez [19][a]	9 (5%)	103 (59%)	38 (22%)	24 (14%)
Total	102 (5%)	827 (41%)	452 (22%)	642 (32%)

[a]Studies that have focused on exclusively surgical patient populations may over represent operable, localized disease stages

from the National Cancer Data Base (NCDB) found that there was no change in initial tumor size or the presence of metastases in patients diagnosed between 1985 and 2005 [22]. These studies contrast with a smaller series of 202 staged patients by Abiven et al., which indicated that since 1989 a higher proportion of patients are being diagnosed at less advanced, more localized stages of disease [17].

That most patients present with advanced disease is especially problematic because stage is a significant predictor of long-term outcome [11, 15, 17, 19, 23–24]. Survival is longer for those diagnosed with localized stage I or II disease, and patients typically live from 23 to 84 months [19, 25–27], with a 5-year survival rate of 33–82% [15–16, 18, 27]. This is considerably longer than survival in patients with advanced disease. Those with stage III ACC generally live from 8 to 28 months [19, 25–27], with a 5-year survival of 18–50% [15–16, 18, 27]. Those with stage IV ACC fare the worst of all, usually living from 9 to 15 months [19, 25–27], with a 5-year survival of 0–13% [15–16, 18].

ACC is an aggressive disease, both locally and distantly. In adults, ACC will often extend outside the adrenal gland, involving the kidney, diaphragm, abdominal wall, or vena cava [12]. The liver and lungs are the two most common sites of disseminated spread. In our own analysis of cumulative data from nine series, involvement of these organs occurs, respectively, in 55 and 50% of patients with metastases [10, 12, 14, 16, 18–22]. Often patients will have lesions at both sites [28].

ACC disseminates via both hematogenous and lymphatic routes [5]. Early lymphatic spread is of particular concern when attempting to establish effective local control. A recent prospective study found that 14.9% of 416 patients had positive lymph nodes at the time of diagnosis [16]. Others have found that lymph nodes are inspected in only 17.6% of all patients [22]. For the minority in whom lymph nodal status was accounted for, 26.5% harbored metastases [22]. Given this incidence, it seems appropriate to consider treating the lymphatic drainage basin of the adrenal gland in the adjuvant setting [29–30].

The predilection of ACC for local invasion makes adequate surgical resections difficult to accomplish. Complete resection occurs mostly in patients with less advanced disease. A summary of survival and recurrence rates in patients who had a complete versus debulking resection is presented in Table 25.2. Although the prognosis for those who undergo debulking procedures is particularly poor, the 5-year survival rates in those with ostensibly complete resections is also not satisfactory [18, 21–22, 27, 31–33]. These rates of recurrence indicate that it is uncommon for resections to be truly complete, despite being labeled as such. Residual disease is often found in an examination of the surgical margins, and an analysis of the NCDB found that 9% of all surgical patients had microscopically positive margins, while an additional 10% were macroscopically positive [22]. This corresponded with a 5-year survival rate of 21 and 10% respectively, which compares unfavorably with the 46% survival rate of those with uninvolved margins [22]. Thus, similar to the experience in other solid malignancies, there appears to be a survival benefit associated with a complete resection, but not with positive resection margins [15–16, 18–19, 25–27]. Tumor stage and resection margin status are likely correlated, and no study to date has adequately disentangled these variables.

Table 25.2 Outcomes in complete versus partial resection

	Patients with complete resection	Survival	Recurrence n (% of those with complete resection) [Note: local recurrence and metastatic recurrence are not mutually exclusive categories]	Patients with debulking resection	Survival
Icard [32][a]	127	42% 5-year	41 (32%) local recurrence 64 (50%) metastatic recurrence	29	9% 1-year
Haak [31][a]	47	49% 5-year	–	37	9% 5-year
Zografos [27]	24	38% 5-year 13 month median	–	17	0% 5-year 2 month median
Bellantone [18][a]	140	45% 5-year	27 (19%) local recurrence 39 (28%) metastatic recurrence	30	5% 5-year
Schulick [21][a]	68	55% 5-year 74 month median	–	45	5% 5-year 12 month median
Kendrick [33][a]	41	51 month median	30 (73%) local and/or metastatic	14	8 month median
Gonzalez [19][a]	174	–	64 (34%) local recurrence 110 (63%) metastatic recurrence	12	–
Bilimoria [22][a]	1670	43% 5-year 39 month median	–	101	36% 5-year 30 month median

[a] A significant portion of patients in these studies were treated with adjuvant chemotherapy, including mitotane

Besides resection margin status, other prognostically significant factors include advanced age at diagnosis, which several investigators have found to be negatively correlated with survival beginning at 35–55 years [15, 17, 22, 28, 32–33]. Tumor functional status is of uncertain consequence, with most reporting that it has no effect on survival [9, 21, 24–26, 28, 31, 34–35], while others have found any type of hormonal activity [32, 36] or cortisol hypersecretion specifically [17, 19] to be a predictor of poor outcomes. This contrasts with a study by Hogan et al. in which functionality was positively associated with survival while nonfunctional tumors were highly correlated with an anaplastic morphology [37]. Lastly, elevated mitotic count is positively correlated with malignancy and poor survival [38–42]. The Weiss criteria, which is commonly used to separate malignant adrenal tumors from benign adenomas, combines mitotic count with eight other histologic features [41], although is it unclear if these add significant information beyond that available from mitotic count alone [35, 38–39].

Among these prognostic indicators, resection margin status remains one of the best predictors of outcome. Regardless, many patients experience a recurrence of their disease even after a resection with uninvolved margins. Local recurrence occurred after 19–34% of complete resections [18–19], and Kendrick et al. found that the adrenal fossa was the single most common site of treatment failure, accounting for 65% of all recurrences [33].

Metastatic recurrence is also common and occurs after 28–63% of complete resections [18–19]. For that reason, systemic adjuvant therapies have been used in an attempt to improve long-term outcomes. One such promising treatment is the adrenolytic agent mitotane. Although some researchers have reported that this agent does not improve outcomes [9, 24–25, 28, 43], a recent multicenter retrospective study by Terzolo et al. makes a strong case that administration of mitotane after complete resection significantly improves survival. Those who received mitotane in addition to surgery survived for a median of 110 months, compared with 52 and 67 months for the two surgery-only cohorts. The 49% rate of recurrence in the surgery plus mitotane group was also considerably better than the 91 and 73% recurrence rates in the groups that did not receive mitotane [35]. To determine the optimal chemotherapeutic regimen in which to utilize mitotane, the First International Randomized Trial in Locally Advanced and Metastatic Adrenocortical Carcinoma Treatment (FIRM-ACT) is currently in the process of recruiting patients for a phase III comparison of etoposide, doxorubicin, cisplatin, and mitotane versus streptozotocin and mitotane [44].

25.2 Radiotherapy for Adrenocortical Carcinoma

Much of the early evidence concerning the utilization of radiotherapy in ACC has been anecdotal in nature. Summarizing the shortcomings of several retrospective series [12, 36, 45–47], such as reliance on small numbers of patients with a heterogeneity of disease status and treatments and inclusion of undocumented results, Percarpio et al. [1] argued that it would be incorrect to infer that radiotherapy is ineffective. Examples include Cohn et al., who stated that irradiation of abdominal

ACC does not improve outcomes, but no patient or treatment details were provided [3]; Schulick et al. who reached the same conclusion but presented no supporting data [21]; and Kasperlik-Zaluska et al. and Pommier et al. who found that radiotherapy is ineffective based on experiences with two and three patients, respectively [26, 48]. Similarly, without offering any treatment details, Bodie et al. reported that radiotherapy did not improve outcomes in five patients with preexisting metastatic disease [24] and another author reported the use of adjuvant radiotherapy in eleven patients, but no results were presented [28].

It is important to recognize that the field of radiation oncology has evolved significantly since the publication of the above series, with dramatic advances in the planning and delivery of radiotherapy. These changes have allowed radiation oncologists to deliver higher, more efficacious, radiation doses with increased accuracy and safety. These developments have led to significant improvements in outcomes in a number of malignancies. For instance, in the treatment of prostate cancer, radiation dose escalation, made safe and feasible by technological advancements, has lead to decreased rates of biochemical and clinical failure [49–52]. Similar advancements have occurred in the management of breast cancer. Radiotherapy after mastectomy has been known since the 1940s to reduce rates of local relapse, but a survival advantage has been documented only recently, after limitations in planning and delivery have been overcome [53–54].

Despite advances in technique, radiotherapy remains remarkably underutilized in the treatment of ACC. An examination of the NCDB, which reports on approximately 75% of all cancer in the United States [55], revealed that only 9.5% of documented ACC treatment regimens utilized radiotherapy [22]. Similarly, analysis of the SEER database, which represents over a quarter of the country's population [56], found that radiotherapy was applied in between 10.4 and 11.7% of cases [11, 20].

In recent years there has been increased recognition of the efficacy of radiotherapy, a fact reflected in emerging consensus opinion documents [57]. Several studies that focused on surgical or chemotherapeutic approaches have reported success in utilizing radiotherapy. Didolkar et al. found that radiotherapy produced tumor regression of 50% or more in four of ten patients [4]. Similarly, Nader et al. found that radiotherapy reduced tumor size or arrested metastatic growth in 22% of treated patients, a rate greater than that achieved with mitotane [8]. King et al. document four patients treated with adjuvant radiotherapy, all of whom survived longer than 5 years [5]. In a study of ACC in children, four patients received adjuvant radiotherapy, only one of whom experienced recurrence within a year [58]. Of particular note, one child experienced such complete regression of her locally invasive tumor that no evidence of cancer was found upon subsequent surgical exploration [58]. Finally, radiotherapy's utility as a palliative therapy has been noted in several series [2–5, 8–9], with one recent study noting the successful relief of symptoms in 22 of 26 patients [10].

Although these reviews were neither large nor specifically designed to evaluate radiotherapy, they nonetheless show that this modality can be effective in treating a substantial portion of patients. This conclusion is bolstered by reviews that have specifically assessed the impact of radiotherapy on ACC. One of the first such studies is the aforementioned report by Percarpio et al., in which all 12 patients given palliative therapy achieved a satisfactory response independent of age, gender, and tumor functional status [1]. Despite this promising result, it was more than 10 years until another study would specifically address the efficacy of radiotherapy. Magee et al. found that of the six patients for whom follow-up data were available, four had a positive response to radiotherapy, consisting of either reduction of tumor or metastatic mass in three cases and a biochemical response in one [6]. Of note, three of these patients survived longer than 10 years [6]. An even more dramatic response was found by Markoe et al. in a retrospective analysis of 13 patients, three of whom were treated with adequate adjuvant radiotherapy [7]. Over the course of 5–7 weeks, these stage III post-surgical patients received 50–60 Gy to the tumor bed and adjacent lymphatics in 1.5–1.8 Gy daily fractions. None of the patients were given adjuvant mitotane or other chemotherapies. Mean survival was greater than 105 months, which is remarkable given that surgical series have found survival rates for stage III disease of between 8 and 28 months [19, 25–27]. This study also found that palliative radiotherapy was successful in several patients [7].

More recently, Fassnacht et al. studied adjuvant radiotherapy in 14 patients who had undergone complete resection and were retrospectively matched to controls for margin status, mitotane treatment, tumor size, and stage [29]. A mean dose of 49 Gy was administered in daily fractions of 1.8–2.0 Gy. Although the use of radiotherapy did not impact survival, it did cause a substantial reduction in the rate of local recurrence at 5 years, which was 14% for those undergoing radiotherapy and 79% in those who did not. The absence of a survival advantage in the experimental group may be related to early disease dissemination [29–30]. Additionally, it may have been due to a lack of statistical power, or the fact the radiotherapy group contained three subjects with stage IV disease, while the control group contained none [29].

Efficacy of radiation has also been demonstrated in preclinical models. Cerquetti et al. compared the effects of radiation and mitotane, independently and in combination, in human-derived functional and non-functional ACC cell lines [59]. Radiotherapy induced G2 cell-cycle arrest in both cell lines, thereby inhibiting growth. However, this effect persisted for only 5 days, after which cellular proliferation resumed. This contrasts with the mitotane only treatment, which did not produce cell cycle arrest or decreased growth in either culture. The best results were achieved with radiotherapy and mitotane in combination. In both cell lines, this produced irreversible cell cycle arrest and inhibition of growth. Since combination treatment was significantly more effective than either therapy alone, this suggests that radiotherapy plus mitotane may offer significant clinical benefit [59].

Although these recent studies demonstrate the efficacy of radiotherapy, it is not appropriate in all contexts. Most studies have focused on patients whose tumors arose sporadically;[19, 21, 24, 27, 31–36] however, ACC can also be found in familial syndromes [60–63]. Of particular concern are those tumors arising in patients with Li-Fraumeni Syndrome, a hereditary condition resulting from germline mutations of the *TP53* tumor suppressor gene, associated with breast cancer, soft-tissue sarcoma, neoplasms of the brain, and leukemia, amongst other malignancies

[64–67]. As it has been well documented that radiation may induce a secondary malignancy in those with this condition [68–71], the use of radiotherapy in this setting cannot be recommended.

25.3 Case Studies

Recent experience treating ACC at the authors' institution has been consistent with the recent evidence for the modality's efficacy. Radiotherapy in the adjuvant setting and for palliation of unresectable primary tumors or metastatic disease has been used with encouraging results. In view of the lack of standardized radiotherapy protocols for ACC and the lack of large patient series, the following representative examples are given from this experience.

25.3.1 Case #1. Adjuvant Radiotherapy

TS is a 48-year-old male who initially presented in early 2008 with the classical stigmata of Cushing's syndrome. He underwent magnetic resonance imaging that revealed an 8.6 cm right adrenal mass, which was completely excised shortly thereafter. Pathology confirmed the diagnosis of stage II ACC and was notable for negative margins, numerous areas of necrosis, and a high mitotic rate.

Approximately 7 weeks after his surgery, TS began a course of radiotherapy. In order to minimize damage to his liver, kidney, and small intestine, intensity-modulated radiation therapy (IMRT) was employed. A total of 52.8 Gy in 2.2 Gy fractions were delivered to the tumor bed. At the same time, 43.2 Gy in 1.8 Gy fractions were delivered to the regional lymph nodes as prophylactic therapy, using 6 MV photon beams. Following treatment, the patient was titrated to a therapeutic level of mitotane. Today, concurrent treatment with mitotane would be recommended, given the in vitro demonstration of its synergistic activity with radiation [59]. Computed tomography (CT) images prior and subsequent to treatment are compared in Fig. 25.1. Radiation dose distributions and a dose volume histogram (DVH) are also provided.

Fig. 25.1 Adjuvant radiotherapy after complete resection of a primary ACC. 1A shows a CT image with a large right-sided adrenal mass (*arrow)* prior to resection. 1B demonstrates the same anatomy 9 months later, after resection, adjuvant IMRT, and mitotane therapy. The right kidney is now visible (*arrow*), and there is no evidence of recurrence. Additional images include radiation dose distributions (1C, 1D axial; 1E coronal; 1F sagittal). A beam display is provided in 1G, which demonstrates gantry angles of 180, 225, 350, 40, 25, 35, and 330°. Finally, 1H is a dose volume histogram (DVH) for the planning target volume (PTV), gross tumor volume (GTV), and relevant vital structures

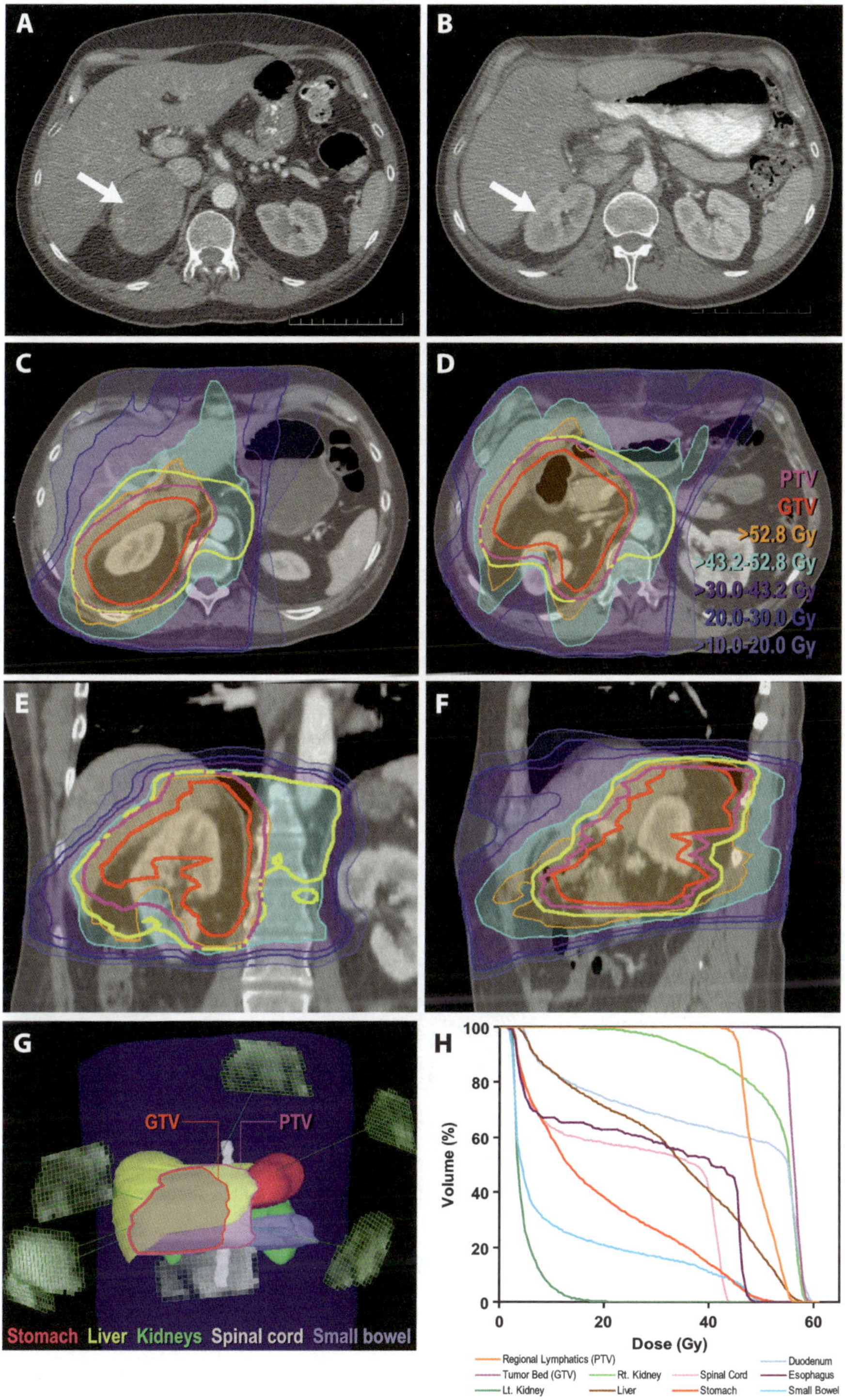

Fig. 25.1 (continued)

25.3.2 Case #2. Adjuvant Radiotherapy After Resection of a Local Recurrence

In late 1997, patient LG, a 47-year-old female, began having symptoms of cortisol hypersecretion, including a 35-pound weight gain, amenorrhea, and moon facies. In March of 1998, a 10 cm adrenal mass was resected; this was not followed by adjuvant therapy. One year later, a 2 cm recurrence in the adrenal fossa was detected on a surveillance CT. This was resected in April of 1999, and adjuvant radiotherapy with concurrent mitotane therapy was initiated in August of that year. In total, 55.8 Gy were delivered to the tumor bed over a 6 week period. At the time, it was not yet our practice to include regional lymphatics within the area of treatment. During radiotherapy, LG suffered from nausea, fatigue, and abdominal cramping, which, in addition to dermatitis, are among the most common side effects of radiation at this anatomical location. However, since fatigue and nausea are also associated with mitotane administration [29, 31, 35], it is unclear whether their presence was in fact due to radiotherapy. Less common but more significant morbidities could include ipsilateral renal impairment, radiation-induced liver disease, and intestinal damage.

Over the course of an 8-year follow-up, LG did not have any recurrence within the radiotherapy target volume, despite having an extremely aggressive tumor as demonstrated by her prior history of local recurrence following initial surgery and her eventual disease relapse with a distant omental metastasis, detected in August of 2006. Figure 25.2 illustrates LG's recurrence-free adrenal fossa and her omental metastasis.

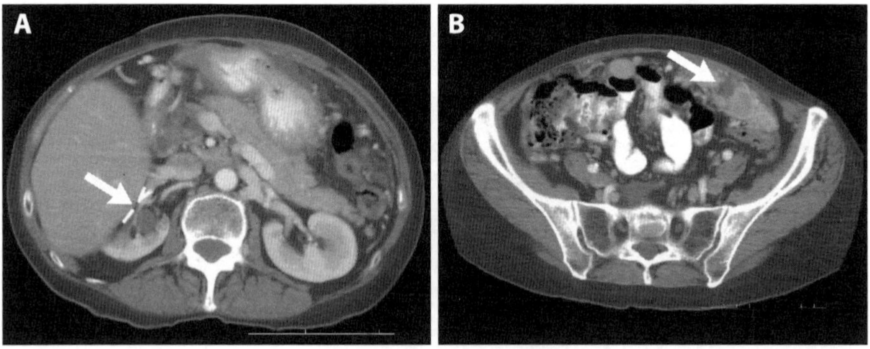

Fig. 25.2 Adjuvant radiotherapy after complete resection of locally recurrent ACC. 2A is a CT image 8 years status post resection and adjuvant radiotherapy. Note the surgical clips at the adrenal fossa (*arrow*) and the lack of local recurrence. 2B, from the same CT sequence 8 years after resection, demonstrates the prominent development of an omental metastasis (*arrow*). This case illustrates disease progression at a distant site, while the tumor bed that has been irradiated remains disease free

25.3.3 Case #3. Palliation of a Bulky Liver Metastasis

Radiotherapy is also efficacious in the palliative treatment of metastatic ACC. In November of 2003, patient KF, a 40-year-old female, presented with a large metastatic lesion in her liver, in addition to several small pulmonary metastases. Three years earlier, she had undergone excision of a large, 25 cm adrenal tumor,

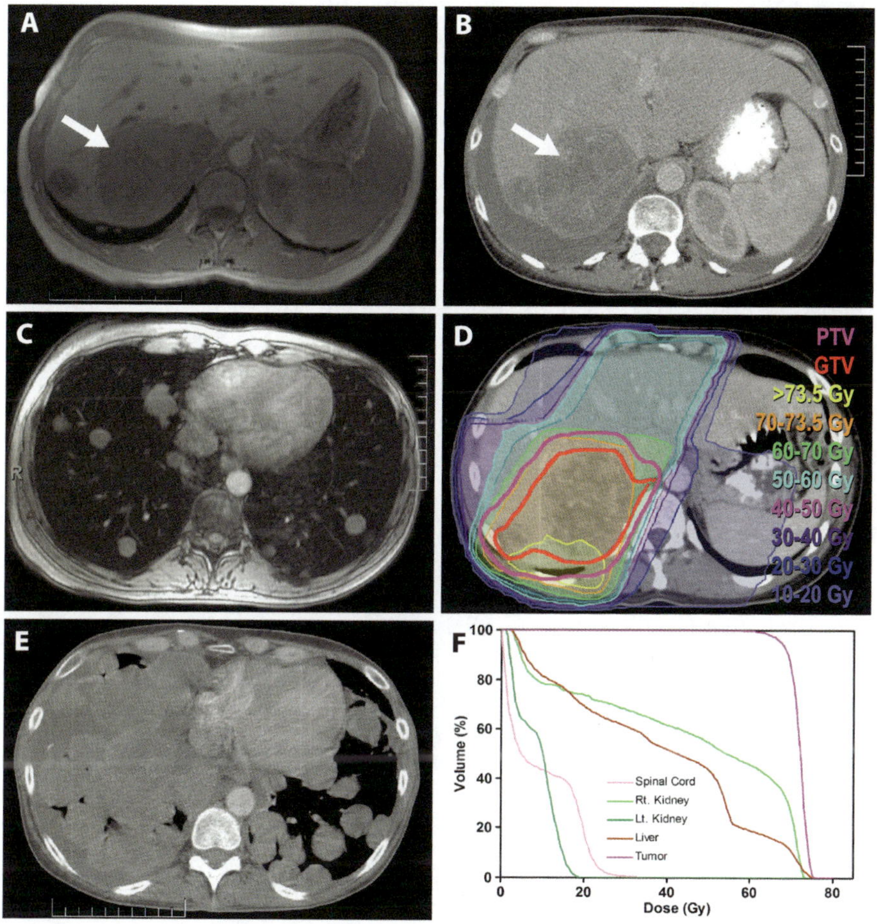

Fig. 25.3 High-dose palliative radiotherapy for an unresectable liver metastasis from ACC. 3A is an MRI image that illustrates the patient's liver lesion (*arrow*) 1 month prior to radiation, while 3C shows her thorax at that same time point. 3B is a CT image demonstrating local control (i.e., arrest of tumor growth) of the patient's liver lesion (*arrow*) 1 year and 9 months after completing radiotherapy. Note the modest reduction in size but the durable lack of progression. This was particularly remarkable given the dramatic progression of the patient's pulmonary lesions, as seen in 3E. 3D is an axial radiation dose distribution. 3F is a DVH showing the dose delivered to the tumor and surrounding vital structures

which was notable for numerous atypical mitotic figures. No adjuvant therapy was provided at that time. Eight months later, her metastases were detected and gradually progressed despite several chemotherapeutic regimens. Radiotherapy was recommended for her unresectable liver lesion, while her pulmonary metastases would later be treated with chemotherapy. A total of 73.5 Gy in 1.5 Gy fractions were delivered to her liver mass over a 5-week period concurrently with the radiosensitizer capecitabine. Following treatment, there was no further progression of her liver metastasis, which was all the more dramatic when contrasted with the aggressive growth of her pulmonary lesions that had not been treated with radiotherapy. Figure 25.3 compares the course of tumor growth at these two sites and demonstrates the benefit of radiotherapy in arresting the growth of metastatic disease. Also shown are radiation dose distributions and a DVH.

25.4 Summary

Rates of local recurrence after surgical resection (with or without adjuvant chemotherapy such as mitotane) are high. Recent experience by a number of investigators has shown that radiation is an effective adjuvant therapy and can reduce local relapse rates. Whether this translates into a survival advantage remains to be tested in a prospective clinical trial. Additionally, radiotherapy is useful as a palliative modality. It can produce tumor regression and long-term freedom from local progression.

The authors utilize radiation routinely as adjuvant therapy for high-risk patients. In our practice, targets include both the tumor bed and the regional lymphatics. Most commonly IMRT is utilized to deliver 45 Gy in 1.8 Gy fractions to the regional lymphatics and 52.5–55 Gy in 2.1–2.2 Gy fractions to the tumor bed. When resection margins are positive we deliver higher tumor bed doses, as permitted by the tolerance of adjacent Organs-at-Risk (OAR). Radiotherapy is also often recommended for palliation of unresectable primary tumors or metastases.

Acknowledgment Grateful acknowledgement is made to Karen Vineberg and Steven Kronenberg for their exceptional assistance with all figures.

References

1. Percarpio B, Knowlton AH (1976) Radiation therapy of adrenal cortical carcinoma. Acta Radiol Ther Phys Biol 15:288–292
2. Bradley III EL (1975) Primary and adjunctive therapy in carcinoma of the adrenal cortex. Surg Gynecol Obstet 141:507–511
3. Cohn K et al (1986) Adrenocortical carcinoma. Surgery 100:1170–1177
4. Didolkar MS et al (1981) Natural history of adrenal cortical carcinoma: a clinicopathologic study of 42 patients. Cancer 47:2153–2161
5. King DR, Lack EE (1979) Adrenal cortical carcinoma: a clinical and pathologic study of 49 cases. Cancer 44:239–244
6. Magee BJ et al (1987) Adrenal cortical carcinoma: survival after radiotherapy. Clin Radiol 38:587–588

7. Markoe AM et al (1991) Radiation therapy for adjunctive treatment of adrenal cortical carcinoma. Am J Clin Oncol 14:170–174
8. Nader S et al (1983) Adrenal cortical carcinoma: a study of 77 cases. Cancer 52:707–711
9. Vassilopoulou-Sellin R et al (1993) Impact of adjuvant mitotane on the clinical course of patients with adrenocortical cancer. Cancer 71:3119–3123
10. Polat B et al (2009) Radiotherapy in adrenocortical carcinoma. Cancer 115:2816–2823
11. Kebebew E et al (2006) Extent of disease at presentation and outcome for adrenocortical caricnoma: have we made progress? World J Surg 30:872–878
12. Macfarlane DA (1958) Cancer of the adrenal cortex: the natural hisotry, prognosis, and treatment in a study of 55 cases. Ann R Coll Surg Engl 23:155–186
13. Sullivan M et al (1978) Adrenal cortical carcinoma. J Urol 120:660–665
14. DeLellis RA et al (eds) (2004) Pathology and genetics of tumours of endocrine organs. International Agency for Research on Cancer, Lyon
15. Icard P et al (2001) Adrenocortical carcinomas: surgical trends and results of a 253-patient series from the French Association of Endocrine Surgeons Study Group. World J Surg 25:891–897
16. Fassnacht M et al (2009) Limited prognostic value of the 2004 International union against cancer staging classification for adrenocortical carcinoma: proposal for a revised TNM classification. Cancer 115:243–250
17. Abiven G et al (2006) Clinical and biological features in the prognosis of adrenocortical cancer: poor outcome of cortisol-secreting tumors in a series of 202 consecutive patients. J Clin Endocrinol Metab 91:2650–2655
18. Bellantone Rl et al (1997) Role of reoperation in recurrence of adrenal cortical carcinoma: results from 188 cases collected in the Italian National Registry for Adrenal Cortical Carcinoma. Surgery 122:1212–1218
19. Gonzalez RJ et al (2007) Response to mitotane predicts outcome in patients with recurrent adrenal cortical carcinoma. Surgery 142:869–875
20. Paton BL et al (2006) Outcomes of adrenal cortical carcinoma in the United States. Surgery 140:914–920
21. Schulick RD, Brennan MF (1999) Long-term survival after complete resection and repeat resection in patients with adrenocortical carcinoma. Ann Surg Oncol 6:719–726
22. Billimoria KY et al (2008) Adrenocortical carcinoma in the United States: treatment utilization and prognostic factors. Cancer 113:3130–3136
23. Soreide JA et al (1992) Adrenal cortical carcinoma in Norway, 1970–1984. World J Surg 16:663–668
24. Bodie B et al (1989) The Cleveland clinic experience with adrenal cortical carcinoma. J Urol 141:257–260
25. Henley DJ et al (1983) Adrenal cortical carcinoma: a continuing challenge. Surgery 94:926–931
26. Pommier RF, Brennan MF (1992) An eleven-year experience with adrenocortical carcinoma. Surgery 112:963–971
27. Zografos GC et al (1994) Adrenal adenocarcinoma: a review of 53 cases. J Surg Oncol 55:160–164
28. Luton JP et al (1990) Clinical features of adrenocortical carcinoma, prognostic factors, and the effect of mitotane therapy. N Engl J Med 322: 1195–1201
29. Fassnacht M et al (2006) Efficacy of adjuvant radiotherapy of the tumor bed on local recurrence of adrenocortical carcinoma. J Clin Endocrinol Metab 91: 4501–4504
30. Kirschner LS (2006) Editorial: paradigms for adrenal cancer: think globally, act locally. J Clin Endocrinol Metab 91:4250–4252
31. Haak HR et al (1994) Optimal treatment of adrenocortical carcinoma with mitotane: results in a consecutive series of 96 patients. Br J Cancer 69:947–951

32. Icard P et al (1992) Adrenocortical carcinoma in surgically treated patients: a retrospective study on 156 cases by the French Association of Endocrine Surgery. Surgery 112:972–980
33. Kendrick ML et al (2001) Adrenocortical carcinoma: surgical progress or status quo? Arch Surg 136:543–549
34. Venkatesh S et al (1989) Adrenal cortical carcinoma. Cancer 64: 765–769
35. Terzolo M et al (2007) Adjuvant mitotane treatment for adrenocortical carcinoma. N Engl J Med 356:2372–2380
36. Hutter Jr AM, Kayhoe DE (1966) Adrenal cortical carcinoma: clinical features of 138 patients. Am J Med 41:572–580
37. Hogan TF et al (1980) A clinical and pathological study of adrenocortical carcinoma. Cancer 45:2880–2883
38. Volante M et al (2008) Pathological and molecular features of adrenocortical carcinoma: an update. J Clin Pathol 61:787–793
39. Berruti A et al (2008) Emerging drugs for adrenocortical carcinoma. Expert Opin Emerg Drugs 13:497–509
40. Harrison LE et al (1999) Pathologic features of prognostic significance for adrenocortical carcinoma after curative resection. Arch Surg 134:181–185
41. Weis LM (1984) Comparitive histologic study of 43 metastasizing and nonmetastasizing adrenocortical tumors. Am J Surg Pathol 8:163–169
42. Weiss LM et al (1989) Pathologic features of prognostic significance in adrenocortical carcinoma. Am J Surg Pathol 13:202–206
43. Barzon L et al (1999) Is there a role for low doses of mitotane (o,p'-DDD) as adjuvant therapy in adrenocortical carcinoma? J Clin Endocrinol Metab 84:1488–1489
44. Skogseid B et al (2008) First International Randomized trial in locally advanced and Metastatic Adrenocortical Carcinoma Treatment. http://www.firm-act.org/. Accessed 11 Dec 2008
45. Hajjar RA et al (1975) Adrenal cortical carcinoma: a study of 32 patients. Cancer 35:549–554
46. Huvos AG et al (1970) Adrenal cortical carcinoma: clinicopathologic study of 34 cases. Cancer 25:354–361
47. Murphy WT (1967) Radiation therapy. WB Saunders, Philadelphia, PA
48. Kasperlik-Zaluska AA et al (1995) Adrenocortical carcinoma: a clinical study and treatment results of 52 patients. Cancer 75:2587–2591
49. Sathya J et al (2005) Randomized trial comparing iridium implant plus external-beam radiation therapy with external-beam radiation therapy alone in node-negative locally advanced cancer of the prostate. J Clin Oncol 23:1192–1199
50. Zietman A et al (2005) Comparison of Conventional-Dose vs High-Dose conformal radiation therapy in clinically localized adenocarcinoma of the prostate a randomized controlled trial. JAMA 294:1233–1239
51. Kuban D et al (2008) Long-term results of the MD Anderson randomized dose-escalation trial for prostate cancer. Int J Radiat Oncol Biol Phys 70:67–74
52. Viani G et al (2009) Higher-than-conventional radiation doses in localized prostate cancer treatment: a meta-analysis of randomized, controlled trials. Int J Radiat Oncol Biol Phys 74:1405–1418
53. Overgaard M et al (1999) Postoperative radiotherapy in high-risk postmenopausal breast-cancer patients given adjuvant tamoxifen: Danish Breast Cancer Cooperative Group DBCG 82c randomised trial. Lancet 353:1641–1648
54. Ragaz J et al (1997) Adjuvant radiotherapy and chemotherapy in node-positive premenopausal women with breast cancer. N Engl J Med 337:956–962
55. Commission on Cancer (2008) The American College of Surgeons Commission on cancer: national cancer data base. http://www.facs.org/cancer/ncdb/index.html. Accessed 9 Dec 2008
56. Surveillance Research Program of the National Cancer Institute (2008) Surveillance, epidemiology, and end results web site. http://seer.cancer.gov/. Accessed 9 Dec 2008

57. Schteingart DE et al (2005) Management of patients with adrenal cancer: recommendations of an international consensus conference. Endocr Relat Cancer 12:667–680
58. Stewart DR et al (1974) Carcinoma of the adrenal gland in children. J Pediatr Surg 9:59–67
59. Cerquetti L et al (2008) Mitotane increases the radiotherapy inhibitory effect and induces G2-arrest in combined treatment on both H295r and SW13 adrenocortical cell lines. Endocr Relat Cancer 15:623–634
60. Li F et al (1988) A cancer family syndrome in twenty-four kindreds. Cancer Res 48:5358–5362
61. Henry I et al (1989) Molecular definition of the 11p15. 5 region involved in Beckwith-Wiedemann syndrome and probably in predisposition to adrenocortical carcinoma. Hum Genet 81:273–277
62. Skogseid B et al (1992) Clinical and genetic features of adrenocortical lesions in multiple endocrine neoplasia type 1. J Clin Endocrinol Metab 75:76–81
63. Painter T, Jagelman D (1985) Adrenal adenomas and adrenal carcinomas in association with hereditary adenomatosis of the colon and rectum. Cancer 55:2001–2004
64. Li F, Fraumeni J (1969) Soft-tissue sarcomas, breast cancer, and other neoplasms: a familial syndrome? Ann Intern Med 71:747–752
65. Li F, Fraumeni J (1982) Prospective study of a family cancer syndrome. JAMA 247: 2692–2694
66. Hartley A et al (1989) Are germ cell tumors part of the Li-Fraumeni cancer family syndrome? Cancer Genet Cytogenet 42:221–226
67. Malkin D et al (1990) Germ line p53 mutations in a familial syndrome of breast cancer, sarcomas, and other neoplasms. Science 250:1233–1238
68. Hisada M et al (1998) Multiple primary cancers in families with Li-Fraumeni syndrome. J Nat Cancer Inst 90:606–611
69. Varley J et al (1999) Are there low-penetrance TP53 alleles? evidence from childhood adrenocortical tumors. Am J Hum Genet 65:995–1006
70. Limacher J et al (2001) Two metachronous tumors in the radiotherapy fields of a patient with Li-Fraumeni syndrome. Int J Cancer 96:238–242
71. Birch J et al (2001) Relative frequency and morphology of cancers in carriers of germline TP 53 mutations. Oncogene 20:4621–4628

Chapter 26
Follow-Up and Monitoring of Adrenocortical Carcinoma

Britt Skogseid and Gerard M. Doherty

Patients with adrenocortical carcinoma (ACC) usually present with (1) symptoms caused by tumor growth and/or (2) hormone production or (3) ACC is discovered incidentally by imaging conducted for reasons other than suspicion of an adrenocortical tumor. Recurrent ACC will therefore mainly be discovered by detection of tumor growth, which can occur at the former resection site or present as distant metastases, by recurrence of symptoms of hormone access, or by biochemical evidence of rising hormone levels produced by the tumor. The only treatment with curative potential is surgical tumor removal. All other treatment modalities, such as cytotoxic chemotherapy, mitotane therapy (in the nonadjuvant setting), antisteroidogenic treatment, or radiation therapy aim towards a reduction of tumor burden or decrease in tumor progression. Therefore, follow-up and surveillance of patients are strongly guided by the intent of the primary treatment approach (curative vs. non-curative), risk stratification, the treatment modality, and the initial pretreatment presentation. Regular office visits also allow for detection and treatment of symptoms related to the disease, such as hypertension, diabetes, and pain.

Surveillance of patients with ACC is extremely important as a significant proportion will face relapse (~50%). There is a large variation regarding the time to tumor recurrence, ranging from weeks to years. The goals of an individualized follow-up and monitoring plan for patients with ACC are to identify disease recurrence to allow further therapy, or to monitor the therapeutic efficacy of treatment for known disease. The follow-up plan should include multiple modalities for disease detection/monitoring, and a carefully considered schedule of evaluation [1, 2]. At present, data to support any specific surveillance program do not exceed the level of expert opinion. As such, any guidelines primarily represent consensus statements generated from national/international working groups [3].

G.M. Doherty (✉)
Department of Surgery, University of Michigan Health System, The University of Michigan, 2920 Taubman Center, 1500 East Medical Center Drive, Ann Arbor, MI 48109, USA
e-mail: gerardd@umich.edu

G.D. Hammer, T. Else (eds.), *Adrenocortical Carcinoma*,
DOI 10.1007/978-0-387-77236-3_26, © Springer Science+Business Media, LLC 2011

26.1 General Modalities for Follow-Up

In general, follow-up of patients should include a careful patient history, physical examination, biochemical evaluation together with general and individualized imaging. Tumor surveillance is guided by clinical findings at initial presentation and staging. Regular visits should also be used to gauge patient expectations that need to be tailored to potential treatment options.

26.2 History

The patient's history and evaluation should be geared towards detection of general symptoms that are caused by side effects of therapy or hormone overproduction by the tumor as well as symptoms which are caused by mass effects of a tumor recurrence at the site of resection or due to distant metastasis.

Interval patient history can reveal recurrent local disease, or new sites of distant cancer spread. Recurrent ACC will mainly lead to symptoms of local tumor growth, such as pain, abdominal fullness, or decreased organ function (e.g., bowel obstruction, ureteral obstruction), as in the case of organ invasion or distant metastasis.

Patients who initially present with hormone overproduction should be screened for recurrent signs and symptoms. It is important though to keep in mind that recurrent tumors do not necessarily present with the same hormonal signs/symptoms as the initial tumor. It is a well-known phenomenon that ACCs that initially led to symptoms and signs of hormone access may recur as a nonfunctional tumor – or switch hormone production from, for example, cortisol production to predominant androgen production. Although less common, a nonfunctioning tumor may recur with hormone excess.

During these visits, systemic symptoms caused by the disease, such as hypertension, diabetes mellitus, psychiatric symptoms, osteoporosis, or pain, can be identified. Patients who have had Cushing's syndrome at their initial presentation, followed by a disease-free interval after treatment, may be quite sensitive in detecting recurrent hormonal symptoms. This seems especially true for women with symptoms of Cushing's syndrome and hirsutism. Complaints reminiscent of original tumor symptoms in a patient with a history of a functional adrenal tumor should always prompt re-evaluation with biochemical testing and potentially imaging. The majority of these issues can be treated medically. Follow-up visits should also include an evaluation of the patient's functional status and wishes regarding therapeutic approaches as these guide current and future therapeutic plans.

26.3 Physical Examination

A focused physical examination is an important part of the follow-up plan for ACC. As with the history, the physical examination can reveal manifestations of the disease and uncover side effects of therapy that could influence future treatment options.

Vital signs should be specifically evaluated as long-term trends in order to detect changes. Weight, blood pressure, and heart rate, in particular, can show changes with progression of disease, e.g., weight can increase with new or recurrent manifestations of Cushing's syndrome or decrease with tumor cachexia, blood pressure can increase with recurrence of Cushing's syndrome or hyperaldosteronism. Standard physical evaluation should include the usual components of a general examination, including an assessment of the functional status, evaluation for signs of hormone excess, and tumor recurrence. Regarding tumor recurrence, a thorough inspection and palpation of lymph nodes, skin, head, neck, chest, abdomen, and pelvis is warranted. Particular areas of focus should include the abdominal wound to evaluate for tumor recurrence or hernia, the abdominal contents for palpable mass or bowel obstruction, the lower extremities for peripheral edema and the cervical and supraclavicular nodal basins for palpable adenopathy. Areas of concern as indicated by the patient history including areas of known disease should receive additional attention, palpating for masses or tenderness.

Although a search for manifestations of hormone excess will guided by any recurrent symptoms in patients with treated functioning tumors, it is worthwhile to watch out for signs of hormone excess that may be discordant with the initial presenting syndrome of hormone excess as shifts of hormone productions as well as de novo and loss of hormone production have been described.

26.4 Laboratory Evaluation

Laboratory evaluation during follow-up is used to detect recurrent or progressive disease, to monitor drug toxicity and tumor-related problems during and after treatment. Following initial resection, a full hormonal evaluation should be initiated to detect persistent disease or the development of subsequent adrenal insufficiency in a patient with a cortisol-producing ACC. In any patient with new adrenal insufficiency, hormone replacement needs to be instituted immediately.

Useful laboratory tests to detect tumor recurrence and progression of ACC depend mainly upon the functional status of the tumor in a particular patient at initial presentation. In addition to electrolytes, LDH and blood counts, biomarkers may include serum levels of cortisol (evening salivary cortisol, or an overnight 1 mg dexamethasone suppression test), androgens (dehydroepiandrosterone sulfate [DHEAS], androstenedione, testosterone), 17-hydroxyprogesterone, and/or 11-deoxycortisol, based on pre-operative hormonal profile [1, 3]. Urine hormone measurements, specifically a 24-h urine-free cortisol are useful.

In patients with functional tumors, blood or urine hormone levels can be used as tumor markers to assess disease recurrence or progression. Patients with cortisol producing ACCs at presentation may be most easily followed with 24-h urine-free cortisol (24-h UFC) measurement. If the patient is taking oral hydrocortisone as replacement therapy for glucocorticoid replacement (either because of HPA axis suppression from treated Cushing's syndrome or during mitotane therapy), then the 24-h UFC will reflect some of the oral replacement dose. To avoid interference with substitution therapy, hydrocortisone replacement dosing can be changed to a bioequivalent dose of dexamethasone for 3 days prior to the 24-h UFC collection. The 24-h UFC collection then reflects only endogenous cortisol production [4]. The follow-up plan for patients with virilizing tumors should include testosterone and other androgen hormone measurements. Patients who initially present with elevated levels of DHEAS will need regular measurement of this steroid. Similarly, patients who present with aldosterone-producing tumors, or mixed tumors that include aldosterone production, should have plasma renin activity and aldosterone included in their plan.

Measurements of hormones is not necessarily mandated, if not elevated at initial presentation. However, it may be included to allow for detection of a tumor recurrence in a patient presenting with symptoms consistent with new hormone excess.

Urinary steroid profiles by HPLC and mass spectrometry have been used in some centers to evaluate both the initial presentation of patients with adrenocortical lesions or as a part of the follow-up evaluation [5, 6]. Patients with adrenal malignancy usually have abnormal urinary steroids components, in some cases even unique for a particular patient and particular tumor. After successful therapy, these profiles often normalize. At the time of recurrence, the urinary steroid profile often becomes abnormal again, but does not always follow the same abnormal pattern as the initial tumor [6]. The assessment of urinary steroid profiles has not been shown to have independent predictive value in the monitoring of ACC patients, at least in part because the availability of the test is limited to specialized centers and the disease is rare.

The assessment of general health and treatment-related effects are similar for ACC patients as for other patients undergoing systemic therapy, with the addition of increased risk of adrenal insufficiency due to surgical resection and mitotane therapy. As a significant number of patients is treated with experimental compounds, for which there is no extensive clinical experience, assessment for side effects is extremely important. Patients should be assessed for anemia and electrolyte imbalances that can cause cancer-related fatigue [7, 8].

26.5 Imaging

Current imaging modalities are so sensitive and specific that it can be tempting to depend upon them entirely during tumor follow-up. The most frequent detection of recurrence is by demonstration on follow-up imaging. However, clinicians must resist the allure of using imaging as the foundation of follow-up in order to avoid discounting important information in the history, physical examination, or laboratory evaluation. Deliberately planning the imaging evaluation in concert with the preceding work-up will help to maintain a balanced, patient-focused approach.

General tumor surveillance by imaging is very similar to the initial staging (see Chapter 4) and may additionally include symptom specific imaging procedures.

26.5.1 Symptom-Specific/Sign-Specific Imaging

Specific symptoms or signs of progression or recurrence should be evaluated by imaging. Potential recurrence in areas that would not typically be included in routine follow-up imaging may necessitate plain films, CNS examinations, bone scans, or FDG-PET scans, which should be arranged when symptoms warrant, or when there is laboratory evidence of disease that is occult on initial studies. Thus, although the follow-up strategy may include planned imaging examinations, the clinicians and patient must anticipate adding additional studies as needed based on up to date information.

26.5.2 Cross-Sectional Imaging

CT scan and MR scan are the mainstays of cross-sectional imaging. The exquisite anatomic detail available has revolutionized our ability to define disease recurrence and progression. For optimal utility, intravenous contrast is necessary, and so patient contrast allergies and renal function are important to the imaging plan, along with actual or potential pregnancy and claustrophobia. The choice of CT or MR scanning as the standard follow-up imaging technique is institution- and clinician-dependent. Many institutions use CT scan as the routine, but incorporate MR for certain patients, or to address specific questions, such as characterization of small liver lesions [1].

CT scans provide rapid, relatively inexpensive and widely available imaging for follow-up examinations (Fig. 26.1). They carry the cumulative risks of ionizing

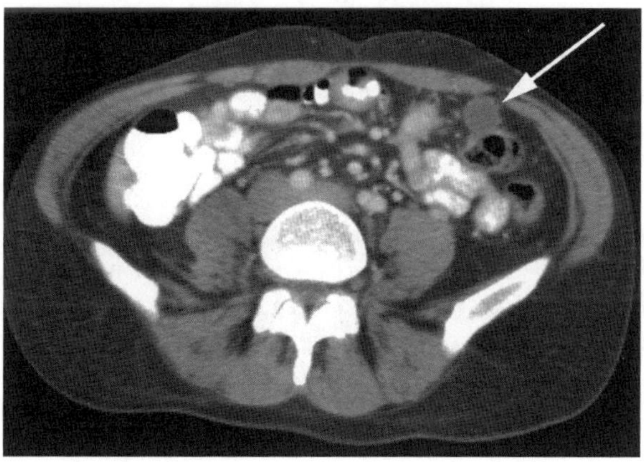

Fig. 26.1 Abdominal CT scan showing intraperitoneal recurrence of ACC (*arrow*)

radiation exposure and the risk of allergic reaction to intravenous contrast dye [9]. They can provide high-quality imaging of the entire body, including the brain, neck, chest, abdomen, and pelvis. High-quality scan equipment is available in or near to most communities, and the images are readily transferable for assessment by clinicians and specialized radiologists. CT scans are also commonly performed in concert with functional studies, such as FDG-PET imaging, in order to provide more detailed anatomic correlates to the functional data (see Chapter 7).

MR scans have some specific areas of advantage over CT scans in the characterization of small liver lesions and subtle brain abnormalities. However, the quality of the scans is equipment- and technique-dependent. High-quality images are not available in many communities, and so follow-up imaging done close to the patient's home can be less than optimal for interpretation. In addition, the interpretation of MR scans can be less directly accessible to clinicians, as CT scans are generally more easily understood by most non-radiologists.

For most patients during follow-up, it is advantageous to select one cross-sectional imaging technique as the standard approach, and then to use that for each examination. This avoids the issue of comparing lesions over time assessed with different techniques, which can interfere with judging subtle changes in disease status.

26.5.3 Functional Imaging

[^{18}F]-fluorodeoxyglucose (FDG)-based positron emission tomography (FDG-PET) is the most commonly performed functional imaging study performed for malignancy (see Chapter 7) (Fig. 26.2). FDG is administered intravenously. The compound is taken up into glucose-metabolizing cells through glucose transporters and phosphorylated. The phosphorylated FDG remains in the cell, but cannot be metabolized as rapidly as normal glucose. ^{18}F releases positrons, which create gamma rays when they intersect with electrons in the tissue. The gamma rays are detected by the scanner, and used to create a tomographic image of the functional utilization of glucose in the body. As many tumors are high metabolizers of glucose, this imaging technique has proved useful for the detection of tumors. When combined with a co-registered cross-sectional imaging study, such as CT scan, the FDG-PET scan can be very sensitive in identifying occult disease [10].

The weakness of FDG-PET scans is false-positive results from other normal or abnormal tissues that can utilize glucose at increased rates, and be mistaken for malignancy. These tissues can include areas of recent trauma (such as surgery), infection, or muscle activity. The images must be carefully interpreted in context of the patient's disease. It can often be critical for definitive decision-making regarding further therapy to biopsy suspicious areas for confirmation.

Other moieties that can be used for PET scans incorporate ^{11}C, ^{13}N, ^{15}O, or ^{18}F into metabolized biological substances to reveal functional tissues. All of these are limited by their short radionuclide half-lives, which is longest for ^{18}F (110 min)

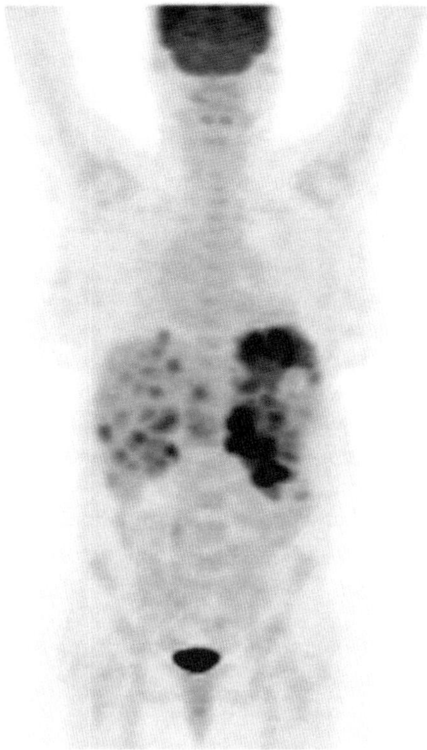

Fig. 26.2 FDG-PET scan demonstrating diffuse upper abdominal ACC dissemination at recurrence of a high-grade tumor. There is no evidence of dissemination outside of the peritoneal cavity

and shortest for ^{15}O (2 min). [^{11}C]-metomidate has been studied for imaging adrenal tumors, including adrenocortical cancers [11, 12]. The limited half-life and availability of this agent have currently limited experience with this.

26.6 Risk-Based Follow-Up Strategies

The risk and likely sites of recurrence or progression of cancer should dictate the frequency and modality of the follow-up strategy [1, 2]. For ACC, the risk varies with the biological aggressiveness of the tumor, the sites of initial disease, the therapy that has been employed, and the response to that therapy. Initial therapy for ACC often includes surgical resection. In general, it is helpful to establish a new baseline imaging profile to compare to during follow-up at some interval after recovery from operation (2–4 months, depending upon the procedure).

Given the rarity of this disease and our lack of definitive knowledge regarding best treatment for the myriad of patient presentations, optimal management of ACC patients may include participation in a clinical trial. For those patients, the follow-up strategy will follow the protocol prescribed by the trial design.

26.6.1 Low-Risk Localized Disease/Complete Resection

A minority of patients, who have a low-grade ACC, with no evidence of capsular invasion, disease extension or metastasis, have a better prognosis than the remainder of the ACC cohort. If these patients have had a resection guided by oncologic principles, with complete resection of the tumor and adjacent soft tissue, and no violation of the tumor capsule, done by an open operative approach, then the risk of recurrence is lower than for most ACC patients. The time to recurrence is likely to be prolonged. In the absence of questionable lesions on baseline scans (that require evaluation at shorter intervals) these patients can be followed carefully, but less frequently.

However, even this best prognosis group is at risk for both local recurrence and distant metastasis. The follow-up plan should include clinical evaluation every 3–6 months with a history, physical examination, biochemical evaluation customized for the patients preoperative findings, cross-sectional imaging of the chest, abdomen, and pelvis, and further evaluation of any symptoms, signs, or study abnormalities [1, 2]. Patients who are on adjuvant therapy in an attempt to decrease the risk of recurrence may require additional monitoring of therapy, such as mitotane levels, and monitoring for side effects of therapy (e.g., thyroid and gonadal axes evaluation, liver function tests, and blood lipid profile). Although the utility of various surveillance regimens has not been formally tested, after some period of time, the frequency of imaging is usually decreased to 6–12 months. Three to five years of semiannual imaging is commonly completed prior to extension of the interval if there has been no recurrence. Some centers extend the surveillance period up to 10 years.

26.6.2 High-Risk Disease/Complete Resection

Patients with high-grade disease, or who had more extensive disease such as local disease extensions, lymph node metastases, or distant metastases, but who have had an apparently complete operative resection, have an increased risk of local or distant recurrence, and a quicker time to recurrence. Their disease risk includes a substantial risk of local or distant recurrence, or both.

The follow-up plan should include clinical evaluation every 3 months with a history, physical examination, biochemical evaluation customized for the patients preoperative findings, cross-sectional imaging of the chest, abdomen, and pelvis, and further evaluation of any symptoms, signs, or study abnormalities [1, 2]. Patients who are on adjuvant therapy in an attempt to decrease the risk of recurrence may require additional monitoring of therapy, but should not require additional monitoring for disease. After some period, typically 1–2 years, if the patient has had no evidence of recurrence, the follow-up interval can be extended to semiannual, and should continue at that frequency until 5–10 years.

26.6.3 Unresectable Localized or Metastatic Disease

Patients with systemic disease should have monitoring as dictated by the tempo of their disease and their current therapy (Fig. 26.3). The monitoring should always include all components of follow-up (history, physical examination, biochemical evaluation, cross-sectional imaging, and further evaluation of any symptoms, signs, or study abnormalities), but the timing should be focused on treatment decisions. For example, in the case of successful cytotoxic therapy with tumor shrinkage, surgery may become an option for symptom control and reduction of tumor burden. Follow-up intervals may be as short as every 2 months (about two cycles for most common cytotoxic chemotherapy regimens), but may also be limited to history, physical examination, and possibly laboratory values to monitor for correctable anemia or electrolyte abnormalities in patients who are receiving solely palliative care.

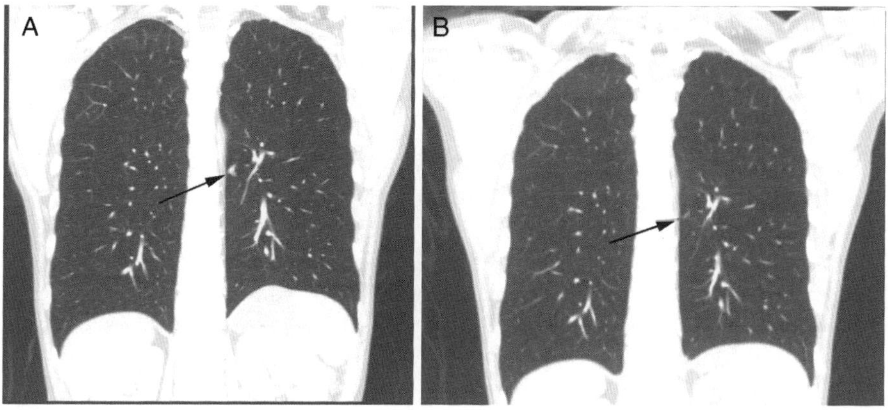

Fig. 26.3 Chest CT scan (**a**) shows a small left lung nodule (*arrow*) that subsequently responded to four cycles of systemic chemotherapy (**b**, tumor remnant *arrow*)

26.7 Risk Modifiers and Follow-Up Strategies

There are some patient characteristics and tumor features that influence the risk of recurrence and hence a modification of the follow-up plan. If the tumor is functional, particularly with Cushing's syndrome, and the initial period of follow-up examinations has shown no evidence of recurrence, the physicians may choose to limit imaging in further follow-up, relying more heavily upon biomarkers of recurrence between less frequent cross-sectional studies. Conversely, if the initial resection was compromised, either by being performed laparoscopically (which carries an increased risk of early intraperitoneal recurrence), or by violation of the tumor capsule during resection, then the imaging surveillance of the peritoneal contents should be increased in frequency and scrutiny (Fig. 26.4) [13].

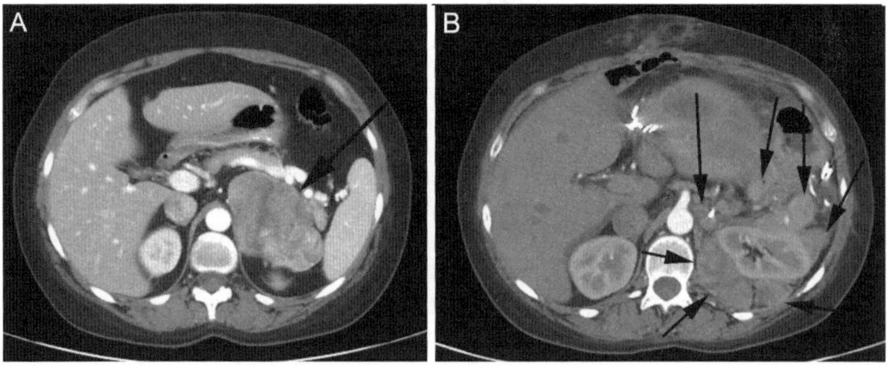

Fig. 26.4 Preoperative (**a**) and 6-month postoperative (**b**) CT scans in a patient with an apparently localized ACC. The operation was marked by fracture and spillage of the tumor, with malignant contamination of the peritoneal cavity. The preoperative scan showed a large but focal process (*large arrow*) while the postoperative scan shows multiple foci of recurrence

26.8 Conclusion

Patients with ACC have a substantial risk of recurrence, but that risk and the likely sites of recurrence are variable for different patient, tumor and treatment characteristics. In addition to general principles, follow-up strategies should always include the complete evaluation of the patient, including history, physical examination, biochemical testing, cross-sectional imaging, and further evaluation of any symptoms, signs, or study abnormalities.

References

1. Strosberg JR et al (2009) Management of adrenocortical carcinoma. J Natl Compr Canc Netw 7(7):752–758; quiz 759
2. Clark OH et al (2009) NCCN clinical practice guidelines in oncology: neuroendocrine tumors. J Natl Compr Canc Netw 7(7):712–747
3. Schteingart DE et al (2005) Management of patients with adrenal cancer: recommendations of an international consensus conference. Endocr Relat Cancer 12(3):667–680
4. Doherty GM et al (1990) Time to recovery of the hypothalamic-pituitary-adrenal axis after curative resection of adrenal tumors in patients with Cushing's syndrome. Surgery 108: 1085–1090
5. Kikuchi E et al (2000) Urinary steroid profile in adrenocortical tumors. Biomed Pharmacother 54(Suppl 1):194s–197s
6. Grondal S et al Steroid profile in urine: a useful tool in the diagnosis and follow up of adrenocortical carcinoma. Acta Endocrinol 122(5):656–663
7. Butt Z et al (2008) Fatigue is the most important symptom for advanced cancer patients who have had chemotherapy. J Natl Compr Canc Netw 6(5):448–455
8. Mock V et al (2007) Cancer-related fatigue. Clinical practice guidelines in oncology. J Natl Compr Canc Netw 5(10):1054–1078

9. Hall EJ, Brenner DJ (2008) Cancer risks from diagnostic radiology. Br J Radiol 81(965): 362–378
10. Podoloff DA et al (2009) NCCN task force: clinical utility of PET in a variety of tumor types. J Natl Compr Canc Netw 7(Suppl 2):S1–26
11. Razifar P et al (2009) Masked volume wise principal component analysis of small adrenocortical tumours in dynamic [11C]-metomidate positron emission tomography. BMC Med Imaging 9:6
12. Khan TS et al (2003) 11C-metomidate PET imaging of adrenocortical cancer. Eur J Nucl Med Mol Imaging 30(3):403–410
13. Miller BS et al (2010) Laparoscopic resection is inappropriate in patients with known or suspected adrenocortical carcinoma. World J Surg 34(6):1380–1385

Part VIII
Unique Cohorts and Future Perspectives

Chapter 27
Aldosterone-Producing Adrenocortical Carcinoma

Anna Patalano, Maria V. Cicala, and Franco Mantero

27.1 Epidemiology

In 1955 Conn described the syndrome of primary hyperaldosteronism (PHA) [1], which has come to be known as "Conn's Syndrome" [2]. PHA is a group of disorders in which aldosterone production is inappropriately high, relatively autonomous from the renin-angiotensin system, and nonsuppressible by sodium loading. Such inappropriate production of aldosterone causes cardiovascular damage, suppression of plasma renin, hypertension, sodium retention, and potassium excretion that if prolonged and severe may lead to hypokalemia. PHA is commonly caused by adenoma (35%), bilateral adrenal hyperplasia (60%), or (rarely) by aldosterone producing adrenocortical carcinoma (APAC) (<1%) (Table 27.1) [3]. The first APAC was reported in 1955 by Foye and Feichtmeir [4] shortly after Conn's original report. Aldosterone hypersecretion in adrenocortical carcinoma (ACC) is rare with only 58 patients being reported in a recent review [5]. The reported numbers of APAC amongst ACCs vary significantly. In one large series of ACCs, only 2.5% had developed hyperaldosteronism [6]. In a single center analysis on ACCs, which were subjected to operative management at the Mayo Clnic, the portion of APACs was 11%. Conversely, it has been estimated that hyperaldosteronism is due to APAC in only 1% of patients with PHA [7].

A main resource is a database created by Seccia et al., containing all reported APAC cases. This database served to delineate the clinical features and characteristics, natural history, and survival of patients with APAC [5]. The peak incidence of APAC is between 40 and 49 years of age (median 44 years, range 17–19 years) with a trend towards a preference for female (57%) vs. male gender (43%). More APAC arise from the right than the left side (58% vs. 42%) (Table 27.2). While the APAC Registry does not include any cases of childhood APAC, analysis of the International Pediatric Adrenocortical Tumor Registry (IPACTR) reports at least two cases [8].

A. Patalano (✉)
Division of Endocrinology, Department of Medical and Surgical Sciences, University of Padua, Via Ospedale 105, 35128 Padova, Italy
e-mail: anna.patalano@libero.it

G.D. Hammer, T. Else (eds.), *Adrenocortical Carcinoma*,
DOI 10.1007/978-0-387-77236-3_27, © Springer Science+Business Media, LLC 2011

Table 27.1 Causes of primary hyperaldosteronism

	Frequency (%)
Aldosterone-producing adenoma (APA)	35%
Bilateral adrenal hyperplasia with idiopathic hyperaldosteronism (IHA)	60%
Unilateral adrenal hyperpalsia	2%
Aldosterone producing adrenal carcinoma (APAC)	<1%
Familial forms of hyperaldosteronism	
– FH – I (GRA)	<1%
– FH – II (APA o IHA)	<2%
Ectopic aldosterone-producing adenomas or carcinomas	<0.1%

Table 27.2 Demographic and clinical features

Variables	Value
Age (years)	44 (17–79)
Gender (M/F/NA) (*n*)	21/27/10
Side of tumour (R/L/NA) (*n*)	26/18/14
Maximum tumor diameter (mm)	70 (25–150)
Tumor mass weight (g)	248 (6.3–1250)
Systolic blood pressure (mmHg)	188±4
Diastolic blood pressure (mmHg)	111 ± 2
Hypertension (*n* of cases; %)	55 (95%)
Plasma potassium levels (mmEq/l)	2.30 ± 0.08
Hypokalemia (present/absent/NA) (*n*, %)	56 (96%)/1 (1.7%)/1 (1.7%)
Low plasma renin activity (present/absent/NA) (*n*, %)	32 (55%)/10 (17%)/16 (27%)
% increase of aldosterone from the upper normal value	+14 (1.1–333)
Adrenalectomy (performed/not performed/NA)	52/4/2

M male, *F* female, *NA* not available, *R* right, *L* left
Source: Reference [5]

However, distinction between malignant and benign cases in this database is not simple (see Chapter 28).

27.2 Clinical and Hormonal Features

Some APACs do not only produce aldosterone, but also secrete other steroid hormones in excess [2, 9–12]. In the analysis by Seccia et al. plasma cortisol was concurrently elevated in 10% of APAC. However, data in this review were insufficient; to draw definitive conclusions on the secretion of other steroid hormones in patients with APAC because data were not always reported in the referenced literature. In a single center study conducted by Kendrick et al., 3 of 15 APACs co-secreted aldosterone and cortisol and another two APAC secreted aldosterone together with both cortisol and androgens. In fact, mineralocorticoid excess as the only biochemical evidence of excessive hormone secretion by ACC is very uncommon [12]. On the contrary, the demonstration of excessive production of multiple steroid hormones by an adrenal tumor is suggestive of an ACC. Therefore, in patients with a known hyperaldosteronism, the measurement of other steroid hormones, mainly cortisol but also adrenal androgens, may be of a potential use to further guide clinical treatment and postoperative tumor surveillance.

In a study series of 105 patients presenting with PHA, Salassa et al. [12] reported six patients with large adrenocortical tumors. Four of these tumors had histological features of malignancy while two had a "benign" histology. This study indicates that although APAC is not a common cause of PHA, 4–5% of patients in a single large series had an APAC as the cause of PHA. In most cases of APAC the clinical picture consists of the classical signs of Conn's syndrome, e.g., hypertension and hypokalemia. The latter, when marked, was reported to be associated with weakness and diffuse muscular pain, cramps, headache, tachycardia, polyuria, polydypsia, and nocturia. All of these signs and symptoms are common in PHA due to any cause (adrenocortical adenoma or hyperplasia) and are therefore not helpful in identifying APACs on a clinical basis [5]. Other electrolyte abnormalities may also be observed. A rare clinical manifestation reported in a few cases was tetany associated with low plasma concentration of calcium and severe hypokalemic alkalosis. Plasma sodium concentration could be normal or high. In general, the magnitude of hypokalemia and hyperaldosteronuria tends to be greater in patients with malignant tumors [12], but these patients cannot be clearly separated from those with benign tumors or hyperplasia on the basis of laboratory values. Moreover, a good response to spironolactone for months does not exclude APAC as cause of PHA [13].

There have been a number of cases of ACC that clinically presented as isolated hypermineralocorticoidism [3, 14–20], arterial hypertension, and hypokalemic metabolic alkalosis. Messer et al. [8] described a case of concomitant secretion of cortisol, androgens, and 11-deoxycorticosterone (DOC) with consequent aldosterone suppression by an ACC, resulting in a clinical picture consistent with Cushing's syndrome, hyperandrogenism, and primary hypermineralocorticoidism. Moreover, in some cases the apparent mineralocorticoid excess as assumed by laboratory evaluation (hypokalemia) and clinical exam (hypertension) is not the result of excessive aldosterone, but rather induced by other steroid metabolites with mineralocorticoid properties, such as 11-deoxycorticosterone (DOC). These observation have led to the recommendation of routine DOC analysis in the setting apparent mineralocorticoid excess levels as elevated DOC levels make ACC a more likely diagnosis.

A rare occurrence is the possibility of a phenotype switch of an APAC to a cortisol-producing ACC. Abma et al. [21] described a case of hypokalemic hypertension due to PHA caused by unilateral APAC. After removal, the aldosterone excess disappeared. The patient's clinical course was uneventful, until she presented with extensive metastases of ACC 4 years later. Biochemical abnormalities were then consistent with glucocorticoid excess without hyperaldosteronism. This finding is consistent with the possibility that the type of ACC-associated hormone production can change during the course of the disease. This phenomenon has been described rarely and is presumably due to modifications in the expression of specific steroidogenic enzymes during tumor dedifferentiation and/or (relative) deficiencies in specific enzymes involved in adrenocortical steroidogenesis [22, 23].

The origin of hyperaldosteronism is almost always an adrenocoritcal neoplasm, namely primary ACC or APAC. However, there are few isolated exceptions of extra-adrenal aldosterone production [24]. Excess aldosterone production by extra-adrenal tissue was first described by Ehrlich et al. [25] in a 9-year-old girl in a case in which aldosterone most probably originated from a gonadal tumor. In another case of a young woman with PHA, a malignant ovarian tumor, was identified as the source of elevated aldosterone levels [26]. This patient presented with severe hypertension, hypokalemia, temporal headaches, muscular weakness, weight loss, polyuria, and occasional tetany crises. Hormone studies revealed extremely high urinary aldosterone, undetectable plasma renin activity, elevated plasma 17-βestradiol and testosterone, as well as low plasma FSH and LH. Autopsy disclosed an ovarian arrhenoblastoma, with polymorphic aspects. Both adrenal glands were normal. Aldosterone and the enzymatic activity responsible for its synthesis were demonstrated in the neoplastic tissue by radioisotopic techniques. Another case in the literature details an ectopic APAC located in the chest [27]. Flanagan and McDonanld [28] reported excess aldosterone due to an adrenal adenoma located at the inferior pole of the right kidney. The underlying cause of ectopic APAC and ACC as well as for ectopic aldosterone production is unclear. Simple explanations would be that these APACs arise from developmentally displaced adrenocortical tissue as it can commonly be found in human beings and confirmed by mouse modelling [29]. Another possibility, specifically in gonad-related aldosterone production, is the process of transdifferentiation. In general, adrenocortical and stromal gonadal tissues are highly related and arise from the same precursor tissue. Therefore, only a few changes may be necessary to acquire the steroidogenic function of the other tissue.

27.3 Pathology

The differentiation between benign and APAC can be difficult on both clinical and morphological grounds [27]. Although several criteria have been proposed to allow discrimination between benign and malignant tumors [30], including some molecular markers such as the DNA index [30, 31], the expression of proliferating cell nuclear antigen (PCNA) [32], p53 protein [33], steroidogenic factor 1 [34], c-Myc protein [31], or insulin-like growth factor 2 gene [30], and telomerase activity [35], to date none of them has gained wide acceptance because of their poor accuracy. The most widely used scoring system for ACC, including APAC, is the Weiss-score (Weiss) (see Chapter 8).

A large tumor size is usually taken as a presumptive sign of malignancy in clinical practice [36, 37]. In contrast, this rule may not apply to APAC. Seccia et al. show in their meta-analysis that very small tumors can be malignant; 9% of all cases were smaller than 3 cm [36, 38–40] and had developed metastases [27, 38, 39].

The site of metastastic spread does not differ markedly for APAC compared to usual ACC. APAC may develop metastases to liver, lung, abdominal lymph nodes, abdomen, vena cava or diaphragm [41]. Interestingly, metastases are not routinely present at diagnosis but usually develop during follow-up [27]. In some cases metastases can be associated with recurrence of hypertension and hypokalemia, but they could be also silent without increase of aldosterone or hypokalemia, further supporting the evolution of an APAC to a nonfunctional ACC. The histological pattern of APAC is variable between cases and even between different portions of the same tumor (Figs. 27.2 and 27.3). In the reported cases, the macroscopic and microscopic examination of the surgical specimens revealed typical signs of malignancy, such as presence of trabecular pattern, high nuclear grade, high mitotic rate, atypical mitosis, calcifications, areas of necrosis and/or invasion of adjacent tissues [31]. Occasionally, APACs may lack overt signs of malignancy, but follow a malignant course of disease. Alternatively APAC may exhibit malignant features but have a benign course [27]. One APAC has been described in the literature representing as an oncocytoma, a rare form of ACC [42].

27.4 Imaging Characteristics

In the study by Seccia et al. only about half of the APACs that were subjected to CT imaging showed at least one sign of malignancy (heterogeneous density, calcifications, capsular invasion, organ displacement, intra-mass hemorrhages), which are also often seen in other ACCs or metastatic neoplasms. Therefore, these signs are nondiagnostic regarding the differential diagnosis ACC vs. APAC, but certainly help to raise the suspicion of a malignant lesion [43]. It remains uncertain whether other imaging modalities, such as MRI, will proof superior to the currently most widely used CT imaging in differentiating APAC from other causes of PHA. As for ACC, enhanced CT imaging can reveal a large, low-attenuation suprarenal mass containing areas of high attenuation that are consistent with hemorrhage. The lesion appears heterogeneous and commonly contains central necrosis and calcifications. Whether the MRI features could be more specific remains unsettled, because of the lack of information on this technology in APAC.

27.5 Prognosis

Generally, the clinical course of APAC is characterized by poor survival, but may be slightly better than for usual ACC. Seccia et al. [5] found that the median survival rate of APAC was 546 days. Cox regression showed that age, hypokalemia, weight, diameter of the adrenal mass, histological signs of malignancy, or metastases at the time of diagnosis did not predict survival (Fig. 27.1). In the study by Kendrick et al. a trend towards increased survival compared to non-aldosterone-secreting ACCs was observed. There are certainly no prospective studies on this extremely rare disease

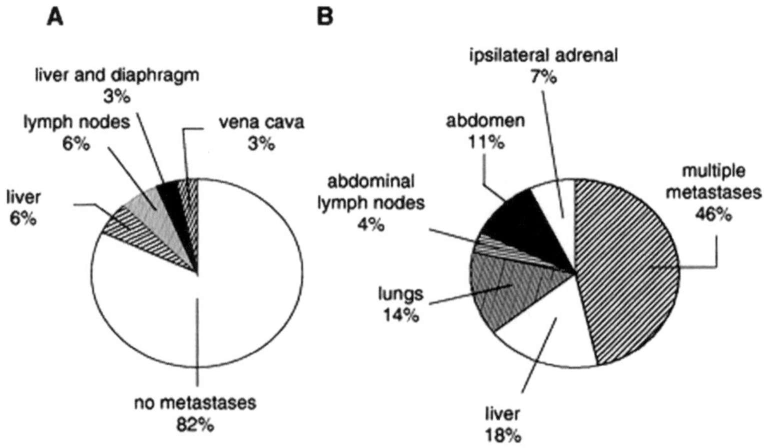

Fig. 27.1 Localization of metastases in APAC. (**a**) Pie graph shows occurrence of metastases at the time of the initial diagnosis. No metastases were observed in 82% of cases. In the remaining cases metastases were localized in liver (6%), lymph nodes (6%), vena cava (3%), or in liver and diaphragm (3%). (**b**) Localization of metastases at the time of the recurrence of the disease. In most cases (46%) they developed in multiple sites. Single localization occurred in liver, lungs, abdomen, ipsilateral adrenal, and abdominal lymph nodes. Values were calculated as percentage of cases developing metastases [5]

entity. Surveillance after initial surgical resection should be identical to the clinical practice guidelines for ACC. The unique feature of potential hormone phenotypic switching suggests that in addition to regular clinical and laboratory follow-up with potassium, aldosterone, plasma renin activity and blood pressure measurements, the clinician should be on the alert for a switch in or loss of hormone production in patients with APAC.

27.6 Treatment

When APAC is suspected, surgical removal should be performed as early as possible. Open adrenalectomy is currently recommended (based on tumor size and imaging features) [44, 45]. While supplemental glucocorticoid therapy should be started after surgical resection of mixed aldosterone-cortisol-secreting tumors to avoid adrenal insufficiency, in general there is no need of mineralocorticoid substitution after removal of aldosterone-secreting tumors. Moreover, spironolactone and K-repletion can be stopped before the tumor removal in anticipation of postoperative hyperkalemia [46]. In patients with large incurable APAC, tumor debulking may also help improve the results of other medical therapies. Surgical removal of limited metastases can also be appropriate. Treatment of patients with APAC has two major challenges; tumor control and protection from the deleterious effects of mineralocorticoid excess. Regarding tumor control, when APAC is suspected or established, therapy follows the same practice as for ACC in general with surgical

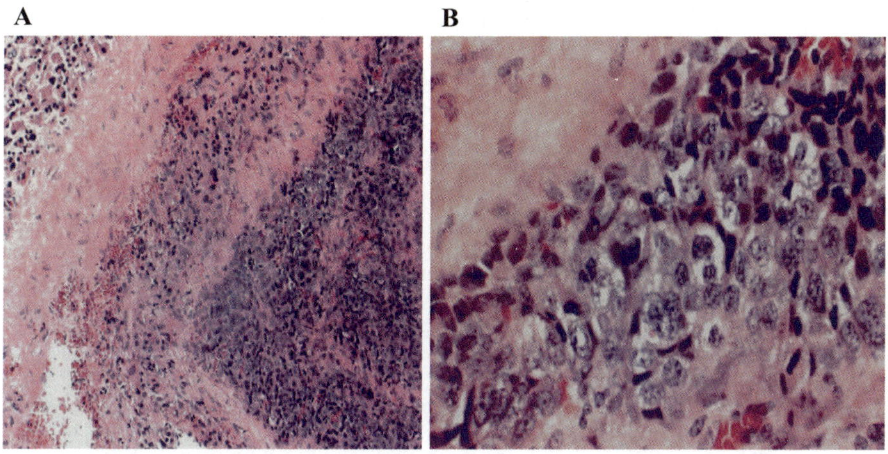

Fig. 27.2 Histopathology of the aldosterone-producing adrenocortical carcinoma (APAC) from case 1. (**a**) The large areas of necrosis and hemorrhage present in the tumor are circumscribed by ill-defined, coarse collagen bands (hematoxylin and eosin staining; Scale bar: 70 μm). (**b**) The nuclei are atypical, hyperchromatic, and pleomorphic with coarse chromatin and two or three prominent nucleoli; the cytoplasms are ill defined, eosinophilic, and pale (hematoxylin and eosin staining; Scale bar: 30 μm) [5]

removal should be performed as early as possible, with potential postoperative adjuvant medical therapy with mitotane and chemotherapy in patients at III–IV stage [47–49].

Interestingly, in a retrospective analysis Kendrick et al. found that perioperative mortality was significantly higher (20%) with APAC when compared to non-aldosterone-producing ACC. All of the patients who died perisurgically had disseminated disease and the surgical approach was palliative. Control of hormone excess is discussed in Chapter 23 and mainly consists of peripheral mineralocorticoid

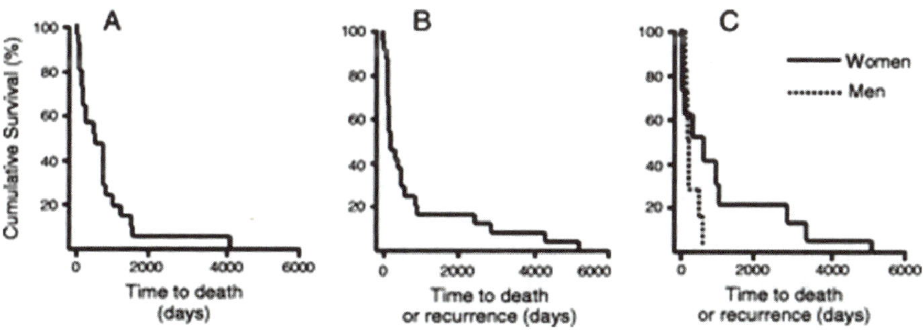

Fig. 27.3 Survival and recurrence-free survival rates in APAC. Kaplan–Meier analysis showed that median survival, considered as time elapsing from diagnosis to death or study end, was 546 days (**a**). The median recurrence-free survival, that was calculated as time elapsing from diagnosis to either recurrence or death, was 212 days (**b**). Recurrence-free survival according to gender showed a worse trend in men than in women (**c**), but this did not attain statistical significance [5]

antagonism through use of agents such as spironolactone. As with all patients with PHA, the clinical challenge is blood pressure control, which can also be achieved with potassium sparing agents like amiloride, triamterene, and calcium antagonists as second line medications.

References

1. Conn JW (1955) Primary aldosteronism. J Lab Clin Med 45:661–664
2. Hajjar RH et al (1975) Adrenal cortical carcinoma- a study of 32 cases. Cancer 35:549–554
3. Funder JW et al (2008) Endocrine society. Case detection, diagnosis, and treatment of patients with primary aldosteronism: an endocrine society clinical practice guideline. J Clin Endocrinol Metab Sep 93(9):3266–3281
4. Foye LV Jr, Feichtmeir TV (1955) Adrenal cortical carcinoma producing solely mineralocorticoid effect. Am J Med 19:966–975
5. Seccia TM et al (2005) Aldosterone-producing adrenocortical carcinoma: an unusual cause of Conn's syndrome with an ominous clinical course. Endocr Relat Cancer 12: 149–159
6. Ng L, Libertino JM (2003) Adrenocortical carcinoma: diagnosis, evaluation and treatment. J Urol 169:5–11
7. Mattsson C, Young WF Jr (2006) Primary aldosteronism: diagnostic and treatment strategies. Nat Clin Pract Nephrol 2:198–208
8. Messer CK et al (2007) Concomitant secretion of glucocorticoid, androgens, and mineralcorticoid by an adrenocortical carcinoma: case report and review of literature. Endocr Pract. Jul–Aug 13(4):408–412
9. Hogan TF et al (1980) A clinical and pathological study of adrenal carcinoma. Cancer 45:2880–2883
10. Libè R et al (2007) Adrenocortical cancer: pathophysiology and clinical management. Endocr Relat Cancer 14(1):13–28
11. Lipsett MB et al (1963) Clinical and pathophysiologic aspects of adrenocortical carcinoma. Am J Med 35:374–383
12. Salassa RM et al (1975) Primary aldosteronism and malignant adrenocortical neoplasia. Trans Am Clin Clin Assoc 86:163–169
13. Levine DS et al (1984) Isolated production of aldosterone by a malignant adrenal carcinoma yale. J Biol Med 57(6):833–841
14. Alterman SL et al (1969) Primary adrenocortical carcinoma causing aldosteronism. Cancer 24:602–609
15. Brooks RV et al (1957) Potassium deficiency of renal and adrenal origin. Am J Med 23: 391–407
16. Crane MG et al (1965) Primary aldosteronism due to adrenal carcinoma. Ann Intern Med 63:494–503
17. Feldman S, Ravera JJ (1961) Arterial hypertension caused by a primary malignant adrenocortical tumor. Thorax Dec 10:284–288
18. Knapton PJ (1965) Hypokalemic alkalosis in adrenal carcinoma. Lancet ii:346
19. Santander S et al (1965) Case of probable mineralcorticoid excess without hypercortisolism due to carcinoma of the adrenal cortex. J Clin Endocrinol 25:1429–1435
20. Zimmerman B et al (1959) Physiologic and surgical problems in the management of primary aldosteronism. Ann Surg 150:653–664
21. Abma EM et al (2008) Malignant aldosterone-producing adrenal tumor: reoccurrence with glucocorticoid excess without hyperaldosteronism. Neth J Med. Jun 66(6):252–255
22. Barzon L et al (1997) Adrenocortical carcinoma: experience in 45 patients. Oncology 54: 490–496

23. Hisamatsu H et al (2002) Adrenocortical carcinoma with primary aldosteronism associated with Cushing syndrome during recurrence. BJU Int 90:971–972
24. Lack EE Adrenal cortical carcinoma. In: Lack EE (ed) Tumors of the adrenal gland and extradrenal paraganglia. Armed Forces Institute of Pathology, Washington, DC, pp 123–147
25. Ehrlich EN et al (1963) J Clin Endocrinol Metab 23:358
26. Todesco S et al (1975) Primary Aldosteronism due to a malignant ovarian tumor. JCEM 41(5):809–819
27. Rossi GP et al (2000) A thoracic mass with hypertension and hypokalaemia. Lancet 356(9241):1570
28. Flanagan MJ, McDonald JH (1967) Heterotopic adrenocortical adenoma producing primary aldosteronism. J Urol 98:133–139
29. Zubair M et al (2009) Transgenic expression of Ad4BP/SF-1 in fetal adrenal progenitor cells leads to ectopic adrenal formation. Mol Endocrinol 23:1657–1667
30. Gicquel C, Le Bouc Y (1997) Molecular markers for malignancy in adrenocortical tumors. Horm Res 47(4–6):269–272
31. Suzuki T et al (1992b) Discerning malignancy in human adrenocortical neoplasms: utility of DNA flow cytometry and immunohistochemistry. Mod Pathol May 5(3): 224–231
32. Ghnassia JP et al (1993) Adrenal cortical tumors. Prognostic evaluation of a series of 12 cases using anti-PCNA antibodies. Ann Pathol 13(5):312–316
33. Reincke M et al (1994) p53 mutations in human adrenocortical neoplasms: immunohistochemical and molecular studies. J Clin Endocrinol Metab Mar 78(3):790–794
34. Sasano H et al (1995) Transcription factor adrenal 4 binding protein as a marker of adrenocortical malignancy. Hum Pathol Oct 26(10):1154–1156
35. Mannelli M et al (2000) Telomerase activity is significantly enhanced in malignant adrenocortical tumors in comparison to benign adrenocortical adenomas. J Clin Endocrinol Metab Jan 85(1):468–470
36. Greathouse DJ et al (1984) Pure primary hyperaldosteronism due to adrenal cortical carcinoma. Am J Med Jun 76(6):1132–1136
37. Young WF Jr (1997) Pheochromocytoma and primary aldosteronism: diagnostic approaches. Endocrinol Metab Clin North Am Dec 26(4):801–827
38. Deckers S et al (1999) Peritoneal carcinomatosis following laparoscopic resection of an adrenocortical tumor causing primary hyperaldosteronism. Horm Res 52(2):97–100
39. Dixon AN, Bing RF (2001) Two cases of adrenocortical carcinoma presenting as Conn's syndrome. J Hum Hypertens Jan 15(1):75–79
40. Weingärtner K et al (1995) Isolated clinical syndrome of primary aldosteronism in a patient with adrenocortical carcinoma. Case report and review of the literature. Urol Int 55(4): 232–235
41. Taylor W et al (1997) Adrenal carcinoma presenting as Conn's syndrome. Aust N Z J Med Apr 27(2):201–202
42. Ali AE, Raphael SJ (2007) Funchonal Oncocytic adrenocortical carcinoma. Endocr Pathol Fall 18(3):187–189
43. Schulick RD, Brennan MF (1999) Adrenocortical carcinoma. World J Urol Feb 17(1):26–34
44. Cobb W et al (2005) Laparoscopic adrenalectomy for malignancy. Am J Surg 189:405–411
45. Paton BL et al (2006) Outcomes of adrenal cortical carcinoma in the United States. Surgery 140:914–920
46. Biglieri EG et al (1966) Postoperative studies of adrenal function in primary aldosteronism. J Clin Endocr 26:553–558
47. Kendrick ML et al (2002) Aldosterone-secreting adrenocortical carcinomas are associated with unique operative risks and outcomes. Surgery 132:1008–1011
48. Skogseid B et al (2008) Experience from an ongoing phase III study: FIRM-ACT. Abstract book of the 2nd annual international adrenal cancer symposium: clinical and basic science. March 14–15
49. Terzolo M et al (2007) Adjuvant mitotane treatment for adrenocortical carcinoma. N Engl J Med 356:2372–2380

Chapter 28
Adrenocortical Cancer in Children

Carlos Rodriguez-Galindo, Gerard P. Zambetti, and Raul C. Ribeiro

Adrenocortical cancer (ACC) is a rare but aggressive childhood endocrine neoplasm. Its incidence in children is extremely low (only 0.2% of pediatric cancers) [1], and most pediatric oncologists see few cases or none. Little is known about this malignancy and most available information has been learned from its more frequent adult counterpart. In recent years, an international registry has provided insight into the clinical characteristics and relevant management issues regarding pediatric ACC and tumor tissue for biological studies. These studies have resulted in the discovery of a novel mechanism of tumorigenesis [2], the gift to science by one of the rarest childhood cancers.

28.1 Epidemiology of Adrenocortical Cancer

ACC appears to follow a bimodal distribution, with peaks during the first and fourth decades [3]. In children, 25 new cases are expected to occur annually in the United States for an estimated annual incidence of 0.2–0.3 cases per million. Internationally, however, the incidence of ACC appears to vary substantially. The incidence of ACC is particularly high in southern Brazil, where it is approximately 10–50 times that observed in the United States. Most cases occur in the contiguous states of Sao Paulo, Paraná, and Santa Catarina [4–7].

Predisposing genetic factors have been implicated in >50% of the cases in North America and Europe, and in 95% of the Brazilian cases. Germline *TP53* mutations are almost always the predisposing factors. In the non-Brazilian cases, relatives of children with ACC often, though not invariably, have a high incidence of other non-ACC cancers (Li-Fraumeni syndrome), and germline mutations usually occur within the region coding for the *TP53* DNA-binding domain (exons 5–8, primarily at highly conserved amino acid residues). In the Brazilian cases, in contrast, the patients'

C. Rodriguez-Galindo (✉)
Department of Pediatric Oncology, Dana-Farber Cancer Institute and Children's Hospital, 44 Binney Street, Boston, MA 02115, USA
e-mail: carlos_rodriguez-galindo@dfci.harvard.edu

G.D. Hammer, T. Else (eds.), *Adrenocortical Carcinoma*,
DOI 10.1007/978-0-387-77236-3_28, © Springer Science+Business Media, LLC 2011

families do not exhibit a high incidence of cancer, and a single, unique mutation at codon 337 in exon 10 of the *TP53* gene is consistently observed (see below) (see Chapters 11, 12 and 13).

Patients with Beckwith-Wiedemann and hemihypertrophy syndromes have a predisposition to cancer, and as many as 16% of their neoplasms are ACC (see Chapter 14) [8]. However, less than 1% of children with ACC have these syndromes [9]. ACC has also been reported in association with other genetic diseases such as congenital adrenal hyperplasia [10].

The differential diagnosis of ACC includes other diseases characterized by adrenal hormone hyper-production. ACTH-independent macronodular adrenal hyperplasia (AIMAH) is a benign proliferative disorder of the adrenal cortex that presents with ACTH-independent Cushing's syndrome. The majority of patients with AIMAH present in the fifth decade of life with sporadic isolated disease; however, in children AIMAH can be associated with McCune-Albright syndrome [11]. A similar macronodular adrenocortical hyperplasia is seen in up to one third of patients with multiple endocrine neoplasia syndrome type 1 (MEN1) and although rare, ACCs have been described in this population, usually in adult age [12]. Primary pigmented nodular adrenocortical disease (PPNAD) is a benign bilateral proliferative disorder characterized by small hyperpigmented nodules, usually associated with the Carney Complex. This is an autosomal dominant syndrome that includes lentiginosis (perioral, ocular or genital), cardiac and peripheral myxomas, melanotic schwannomas, and endocrine overactivity. Clinically evident PPNAD is seen in up to 30% of patients with Carney Complex and usually presents in childhood, late adolescence, or early adulthood [11].

28.2 Biology of Adrenocortical Carcinoma

The molecular mechanisms of tumorigenesis of the adrenal cortex are not well understood [13, 14]. Carcinogenesis is a multistep process, and the pathogenesis of ACC may combine dedifferentiation and unchecked proliferation induced through the activation of hormonal or growth factor signaling receptors. The insulin-like growth factor (IGF) system is well characterized for its contribution to normal and pathological adrenocortical growth. Clues to the role of this pathway in the development of ACC also came through the recognition of the increased incidence of ACC in children with Beckwith-Wiedemann syndrome (BWS) [9]. Genetic alterations associated with BWS are mapped to regions of chromosome band 11p15 designated BWS chromosomal regions (*BWSCR*) 1, 2, and 3 [9]. *IGF2* is mapped to *BWSCR1*. The strong association of BWS, *IGF2*, and ACC suggests that IGF2 participates in tumorigenesis, and studies have shown increased IGF2 protein and mRNA in ACC [15, 16]. Sporadic ACC also show striking overexpression of *IGF2*, and studies in adults have documented >100-fold higher expression levels in carcinomas in comparison to adenomas and normal adrenal tissue [17]. This differential *IGF2* expression between adenomas and carcinomas does not seem to be observed in pediatric tumors (see below) [18, 19]. Interestingly, the antiproliferative effect of ACTH is blunted in ACC cell lines overexpressing *IGF1R* [20]. Further, transgenic mice expressing *IGF2* postnatally develop adrenal hyperplasia (although not frank malignancy) [21]. Taken together, the evidence strongly suggests that the IGF system is involved in adrenal growth and tumorigenesis. High local IGF2 levels combined with elevated *IGF1R* expression would provide a significant growth advantage, but additional steps are required for neoplastic transformation [13, 14, 20]. Studies in several model organisms indicate the presence of undifferentiated multipotent adrenocortical cells, and a few molecular studies have implicated Wnt signaling pathway activation in ACC [22]. Further investigations are necessary to elucidate the contributions of developmental signaling pathways like Wnt in adrenal tumorigenesis (see Chapter 16).

The hypothetical multistep transformation process also requires intracellular signaling abnormalities other than dedifferentiation- and proliferation-inducing signals. *TP53* mutations appear to underlie such abnormalities in most cases, and ACCs are strongly associated with germline *TP53* mutations (see Chapters 11, 12 and 29). ACCs are among the tumors most increased in frequency in families with Li-Fraumeni syndrome [23–25], suggesting that germline *TP53* mutations exert tissue-specific effects. The diagnosis of ACC in a young patient should be considered a strong indicator of a germline *TP53* mutation, regardless of the family history [25]. A wide spectrum of germline *TP53* alterations have been described in ACC, and these mutations may contribute to the etiology of more than 80% of cases in children [26, 27]. Consistent with the presence of a germline *TP53* mutation, relatives of children with ACC often have a high incidence of cancer; however, the lack of family history should not preclude investigation of *TP53* germline status [26–30]. In North American children, the spectrum of germline *TP53* mutations in ACC is quite diverse, although germline mutations occur primarily in the *TP53* DNA-binding domains (exons 4 to 8) [26, 27, 31]. In the Brazilian cases, by contrast, the patients' families do not have a high incidence of cancer, and a single mutation in exon 10 of the *TP53* gene is consistently observed. This mutation encodes an arginine in place of histidine at codon 337 (*TP53*-R337H) within the tetramerization domain. The families of these children do not share common ancestry. Recent studies have indicated that the R337H mutation is a relatively common polymorphism among southern Brazilians. Further, the penetrance of this mutation is low (only 10–15% of carriers develop ACC), and it appears not to predispose carriers to other malignancies later in life [4]. The wild-type allele is deleted in these tumors, and the mutant p53 protein accumulates in the nucleus. Functional analyses have shown that the mutant p53 retains transactivation function and can induce apoptosis [2]. However, the mutant tetramerization domain is less stable than the wild-type domain and is sensitive to slightly increased pH, suggesting that a unique physiological condition within adrenocortical cells may contribute to the observed tissue-restricted pathogenesis [32]. Thus, this inherited unique *TP53* mutation represents a low-penetrant, hypomorphic allele that contributes to the development of ACC in a tissue specific manner [2]. Other *TP53* mutations, such as the *TP53*R157L, with sufficient activity to suppress Li-Fraumeni syndrome but not ACC, have been described [33], thus the importance of in-depth evaluation and genetic counseling of children with ACC and their families.

Additional genetic alterations may be necessary for malignant transformation. ACCs are characterized by a high frequency of chromosomal gains and amplifications, and several chromosomal subregions containing candidate proto-oncogenes are affected (see Chapter 9) [34–36]. Interestingly, the pattern of genomic imbalances in pediatric ACC appears to be different from their adult counterparts. In a series of nine cases in Southern Brazil, the most consistent findings were a gain of all or part of chromosome arm 9q (eight cases) and amplification of band 9q34 (five cases) [35]. Loncarevic et al. analyzed 14 pediatric ACCs by comparative genomic hybridization. Recurring genomic changes included gains of 1q, 12p, 12q, 1p, 7q, 9q, and 15q; and losses of 4q, 11q, 4p, and 16q [36]. Of particular interest is the consistent finding of gain of 9q in both series. The steroidogenic factor 1 gene (*SF1*, *NR5A1*) is located within this region and has been shown to be overexpressed in nearly all childhood ACC [37]. Enforced expression of *SF1* increases human adrenocortical cell proliferation and promotes adrenocortical tumorigenesis in transgenic mouse models. Collectively, these findings strongly implicate *SF1* as a driver in the initiation and/or progression of ACC. Additional studies are required to determine whether deregulation of *SF1* cooperates with *TP53* loss in ACC.

Microarray studies in childhood ACC show distinct patterns of gene expression that distinguish normal adrenal tissue, adenomas, and carcinomas [19]. A significantly increased expression of *FGFR4* and *IGF2* was found in childhood ACC, although the degree of *IGF2* expression seems to be lower than adult tumors, and in contrast to adult ACC, this expression does not distinguish childhood adrenocortical adenoma from ACC. Also, there was a remarkable correlation in gene expression profiles between normal fetal adrenal tissue and pediatric ACC. There were very significant differences in gene expression between pediatric adenomas and carcinomas; remarkably, expression of major histocompatibility class II genes was lower in carcinomas than in adenomas, suggesting that malignant tumors may have evolved mechanisms to evade recognition by the immune system [19].

The distinctive clinical features suggest that ACC arises from the fetal zone of the fetal adrenal cortex. The fetal zone represents 85% of the adrenal cortex during fetal development, and it is oriented towards dehydroepiandrosterone production. It is thus possible that the presence of a constitutional *TP53* mutation increases the penetrance of ACC in the fetal adrenal cortex with lower risk for the remaining layers. Disruption of the *TP53* pathway under certain conditions may result in abnormalities of other cellular pathways, leading to tumor formation.

28.3 Clinical Characteristics of Pediatric Adrenocortical Carcinoma

The clinical characteristics, treatment, and outcome of ACC have been described mainly in adults; because there are few reports about pediatric ACC, it is difficult to discriminate features unique to either age group. The degree and type of endocrine disturbance appear to be related to patient age [3, 38]. Older patients tend to have a much higher incidence of nonfunctional tumors, whereas more than 90% of childhood ACT are functional [38–41]. Adults usually have mixed virilization-hypercortisolism syndromes, whereas virilization syndrome is the most common presentation in children [38–41].

Despite the rarity of childhood ACC, its clinical and pathologic characteristics have been well characterized in recent years [6, 7, 39–45]. Significant information has been obtained from the International Pediatric Adrenocortical Tumor Registry (IPACTR) (www.stjude.org/ipactr), established in 1990 by the St. Jude Children's Research Hospital International Outreach Program, and institutions in Brazil. The registry has served as an information-exchange web site, and more than 300 patients have been registered to date [46]. The registry now also includes a tumor bank component to collect from international sites both normal and adrenal tumor tissue for detailed biological studies.

Childhood ACC typically present during the first 5 years of life (median age, 3–4 years), although there is a second, smaller peak during adolescence [39, 40, 42, 43, 45–47]. Female sex is consistently predominant in most studies, with a female to male ratio of 1.6:1 [40, 42, 43, 46, 47, 48]. According to the IPACTR data, the female predominance is more significant for patients younger than 3 years of age (1.7:1) and for patients older than 13 years (6.2:1), but not for patients between 3 and 12 years [46]. Because pediatric ACCs are almost universally functional, they cause endocrine disturbances, and a diagnosis is usually made 5–8 months after the first signs and symptoms emerge [40, 42, 46]. Virilization (pubic hair, accelerated growth, enlarged penis, clitoromegaly, hirsutism and acne) due to excess of androgen secretion is seen, alone or in combination with hypercortisolism, in more than 80% of patients (Fig. 28.1). Isolated Cushing's syndrome is very rare (5% of

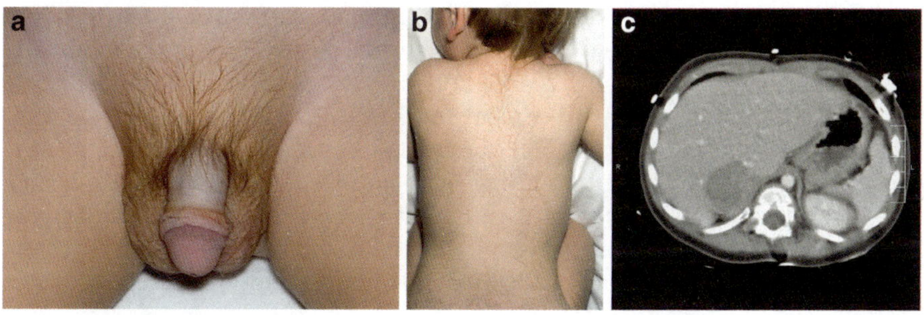

Fig. 28.1 A 2-year-old boy presenting with virilization (**a**, **b**). CT scan demonstrated a right adrenal mass (**c**)

patients), and it appears to occur more frequently in older children (median age 12.6 years in the IPACTR) [40, 42, 45, 46, 48]. Likewise, nonfunctional tumors are rare (less than 10%) and tend to occur in older children [46]. Half of the patients have severe hypertension at presentation, and hypertensive crisis resulting in seizures is the presenting feature in 10% of cases [39, 42, 43, 46, 49]. However, isolated Conn's syndrome with hypertension, hypokalemia, and pseudoparalysis resulting from hyperproduction of aldosterone or deoxycorticosterone is extremely rare (less than 1% in the IPACTR data) but has been described [46, 47]. An abdominal mass can be palpated in approximately half the patients [40, 45].

At the time of diagnosis, two thirds of pediatric patients have limited disease (tumors are completely resected), and the remaining patients have either unresectable or metastatic disease [46]. In up to 20% of the cases intracaval extension of the tumor is present [46, 50]. Unlike adult ACC, histologic differentiation of adenomas and carcinomas is difficult. However, approximately 10–20% of pediatric cases are adenomas [42, 46].

28.4 Diagnosis of Adrenocortical Carcinoma

Children with ACC usually present with striking endocrine syndromes, most commonly virilization, and thus are usually diagnosed earlier than adults. Because of the hormone hypersecretion, it is possible to establish an endocrine profile for each particular tumor, which may facilitate the evaluation of response to treatment and monitor for tumor recurrence. Laboratory evaluation can also help distinguish physiological adrenarche or congenital adrenal hyperplasia from ACC. Patients with adrenarche have elevated basal concentration of DHEAS and androstenedione, while those with congenital adrenal hyperplasia may show increased basal or ACTH-stimulated peak concentration of 17-OH-progesterone [6]. While the diagnosis of ACC is usually clinical, imaging studies are important to complete staging and for surgical planning. Magnetic resonance imaging (MRI) and computed tomography (CT) are needed for evaluation of the size and location of the primary tumor, the degree of invasion to surrounding structures, the presence of metastases, and involvement of venous structures. Although bone metastases at diagnosis are extremely rare, scintigraphic studies are recommended. On CT, large tumors usually have a central area of stellate appearance caused by hemorrhage, necrosis, and fibrosis; this central area is usually hyperintense on T2-weighted MRI and STIR images. Calcifications are also common [51]. In order to evaluate tumor extension into the vena cava ultrasound or MRI are always recommended, and a careful evaluation of the presence of a tumor thrombus must always be performed prior to surgery [6, 50]. Because ACCs are metabolically active whole-body fluorodeoxyglucose (FDG) positron-emission tomography (PET) is being increasingly used. Although the experience in pediatrics is limited, available information suggests that this may be a very useful technique in the imaging of the regional and metastatic extension, and in the diagnosis of recurrences in areas not typically imaged [52, 53].

The distinction between benign (adenomas) and malignant (carcinomas) tumors can be problematic. In fact, adenoma and carcinoma appear to share multiple genetic aberrations and may represent points on a continuum of cellular transformation (see Chapter 9) [34, 35]. Macroscopically, adenomas tend to be well defined and spherical, and they never invade surrounding structures. They are typically small (usually <200 cm^3), and some studies have included size as a criterion for adenoma. Microscopically, they may resemble normal adrenal cortex. By contrast, carcinomas have macroscopic features suggestive of malignancy; they are larger, and they show marked lobulation with extensive areas of hemorrhage and necrosis. Microscopically, carcinomas comprise larger cells with eosinophilic cytoplasm, arranged in alveolar clusters. Several authors have proposed histologic criteria that may help to distinguish the two types of neoplasm [54, 55] However, morphologic criteria may not allow reliable distinction of benign and malignant ACC. Mitotic rate is consistently reported as the most important determinant of aggressive behavior [56–59]. *IGF2* expression also appears to discriminate between carcinomas and adenomas in adults, but not in children [18, 19, 60, 61]. Other histopathologic variables are also important, and risk groups may be identified on the basis of a score derived from characteristics, such as venous, capsular, or adjacent organ invasion, tumor necrosis, mitotic rate, and the presence of atypical mitoses [58]. Two retrospective studies have investigated the histological criteria of malignancy in pediatric ACC. Bugg et al. analyzed the histology, ploidy, proliferative index, and tumor size in 54 cases [44]. The histologic criteria for malignant tumors were the mitotic index, the presence of confluent necrosis and atypical mitoses, and the nuclear grade, as previously defined by Weiss [54, 56]. The most statistically significant predictors of outcome were tumor histology and tumor weight (<100 vs. >100 g). Ploidy and proliferative index were not predictive of outcome [44]. More recently, Wienecke et al. analyzed features associated with increased probability of a malignant behavior in a series of 83 pediatric ACCs [42]. Tumor weight >400 g, tumor size >10.5 cm in the largest diameter, vena cava, capsular or vascular invasion, extension into periadrenal soft tissues, confluent necrosis, presence of severe nuclear atypia, atypical mitoses, and presence of >15 mitotic figures per 20 high-power field were all associated with adverse outcome. However, on multivariate analysis, only vena cava invasion, presence of necrosis, and high mitotic rate retained prognostic significance. The incorporation of gene expression techniques to the diagnostic evaluation of adrenocortical tumors may provide additional means to anticipate the clinical and biological behavior, both in adult [62] and in pediatric [19] tumors. However, still unknown biological events rather than histopathologic tumor characteristics are likely to dictate clinical behavior.

28.5 Prognostic Factors

In an analysis of 40 cases in Southern Brazil, Ribeiro et al. [39] found tumor volume >200 mL or weight >80 g, and age >3.5 years to be associated with worse outcome, although only tumor size was independently predictive. In the IPACTR data, several clinical features, including age, sex, clinical syndrome, interval between first symptoms and diagnosis, blood pressure, disease stage, tumor spillage, tumor thrombus, and tumor weight were examined for their association with outcome. In patients with localized disease, age between 0 and 3 years, virilization alone, normal blood pressure, disease stage I, absence of spillage during surgery, and tumor weight ≤200 g were associated with a greater probability of survival. In a Cox regression model analysis, only stage I, virilization alone, and age 0 to 3 years were independently associated with a better outcome [46] (Figs. 28.2 and 28.3).

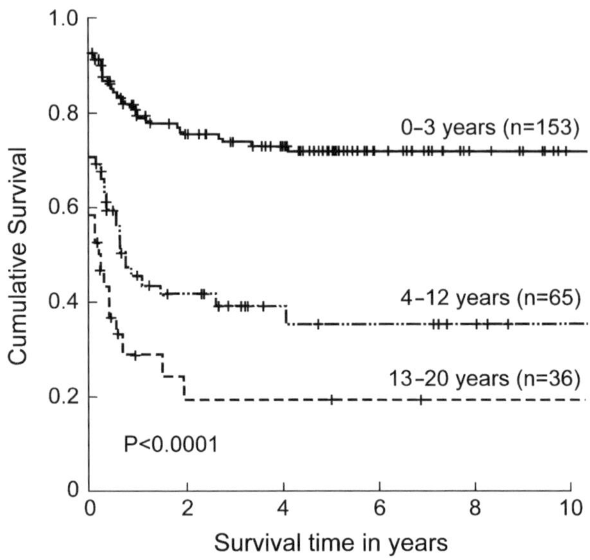

Fig. 28.2 Probability of 5-year event-free survival according to age at the time of diagnosis in 254 children with ACT (from Michalkiewicz et al. [46] with permission)

Thus, available data suggest that tumor size is especially important in children; patients with small tumors have an excellent outcome with surgery alone, regardless of histologic features [39, 42, 44, 46, 63]. A staging system based on disease extent and tumor size has been proposed on the basis of these findings (Table 28.1) [7, 43]. The overall probability of 5-year survival for children with ACC is reported to be 54–74% [40, 42, 43, 45, 46, 48, 50]. Data from the IPACTR and other series show the staging system to be highly predictive of outcome in children with stage I or stage IV disease: more than 90% of patients with stage I disease, but only 10% of those with stage IV disease, are long-term survivors (Fig. 28.3). Determining the prognosis of patients with intermediate-stage disease is much more difficult. Despite presumed complete tumor resection, local recurrence is the most common adverse event in patients with stage II disease (30–50% of cases) [46, 50].

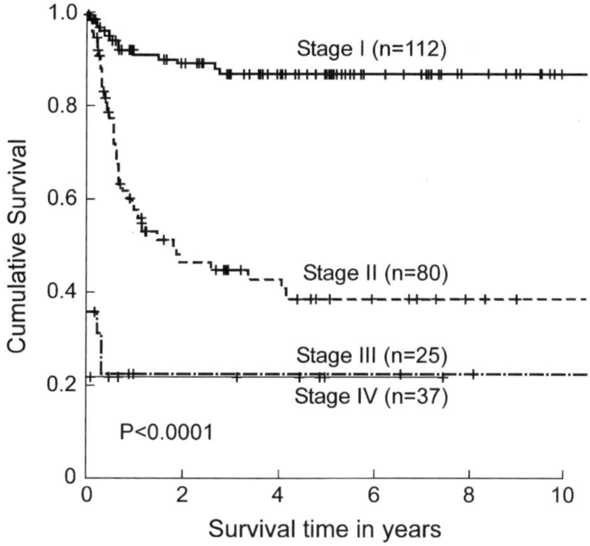

Fig. 28.3 Probability of 5-year event-free survival according to disease stage at the time of diagnosis in 254 children with ACT (from Michalkiewicz et al. [46] with permission)

28.6 Treatment of Pediatric Adrencortical Carcinoma

Treatment of ACC is extensively reviewed in Chapters 20–26. Treatment of childhood ACC has evolved from the data derived from the adult studies, and same guidelines are used; surgery is the most important mode of therapy, and mitotane and cisplatin-based regimens are recommended for patients with advanced disease [6, 7, 64, 65]. An aggressive surgical approach of the primary tumor and all metastatic sites is recommended when feasible [50, 66]. Because of tumor friability, rupture of the capsule with resultant tumor spillage is frequent (approximately 20% of

Table 28.1 Proposed staging of adrenocortical tumors in children

- **STAGE I –**
  - o Completely resected, small tumors (<100 g and <200 cm^3) with normal post-operative hormone levels
- **STAGE II –**
  - o Completely resected, large tumors (≥ 100 g or ≤ 200 cm^3) with normal post-operative hormone levels
- **STAGE III –**
  - o Unresectable, gross or microscopic residual disease
  - o Tumor spillage
  - o Patients with stage I and II tumors who fail to normalize hormone levels after surgery
  - o Patients with retroperitoneal lymph node involvement
- **STAGE IV –**
  - o Presence of distant metastases

Source: Modified from Sandrini et al. [43]

initial resections and 43% of resections after recurrence) [43, 46]. In fact, spontaneous tumor rupture resulting in acute abdomen as presentation of a pediatric ACC has been described [67]. When the diagnosis of ACC is suspected, laparotomy and a curative procedure are recommended rather than fine-needle aspiration to avoid the risk of tumor rupture [68]. Laparoscopic resection is associated with a high risk of rupture and peritoneal carcinomatosis; thus, open adrenalectomy remains the standard of care [69]. The lymph node drainage of the adrenal gland is complex. There is an extensive subserosal network of lymphatic channels around the gland, crossing several levels in different directions inside the fascia and connective tissue involving the adrenal gland. The incidence of lymph node involvement is not known, although some studies report it to be close to 40% in adults [70, 71]. In children, available data suggest that nodal involvement is present in approximately 30% of the cases [66]. Whether ipsilateral retroperitoneal lymph node dissection may improve local control is a matter of debate, and a question currently being investigated in the Children's Oncology Group ARAR0332 study (see below).

Chemotherapeutic regimens used for patients with advanced disease have derived from the standard treatments used in adults. A cisplatin-based combination, usually incorporating doxorubicin and etoposide, is most commonly used [6, 7, 40, 45, 46, 64]. Because of cisplatin's renal dose-limiting toxicity, Ayass and coworkers substituted carboplatin for cisplatin given in combination with etoposide to a 17-month-old boy with ACC that had metastasized to the brain and chest. After complete resection of the primary tumor and eight cycles of etoposide and carboplatin, the metastatic disease responded completely and the patient survived long-term [72].

Little information is available about the use of mitotane in children, although response rates appear to be similar to those seen in adults [6, 64]. There have been several reports of complete responses in children with advanced or metastatic ACC, but these appear to be rare events [73, 74]. In a review of 11 children with advanced ACC treated with mitotane and a cisplatin-based chemotherapeutic regimen, measurable responses were seen in seven patients. The mitotane daily dose required for therapeutic levels was around 4 g/m^2, and therapeutic levels were achieved after 4–6 months of therapy [64]. Compliance with daily mitotane administration is a major limitation to therapy in young children; nausea, vomiting, diarrhea, and neurologic alterations are common [64]. Monitoring for neurotoxicity is particularly important in young patients as the use of mitotane has been associated with motor and speech developmental delays [75].

The use of radiotherapy in pediatric ACC has not been consistently investigated. ACC are generally considered to be radioresistant [38]. Furthermore, because many children with ACC carry germline *TP53* mutations that predispose to cancer, radiation may increase the incidence of secondary tumors. Driver et al. reported that 3 of 5 long-term survivors of pediatric ACC died of secondary sarcoma that arose within the radiation field [41]. For most patients with metastatic or recurrent disease that is unresponsive to mitotane and chemotherapy, repeated surgical resection is the only alternative. However, given the infiltrative nature of the disease, complete resection is difficult to achieve. Image-guided tumor ablation with radiofrequency currently offers a valid alternative for these patients. Radiofrequency ablation is a minimally invasive and safe treatment for patients in whom surgery may not be possible. Using this technique, Wood et al. reported responses in 53% of the adult patients treated; these results suggest that radiofrequency ablation has a role in the management of this aggressive malignancy [76]. Data regarding the use of this treatment modality in children are limited; however, it appears to offer a valid alternative for children with unresectable ACC [77].

Finally, advances in our understanding of ACC biology may lead to the identification of new molecular targets [78]. In particular, new developments in IGF pathway inhibition, such as monoclonal antibodies against the IGF1R, may provide effective alternatives and are currently being investigated [18, 79].

28.7 A Collaborative Research Initiative for Childhood Adrenocortical Carcinoma

Cooperative multi-institutional efforts have been pivotal in the advancement of pediatric oncology during the past several decades. Rare pediatric tumors, however, have remained research orphans, and children with these rare malignancies have yet to benefit from group-wide initiatives. In recent years, the Children's Oncology Group (COG) has made a commitment to develop research programs in rare childhood malignancies. Part of this effort is a collaboration between COG and Brazilian institutions to develop a study protocol for childhood ACC (ARAR0332) (Table 28.2). This protocol investigates three main clinical questions: (1) the efficacy of surgery alone for stage I tumors; (2) the role of retroperitoneal lymph node resection in reducing local recurrence of stage II tumors; and (3) the impact of mitotane and cisplatin-based chemotherapy for unresectable and metastatic disease.

Table 28.2 Treatment on the COG ARAR 0332 protocol

Stage	Treatment
Stage I	• Surgery alone
Stage II	• Surgery • RPLN dissection
Stage III	• Mitotane • CDDP/ETO/DOX • Surgery + RPLN dissection
Stage IV	• Mitotane • CDDP/ETO/DOX • Surgery + RPLN dissection

Abbreviations: *RPLN* retroperitoneal lymph node, *CDDP* cisplatin, *ETO* etoposide, *DOX* doxorubicin

The ARAR0332 protocol also attempts to provide further insight into the biology of ACC and the different patterns of *TP53* mutations. In addition to the near-requisite germline *TP53* mutations, a number of consistent chromosomal gains and losses have been observed in childhood ACC. These genetic alterations presumably favor the expression of tumor-promoting oncogenes while eliminating potential tumor suppressors. Genomic DNA analyses used with microarray gene expression profiling should allow the identification of the genes that cooperate with p53 inactivation to promote development of ACC.

References

1. Bernstein L, Gurney JG (1999) Carcinomas and other malignant epithelial neoplasms. In: Ries LAG et al (eds) Cancer and survival among children and adolescents: United States SEER program 1975–1995. National Cancer Institute, SEER program, Bethesda, MD, pp 139–147
2. Ribeiro RC et al (2001) An inherited p53 mutation that contributes in a tissue-specific manner to pediatric adrenal cortical carcinoma. Proc Natl Acad Sci USA 98:9330–9335
3. Wooten MD, King DK (1993) Adrenal cortical carcinoma. Epidemiology and treatment with mitotane and a review of the literature. Cancer 72:3145–3155
4. Figueiredo BC et al (2006) Penetrance of adrenocortical tumours associated with the germline *TP53* R337H mutation. J Med Genet 43:91–96
5. Pianovski MAD et al (2006) Mortality rate of adrenocortical tumors in children under 15 years of age in Curitiba, Brazil. Pediatr Blood Cancer 47:56–60
6. Ribeiro RC, Figueiredo B (2004) Childhood adrenocortical tumours. Eur J Cancer 40: 1117–1126
7. Rodriguez-Galindo C et al (2005) Biology, clinical characteristics, and management of adrenocortical tumors in children. Pediatr Blood Cancer 45:265–273
8. Hoyme HE et al (1998) Isolated hemihyperplasia (Hemihypertrophy): report of a prospective multicenter study of the incidence of neoplasia and review. Am J Med Genet 79:274–278
9. Steenman M et al (2000) Genetics of Beckwith-Wiedeman syndrome-associated tumors: common genetic pathways. Genes Chromosomes Cancer 28:1–13
10. Varan A et al (2000) Adrenocortical carcinoma associated with adrenogenital syndrome in a child. Med Pediatr Oncol 35:88–90
11. Sutter JA, Grimberg A (2006) Adrenocortical tumors and hyperplasias in childhood – etiology, genetics, clinical presentation and therapy. Pediatr Endocrinol Rev 4:32–39
12. Langer P et al (2002) Adrenal involvement in multiple endocrine neoplasia type 1. World J Surg 26:891–896
13. Kirschner LS (2002) Signaling pathways in adrenocortical cancer. Ann N Y Acad Sci 968:222–239
14. Barlaskar FM, Hammer GD (2007) The molecular genetics of adrenocortical carcinoma. Rev Endocr Metab Disord 8:343–348
15. Ilvesmaki V et al (1993) Insulin-like growth factors (IGFs) and their receptors in adrenal tumors: high IGF-II expression in functional adrenocortical carcinomas. J Clin Endocrinol Metab 77:852–858
16. Boulle N et al (1998) Increased levels of insulin-like growth factor II (IGF-II) and IGF binding protein-2 are associated with malignancy in sporadic adrenocortical tumors. J Clin Endocrinol Metab 83:1713–1720
17. Gicquel C et al (2001) Molecular markers and long-term recurrences in a large cohort of patients with sporadic adrenocortical tumors. Cancer Res 61:6762–6767
18. Almeida MQ et al (2008) Expression of insulin-like growth factor-ii and its receptor in pediatric and adult adrenocortical tumors. J Clin Endocrinol Metab 93:3524–3531
19. West AN et al (2007) Gene expression profiling of childhood adrenocortical tumors. Cancer Res 67:600–608
20. Weber MM et al (2000) The role of the insulin-like growth factor system in adrenocortical tumorigenesis. Eur J Clin Invest 30(Suppl 3):69–75

21. Weber MM et al (1999) Postnatal overexpression of insulin-like growth factor II in transgenic mice is associated with adrenocortical hyperplasia and enhanced steroidogenesis. Endocrinology 140:1537–1543
22. Tissier F et al (2005) Mutations of {beta}-catenin in adrenocortical tumors: activation of the Wnt signaling pathway is a frequent event in both benign and malignant adrenocortical tumors. Cancer Res 65:7622–7627
23. Birch J et al (2001) Relative frequency and morphology of cancers in carriers of germline TP53 mutations. Oncogene 20:4621–4628
24. Kleihues P et al (1997) Tumors associated with *p53* germline mutations. A synopsis of 91 families. Am J Pathol 150:1–13
25. Gonzalez KD et al (2009) Beyond Li Fraumeni syndrome: clinical characteristics of families with p53 germline mutations. J Clin Oncol 27:1250–1256
26. Varley JM et al (1999) Are there low-penetrance *TP53* alleles? Evidence from childhood adrenocortical tumors. Am J Hum Genet 65:995–1006
27. Wagner J et al (1994) High frequency of germline p53 mutations in childhood adrenocortical cancer. J Natl Cancer Inst 86:1707–1710
28. Ariffin H et al (2008) Li-Fraumeni syndrome in a Malaysian kindred. Cancer Genet Cytogenet 186:49–53
29. Khayat CM, Johnston DL (2004) Rhabdomyosarcoma, osteosarcoma, and adrenocortical carcinoma in a child with a germline p53 mutation. Pediatr Blood Cancer 43:683–686
30. Rossbach H-C et al (2008) Composite adrenal anaplastic neuroblastoma and virilizing adrenocortical tumor with germline TP53 R248W mutation. Pediatr Blood Cancer 50: 681–683
31. Reincke M et al (1994) p53 mutations in human adrenocortical neoplasms: immunohistochemical and molecular studies. J Clin Endocrinol Metab 78:790–794
32. DiGiammarino EL et al (2001) A novel mechanism of tumorigenesis involving pH-dependent destabilization of a mutant p53 tetramer. Nat Struct Biol 9:12–16
33. West AN et al (2006) Identification of a novel germ line variant hotspot mutant p53-R175L in pediatric adrenal cortical carcinoma. Cancer Res 66:5056–5062
34. Dohna M et al (2000) Adrenocortical carcinoma is characterized by a high frequency of chromosomal gains and high-level amplifications. Genes Chromosomes Cancer 28: 145–152
35. Figueiredo BC et al (1999) Comparative genomic hybridization analysis of adrenocortical tumors of childhood. J Clin Endocrinol Metab 84:1116–1121
36. Loncarevic IF et al (2008) Number of genomic imbalances correlates with the overall survival for adrenocortical cancer in childhood. Pediatr Blood Cancer 51:356–362
37. Doghman M et al (2007) Increased steroidogenic factor-1 dosage triggers adrenocortical cell proliferation and cancer. Mol Endocrinol 21:2968–2987
38. Wajchenberg BL et al (2000) Adrenocortical carcinoma: clinical and laboratory observations. Cancer 88:711–736
39. Ribeiro RC et al (1990) Adrenocortical carcinoma in children: a study of 40 cases. J Clin Oncol 8:67–74
40. Ciftci AO et al (2001) Adrenocortical tumors in children. J Pediatr Surg 36:549–554
41. Driver CP et al (1998) Adrenal cortical tumors in childhood. Pediatr Hematol Oncol 15: 527–532
42. Wieneke JA et al (2003) Adrenal cortical neoplasms in the pediatric population: a clinicopathologic and immunophenotypic analysis of 83 patients. Am J Surg Pathol 27:867–881
43. Sandrini R et al (1997) Childhood adrenocortical tumors. J Clin Endocrinol Metab 7: 2027–2031
44. Bugg MF et al (1994) Correlation of pathologic features with clinical outcome in pediatric adrenocortical neoplasia. Am J Clin Pathol 101:625–629
45. Teinturier C et al (1999) Clinical and prognostic aspects of adrenocortical neoplasms in childhood. Med Pediatr Oncol 32:106–111

46. Michalkiewicz E et al (2004) Clinical and outcome characteristics of children with adrenocortical tumors. An analysis of 254 cases from the international pediatric adrenocortical tumor registry. J Clin Oncol 22:838–845
47. Narasimhan KL et al (2003) Adrenocortical tumors in childhood. Pediatr Surg Int 19:432–435
48. Hanna AM et al (2008) Outcome of adrenocortical tumors in children. J Pediatr Surg 43: 843–849
49. Wang X et al (2007) Nine cases of childhood adrenal tumour presenting with hypertension and a review of the literature. Acta Paediatr 96:930–934
50. Tucci JR et al (2005) The impact of tumor stage on prognosis in children with adrenocortical carcinoma. J Urol 174:2338–2342
51. Ribeiro J et al (2000) Imaging findings in pediatric adrenocortical carcinoma. Pediatr Radiol 30:45–51
52. Mackie GC et al (2006) Use of [18F]fluorodeoxyglucose positron emission tomography in evaluating locally recurrent and metastatic adrenocortical carcinoma. J Clin Endocrinol Metab 91:2665–2671
53. Murphy JJ et al (2008) Early experience with PET/CT scan in the evaluation of pediatric abdominal neoplasms. J Pediatr Surg 43:2186–2192
54. Weiss LM (1984) Comparative histologic study of 43 metastasizing and nonmetastasizing adrenocortical tumors. Am J Surg Pathol 8:163–169
55. Slooten HV et al (1985) Morphologic characteristics of benign and malignant adrenocortical tumors. Cancer 55:766–773
56. Weiss LM et al (1989) Pathologic features of prognostic significance in adrenocortical carcinoma. Am J Surg Pathol 13:202–206
57. Kendrick ML et al (2001) Adrenocortical carcinoma: surgical progress or status quo? Arch Surg 136:543–549
58. Stojadinovic A et al (2002) Adrenocortical carcinoma: clinical, morphologic, and molecular characterization. J Clin Oncol 20:941–950
59. Harrison LE et al (1999) Pathologic features of prognostic significance for adrenocortical carcinoma after curative resection. Arch Surg 134:181–185
60. Rosati R et al (2008) High frequency of loss of heterozygosity at 11p15 and IGF2 overexpression are not related to clinical outcome in childhood adrenocortical tumors positive for the R337H TP53 mutation. Cancer Genet Cytogenet 186:19–24
61. Erickson LA et al (2001) Pathologic features and expression of insulin-like growth factor-2 in adrenocortical neoplasms. Endocr Pathol 12:429–435
62. de Reynies A et al (2009) Gene expression profiling reveals a new classification of adrenocortical tumors and identifies molecular predictors of malignancy and survival. J Clin Oncol 27:1108–1115
63. Michalkiewicz EL et al (1997) Clinical characteristics of small functioning adrenocortical tumors in children. Med Pediatr Oncol 28:175–178
64. Zancanella P et al (2006) Mitotane associated with cisplatin, etoposide, and doxorubicin in advanced childhood adrenocortical carcinoma. Mitotane monitoring and tumor regression. J Pediatr Hematol Oncol 28:513–524
65. Hovi L et al (2003) Adrenocortical carcinoma in children: a role for etoposide and cisplatin adjuvant therapy? Preliminary report. Med Pediatr Oncol 40:324–326
66. Stewart JN et al (2004) A surgical approach to adrenocortical tumors in children: the mainstay of treatment. J Pediatr Surg 39:759–763
67. Leung LYJ et al (2002) Ruptured adrenocortical carcinoma as a cause of paediatric acute abdomen. Pediatr Surg Int 18:730–732
68. Kardar AH (2001) Rupture of adrenal carcinoma after biopsy. J Urol 166:984
69. Gonzalez RJ et al (2005) Laparoscopic resection of adrenal cortical carcinoma: a cautionary note. Surgery 138:1078–1086
70. Crucitti F et al (1996) the Italian registry for adrenal cortical carcinoma: analysis of a multiinstitutional series of 129 patients. The ACC Italian registry study group. Surgery 119:161–170

71. Lee JE et al (1995) Surgical management, DNA content, and patient survival in adrenal cortical carcinoma. Surgery 118:1090–1098
72. Ayass M et al (1991) High-dose carboplatinum and VP-16 in treatment of metastatic adrenal carcinoma. Am J Pediatr Hematol Oncol 13:470–472
73. Coelho Netto AS et al (1963) Treatment of adrenocortical cancer with o,p′ -DDD. Ann Intern Med 59:74–78
74. Ostuni JA, Roginsky MS (1975) Metastatic adrenal cortical carcinoma: documented cure with combined chemotherapy. Arch Intern Med 135:1257–1258
75. De Leon DD et al (2002) Long-Term (15 Years) outcome in an infant with metastatic adrenocortical carcinoma. J Clin Endocrinol Metab 87:4452–4456
76. Wood BJ et al (2003) Radiofrequency ablation of adrenal tumors and adrenocortical carcinoma metastases. Cancer 97:554–560
77. Hoffer FA et al (2009) A phase 1/pilot study of radiofrequency ablation for the treatment of recurrent pediatric solid tumors. Cancer 115:1328–1337
78. Kirschner LS (2006) Emerging treatment strategies for adrenocortical carcinoma: a new hope. J Clin Endocrinol Metab 91:14–21
79. Barlaskar FM et al (2009) Preclinical targeting of the type I insulin-like growth factor receptor in adrenocortical carcinoma. J Clin Endocrinol Metab 94:204–212

Chapter 29
Genome-Wide Studies in Adrenocortical Neoplasia

Thomas J. Giordano

29.1 Introduction and the Potential of Genomic Studies

In the not too distant past, there existed a mystique amongst pathologists, radiologists, and clinicians regarding neoplasms of the adrenal cortex. Specifically, there was a belief by some that it was not possible to accurately classify adrenal tumors into benign and malignant categories in the absence of metastatic disease. It was this mystical quality that led Larry Weiss and his colleagues to systematically examine the histopathology of a series of adrenocortical tumors and thus derive the evaluation system that bears his name [1, 2]. Despite elegant work by him and others [3], in some respects, this mystical notion regarding the clinical behavior of adrenocortical tumors persists today.

Over the past 8 years, genomic studies of adrenocortical tumors have shed much light on these tumors and made much progress towards dismantling their mystique. Genome-wide gene expression studies have improved our understanding of the pathobiology of these neoplasms, supported and refined their pathologic classification, and have laid the foundation for molecular prognostication and prediction of clinical behavior. This chapter will review those primary genomic studies focused on neoplasms of the adrenal cortex. Studies focused on adrenocortical hyperplasias are not discussed.

29.2 Genome-Wide Gene Expression Studies

In North America, The Director's Challenge Program of the National Cancer Institute was responsible for initiating many DNA microarray-based gene expression profiling studies of common tumor types. While none of these funded programs were for adrenal tumors, the infrastructure provided by a grant to the University

T.J. Giordano (✉)
Departments of Pathology and Internal Medicine, University of Michigan Health System, University of Michigan, 1500 East Medical Center Drive, Ann Arbor, MI 48109, USA
e-mail: giordano@med.umich.edu

G.D. Hammer, T. Else (eds.), *Adrenocortical Carcinoma*,
DOI 10.1007/978-0-387-77236-3_29,

of Michigan facilitated one of the first gene expression studies using a cohort of adrenocortical tissues that included normal cortex (NC), adrenocortical adenoma (ACA), and adrenocortical carcinoma (ACC) [4]. Despite the relatively small cohort and a DNA microarray that represented about a third of the transcriptome, the results were clear and striking. Using principal component analysis (PCA) and hierarchical clustering (HC) of the expression data set, ACCs were clearly shown to be different from NCs and ACAs and thus ACCs consistently expressed a distinct set of genes. Interestingly, a low-grade ACC was intermediate between the NC/ACA and ACC cohorts, a finding that would fit with the notion of histologic progression from ACA to low-grade ACC to high-grade ACC and also illustrated the relationship between histopathology and gene expression profiles. In addition to these global results, relative overexpression of *IGF2* was one of the most dominant transcriptional changes present in the ACC cohort compared to NC and ACA. This finding was entirely consistent with a large body of research that elucidated the role of alterations at the *IGF2* locus as one of the major genetics events present in ACC [reviewed in 5, 6, 7, 8]. Equally interesting was the lack of expression in ACC of other common molecular targets commonly present in other epithelial tumors, such as *EGFR*. Another interesting aspect of this study was the finding of increased expression of angiogenic factors, such as angiopoietin 2 (*ANGPT2*), that highlights the potential importance of angiogenesis in the development of ACC. The two major limitations of this study were the small size of the ACC cohort, thereby preventing a subclassification of ACC, and the lack of outcome data, thereby preventing all types of survival analyses.

Several subsequent DNA microarray studies of adrenocortical tumors have been performed. De Fraipont et al. [9] used a limited cDNA microarray with 230 selected probes to study a set of 57 tumors. Using hierarchical clustering, they separated ACA and ACC and defined several differentially expressed gene sets, i.e., an *IGF2* cluster and a steroidogenesis cluster. This study was the first to incorporate clinical outcome data, permitting identification of genes whose expression discriminated recurring and nonrecurring ACCs.

Slater et al. [10] used a cDNA microarray with 11,540 probes to examine gene expression in 10 ACAs and 10 ACCs. This study, largely confirmatory, identified differentially expressed genes, including *IGF2*. Likewise, Velazquez-Fernandez et al. [11] profiled a small cohort of 13 ACAs and 7 ACCs with a cDNA microarray with 29,760 probes and identified a set of differentially expressed genes.

Two studies in close agreement were recently published [12, 13], an encouraging finding given distinct patient populations (i.e., France and North America). These studies used similar-sized cohorts of benign and malignant adrenocortical tumors and identical oligonucleotide microarrays with near-complete genomic coverage. Both studies showed that benign tumors (ACA or tumors with low Weiss scores) could easily be separated from malignant tumors (ACC or tumors with high Weiss scores) (Figs. 29.1 and 29.2) and further confirmed that ACCs could be separated into two distinct subtypes that reflected tumor grade (i.e., rate of proliferation) in one of the studies (Figs. 29.2 and 29.3) [13] but was not associated with histological changes in the other study, although tumor mitotic rates were not assessed in

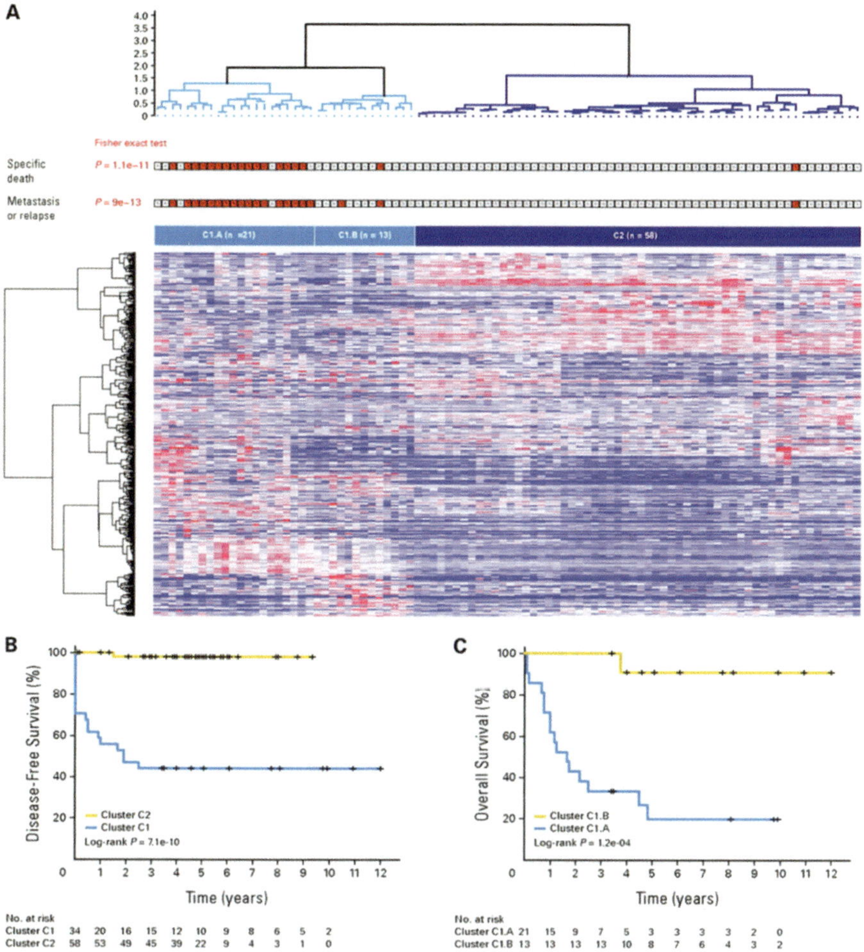

Fig. 29.1 **(a)** Molecular classification of 92 adrenocortical tumors by unsupervised hierarchical clustering. Tumors were broadly divided into benign and malignant groups, and malignant tumors were further divided into two subgroups. **(b, c)** All clusters were associated with difference in overall survival. Reproduced with permission from de Reynies et al. [12]

this study. Importantly, the two ACC subtypes corresponded to differences in survival (Figs. 29.1 and 29.4). One of the studies [12] distilled the gene expression data to two genes (*BUB1B* and *PINK1*), whose expression predicted overall survival even after adjusting for tumor stage (but not mitotic grade). The other study [13] showed that gene expression data, in the form of the Principal Component 1 measurement, contained significant independent prognostic information in Cox models that included stage and mitotic grade. Collectively, these studies nicely illustrate the potential role of gene expression profiling as an adjunctive diagnostic and prognostic tool for the assessment of adrenocortical tumors.

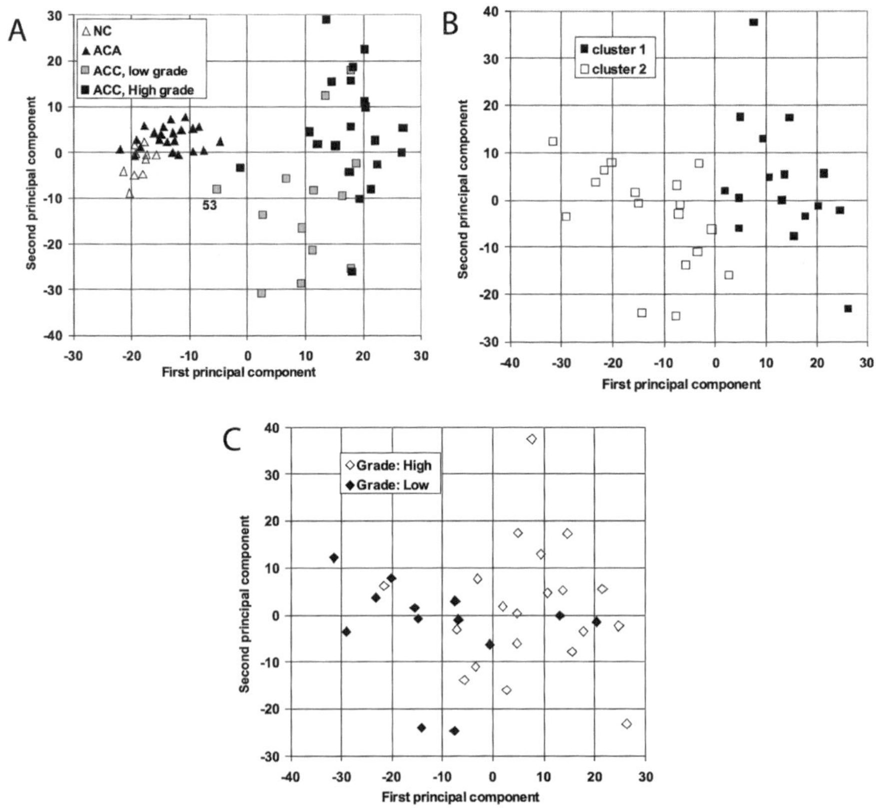

Fig. 29.2 Molecular classification of 55 adrenocortical tumors and 10 normal cortex samples. **(a)** ACC samples were disctinctly different from ACA and NC samples using prinicial component analysis. **(b, c)** ACC samples were separated into two subtypes that reflected ACC tumor grade as determined by mitotic count. Reproduced with permision from Giordano et al. [13]

A recently published report by Laurell et al. [14], a follow-up study of Velazquez-Fernandez et al. [11], used a cDNA microarray to examine expression of 29,760 genes in a cohort of 4 NCs, 17 ACAs, and 11 ACAs. Unsupervised analyses showed clear discrimination of NC/ACA from ACC samples, with the exception of one ACC that profiled with the NC/ACA group. This tumor was associated with an excellent outcome and thus may represent an ACA rather than ACC. This study confirmed the importance of the IGF signaling pathway and the ubiquitination pathway in ACC. Finally, although the ACC cohort was small, the authors suggested that *BUB1B* and *PINK1* (the genes identified by de Reynies et al. [12]) might be useful predictors of survival.

A few studies have specifically addressed the issue of adrenocortical neoplasms in pediatric patients. The study by West et al. [15] examined gene expression profiles in a series of pediatric tumors (5 ACA, 18 ACC, and one tumor of uncertain malignant potential) and NC. Distinct gene expression profiles were determined, although

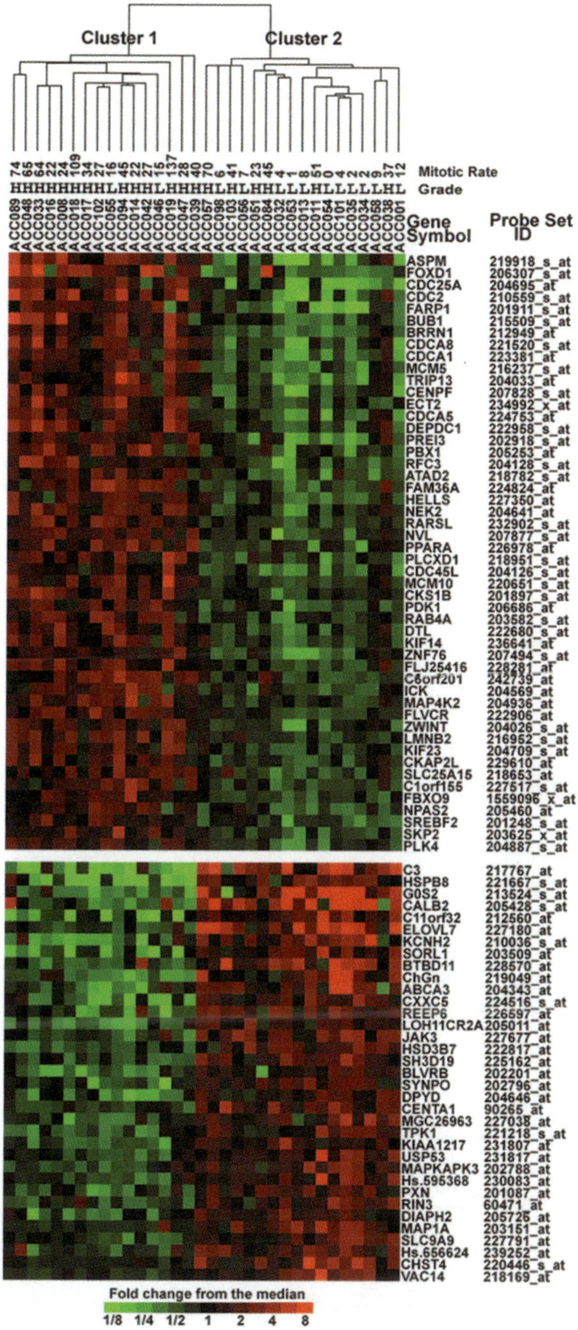

Fig. 29.3 Primary gene expression differences between two ACC clusters that reflect tumor grade as determined by mitotic count. Reproduced with permision from Giordano et al. [13]

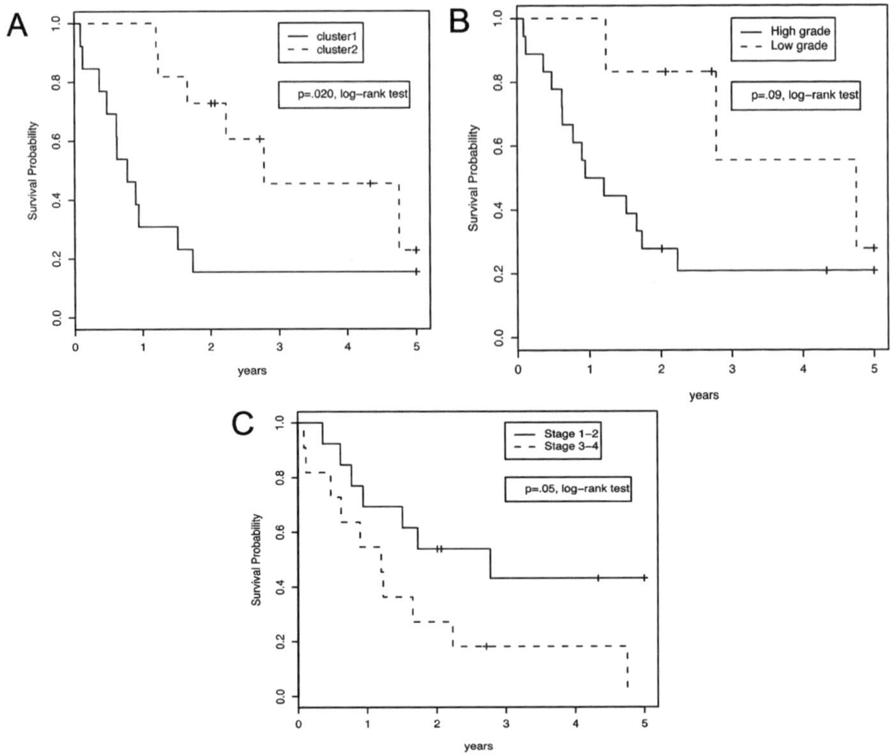

Fig. 29.4 Survival differences between ACC clusters **(a)**, tumor grade **(b)**, and stage **(c)**. Reproduced with permision from Giordano et al. [13]

with not the same false discovery rates seen in studies of adult tumors. There was some similarity among the differentially expressed genes compared to adult tumors. The most recent study by Giordano et al. [13] did include a few pediatric tumors that were indistinguishable from the adult cases. Defining diagnostic biomarkers for pediatric tumors would represent a true advance, as determining malignant potential in these tumors can be difficult.

29.3 Array-Based Comparative Genomic Hybridization

Recent advances in microarray technology have permitted assessment of acquired copy number changes in tumors [16, 17]. Using one such technology, array-based comparative genomic hybridization, Stephan et al. [18] identified recurrent copy number changes in cohort of 25 ACC samples. Interestingly, some of the alterations (amplification of 6q, 7q, 12q, and 19p and deletions of 3, 8, 10p, 16q, 17q, and 19q) were associated with differential survival. These results represent a starting point for the investigation of these potentially important chromosomal regions, although a particular challenge is the distinction of general tumoral aneuploidy from specific genetic alterations. As observed in one of the recent gene expression profiling studies [13], many ACCs, particularly high-grade tumors, share a gene expression pattern associated with aneuploidy.

29.4 MicroRNA Profiling

A recently published microRNA (miRNA) profiling study of 36 adrenocortical tissues and tumors revealed differentially expressed miRNAs and that the difference between two miRNAs (miR-511 and miR-503) could distinguish ACA from ACC with high sensitivity and specificity [19]. While the results need to be validated by other groups and with larger ACC sets, the date are is diagnostically exciting as miRNAs are relatively stable and thus better survive routine pathology processing compared to mRNAs.

29.5 Molecular Profiling and Its Potential Impact on Adrenal Pathology and Management of Patients with Adrenal Cancer

Genomic evaluation of adrenocortical tumors has great potential to favorably impact their evaluation in several regards, including diagnosis, prognosis, prediction of behavior, and response to therapy, as discussed below.

29.5.1 Diagnosis

It is clear from the studies performed to date that gene expression studies have the potential to classify adrenocortical tumors into groups with and without the ability to invade and metastasize (i.e., malignant potential). However, pathologists with experience in these rare tumors also possess accurate diagnostic skills in this regard. Thus, the essential question becomes in which clinical setting does DNA microarray analysis have potential as a clinical diagnostic. It can be surmised that patients with tumors in which experienced pathologists classify as having "uncertain malignant potential" stand to benefit from this technology. Beyond those cases, traditional histopathologic evaluation will likely remain the mainstay of diagnostic classification. More simply stated, pathologic evaluation is and will continue to be adequate for the diagnosis of the 1.5 cm lipid-rich ACA and the 10 cm high-grade ACC.

29.5.2 Prognosis

The most recent gene expression studies, outlined above, have illustrated the potential of defining gene expression profiles that are associated with patient survival. Some of the remaining questions include the following: Which genes are most informative? Are they informative in all cases of ACC or some histologic or molecular subset yet to be defined (i.e., tumors with WNT pathway activation)? How well do expression profiles compete with traditional histopathologic grading such as mitotic figure counting? In ACCs with multiple histologic clones, which is the appropriate clone for molecular profiling? Once these questions and others have been addressed, it is likely that a gene expression assay and future genomic/epigenomic profiles can be routinely offered to ACC patients to further refine their prognosis.

29.5.3 Prediction

There is great enthusiasm that molecular profiles of tumors will be shown to possess significant predictive power for a whole range of clinical parameters, such as metastatic patterns and response to cancer therapy. Much work needs to be done in this area regarding adrenocortical tumors, yet work from other tumor types is encouraging [20, 21, 22].

29.6 Conclusion

In summary, it is possible to envision a not-too-distant future in which patients with adrenocortical tumor will have their tumors molecularly profiled to (1) confirm the diagnosis in diagnostically difficult cases, (2) provide a more refined assessment of their prognosis, and (3) assist in management by guiding the clinical workup and choice of therapies. However, much work yet remains to be done before we can realize this exciting and promising future of personalized care for patients with adrenal cancer.

References

1. Lau SK, Weiss LM (2009) The Weiss system for evaluating adrenocortical neoplasms: 25 years later. Hum Pathol 40:757–768
2. Weiss LM (1984) Comparative histologic study of 43 metastasizing and nonmetastasizing adrenocortical tumors. Am J Surg Pathol 8:163–169
3. van Slooten H et al (1985) Morphologic characteristics of benign and malignant adrenocortical tumors. Cancer 55:766–773
4. Giordano TJ et al (2003) Distinct transcriptional profiles of adrenocortical tumors uncovered by DNA microarray analysis. Am J Pathol 162:521–531
5. Barlaskar FM, Hammer GD (2007) The molecular genetics of adrenocortical carcinoma. Rev Endocr Metab Disord 8:343–348

6. Bertherat J, Gimenez-Roqueplo AP (2005) New insights in the genetics of adrenocortical tumors, pheochromocytomas and paragangliomas. Horm Metab Res 37:384–390
7. Libe R, Bertherat J (2005) Molecular genetics of adrenocortical tumours, from familial to sporadic diseases. Eur J Endocrinol 153:477–487
8. Stratakis CA (2003) Genetics of adrenocortical tumors: gatekeepers, landscapers and conductors in symphony. Trends Endocrinol Metab 14:404–410
9. de Fraipont F et al (2005) Gene expression profiling of human adrenocortical tumors using complementary deoxyribonucleic acid microarrays identifies several candidate genes as markers of malignancy. J Clin Endocrinol Metab 90:1819–1829
10. Slater EP et al (2006) Analysis by cDNA microarrays of gene expression patterns of human adrenocortical tumors. Eur J Endocrinol 154:587–598
11. Velazquez-Fernandez D et al (2005) Expression profiling of adrenocortical neoplasms suggests a molecular signature of malignancy. Surgery 138:1087–1094
12. de Reynies A et al (2009) Gene expression profiling reveals a new classification of adrenocortical tumors and identifies molecular predictors of malignancy and survival. J Clin Oncol 27:1108–1115
13. Giordano TJ et al (2009) Molecular classification and prognostication of adrenocortical tumors by transcriptome profiling. Clin Cancer Res 15:668–676
14. Laurell C et al (2009) Transcriptional profiling enables molecular classification of adrenocortical tumours. Eur J Endocrinol 161:141–152
15. West AN et al (2007) Gene expression profiling of childhood adrenocortical tumors. Cancer Res 67:600–608
16. Higgins RA et al (2008) Clinical application of array-based comparative genomic hybridization for the identification of prognostically important genetic alterations in chronic lymphocytic leukemia. Mol Diagn Ther 12:271–280
17. Mantripragada KK et al (2004) Genomic microarrays in the spotlight. Trends Genet 20:87–94
18. Stephan EA et al (2008) Adrenocortical carcinoma survival rates correlated to genomic copy number variants. Mol Cancer Ther 7:425–431
19. Tombol Z et al (2009) Integrative molecular bioinformatics study of human adrenocortical tumors: microRNA, tissue-specific target prediction, and pathway analysis. Endocr Relat Cancer 16:895–906
20. Kunz M (2008) Genomic signatures for individualized treatment of malignant tumors. Curr Drug Discov Technol 5:9–14
21. Potti A, Nevins JR (2008) Utilization of genomic signatures to direct use of primary chemotherapy. Curr Opin Genet Dev 18:62–67
22. Wulfkuhle J et al (2004) Genomic and proteomic technologies for individualisation and improvement of cancer treatment. Eur J Cancer 40:2623–2632

Chapter 30
New Strategies for the Treatment of Adrenocortical Carcinoma

Lawrence S. Kirschner

As detailed elsewhere in this volume, ACC is a rare disease with a poor prognosis [1]. Although advances have been made in the identification of cytotoxic chemotherapy regimens that produce some benefit in ACC, these cancers remain poorly responsive to standard treatments and the incidence of complete remission is very low.

Over the past 10 years, significant progress has been made in characterizing the biology of ACC and other tumor types at the molecular level. These advances parallel improvements in the ability to target specific signaling pathways within the cell, providing the hope that these two areas of investigation may eventually be merged and used to design better treatment strategies that will attack tumors at their most vital points. Even though this subject was reviewed as recently as 2006 [2], the field has continued to evolve rapidly with new drugs and new concepts.

This chapter will give insights into some of the developments in this field that have continued to be of value in considering the therapy of ACC, and also attempt to identify new strategies that may play a role in the future treatment of this cancer (Fig. 30.1, Table 30.1).

30.1 Therapy Targeted Towards Altered Signaling Pathways in Adrenocortical Carcinoma Cells

30.1.1 Identification of Potential Signaling Targets

In the pre-genomic era, studies of tumor signaling generally relied on the study of candidate proteins and their signaling effects. Although this led to the identification of altered pathways [3], the work was limited in scope and effectiveness. In the

L.S. Kirschner (✉)
Division of Endocrinology, Diabetes and Metabolism, Department of Internal Medicine and Department of Molecular Virology, Immunology and Medical Genetics, The Ohio State University, Columbus Enarson Hall 154 W. 12th Avenue, Columbus, OH 43210, USA
e-mail: lawrence.kirschner@osumc.edu

G.D. Hammer, T. Else (eds.), *Adrenocortical Carcinoma*,
DOI 10.1007/978-0-387-77236-3_30, © Springer Science+Business Media, LLC 2011

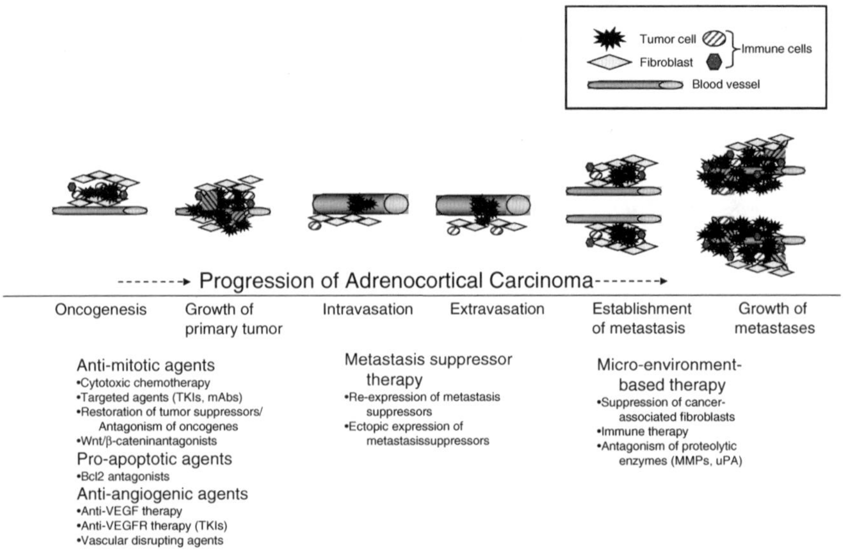

Fig. 30.1 Progression of adrenocortical carcinoma and sites for emerging therapies. The figure shows a schematic representation of the development and progression of a typical ACC tumor. Beneath is shown potential mechanisms for each of the potential therapies described in the text. The legend at the upper right shows the different cell types found in the tumor and its microenvironment

current era, the use of both human and model animal genetics, coupled with high-throughput analyses of gene expression (e.g., cDNA microarray or serial analysis of gene expression [SAGE]), has enabled a much improved understanding of tumor genetics and tumor signaling, allowing an improved focus on the identification of pathways potentially suitable for therapeutic targeting.

30.1.1.1 Target Identification from the Study of Genetic Syndromes

ACC has been classically associated with Li-Fraumeni syndrome (LFS) and Beckwith-Wiedemenn syndrome (BWS), although more intensive family studies have also suggested it may occur occasionally in the setting of adenomatous polyposis of the colon (APC, also known as familial adenomatous polyposis, FAP) and multiple endocrine neoplasia type I (MEN1) (see Chapter 10).

LFS is an autosomal dominant tumor syndrome characterized by the development of malignant sarcomas, breast and brain cancer, and other types of tumors, including ACC in approximately 1% of cases ([OMIM] [4] #151623) (see Chapter 11). The predominant variant of this disease is caused by mutations in the *TP53* tumor suppressor gene, a DNA-binding protein that is activated by cellular stresses to trigger cell cycle arrest. Loss of TP53 function, or the presence of dominant negative mutations, appears to be important for a wide variety of human cancers [5]. LFS can also be caused by mutations in the CHEK2 protein kinase

Table 30.1 Examples of new agents with potential use in ACC[a]

CATEGORY		TARGET	CLASS[b]	AGENTS[c]	
		IGF1R	SM	OSI-906	
			SM	NVP-AEW541	
			SM	BMS-536942	
			Ab	IMC-A12	
			Ab	CP-751,871	
		FGFR	SM	TKI258	
			Ab	FP-1039	*Antibody chimera
		EGFR	SM	Gefitinib	
			SM	Erlotinib	
	Specific pathway inhibitors		Ab	Trastuzumab	
			Ab	Cetuximab	
Kinase inhibitors		PDGF	SM	Leflunomide	
			SM	PKC412	
		VEGR	SM	Vatalanib	
			SM	CEP-701	
			Ab	Bevacizumab	
			Ab	IMC-1121B	
		P38 (MAPK14)	Ab	SB203580	
			Ab	BIRB-796	
		VEGFR/EGFR	SM	Vandetanib (ZD-6474)	
			SM	AEE788	
	Multi-kinase inhibitors	RAF-1/VEGFR/PDGFR	SM	Sorafenib (BAY43-9006)	
		PDGF/VEGFR/KIT	SM	Sunitinib (SU11248)	
Other emerging treatment strategies	Wnt inhibitors		SM	PKF115-584	
	Reversal of drug resistance		SM	Tariquidar (XR9576)	
	Pro-apoptotic	BCL2	SM	AT-101	
		Vasculature	SM	Combretastatin A-4-P	
			SM	DMXAA (dimethyl-xanthrone acetic acid)	
			SM	Rapamycin	
			SM	Temsirolimus (CCI-779)	
			SM	Temsirolimus (CCI-779)	

Table 30.1 (continued)

CATEGORY		TARGET	CLASS[b]	AGENTS[c]
	Microenvironment modifying agents		Ab	anti fibronectin EDB conjugates
			Peptide	Endostatin
			Peptide	Angiostatin
			Ab	TRC105
		HGF/MET	SM	PF-02341066
			SM	PHA-665752
			SM	GSK1363089 (XL880)
			Ab	AMG102
			Ab	DN30
		Cytokines	Ab	GC1008
			ODN	AP12009
			SM	MSX-122
		Inhibitors of proteolytic enzymes	SM	Marimastat
			SM	Prinomastat
			Peptide	rhPAI-1
	Metastasis suppres-sors		Hormone	medroxyprogesterone
			Peptide	KISS-1

[a]This table provides example only, and is not intended to be encyclopedic
[b]SM small molecule agent, Ab therapeutic antibody, ODN therapeutic nucleotide
[c]Agents in active clinical trials (as of Sept 1, 2009) are highlighted in red

(LFS2, OMIM #609265). *CHEK2* is the homolog of yeast (*S. cerevisiae*) *rad53*, a well-described kinase that triggers cell arrest at the DNA checkpoint. CHEK2 phosphorylates TP53, causing its release from its binding partner MDM2, and also phosphorylates BRCA1, another protein involved in cell cycle control. Like *TP53*, *CHEK2* acts as a tumor suppressor, such that disease-associated mutations cause loss of the protein function, and thereby prevent TP53 from functioning normally. Due to the fact that disease-associated mutations produce a loss of function, therapies aimed at targeting this molecular defect would likely involve replacing the function of the missing genes. Because gene therapy for cancer involves a specific set of issues, this topic will be discussed for all applications below (see Section 30.5).

BWS (OMIM #130650) is typically seen as a sporadic disease, and extensive genetic studies have identified a defect in chromosomal region 11p15.5 (see Chapter 14). This disease is characterized by exomphalos (abdominal wall defects), macroglossia, and overgrowth. These patients are at risk for various cancers, including Wilm's tumor, hepatoblastoma, and ACC. At the genetic level, these patients exhibit abnormalities of the 11.p15 region, which can include deletions, duplications, or imprinting defects of this region, which includes the coding genes *IGF2* and *CDKN1C* ($p57^{Kip2}$) *and KCNQ1*, as well non-coding genes such as *H19 and KCNQ1OT1 (LIT1)*. The exact mechanism of disease remains somewhat elusive, although a fair amount of evidence supports overexpression of the imprinted *IGF2* gene in the process. These observations have suggested that IGF2 signaling may play a role in the pathogenesis of both BWS as well as non-syndromic ACC.

APC (OMIM #175100) is a syndrome mainly associated with colon cancer caused by inactivating mutations in the *APC* tumor suppressor gene. This mutation affects signaling through the Wnt/β-catenin pathway, which will be discussed below. In patients with MEN1 (OMIM #131100), adrenocortical tumors are observed in about 30% of patients [6]. These lesions have generally been considered benign, although recent reports have indicated this may not always be the case [7]. As the signaling pathways involving the MEN1 protein remain unclear, this topic will not be addressed further in this chapter.

30.1.1.2 Targets Identified from Gene Expression Analysis

The initial microarray expression analysis from ACC was performed by Giordano and colleagues in 2003 [8]. In that study, the authors identified overexpression of *IGF2* as the most consistent signaling abnormality that differentiated ACC from either benign tumors or normal adrenal tissue. This observation paralleled earlier studies of IGF2 signaling done in isolation [9, 10]. The finding of elevated *IGF2* expression has been confirmed in subsequent expression analysis studies [11, 12, 13], confirming the genetic data of BWS patients.

Another growth factor receptor that was observed to exhibit elevated expression was the fibroblast growth factor receptor 1 (*FGFR1*), another member of the receptor tyrosine kinase (RTK) family of signaling proteins. Elevations in FGF1R and/or FGF4R have been confirmed in independent studies [8, 11, 12]. In one of these studies, elevation of FGFR1 was one of the most prominent changes that discriminated between benign and malignant adrenal tumors [12].

30.1.2 Targeting the IGF2-IGF1R Pathway

Efforts to target this pathway have fallen along two different lines. As one means of inhibiting the IGF1R, small molecular tyrosine kinase inhibitors (TKIs) have been developed and studied. As an alternative approach, humanized antibodies that bind but do not activate the receptor are in development.

30.1.2.1 Small Molecule TKIs

Because of close similarity between the IGF1R and the insulin receptor (IR), small molecules targeted against this pathway must be evaluated for cross-binding and producing side effects resulting from the inhibition of the IR (e.g., hyperglycemia).

Novartis Pharmaceuticals was the first to describe compounds targeted to this pathway with agents NVP-ADW742 and NVP-AEW541. The former showed modest selectivity against the IGF1R compared to the IR (15-fold). It also showed effects in inhibiting the growth of cancer cells [14, 15]. The latter showed slightly better targeting specificity, with an approximately 25-fold selectivity for IGF1R over IR in cell-based studies [16]; however, neither of these compounds has been pursued for clinical studies

Other small molecule TKIs targeted to the IGF1R have been synthesized (e.g., BMS-536942, NVPAEW541, AG1024, PQIP, picropodophyllin PPP, Nordihydroguaiaretic acid Insm-18/NDGA, and OSI-906) and are currently in the process of pre-clinical studies [17]. One of these agents (OSI-906) is currently beginning phase I trials for advanced solid tumors, either as single-agent therapy or in combination with the EGFR inhibitor erlotinib (Tarceva).

30.1.2.2 Anti-IGF1R Antibodies

Therapeutic antibodies have been shown to be effective in clinical situations, and examples in use in other cancers include trastuzumab (Herceptin, Anti-ErbB2/Her2) and cetuximab (Erbitux, anti-ErbB1/EGFR) among many others. Existing anti-IGF1R antibodies include CP-751,871, AVE1642/EM164, IMC-A12, SCH-717454, BIIB022, AMG 479, and MK-0646/h7C10. IMC-A12 has demonstrated effectiveness in vitro [18, 19] and in pre-clinical models [20], as well as in early clinical studies [19]. Clinical trials of this agent for ACC are currently underway. Similar findings for the CP-751,871 have also been generated in pre-clinical [21] and early clinical studies for lung and other solid tumors [22, 23, 24] although no adrenal-specific trial has yet been presented.

30.1.3 Targeting the FGF Receptor

Although the *FGFR* seems to be expressed at elevated levels in ACC, no clinical trials targeting this pathway have yet been started in ACC. Unlike the IGF1R, which has been targeted by multiple agents in development, agents aimed at the FGFRs are uncommon. Initial studies have been focused on targeting this pathway in multiple myeloma, owing to the fact that the t(4:14) translocation in this disease causes ectopic expression of *FGFR3* [25]. The initial drug was developed by Chiron, and was known as CHIR-258, now renamed as TKI258, and was shown to have activity against multiple RTKs, including FGFR, VEGFR, PDGFR, C-KIT, and FLT3. Pre-clinical studies aimed at either FGFR3 [26] or FGFR1 [27] were promising, as was a study in glioblastoma cells expressing multiple FGFR isoforms [28]. A phase I clinical trial of this agent in multiple myeloma showed good tolerability although response rates were low [29]. This agent is currently in clinical trials for cancers of the kidney, prostate, bladder, and for melanoma.

In addition to this agent, a recently developed chimeric molecule consisting of the ligand-binding domain of FGFR1 fused to the Fc portion of IgG was developed as a means to prevent bind FGFR1 agonists and prevent signaling. This molecule, known as FP-1039, is able to inhibit FGF-dependent activities, including growth and angiogenesis in pre-clinical models [30]. Phase I trials of this agent are also currently underway.

30.1.4 Targeting the EGF Receptor

EGFR expression is observed in over 90% of ACC, although levels do not tend to be elevated when compared to normal adrenal tissue [31, 32, 33]. Immunohistochemical date also suggest that EGF is likely not the ligand for the receptor in ACC tumors, but that the receptor can promote growth by binding TGFα [33]. In a single trial, the EGFR inhibitor gefitinib (Iressa) was shown to be ineffective in a pilot study, and plans to proceed with further patient enrollment were scrapped when no responses were observed after the first 18 subjects [32]. At this point, it seems unlikely that single agent trials targeted to the EGFR will be fruitful.

30.1.5 Multi-kinase Inhibition Strategies

Although early trials have focused on the use of signaling inhibitors as monotherapy, it seems more productive to focus on blockade of multiple pathways, in analogy to the use of multiple cytotoxic agents with different mechanisms of actions. This can be accomplished by the use of a single-agent targeting multiple kinases (e.g., sunitinib or TKI258 (as described above)) or by the use of multiple more specific inhibitors. As a trial of Sunitinib for ACC is already underway (http://www.clinicaltrials.gov/ Trial ID NCT00453895), the effectiveness of this agent for ACC may become known in the next few years.

Recent data have suggested that there is significant crosstalk between the EGFR and the IGF1R, and that inhibitors of both pathways may produce synergistic benefits when used together [34, 35, 36, 37]. Because of this, consideration for combination therapy with IGF1R in combination with EGFR inhibitors (e.g., Erlotinib) is underway with clinical trials of combinations along these lines to begin soon.

30.1.6 Targeting the Wnt Signaling Pathway

Wnt signaling has been identified as a key oncogenic pathway, initiating from the identification in the early 1990s of the *APC* gene, which causes the clinical syndrome of adenomatous polyposis of the colon (APC) [38, 39]. Analysis of the function of this gene demonstrated that it is a negative regulator of the Wnt/β-catenin pathway, which is involved in cancers of the colon and many other tissues [40]. In the adrenal gland, the connection between aberrant Wnt signaling and adrenal cancer was suggested by reports of ACC arising in APC patients [41, 42, 43]. In each of these cases, the tumors were associated with loss of the normal *APC* allele. Additionally, somatic mutations in the β-catenin gene (*CTNNB1*) have been detected in a substantial fraction of adrenocortical tumors, including both benign and malignant lesions [44, 45, 46, 47]. Finally, gene expression analyses in adrenal tumors have shown alterations in this pathway in both adrenal macro- and micronodular hyperplasia [48, 49] (see Chapter 16).

These observations suggest that activation of the tumorigenic Wnt/β-catenin pathway is a frequent event in adrenal tumors, making it another potential area for therapeutic intervention. Because of the fact that mutations in this pathway cause many types of tumors, there has been substantial interest in drug development targeting these proteins [40, 50]. Although clinical trials involving ACC with these agents have not yet started, pre-clinical data have shown that a small-molecule inhibitor of Wnt signaling (PKF115-584) is able to suppress the growth of adrenocortical tumor cells in vitro [51]. Further studies of this strategy will likely be of value in the future.

30.2 Enhancing the Effectiveness of Cytotoxic Chemotherapy

It has been known for a long time that the adrenal cortex is a rich source of P-glycoprotein, encoded by the multidrug resistance 1 (*ABCB1/MDR1)* gene [52, 53]. This membrane protein functions at the cell membrane to extrude from the cell cytotoxic hydrophobic agents, including doxorubicin, taxanes, and other alkaloids (e.g., vinblastine, VP-16). Although the encoded P-glycoprotein (PGP) plays a role in the resistance of cancer cells to hydrophobic cytotoxic agents, there are also MDR1-independent drug resistance mechanism that may explain the resistance of ACC cells to water-soluble cytotoxic agents [54, 55].

Because of high *MDR1* expression, significant effort from the group of Fojo has gone into the study of MDR reversing agents in enhancing the effectiveness of cytotoxic agents. Early studies were focused on the use of non-toxic PGP inhibitors such as D-verapamil, which is inactive as a calcium channel blocker [54]. Although these agents were able to enhance drug accumulation in vitro, clinical benefit was not demonstrated. A second generation (PSC833, or Valspodar) showed a similar profile, with good in vitro effects, which did not translate to patients [56]. Most recently a similar approach has been taken with a third-generation compound known as Tariquidar (XR9576). This compound led to significant and sustained inhibition of the PGP efflux pump. Although in this trial no benefit on overall survival was observed, 2/44 evaluable patients obtained a complete remission lasting >3 years [57]. Based on this trial, it has been suggested that Tariquidar may have usefulness as an adjunct for ACC therapy in the proper setting.

30.3 Proapoptoic Strategies

Resistance to apoptosis is a key feature of cancers, and advances in this area have been significant. Apoptosis appears to be mediated in many cell types by members of the BCL family of proteins, and agents targeting this pathway have been in development.

Gossypol is a natural product derivative that has been used as an herbal remedy in China, and studies had suggested it had anti-adrenal properties [58]. A trial of this agent in ACC demonstrated that 3/18 treatment-refractory patients achieved a partial response with this agent [59]. However, a better understanding of the chemistry of this agent revealed that it is a racemic mixture with differential effects of (+) and (–) stereoisomers [60, 61, 62]. Analysis of the anti-cancer action of the compound suggested that this resided in the (–) isomer [63], and that the action of this compound is mediated through alteration of BCL2, BCLxL, and BAX levels to promote apoptosis [64, 65] The (–) stereoisomer has now been prepared as a potential treatment agent (renamed AT-101), and this agent will be entering clinical trials to examine its effectiveness. Aside from this compound, other agents directly designed for inhibiting pro-survival BCL2 family members have been developed. Alternately, agents that are mimetics of the pro-apoptotic members of the family (BIM, BAD) have also been developed, providing another means of potentially targeting this cell survival pathway.

30.4 Novel Strategies

30.4.1 Targeting Tumor Vasculature

Like most endocrine tissues, the adrenal gland is highly vascular, perhaps providing some rationale why metastatic spread occurs early in these tumors. As shown by the pioneering work of Folkman [66], tumors require nutrients and oxygen, and targeting the blood supply is one potential mechanism to inhibit tumor growth and/or inhibit tumor spread. Vascular targeted therapies can be divided into two different categories: those that are aimed at the prevention of new blood vessels (anti-angiogenic agents) and those that disrupt the existing tumor vasculature [67].

A large part of the signal for blood vessel formation is mediated by various forms of the vascular endothelial growth factor (VEGF). VEGF has three receptors, known as the VEGFR1 (Flt1), VEGFR2 (Flk1/KDR), and VEGFR3 (Flt4). Of these, VEGFR2 is thought to be the major mediator of blood vessel growth, although VEGFR1 may also play a role. VEGFR3 appears to function normally in lymphangiogenesis, which is a different physiological process, although newer work has also indicated a possible role for this family member in tumor angiogenesis as well [68].

Significant amounts of work have been spent trying to develop anti-angiogenic therapies, and initial modest successes led to the approval of bevacizumab (Avastin), a monoclonal antibody targeting VEGF, as part of therapy for colon cancer [69]. Subsequent studies have also seen the approval of this agent for non-small cell lung cancer and breast cancer as well [70].

Overall, the response rate of tumors to bevacizumab, as well as to the TKIs sorafenib (Nexavar) and sunitinib (Sutent) which target (at least in part) the VEGFRs, has been modest, and the frequency of escape from this treatment is very high. This effect may be mediated by a number of potential mechanisms, including the elucidation of other angiogenic factors (e.g., fibroblast growth factors [FGFs], placental growth factor [PlGF], or the cytokine CXC12/SDF1) [70, 71].

Of more potential concern is the fact that two recent reports suggest that treatment with anti-angiogenic agents can lead to a more aggressive phenotype when the tumor returns [72, 73]. The mechanism of these findings is unclear as of yet, but these observations raise specific concerns about the use of the agents in isolation. Whether or not these same types of effects will be observed with combination therapy is unknown. Also, whether or not the balance of future behavior may be tipped by combination therapy is an open question that needs to be addressed.

In order to overcome this resistance to single anti-angiogenic agents, it seems likely that agents targeting not only VEGF, but these other signaling systems as well, will be required. This paradigm echoes the evolution of cytotoxic chemotherapy from one-drug regimens to today's complex multi-drug/multi-target regimens. For example, such a cocktail might include an anti-VEGF/VEGFR agent in combination with anti-FGF and/or anti-CXC12 therapies (and potentially others). Given the current understanding of the problems, it seems likely that the angiogenic signal could be successfully blocked; however, the consequences of this procedure for normal physiology would need to be considered very carefully, including the possibility for significant bleeding and/or clotting.

Although therapy directed against angiogenic signals may play a part of treatment, blood vessels are lined by pericytes, which are tightly linked to the endothelial cells and support them structurally. Disruption of pericyte architecture may render the tumor blood vessels more susceptible to damage so that targeting of this cell type, for example, by PDGF antagonists, may also provide a therapeutic benefit [70].

In addition to synthetic anti-angiogenics, further development of endogenous anti-angiogenic compounds has been pursued as another therapeutic modality. Examples of this type of protein include both endostatin and angiostatin. Combination of these therapies with traditional cytotoxic agents has shown some promise [74, 75], but further studies are needed.

An alternative approach to interfering with the tumor vasculature involves taking advantage of the unique properties of tumor blood vessels to develop agents specifically targeted to these cells. In general, tumor vessels lack a well-formed basement membrane and hence have significantly increased vascular permeability compared to normal vessels [76]. Although it was initially thought that it might be possible to identify specific ligands on the walls of these abnormal blood vessels and thus target them for destruction, this concept has not played out well to date. There has been some recent interest in targeting the CD105 (Endoglin) protein. This protein is expressed on normal endothelial cells, but it appears to be present at significantly higher levels on tumor endothelial cells (TECs). A humanized monoclonal antibody targeting this protein has been developed and has shown promise in preclinical studies [77, 78]. A phase I trial of this agent (TRC105) for advanced solid malignancies has just begun. The other approach to targeting the tumor vasculature relies on the altered physical properties of these vessels, including enhanced leakiness and a reduction in loss of tight junctions among endothelial and perivascular cells.

Specific drug therapy aimed at disrupting the tumor vasculature has included the use of synthetic flavinoids such as flavone acetic acid (FAA) or dimethyl-xanthrone acetic acid (DMXAA). These compounds were shown to have good activity in animal models, but similar effectiveness has not been observed in human studies to date. Combretastatins (e.g., combretastatin A4) also seem to function via disrupting the blood supply of tumors. Although the exact mechanism of action remains elusive, these agents seem to work by disrupting microtubule formation in the vascular compartment. Studies of this agent in a variety of tumors either as single agent or in combination are underway; for solid tumors the place of these agents in therapy is determined.

30.4.2 Targeting the Microenvironment

Although the mainstay of therapeutic intervention has been targeted towards proliferating abnormal cells (i.e., tumor cells), it has recently been recognized that tumors do not grow in isolation. The so-called microenvironment consists of blood and lymphatic vessels, fibroblasts, immune cells, and many other cell types, all of which exist in the context of an extracellular matrix. As tumors grow, they are influenced by the components of the microenvironment, and in turn affect the composition and function of these neighboring cells. These interactions are true not only for the establishment and growth of a primary tumor but also significant for understanding the process of metastasis development. This latter concept was crystallized many years ago by Paget as the so-called "seed-and-soil" hypothesis, by which the nature of specific target organs was proposed to affect the localization of metastatic deposits (see [79]). The earliest demonstration of this type was from Mintz's classic experiment in the mid-1970s, showing that teratocarcinoma cells could be reprogrammed into normal mouse cells when placed in the environment of a normal mouse blastocyst [80].

It is beyond the scope of this review on ACC to address this topic in full, and interested readers are referred to any number of recent reviews on this topic [81, 82, 83, 84].

In addition to being a potential target for therapy, it is important to consider the role of the microenvironment in considering response to therapy, as there is good evidence that the microenvironment structure will affect the effectiveness of chemotherapy, as has already been shown for anti-angiogenic therapy, which is strongly affected by the presence of myeloid cells within the stroma [84].

Although these cells are technically not malignant and do not show enhanced proliferation or genetic instability, they are just as important part of understanding tumor biology as the malignant cells themselves.

30.4.2.1 Fibroblasts of the Microenvironment

In most tissues and tumors, fibroblasts make up a substantial portion of the cell mass. This may or may not be true of ACCs, as these tumors tend to be fairly dense collections of mono- or dimorphic malignant cells. However, fibroblasts form an important part of the stroma, and thus likely play an important role in the early stages of development of metastatic disease.

In cancers where they have been studied, cancer-associated fibroblasts (CAFs) exhibit an "activated" behavior compared to normal cells. In normal physiology, fibroblasts assume an activated state when they are actively dividing or migrating, such as in the process of wound healing. Whereas normal cells will return to the quiescent stage after the acute insult is resolved, CAFs never return to the basal state [83]. The exact reason why CAFs exhibit this behavior is not well established, but it likely includes response to the presence of cytokines such as hepatocyte growth factor (HGF) or transforming growth factor-β (TGFβ), which can be produced either by the tumor or by other stromal cells. There has also been evidence suggesting that the CAFs arise from bone marrow derived cells and migrate into the tumor during the establishment of a primary or metastatic tumor deposit. Signals for the migration of these cells to the tumor may come from pre-existing CAFs or may represent a response to tumor hypoxia.

Therapy targeted at fibroblasts has the potential for significant side effects, as any type of treatment along these lines would need to target CAFs but leave normal fibroblasts unaffected. As noted above, CAFs appear to be stimulated by specific growth factors, so targeting these pathways provides potential avenues for treatment development. There have been a number of agents developed targeting the pathway stimulated by HGF and its receptor, c-MET [85]. These include both TKIs targeted to c-MET (e.g., PHA-665752, SU11274), anti-HGF neutralizing antibodies (AMG 102), and other agents that prevent HGF processing or binding (e.g., NK4, DN30). Although most of these agents are in the pre-clinical phase, the anti-HGF antibody AMG102 is currently in phase I and II trials for a variety of advanced neoplasms, including gliomas, colon cancer, and NSCLC. A newer c-MET TKI, PF-02341066, has also recently entered phase I clinical trials for advanced cancer, as has ARQ 197 [86]. Another agent GSK1363089 (Formerly XL880) appears to have both anti-MET and anti-VEGF properties, and is currently in trials for head and neck cancer.

Therapies against TGFβ are also being tried in advanced cancers, including both monoclonal antibodies against this protein (GC1008) as well as anti-sense nucleotides for TGFβ (AP12009), in a trial targeted to patients with tumors known to overproduce this cytokine.

It may also be possible to target factors produced by CAFs, such as CXCL12 (SDF1). A phase I trial of MSX-122, a small molecule inhibitor which blocks receptor binding of this cytokine, was begun; however, this trial is currently suspended and no further information is currently available.

30.4.2.2 Immune Cells of the Microenvironment

The understanding of the role of immune cells in the tumor microenvironment is one that is changing rapidly as new data are integrating into existing frameworks. It has been well established that immune cells are an important part of the tumor stroma. Both macrophages (tumor-associated macrophages, TAMs) and monocytes (typically TIE-2 expressing monocytes, TEMS) are present in tumor stroma, and these appear to secrete a variety of cytokines, which not only affect the behavior of tumor cells, but also have potent effects on other cells of the microenvironment. These include products like VEGF, FGFs, TNFα, as well as a variety of classical cytokines, including IL1β, IL10, IL12, and others. These cytokines establish a self-reinforcing loop leading to recruitment of other cells of the hematopoetic lineage, including neutrophils, eosinophils, mast cells, dendritic cells, and others [87].

Additionally, one of the curious features of malignancies is the fact that they are able to evade immune surveillance as they progress and grow. Significant work has gone in to understanding this phenomenon. Most current data indicate that these effects are due to the presence of marrow-derived suppressor cells (MDSCs), which alter the balance of T lymphocytes to cause predominance of regulatory T cells (Tregs), which are capable of suppressing the surveillance function of other immune cells [88].

Therapy targeting immune cells and their role in cancer also has the potential to be of significant benefit, although again the issue of targeting specificity will need to be overcome; otherwise, the result may be global immune suppression. There has been interest in therapy aimed at the MDSC population, which appear to account for significant amounts of the immune privileged status of tumors. For reasons that are not well defined, sunitinib appears to specifically target tumor-associated MDSCs in renal cell cancer for apoptosis [89]. Understanding the basis of this observation may lead to further advances in this area. There is also some evidence that SCF and its receptor c-KIT may play a role in immune tolerance. This receptor is already targeted by imatinib (Gleevec), so combination use of this agent may also play a role.

As immune cells appear to interact with other stromal cells to promote tumorigenesis/metastasis, therapies aimed at inhibiting a variety of cytokines, including IL15, IL2, IL12, and Fractalkine (FKN) may have some value but little is currently known about them. This has the potential to be relevant in the adrenal literature, particularly given the prior report of at least one case of an adrenal tumor whose growth was stimulated by IL1 [90].

30.4.2.3 Proteolytic Enzymes in the Microenvironment

In order for a tumor to grow and spread, it must degrade, at least partially, the ECM. Not only does this have the effect of releasing ECM-bound growth factors (e.g., FGFs), but this process also creates the tracks via which these tumors can invade into tissue. In most tumor types, there is upregulation of various members of the matrix metalloproteinase (MMP) family of proteins, which serve this purpose, the most common being MMP2 and MMP9. These proteins are zinc-dependent endopeptidases, which have been known for many years to degrade the ECM.

Another enzyme of the same class is the urinary-type plasminogen activator (uPA), which is a serine protease also known to degrade the ECM. uPA has a specific receptor (uPAR) that tethers the protein to the outer cell membrane of cells expressing the receptor, allowing for localized function of this protease, often leading to the localized release of matrix-embedded growth factors such as FGF, VEGF, and HGF [85].

Because of the widespread nature of the overexpression of these enzymes, the MMPs serve as a prominent target for the development of drugs. Many drugs targeted to the MMPs have been developed (e.g., Marimastat, Prinomastat, Tannomastat, etc). These agents have been used in clinical trials in lung cancer, pancreatic cancer, and others [85]. Although the concept of using MMP inhibitors to treat aggressively metastatic cancers seems reasonable, clinical results to date have been somewhat disappointing [91], suggesting that we have not yet come up with the most effective means of utilizing these agents. Similar agents targeted to the uPA system are in development or in early stage clinical trials, including recombinant plasminogen activator inhibitor-1 (PAI-1).

30.4.3 Therapy Aimed at Metastasis Suppression

Although the role of oncogenes has been appreciated for many years, an emerging concept in the field of oncogenesis is the concept of metastasis suppressing or promoting factors. This approach may pay significant dividends in ACC as metastatic disease, which may occur either at presentation or after "complete" resection, remains a significant cause of morbidity and mortality in this disease. In general, metastasis promoters and suppressors are proteins whose presence does not affect the growth rate of cells but appears to alter their ability to metastasize. This effect can occur anywhere in the process of metastasis, including enhancing invasiveness of the primary tumor, enhancing the ability to invade and survive in the bloodstream, as well as to extravasate and form a new tumor in a metastatic location. There is little known about proteins that promote metastasis; however, there is already a good literature about proteins that suppress metastasis, as loss of these proteins has been observed in metastatic tumors (typically identified by genome-wide approaches) and have been verified to suppress metastasis in experimental models. In general, downregulation of these genes occurs at the transcription level, as mutations in the genes are generally not observed.

The first of these genes to be discovered was *NM23* (also known as *NME1)*, which is a member of a multi-gene family of histidine kinases, some of which have metastasis suppressor activity. NM23 appears to be able to down-regulate the RAS-signaling pathway, providing a potential mechanism for its effects. Small G-protein signaling pathways appear to be targeted by other proteins with metastasis suppressor function, including RKIP (Raf kinase inhibitor protein), RhoGDI2 and MKK4. Upstream from these signaling proteins, the KAI1 metastasis suppressor appears to suppress metastasis by downregulating signaling from the EGFR and other cell surface proteins. The BRMS1 (breast cancer metastasis suppressor 1) protein has a different mechanism of action, appearing to be directly involved in causing anoikis, the process by which cells die when they lose contact with the ECM. Loss of this function allows the cells to survive in the bloodstream, a key component of vascular metastasis.

By definition, these genes were characterized by the fact that their expression is lost in metastasis. Therapeutic approaches to restore their function would need to be aimed either at allowing re-expression of these genes in the tumors, or by re-introducing these genes exogenously (i.e., via gene therapy vectors [92]. Given the fact that metastasis is not uncommon at presentation, this latter approach does not seem likely to succeed. However, there has been interest in the former, spurred by the observation that the *NME1* promoter appears to be reactivated by medroxyprogesterone acetate (MPA) [93], which may provide some rationale for the use of this agent in advanced tumors [94].

In addition to these intracellular metastasis suppressor proteins, there are also soluble metastasis suppressors that appear to function by liganding signaling receptors to suppress tumor spread. Perhaps the best example of this is the KISS1 protein, which signals through the G-protein coupled receptor (GPCR) GPR54 to suppress cell mobility and migration [95]. Other molecules in this class include BMP4 and CTGF (connective tissue growth factor). For these agents, administration of the agent by traditional routes may be a viable approach, but their effectiveness as the likely need for continued administration may present technical difficulties in using these agents to treat patients.

30.5 Delivery of Newer Modes of Therapy

With the identification of newer targets for therapy, the next challenge (in addition to target validation) will arise in the implementation of these new therapeutic modalities to the tumors. Gene therapy as a concept has been around for many years, but clinical trials of gene therapies have been fraught with technical problems in gene delivery [96]. Additionally, trials of gene therapy for the correction of metabolic defects were dealt a significant blow when well-publicized cases of leukemia developed in patients during a gene therapy trial for X-linked severe combined immunodeficiency (SCID) as a result of vector integration into a proto-oncogene locus [97, 98, 99].

Despite this setback, efforts into the development of gene transduction vectors have continued. For a tumor like ACC, which exhibits rapid and early dissemination, systemic therapy would appear to be required, as compared to more localized treatment in tumors such as glioblastoma multiforme, a tumor which invades aggressively but does not produce distant metastases [100]. For these purposes, a variety of viral vectors have been pursued, including adenovirus and the related adeno-associated virus (AAV), with newer programs aimed at exploiting other viruses including poxviruses and lentiviruses [101, 102, 103, 104], as well as non-viral gene transduction [105, 106].

If the problem of gene delivery can be overcome, gene therapy could be targeted in the same fashion as more traditional drug therapy implicated above. For example, gene therapy could be used to enhance expression of a growth-arrest promoting protein or to suppress expression of an oncogene, e.g., via siRNA expression [107]. As described in Section 30.4, the tumor stroma plays and important role in tumor behavior, so it is not necessary to target tumor cells themselves; but targeting expression to the stroma may provide benefit with surer targeting, as the tumor stroma cells tend to exhibit more stable genetic and mRNA expression behavior. This same strategy could be applied to the re-expression of proteins capable of metastasis suppression, which may play important roles in the progression of ACC, as discussed above.

The other new concept in therapeutic delivery lies in modulating the immune response in order to provide therapeutic benefit [108]. As the understanding of the role of immune cells in the tumor microenvironment has expanded (see above), the conceptualization of the potential sites for therapy in this realm has also continued to evolve and improve. This approach includes the development of cancer vaccines [109, 110], as well as treatment aimed at using dendritic cells to initiate or enhance an innate anti-tumor response [111, 112, 113]. As of yet, these therapies are only in their infancy, and further trials in a variety of diseases (some of which are ongoing) will be required to determine if the promise of these modalities can be brought into practice.

30.6 Summary and Future Directions

Although efforts to improve on targeted therapies that take advantage of the signaling pathways known to be disrupted in ACC are valuable, clinical progress along these lines has been slow. Some of the agents predicted to be effective in this area are currently underway, so that in a few years' time we may know which one of them provides clinical promise. However, it seems unlikely that the use of single-agent "magic bullets" is likely to provide frequent and durable cure to ACC patients.

In this regard, this chapter has attempted to identify areas of emerging research into new modalities that may prove to be of use for these aggressive cancers. In all likelihood, it will be an enhanced knowledge of tumor behavior and the interaction of the tumor with its microenvironment that will allow identification of an appropriate set of therapeutic targets. Although it is likely that the specific agents required to treat ACC may be different than those used to treat, for example, lung or breast cancer, the therapeutic lessons learned from these more common malignancies should illuminate future strategic development. This concept requires those in the field of ACC therapy not only to continue to make progress by studying ACC patients but also to make progress by studying therapeutic successes in other cancers, particularly as it applies to emerging therapies.

References

1. Allolio B, Fassnacht M (2006) Clinical review: Adrenocortical carcinoma: Clinical update. J Clin Endocrinol Metab 91:2027–2037
2. Kirschner LS (2006) Emerging treatment strategies for adrenocortical carcinoma: a new hope. J Clin Endocrinol Metab 91:14–21
3. Kirschner LS (2002) Signaling pathways in adrenocortical cancer. Ann N Y Acad Sci 968:222–239
4. Online Mendelian Inheritance in Man, OMIM^{TM}. Johns Hopkins University, Baltimore, MD. Accessed May 1, 2009. URL: http://www.ncbi.nlm.nih.gov/omim/
5. Benard J et al (2003) TP53 family members and human cancers. Hum Mutat 21:182–191
6. Skogseid B et al (1995) Adrenal lesion in multiple endocrine neoplasia type 1. Surgery 118:1077–1082
7. Langer P et al (2002) Adrenal involvement in multiple endocrine neoplasia type 1. World J Surg 26:891–896
8. Giordano TJ et al (2003) Distinct transcriptional profiles of adrenocortical tumors uncovered by DNA microarray analysis. Am J Pathol 162:521–531
9. Gicquel C et al (1994) Rearrangements at the 11p15 locus and overexpression of insulin-like growth factor-II gene in sporadic adrenocortical tumors. J Clin Endocrinol Metab 78: 1444–1453
10. Gicquel C, Le Bouc Y (1997) Molecular markers for malignancy in adrenocortical tumors. Horm Res 47:269–272
11. de Fraipont F et al (2005) Gene expression profiling of human adrenocortical tumors using complementary deoxyribonucleic acid microarrays identifies several candidate genes as markers of malignancy. J Clin Endocrinol Metab 90:1819–1829
12. Slater EP et al (2006) Analysis by cDNA microarrays of gene expression patterns of human adrenocortical tumors. Eur J Endocrinol 154:587–598
13. Velazquez-Fernandez D et al (2005) Expression profiling of adrenocortical neoplasms suggests a molecular signature of malignancy. Surgery 138:1087–1094
14. Warshamana-Greene GS et al (2005) The insulin-like growth factor-I receptor kinase inhibitor, NVP-ADW742, sensitizes small cell lung cancer cell lines to the effects of chemotherapy. Clin Cancer Res 11:1563–1571
15. Warshamana-Greene GS et al (2004) The insulin-like growth factor-I (IGF-I) receptor kinase inhibitor NVP-ADW742, in combination with STI571, delineates a spectrum of dependence of small cell lung cancer on IGF-I and stem cell factor signaling. Mol Cancer Ther 3: 527–535
16. Garcia-Echeverria C et al (2004) In vivo antitumor activity of NVP-AEW541-A novel, potent, and selective inhibitor of the IGF-IR kinase. Cancer Cell 5:231–239
17. Hewish M et al (2009) Insulin-like growth factor 1 receptor targeted therapeutics: novel compounds and novel treatment strategies for cancer medicine. Recent Pat Anticancer Drug Discov 4:54–72
18. Barlaskar FM et al (2009) Preclinical targeting of the type I insulin-like growth factor receptor in adrenocortical carcinoma. J Clin Endocrinol Metab 94:204–212
19. Barnes CJ et al (2007) Insulin-like growth factor receptor as a therapeutic target in head and neck cancer. Clin Cancer Res 13:4291–4299
20. Rowinsky EK et al (2007) IMC-A12, a human IgG1 monoclonal antibody to the insulin-like growth factor I receptor. Clin Cancer Res 13:5549s–5555s

21. Cohen BD et al (2005) Combination therapy enhances the inhibition of tumor growth with the fully human anti-type 1 insulin-like growth factor receptor monoclonal antibody CP-751,871. Clin Cancer Res 11:2063–2073
22. Haluska P et al (2007) Phase I dose escalation study of the anti insulin-like growth factor-I receptor monoclonal antibody CP-751,871 in patients with refractory solid tumors. Clin Cancer Res 13:5834–5840
23. Karp DD et al (2009) Phase II study of the anti-insulin-like growth factor type 1 receptor antibody CP-751,871 in combination with paclitaxel and carboplatin in previously untreated, locally advanced, or metastatic non-small-cell lung cancer. J Clin Oncol 27:2516–2522
24. Lacy MQ et al (2008) Phase I, pharmacokinetic and pharmacodynamic study of the anti-insulinlike growth factor type 1 Receptor monoclonal antibody CP-751,871 in patients with multiple myeloma. J Clin Oncol 26:3196–3203
25. Trudel S et al (2005) CHIR-258, a novel, multitargeted tyrosine kinase inhibitor for the potential treatment of t(4;14) multiple myeloma. Blood 105:2941–2948
26. Xin X et al (2006) CHIR-258 is efficacious in a newly developed fibroblast growth factor receptor 3-expressing orthotopic multiple myeloma model in mice. Clin Cancer Res 12:4908–4915
27. Chase A et al (2007) Activity of TKI258 against primary cells and cell lines with FGFR1 fusion genes associated with the 8p11 myeloproliferative syndrome. Blood 110:3729–3734
28. Loilome W et al (2009) Glioblastoma cell growth is suppressed by disruption of fibroblast growth factor pathway signaling. J Neurooncol 94:359–366
29. Lonial S et al (2006) Phase I trial of chir-258 in multiple myeloma. J Clin Oncol 24:17502
30. Zhang H et al (2007) FP-1039 (FGFR1:Fc), A soluble FGFR1 receptor antagonist, inhibits tumor growth and angiogenesis. Paper presented at: AACR-NCI-EORTC international conference molecular targets and cancer therapeutics discovery, biology and clinical applications, San Francisco, CA
31. Kamio T et al (1990) Immunohistochemical expression of epidermal growth factor receptors in human adrenocortical carcinoma. Hum Pathol 21:277–282
32. Samnotra V et al (2007) A phase II trial of gefitinib monotherapy in patients with unresectable adrenocortical carcinoma (ACC). J Clin Oncol 25:15527
33. Sasano H et al (1994) Transforming growth factor alpha, epidermal growth factor, and epidermal growth factor receptor expression in normal and diseased human adrenal cortex by immunohistochemistry and in situ hybridization. Mod Pathol 7:741–746
34. Buck E et al (2008) Feedback mechanisms promote cooperativity for small molecule inhibitors of epidermal and insulin-like growth factor receptors. Cancer Res 68:8322–8332
35. Cunningham MP et al (2008) Co-targeting the EGFR and IGF-IR with anti-EGFR monoclonal antibody ICR62 and the IGF-IR tyrosine kinase inhibitor NVP-AEW541 in colorectal cancer cells. Int J Oncol 33:1107–1113
36. Huang F et al (2009) The mechanisms of differential sensitivity to an insulin-like growth factor-1 receptor inhibitor (BMS-536924) and rationale for combining with EGFR/HER2 inhibitors. Cancer Res 69:161–170
37. Jin Q, Esteva FJ (2008) Cross-talk between the ErbB/HER family and the type I insulin-like growth factor receptor signaling pathway in breast cancer. J Mammary Gland Biol Neoplasia 13:485–498
38. Groden J et al (1991) Identification and characterization of the familial adenomatous polyposis coli gene. Cell 66:589–600
39. Nishisho I et al (1991) Mutations of chromosome 5q21 genes in FAP and colorectal cancer patients. Science 253:665–669
40. Takahashi-Yanaga F, Sasaguri T (2007) The Wnt/beta-catenin signaling pathway as a target in drug discovery. J Pharmacol Sci 104:293–302
41. Blaker H et al (2004) Analysis of somatic APC mutations in rare extracolonic tumors of patients with familial adenomatous polyposis coli. Genes Chromosomes Cancer 41:93–98
42. Seki M et al (1992) Loss of normal allele of the APC gene in an adrenocortical carcinoma from a patient with familial adenomatous polyposis. Hum Genet 89:298–300

43. Wakatsuki S et al (1998) Adrenocortical tumor in a patient with familial adenomatous polyposis: a case associated with a complete inactivating mutation of the APC gene and unusual histological features. Hum Pathol 29:302–306
44. Gaujoux S et al (2008) Wnt/beta-catenin and 3′,5′-cyclic adenosine 5′-monophosphate/protein kinase A signaling pathways alterations and somatic beta-catenin gene mutations in the progression of adrenocortical tumors. J Clin Endocrinol Metab 93:4135–4140
45. Tadjine M et al (2008a) Frequent mutations of beta-catenin gene in sporadic secreting adrenocortical adenomas. Clin Endocrinol (Oxf) 68:264–270
46. Tadjine M et al (2008b) Detection of somatic beta-catenin mutations in primary pigmented nodular adrenocortical disease (PPNAD). Clin Endocrinol (Oxf) 69:367–373
47. Tissier F et al (2005) Mutations of beta-catenin in adrenocortical tumors: activation of the Wnt signaling pathway is a frequent event in both benign and malignant adrenocortical tumors. Cancer Res 65:7622–7627
48. Bourdeau I et al (2004) Gene array analysis of macronodular adrenal hyperplasia confirms clinical heterogeneity and identifies several candidate genes as molecular mediators. Oncogene 23:1575–1585
49. Horvath A et al (2006) Serial analysis of gene expression in adrenocortical hyperplasia caused by a germline PRKAR1A mutation. J Clin Endocrinol Metab 91:584–596
50. Lepourcelet M et al (2004) Small-molecule antagonists of the oncogenic Tcf/beta-catenin protein complex. Cancer Cell 5:91–102
51. Doghman M et al (2008) The T cell factor/beta-catenin antagonist PKF115-584 inhibits proliferation of adrenocortical carcinoma cells. J Clin Endocrinol Metab 93:3222–3225
52. Cordon-Cardo C et al (1990) Expression of the multidrug resistance gene product (P-glycoprotein) in human normal and tumor tissues. J Histochem Cytochem 38:1277–1287
53. Thiebaut F et al (1987) Cellular localization of the multidrug-resistance gene product P-glycoprotein in normal human tissues. Proc Natl Acad Sci USA 84:7735–7738
54. Fridborg H et al (1994) P-glycoprotein expression and activity of resistance modifying agents in primary cultures of human renal and adrenocortical carcinoma cells. Anticancer Res 14:1009–1016
55. Haak HR et al (1993) Expression of P-glycoprotein in relation to clinical manifestation, treatment and prognosis of adrenocortical cancer. Eur J Cancer 29A:1036–1038
56. Bates S et al (2001) A Phase I study of infusional vinblastine in combination with the P-glycoprotein antagonist PSC 833 (valspodar). Cancer 92:1577–1590
57. Menefee ME et al (2008) Effects of the P-glycoprotein (Pgp) antagonist tariquidar (XR-9576; TQD) on Pgp function as well as the toxicity and efficacy of combined chemotherapy in patients with metastatic adrenocortical cancer (mACC). J Clin Oncol 26:2543
58. Wu YW et al (1991) Inhibitory effects of gossypol on adrenal function. Acta Endocrinol (Copenh) 124:672–678
59. Flack MR et al (1993) Oral gossypol in the treatment of metastatic adrenal cancer. J Clin Endocrinol Metab 76:1019–1024
60. Den Boer PJ, Grootegoed JA (1988) Differential effects of (+)- and (–)-gossypol enantiomers on LDH-C4 activity of hamster spermatogenic epithelium in vitro. J Reprod Fertil 83: 701–709
61. Joseph AE et al (1986) Cytotoxicity of enantiomers of gossypol. Br J Cancer 54:511–513
62. Wu DF et al (1988) Determination of gossypol enantiomers in plasma after administration of racemate using high-performance liquid chromatography with precolumn chemical derivatisation. J Chromatogr 433: 141–148
63. Liu S, et al (2002) The (–)-enantiomer of gossypol possesses higher anticancer potency than racemic gossypol in human breast cancer. Anticancer Res 22:33–38
64. Huang YW et al (2006) Molecular mechanisms of (–)-gossypol-induced apoptosis in human prostate cancer cells. Anticancer Res 26:1925–1933
65. Oliver CL et al (2005) (–)-Gossypol acts directly on the mitochondria to overcome Bcl-2- and Bcl-X(L)-mediated apoptosis resistance. Mol Cancer Ther 4:23–31

66. Zetter BR (2008) The scientific contributions of M. Judah Folkman to cancer research. Nat Rev Cancer 8, 647–654
67. Cao Y (2009) Tumor angiogenesis and molecular targets for therapy. Front Biosci 14: 3962–3973
68. Laakkonen P et al (2007) Vascular endothelial growth factor receptor 3 is involved in tumor angiogenesis and growth. Cancer Res 67:593–599
69. Ellis LM, Hicklin DJ (2008) VEGF-targeted therapy: mechanisms of anti-tumour activity. Nat Rev Cancer 8:579–591
70. Bergers G, Hanahan D (2008) Modes of resistance to anti-angiogenic therapy. Nat Rev Cancer 8:592–603
71. Paez-Ribes M et al (2009) Antiangiogenic therapy elicits malignant progression of tumors to increased local invasion and distant metastasis. Cancer Cell 15:220–231
72. Ebos JM et al (2009) Accelerated metastasis after short-term treatment with a potent inhibitor of tumor angiogenesis. Cancer Cell 15:232–239
73. Quesada AR et al (2007) Playing only one instrument may be not enough: limitations and future of the antiangiogenic treatment of cancer. Bioessays 29:1159–1168
74. Folkman J (2006) Antiangiogenesis in cancer therapy–endostatin and its mechanisms of action. Exp Cell Res 312:594–607
75. Kurup A et al (2006) Recombinant human angiostatin (rhAngiostatin) in combination with paclitaxel and carboplatin in patients with advanced non-small-cell lung cancer: a phase II study from Indiana University. Ann Oncol 17:97–103
76. Chan LS et al (2008) Selective targeting of the tumour vasculature. ANZ J Surg 78:955–967
77. Shiozaki K et al (2006) Antiangiogenic chimeric anti-endoglin (CD105) antibody: pharmacokinetics and immunogenicity in nonhuman primates and effects of doxorubicin. Cancer Immunol Immunother 55:140–150
78. Tsujie M et al (2008) Anti-tumor activity of an anti-endoglin monoclonal antibody is enhanced in immunocompetent mice. Int J Cancer 122:2266–2273
79. Mendoza M, Khanna C (2009) Revisiting the seed and soil in cancer metastasis. Int J Biochem Cell Biol 41:1452–1462
80. Mintz B, Illmensee K (1975) Normal genetically mosaic mice produced from malignant teratocarcinoma cells. Proc Natl Acad Sci USA 72:3585–3589
81. Hofmeister V et al (2008) Anti-cancer therapies targeting the tumor stroma. Cancer Immunol Immunother 57:1–17
82. Joyce JA, Pollard JW (2009) Microenvironmental regulation of metastasis. Nat Rev Cancer 9:239–252
83. Li H, et al (2007) Tumor microenvironment: the role of the tumor stroma in cancer. J Cell Biochem 101:805–815
84. Shojaei F, Ferrara N (2008) Role of the microenvironment in tumor growth and in refractoriness/resistance to anti-angiogenic therapies. Drug Resist Updat 11: 219–230
85. Iiizumi M et al (2008) Drug development against metastasis-related genes and their pathways: a rationale for cancer therapy. Biochim Biophys Acta 1786:87–104
86. Garcia A et al (2007) Phase 1 study of ARQ 197, a selective inhibitor of the c-Met RTK in patients with metastatic solid tumors reaches recommended phase 2 dose. J Clin Oncol 25:3525
87. Murdoch C et al (2008) The role of myeloid cells in the promotion of tumour angiogenesis. Nat Rev Cancer 8:618–631
88. Ko JS et al (2009a) Myeloid-derived suppressor cells: a novel therapeutic target. Curr Oncol Rep 11:87–93
89. Ko JS et al (2009b) Sunitinib mediates reversal of myeloid-derived suppressor cell accumulation in renal cell carcinoma patients. Clin Cancer Res 15:2148–2157
90. Willenberg HS et al (1998) Aberrant interleukin-1 receptors in a cortisol-secreting adrenal adenoma causing Cushing's syndrome. N Engl J Med 339:27–31

91. Coussens LM et al (2002) Matrix metalloproteinase inhibitors and cancer: trials and tribulations. Science 295:2387–2392
92. Takeda T et al (2007) Adenoviral transduction of MRP-1/CD9 and KAI1/CD82 inhibits lymph node metastasis in orthotopic lung cancer model. Cancer Res 67:1744–1749
93. Palmieri D et al (2005) Medroxyprogesterone acetate elevation of Nm23-H1 metastasis suppressor expression in hormone receptor-negative breast cancer. J Natl Cancer Inst 97:632–642
94. Steeg PS et al (2008) Clinical-translational approaches to the Nm23-H1 metastasis suppressor. Clin Cancer Res 14:5006–5012
95. Ohtaki T et al (2001) Metastasis suppressor gene KiSS-1 encodes peptide ligand of a G-protein-coupled receptor. Nature 411:613–617
96. Sinkovics JG, Horvath JC (2008) Natural and genetically engineered viral agents for oncolysis and gene therapy of human cancers. Arch Immunol Ther Exp (Warsz) 56(Suppl 1): 3s–59s
97. Hacein-Bey-Abina S et al (2002) Sustained correction of X-linked severe combined immunodeficiency by ex vivo gene therapy. N Engl J Med 346:1185–1193
98. Hacein-Bey-Abina S et al (2003) LMO2-associated clonal T cell proliferation in two patients after gene therapy for SCID-X1. Science 302:415–419
99. McCormack MP, Rabbitts TH (2004) Activation of the T-cell oncogene LMO2 after gene therapy for X-linked severe combined immunodeficiency. N Engl J Med 350:913–922
100. Grandi P et al (2009) Design and application of oncolytic HSV vectors for glioblastoma therapy. Expert Rev Neurother 9:505–517
101. Bachtarzi H et al (2008) Cancer gene therapy with targeted adenoviruses. Expert Opin Drug Deliv 5, 1231–1240
102. Breckpot K et al (2008) Lentiviral vectors for anti-tumor immunotherapy. Curr Gene Ther 8:438–448
103. Kirn DH, Thorne SH (2009) Targeted and armed oncolytic poxviruses: a novel multi-mechanistic therapeutic class for cancer. Nat Rev Cancer 9:64–71
104. Ribacka C et al (2008) Cancer, stem cells, and oncolytic viruses. Ann Med 40:496–505
105. Chen Y, Huang L (2008) Tumor-targeted delivery of siRNA by non-viral vector: Safe and effective cancer therapy. Expert Opin Drug Deliv 5:1301–1311
106. Li SD, Huang L (2008) Targeted delivery of siRNA by nonviral vectors: lessons learned from recent advances. Curr Opin Investig Drugs 9:1317–1323
107. Aharinejad S et al (2009) Targeting stromal-cancer cell interactions with siRNAs. Methods Mol Biol 487:243–266
108. Chaudhuri D et al (2009) Targeting the immune system in cancer. Curr Pharm Biotechnol 10:166–184
109. Chen X et al (2009) Novel strategies for improved cancer vaccines. Expert Rev Vaccines 8:567–576
110. Itoh K et al (2009) Recent advances in cancer vaccines: an overview. Jpn J Clin Oncol 39:73–80
111. Engell-Noerregaard L et al (2009) Review of clinical studies on dendritic cell-based vaccination of patients with malignant melanoma: assessment of correlation between clinical response and vaccine parameters. Cancer Immunol Immunother 58: 1–14
112. Melief CJ (2008) Cancer immunotherapy by dendritic cells. Immunity 29:372–383
113. Santegoets SJ et al (2008) Human dendritic cell line models for DC differentiation and clinical DC vaccination studies. J Leukoc Biol 84:1364–1373

Part IX
Adrenal Cancer Networks and Registries

Chapter 31
The Dutch Adrenal Network

Ilse G.C. Hermsen, Yvonne E. Groenen, and Harm R. Haak

The incidence of ACC in the Netherlands, a small country in Western Europe with a population of 16.5 million people, is about 20–30 patients a year. Because of the rarity of the disease, the chance of encountering an inexperienced doctor is high. The diagnosis of ACC is often delayed or missed, and patients may be treated incorrectly. The Dutch Adrenal Network is a national cooperation which was founded to gather knowledge and experience in order to improve the quality and efficiency of ACC patient care in the Netherlands.

31.1 The Dutch Adrenal Network

The Dutch Adrenal Network was created of 2004. This national cooperation of endocrinologists, oncologists, surgeons, pathologists and basic scientists includes all university hospitals (LUMC Leiden, AMC Amsterdam, VU Amsterdam, UMCG Groningen, UMC Utrecht, UMCN Nijmegen, and UMC Maastricht) and Máxima Medical Centre in Eindhoven. The Dutch Adrenal Network aims to improve patient care in ACC and stimulate scientific research and (inter)national trial participation. In clinical practice, the Dutch Adrenal Network participates in telephone consultation with local doctors, referral of patients to one of the regional centers for diagnosis and therapy, and referral of patients from regional centers to trial centers (for example, FIRM-ACT study: LUMC Leiden, AMC Amsterdam, VU Amsterdam, UMCG Groningen, MMC Eindhoven).

The Network launched a website (www.bijniernetwerk.nl) for health care professionals and patients providing information about the disease epidemiology, treatment options and trial information. National adrenal meetings are organized twice a year and a newsletter is disseminated four times a year. In addition to national cooperation, the Network participates in international trials like FIRM-ACT (First

I.G.C. Hermsen (✉)
Department of Internal Medicine, Máxima Medical Centre, Ds. Th. Fliednerstraat 1,
PO Box 90052, 5600 PD Eindhoven, Leiden University Medical Centre, Leiden, The Netherlands
e-mail: i.hermsen@mmc.nl

G.D. Hammer, T. Else (eds.), *Adrenocortical Carcinoma*,
DOI 10.1007/978-0-387-77236-3_31, © Springer Science+Business Media, LLC 2011

International Randomized Trial in locally advanced and Metastatic Adrenocortical Cancer Treatment) and Pk study (Study of the Pharmacokinetics of Oral Lysodren).

31.2 The Dutch Adrenal Registry

Since the beginning of 2007 patients can be enrolled in the Dutch ACC Registry. With the collection of data of as many patients as possible, the Network will gain more insight into Dutch patient care, prognostic markers, and new treatment options. Until January 2008, the registration of the ACC patients in the Netherlands resulted in the collection of data of 204 patients. The registry consists of two components, a retrospective part, which contains information of patients diagnosed before 2004, and a prospective part, containing information of patients diagnosed since the foundation of the Network in 2004.

The data include information regarding clinical presentation, stage at diagnosis, surgery, pathology, chemotherapy, mitotane therapy, responses to treatment, survival, etc. Simultaneously, the availability of tumor tissue (paraffin embedded and fresh frozen tumors) is registered.

31.3 Results

The Dutch ACC population does not differ significantly from the patient characteristics described in the literature. With peak prevalence in the 3rd to the 5th decade, the mean age at diagnosis was 50 (range 18–81 year). A slight predominance for female vs. male gender was seen. The majority of tumors are functional. Women developed functional ACC more often than men, while men were more likely to develop nonfunctioning tumors.

Patients often present with late stage of disease; 41% of the patients had stage IV (ENS@T) disease at presentation, 37% presented with stage III, 23% with stage II, and 0% with stage I disease. The stage at diagnosis is an important prognostic factor. In our series, patients with stage II and stage III disease survived significantly longer than patients with stage IV disease, with 5-year survival rates of 85, 60, 10%, respectively. Besides stage at diagnosis, complete tumor removal is also an important prognostic factor. R0 resection offers the best chance of survival. The completeness of the surgery is, however, not always discovered in our cohort because of incomplete pathological and surgical reports. Fifty one patients underwent R0 resection, and Kaplan Meier analysis showed significant better survival compared to patients with incomplete or no surgery. In addition to surgery, mitotane and chemotherapy were the main treatments used. Adjuvant treatment with mitotane is given as a standard therapy in only one centre. The role of adjuvant mitotane treatment remains unclear. In this Dutch series patients with adjuvant mitotane did not show a significant longer survival or disease-free survival compared to patients without adjuvant treatment. The most often used chemotherapy regimens are those used in FIRM-ACT (doxorubicin, etoposide, cisplatin plus mitotane and streptozotocin in combination with mitotane). Until March 2009, 26 Dutch patients were included in this trial.

Unfortunately, not all tumors of patients included in the registry have been available for tissue banking, because tissues derived from surgery performed in local hospitals are routinely destroyed after 10 years and many of the Dutch patients receive surgical care at centers without consultation of regional centers. Thus far tissue has been collected from 125 of the 204 ACC patients in the registry. This collection will be used for scientific research.

31.4 Future Goals

The Dutch Adrenal Network aims at the following goals:

- Further improvement of patient care in the field of organization, logistics, and knowledge.
- Making progress in detection of the disease in early stage.
- Improve primary surgery, strive towards for R0 resections.
- Standardization of surgery and pathology reporting.
- Participation in adjuvant therapy trials and future chemotherapy trials.
- International cooperation and trial participation.

31.5 Conclusion

To improve the treatment of adrenocortical carcinoma, national and international alliances have been organized. The Dutch Adrenal Network is a national cooperation with a primary goal of predicting patients with the best possible treatment, by bringing together knowledge and expertise and trying to implementing care guidelines regionally and nationally. The foundations for patient care improvement have facilitated by the establishment of the Dutch Network, which has contributed to basic (ACC Registry and tissue-banking) and clinical research (FIRM-ACT, PK-study).

Chapter 32
The ENS@T Initiative

Xavier Bertagna

There are special circumstances related to the study of rare disease entities, such as ACC. It is crucial to combine clinical forces, if not simply to collect enough clinical material. There is no other way to (1) engage enough patients in clinical trials to establish genotype–phenotype correlations, (2) to catalogue a library of mutations and (3) to establish new prognostic markers. However, the ultimate goal of a network goes far beyond bringing together clinicians and scientists from different countries with various technical skills, dedicated to research and care of patients with the same disease. The goal is to share ideas, biological materials, techniques, and research projects – and finally to add clinical value.

But the ultimate goal of a network goes far beyond these issues: bringing together clinicians and scientists, from different countries, with various technical skills, which are all dedicated to research and care of the same disease, is indeed the real challenge. The goal is to share ideas, biological materials, techniques, and research projects – and finally to add value.

A young Network dedicated to adrenal tumors was recently established in Europe, ENS@T, the European Network for the Study of @drenal Tumors.

32.1 The History: From National Networks to ENS@T

Three national networks on adrenal tumors had initially been active in three European countries:

COMETE (COrtico- MEdullo- Tumors Endocrines) in France; NISGAT (National Italian Study Group on Adrenal Tumors) in Italy; and GANIMED (German Adrenal Network Improving Medical research and EDucation) in Germany. These national networks, with teams from the Universities of Birmingham

X. Bertagna (✉)
Endocrinology Department, Cochin Hospital, Paris, France; National Network COMETE, INCa, Paris, France; European Network for the Study of @drenal Tumors (ENS@T), 27 Rue du Faubourg Saint-Jacques, 75014 Paris, France
e-mail: xavier.bertagna@cch.aphp.fr

G.D. Hammer, T. Else (eds.), *Adrenocortical Carcinoma*,
DOI 10.1007/978-0-387-77236-3_32, © Springer Science+Business Media, LLC 2011

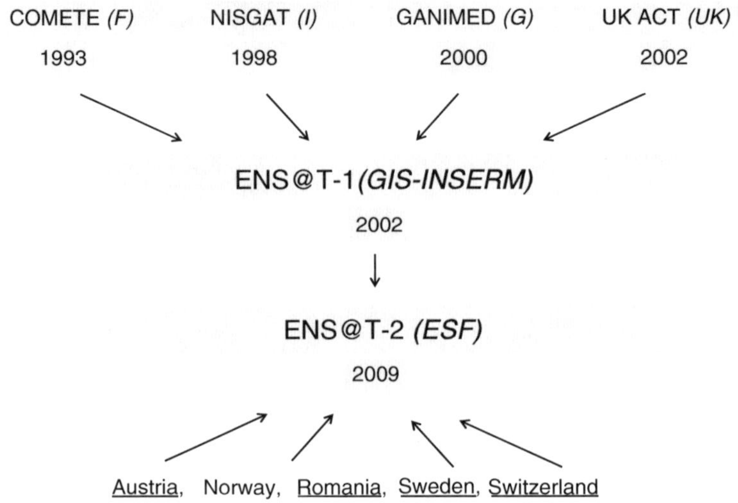

Fig. 32.1 The origin and present development of the ENS@T .COMETE (COrtico MEdullo Tumeurs Endocrine), NISGAT (National Italian Study Group on Adrenal Tumors), GANIMED (German Adrenal Network Improving Medical research and Education), UKACT (UK Adrenal Cortical Tumors). The roles of INSERM (Institut National de la Recherche Française), and ESF (European Science Foundation)

and Glasgow (UK), came together to build the European Network for the Study of @drenal Tumors (ENS@T, see Fig. 32.1): at a 2002 Paris meeting, friendly colleagues decided that they would be stronger if they would join their clinical and scientific forces.

The original ENS@T Steering Committee (SC) comprised B Allolio (Germany), X Bertagna (Chair, France), M Mannelli (Italy), F Mantero (Italy), PF Plouin (France), M Reincke (Germany), and P Stewart (UK), under the financial support of a grant from "Maladies Rares GIS-INSERM".

32.2 Increasing the Patient Number

Adrenal tumors comprise adrenocortical adenomas and carcinomas, and benign or malignant chromaffin tumors derived from the adrenal medulla, pheochromocytomas. Paragangliomas arise from extra-adrenal chromaffin tissue; yet, they share most of the phenotypic and genotypic traits of pheochromocytomas, and patients with pheochromocytomas may also harbor paragangliomas and vice versa.

Patients with adrenocortical tumors, pheochromocytomas, and paragangliomas often present with hypersecretory syndromes (hypercortisolism or Cushing's syndrome, hyperaldosteronism, hyperadrenergic states, etc.) and hypertension. Because they are relatively rare and have a variable or nonspecific presentation, there is frequently a long delay between the onset of symptoms and signs and the diagnosis of the tumor. For instance, the average duration of hypertension before the diagnosis of the underlying tumor is 8 years in aldosterone-producing adenomas (Conn's adenomas) and 3 years in pheochromocytomas and paragangliomas.

Some adrenal tumors, mainly pheochromocytomas, but also adrenocortical tumors, are inherited. The identification of the causative mutation in an index case allows genetic screening to be proposed to relatives, enabling early detection of asymptomatic disease in mutation carriers and finally probably increase survival.

Adrenal tumors can also be found incidentally during imaging procedures for clinical conditions not related to adrenal disease.

Adrenal tumors have long been considered rare, and many actually are. However, advances in biochemical tests and imaging techniques have increased the number of diagnosed cases to several percent of the population referred to hospitals; most are non-functional adrenal cortical adenomas that bear little or no threat to health. Conn's adenomas are also benign tumors that can be found in up to 1–3% of hypertensive patients. In contrast, pheochromocytomas/paragangliomas and other adrenal tumors responsible for Cushing's syndrome, and their malignant counterparts, are extremely rare. They are tumors that bear the high risk with high morbidity and/or mortality.

In many countries in Europe, Networks already existed that were working in the field of adrenal tumors. ENS@T is the fusion between these national networks. It is predicted that further European extension will optimize research in the field, simply by combining patient registries will result to increase the number of patients available for analysis.

32.3 Increasing Technical and Methodological Exchange

The Network also brings together laboratory forces that aim to understand the biology of adrenal tumors.

Little is known about (1) the pathophysiological mechanisms leading to adrenal tumorigenesis, (2) molecular markers that allow to distinguish between benign and malignant adrenal tumors and (3) predictors of outcome or therapeutic response. No targeted therapy exists today that can specifically control the growth of these tumors.

However, clues have emerged that stress the roles of various signaling pathways in adrenal cortical tumors (e.g., the cAMP pathway, the IGF2 signaling pathway, the Wnt/β-catenin pathway). In pheochromocytomas/paragangliomas the roles of SDH complex, the mitochondrial respiration and angiogenic factors are being investigated.

New general approaches to the study of cellular growth, directed towards the assessment of gene profiling, angiogenic pathways, factors involved in the control of cell cycle are increasingly employed in the study of adrenal tumors.

Several ENS@T partners have access to cell imaging platforms, molecular biology platforms (proteomics, tissue arrays, and peptide synthesis), mouse tumor models, and modified adrenocortical carcinoma cell lines for genetic and genomic studies.

The European collaborations use a network of Biological Resource Centers sharing common quality standards, handling procedures, and catalogues complying with European ethical regulations. It will implement common platforms providing the tools for the investigation of patients and their tumors.

These techniques allow state-of-the-art genomic and proteomic approaches (microarray analysis, serial analysis of gene expression, tissue array) and other technical approaches (in situ hybridization, laser cell capture, and tissue or cell culture perfusion) where necessary animal models are used (transgenic mice, gene knockout, transplantation of pathological or transformed adrenal cells into SCID mice), with the view of optimizing the 3 Rs (Replacement, Reduction, Refinement) and thereby reducing the number of animal experiments.

To this end, a multidisciplinary approach encompassing endocrinology, genetics, molecular and cell biology, informatics, epidemiology, pathology, and radiology is planned, ultimately bridging back from bench to bedside with the implementation of translational studies. Ethical approval for tissue collection, storage, and research is in place in each participating center.

32.4 The Idea of "Exchange"

32.4.1 Harmonization

A common ENS@T procedure has been set for the optimal freezing/storage of adrenal tissue in view of studying DNA, RNA, and proteins.

32.4.2 Material

All clinical teams of the Network have patient registries. Many have germinal DNA collections, and several have adrenal-specific imaging facilities including PET-scan, Clinical Investigation Centers, and Biological Resource Centers (e.g., about 1,000 tumor samples plus lymphocyte DNA and pertinent annotations in COMETE).

Harmonized databases have been constructed for four different types of adrenal tumors: NAPACA (non-aldosterone-producing adrenal adenoma), APA (aldosterone-producing adenoma), ACC (adrenal cortical carcinoma), and PHE/PGL (pheochromocytoma/paraganglioma). By using a common nomenclature and standardized phenotypic descriptions in electronic databases, this Network enables reliable estimates of the prevalence of a series of sporadic or familial diseases. It will provide European patients and physicians with access to state-of-the-art diagnostic and prognostic tests.

32.4.3 Science

ENS@T Scientific Meetings are organized yearly and have focused, so far, on the member teams of ENS@T. The goals have been to identify individual and cooperative projects of each team, the need for European collaborations have focused on collecting and sharing more patients, more biological specimen and/or technical help: The meetings have been organized in the members countries: Paris, Padova, Birmingham, Wurzburg, Firenze, Munich. In parallel, short visits between members of ENS@T have been also organized.

32.5 Examples of Research Advancements

The ultimate aim of the ENS@T Network is to develop research in the field of adrenal tumors to improve our diagnosis and treatment abilities, at both clinical and basic levels. The Network facilitates the recruitment of a sufficient number of patients with rare disorders in a number of European centers to harmonize diagnosis criteria and to standardize procedures to (1) collect blood and tissues in Biological Resource Centers (BRC), (2) share databases, and (3) use the various technological approaches of a number of laboratories.

The "added value" provided by ENS@T is to make possible research projects that would not be feasible at the sole national level. The multinational dimension was indeed seminal for some recent, paradigmatic achievements of ENS@T members.

The recent initiation of the "First International Randomized trial in locally advanced and Metastatic Adrenocortical Carcinoma Treatment (FIRM-ACT)" is an example where ENS@T can be involved at the European and indeed global level. This worldwide trial was initiated by ENS@T researchers and is funded by various national grants (e.g., BMBF grant in Germany). It highlights, therefore, both the success of ENS@T and the problems of current fragmentation in research funding.

The Eurine-ACC protocol has in a short time period allowed for the collection of numerous urine samples from well-characterized patients with various types of adrenal cortical tumors from Germany, England, France, and Italy, and to establish the first steroid profile signature for a highly efficient diagnosis of malignant tumors [1].

The Italian and German Networks, NISGAT and GANIMED, jointly designed a protocol that established the potential protective effect of Mitotane as an adjuvant treatment of ACCs after curative surgery. The results, for the first time, were strengthened by comparing two cohorts in two different countries [2] (Fig. 32.2).

The search of prognostic molecular markers in adrenal cortical tumors is commonly compared in patient's cohorts of different countries within ENS@T: the Network is essential to this approach where "validation" cohorts are needed. In the same field of prognosis assessment a new classification of ACCs has been proposed [3].

Phenotype–genotype studies in familial pheochromocytoma/paragangliomas have been amplified by adding the data of different countries [4].

Some on-going research projects:

Clinical

– Lysodren as adjuvant treatment: a randomized study (ADIUVIO trial)
– New compounds in advanced ACCs.

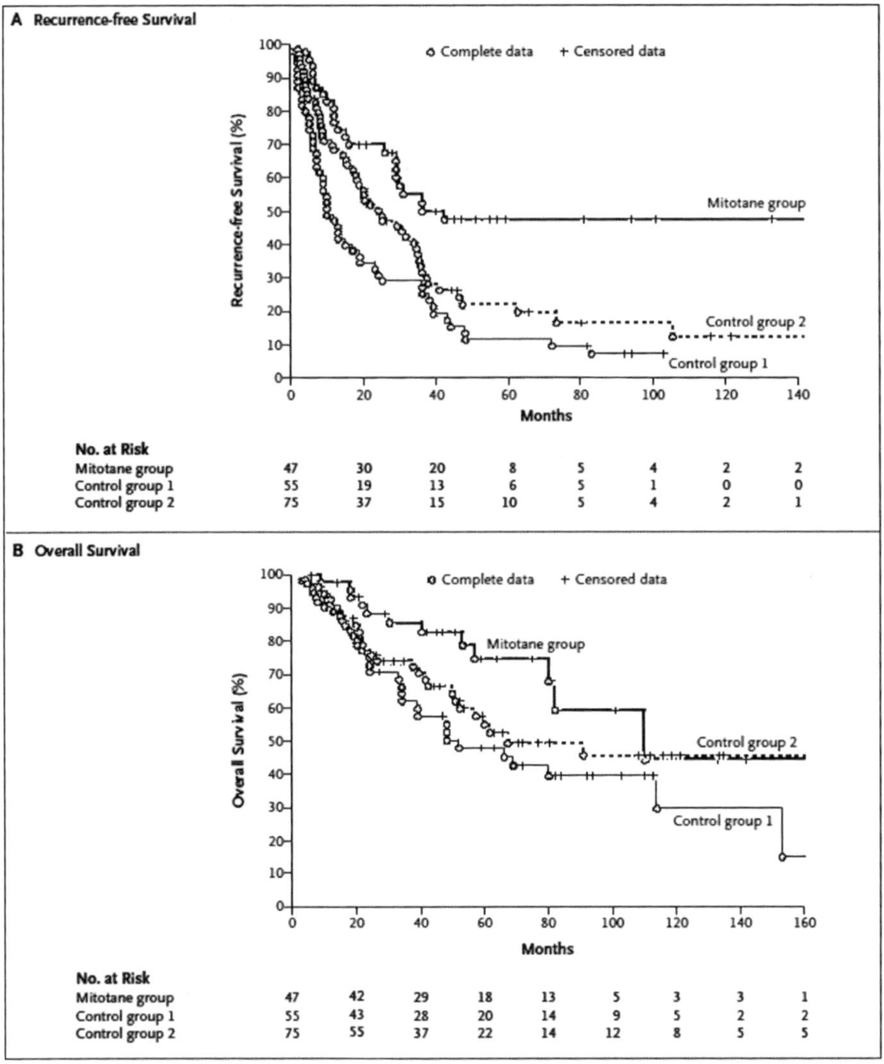

Fig. 32.2 Adjuvant O,p'DDD treatment after complete surgery of localized ACC. Patients cohorts were retrospectively analyzed within the German (GANIMED) and Italian (NISGAT) networks, showing that O,p'DDD administration prolongs Disease Free Survival in ACC patients after complete surgery (Terzolo et al. [2])

- Epidemiology of Conn's syndrome
- Improving diagnostic procedures for the diagnosis of hypersecretory adrenal cortical tumors (Conn, Cushing, ACC)
- A European cohort of familial Pheo/PGL
- A European cohort of Carney complex patients
- Families with ACTH-independent macronodular adrenal hyperplasia

- Families with the Carney complex.
- Salivary aldosterone
- Subclinical adrenal Cushing's

Basic

- Molecular markers of prognostic in adrenocortical tumors
- Molecular markers of malignant Pheo/PGL
- Signaling pathways in adrenal tumorigenesis (cAMP, IGF1,Wint, BMPs, etc)
- Animal models of adrenal tumors
- Gene profiling in tumors
- PDEs in ACTs
- New classification of ACCs
- Transcriptome analysis in ACCs
- New imaging techniques in adrenal cortical tumors
- Adjuvant mitotane in ACC
- Genetics of hyperaldosteronism
- Proteomics of ACC
- Stem cells in ACC

32.6 Organizing the Network

32.6.1 The Steering Committee

Six members are present in the ENS@T-Steering Committee, from France, Germany, Italy, and UK.

32.6.2 The Working Groups

Four working groups have been designed that deal specifically with different tumor types.

- Non-Aldosterone-Producing AdrenoCortical Adenomas (NAPACA): Working Group (WG) members: W Arlt, X Bertagna, S Hahner, F Mantero, P Stewart (Chair), and M Terzolo
- Pheochromocytomas and paragangliomas (Pheo): WG members: AP Gimenez-Roqueplo, H Lehnert, M Mannelli, H Neumann, G Opocher, E Maher, and PF Plouin (chair)
- Primary Aldosteronism (PAL): WG members: J Connell, F Mantero (chair), PF Plouin, M Reincke, GP Rossi, and M Quinkler
- Adrenocortical Carcinoma (ACC): WG members: B Allolio (chair), E. Baudin, J Bertherat, F Beuschlein, M Fassnacht, M Mannelli, and M Terzolo

32.6.3 ENS@T Website

An "ENS@T" website was created (www.ensat.org) (Fig. 32.3).

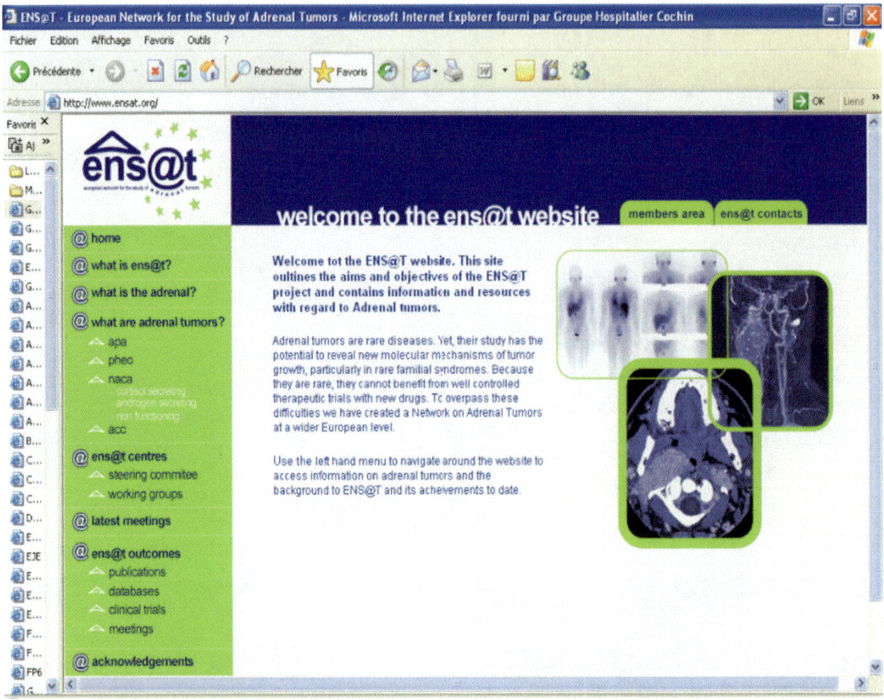

Fig. 32.3 The website page of ENS@T

32.7 Financing the Network

ENS@T was able to obtain institutional supports from National and European organizations.

- GIS-Maladies Rares INSERM (2002)
- Italian Ministry of Research (2006)
- European Science Foundation (ESF, 2009)

Industrial support has been obtained with the HRA pharmaceutical company, providing the human resource that will help implement the ENS@T ACC Data Base in the European countries.

32.8 Perspectives

The continuous search for financial support of the ENS@T Network eventually succeeded with the ESF Call for Research Network Program (RNP) 2007. The ESF

(European Science Foundation) had selected the ENS@T project, within 19 among 122 projects, for its organization and research objectives. Nine European countries now contribute to ENS@T through this ESF RNP: France, Germany, UK, Austria, Switzerland, Romania, Sweden, Norway, and Italy. The budget is 600 KEuro for the next 5 years, starting 2009. This ESF boost has two major implications: enlarging ENS@T to other European counties, and providing the budget for Web-based databases. It will also allow the financing for ENS@T scientific meetings and scientific exchanges.

The year 2009 did see changes in ENS@T:

- A new, younger, Steering Committee is formed. Wiebke Arlt, UK; Felix Beuschlein, Germany (Chair); Jérôme Bertherat, France; Massimo Mannelli, Italy; Massimo Terzolo, Italy; Pierre François Plouin, France.
- ENS@T was recognized as a legal entity (Association Loi de 1901).
- ENS@T will open the membership to all individuals interested in research in adrenal tumors in Europe.

In addition, the Network will promote continuous medical education using electronic platforms such as CASUS, which have already been developed by ENS@T partners. These measures will be orchestrated by other teaching initiatives, such as postgraduate courses in adrenal diseases. In addition, young researchers from participating centers will have the opportunity to visit and study centers in other European countries, thereby increasing intra-European researcher mobility and cross-disciplinary training.

Patient education will be improved through close liaison with patient support groups (*Cushy*, *Climb*, *Addison Self-Help Group (ADSHG)* in the United Kingdom, Association *Surrénales* in France, *and Glandula* in Germany). The first European course of adrenal diseases was held in Hamburg in 2005. Born out of this meeting pathologists from six European countries started an initiative for a standardized grading of adrenal tumors.

32.8.1 Integrational and Disseminative Effects of a European Network

By using a common nomenclature and standardized phenotypic descriptions in electronic databases, this Network will enable reliable estimates of the prevalence of a series of sporadic or familial adrenal diseases. It will provide European patients and physicians with access to state-of-the-art diagnostic and prognostic tests. It will create a European Adrenal Tumor Bank through a Biological Resource Centers network complying with national and European regulations. Common platforms will enable fruitful personal exchanges, the training of young researchers, and the organization of teaching or research seminars. The European dimension of patient cohorts and the Biological Resource Centers network will improve the statistical power and external validity of clinical and pathophysiological analyses. Overall, this network will establish high-quality standards for clinical care and European research on adrenocortical adenomas and carcinomas, pheochromocytomas, and paragangliomas, and will avoid duplication at national levels, which would be a drain on limited resources and facilities. A simplified presentation of the projected structure is shown below.

The ultimate goal of ENS@T is to improve the care of patients with adrenal tumors, through science and organization of patient management (Fig. 32.4). The major hope is to make discoveries that will increase our understanding of adrenal tumors and their treatment. There is also the hope that research results from studying this rare disease entity may have an impact on other tumors, and create larger concepts useful in a much broader field. The IGF2, β-catenin and cAMP pathways, which are important in adrenal tumor biology, may well be involved in many other types of tumors.

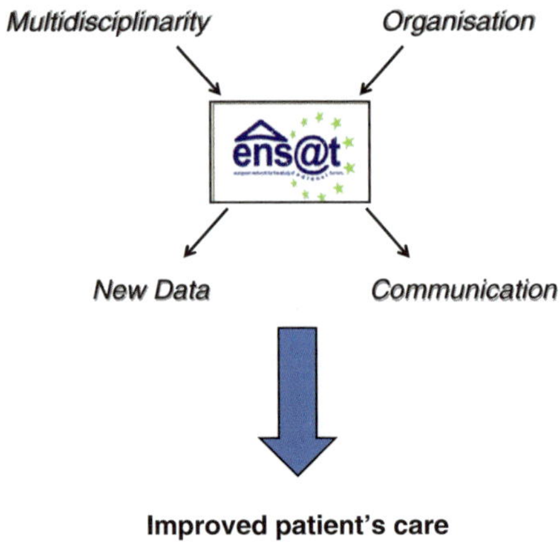

Fig. 32.4 Means and objectives of ENS@T

Ultimately the Network hopes to disseminate emerging knowledge surrounding adrenal tumors. ENS@T hopes to set an example in (1) how to organize locally the multidisciplinary management of the patients, (2) how to avoid dangerous and/or suboptimal surgery of an adrenal tumor that secondarily proves to be an unanticipated pheochromocytoma or ACC, (3) how to improve the difficult diagnosis of ACC through national programs with pathologists and (4) how to spread the availability of genotyping patients nationally and internationally.

References

1. Arlt W et al (2008) Steroid profiling in the diagnosis and monitoring of adrenocortical cancer – results of the EURINE ACC study of the European Network for the study of adrenal tumors (ENS@T). The endocrine society's 90th annual meeting 2008, San Francisco
2. Terzolo M et al (Jun 2007) Adjuvant mitotane treatment for adrenocortical carcinoma. N Engl J Med 356(23):2372–2380

3. Fassnacht M et al (2009) For the German adrenocortical carcinoma registry group and the European Network for the study of adrenal tumors members of the german ACC registry group members of the ENSAT ACC working group (in alphabetical order): Bruno Allolio (University of Würzburg, Würzburg, Germany), Eric Baudin (Institut Gustave Roussy, Paris, France), Jerome Bertherat (Institut Cochin, Paris, France), Felix Beuschlein (University of Munich, Munich, Germany), Martin Fassnacht (University of Würzburg, Würzburg, Germany), Massimo Mannelli (University of Florence, Florence, Italy), and Massimo Terzolo (University of Turin, Turin, Italy). Limited prognostic value of the 2004 International Union Against Cancer staging classification for adrenocortical carcinoma: proposal for a Revised TNM Classification. Cancer 115:243–250
4. Gimenez-Roqueplo AP et al (Dec 2006) European Network for the study of adrenal tumours (ENS@T) pheochromocytoma Working Group. Phaeochromocytoma, new genes and screening strategies. Clin Endocrinol (Oxf) 65(6):699–705

Index

G.D. Hammer, T. Else (eds.), *Adrenocortical Carcinoma*,
DOI 10.1007/978-0-387-77236-3, © Springer Science+Business Media, LLC 2011

L

M

N